Neuroscience for Rehabilitation

Neuroscience for Rehabilitation

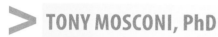 **TONY MOSCONI, PhD**

Associate Professor
Department of Physical Therapy
Crean College of Health and Behavioral Sciences
Chapman University
Irvine, California

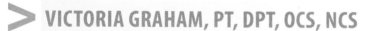 **VICTORIA GRAHAM, PT, DPT, OCS, NCS**

Assistant Professor, Department of Physical Therapy
College of Health and Human Development
California State University, Northridge
Northridge, California

New York / Chicago / San Francisco / Athens / London / Madrid
Mexico City / Milan / New Delhi / Singapore / Sydney / Toronto

Neuroscience for Rehabilitation

1 2 3 4 5 6 7 8 9   LWI   22 21 20 19 18 17

ISBN: 978-0-07-182888-8
MHID: 0-07-182888-5

This book was set in Chaparral pro by MPS Limited.
The editors were Michael Weitz, Brian Kearns, and Peter J. Boyle.
The production supervisor was Richard Ruzycka.
Production management was provided by Gaurav Prabhu, MPS Limited.
The cover designer was Randomatrix.
The designer was Marsha Cohen.

Cover photos: We are pleased to display pictures of three of the generous contributors to our book. We watched Miles grow from infancy to toddler through all of his developmental milestones (Chapter 4); his future is full of promise because his parents have given him a rich, loving home. Bobby overcame an enormous challenge in his young life (Chapter 5); he is living proof that a man of fortitude and focus will not be limited. Tabitha shared the story of her cerebellar tumor (Chapter 7); she demonstrates the therapeutic value of a loving family and strong faith.

Library of Congress Cataloging-in-Publication Data

Names: Mosconi, Tony, author. | Graham, Victoria, active 2017, author.
Title: Neuroscience for rehabilitation / Tony Mosconi, Victoria Graham.
Description: New York: McGraw-Hill, [2017]
Identifiers: LCCN 2017001639| ISBN 9780071828888 (pbk: alk. paper) | ISBN 0071828885 (pbk: alk. paper)
Subjects: | MESH: Physical Therapy Modalities | Nervous System—Anatomy & Histology | Case Reports
Classification: LCC RM700 | NLM WB 460 | DDC 615.8/2—dc23

McGraw-Hill Education books are available at special quantity discounts to use as premiums and sales promotions or for use in corporate training programs. To contact a representative, please visit the Contact Us pages at www.mhprofessional.com.

To my talented child, Jamie Graham.
It has been a pleasure to collaborate, and
I look forward to many more projects in the years ahead.
I love you.

VG

To Gabriele, for your unwavering love, support, and confidence.

TM

Contents

Preface

When McGraw Hill first approached me (Tony Mosconi) to write a neuroanatomical and neurophysiological text aimed at students of physical therapy, I was both intrigued and intimidated. Despite many years' experience teaching neuroanatomy and neurophysiology to these students, I was no clinician. Knowing a bit about the psychology of clinically oriented students, I recognized this as a major impediment to my ability to compose such a text.

At this time of grim self-reflection, I recalled the time my colleague, a physical therapist, accosted me in the hall between our offices, grilling me on the presentation of patients with a lesion of the hypoglossal nerve. It was the first time for either of us to directly compare differences in basic scientific and clinical descriptions of neuroscience and pathology. It was the beginning of a beautiful friendship (and collaboration).

We spent a long time discussing how we could combine disciplines to create a format that was different from the current texts in the field. It became clear that the available texts were aimed at the educational needs of medical students, who would be using the information for medical differential diagnosis, and lacked the basic science that forms the foundation of modern rehabilitative health care. Herein, we tried to find a common clinical-scientific ground, emphasizing the science necessary to conceptualize the conditions that physical therapists see in their practices. Further, we wanted it to be readable and stimulating, mindful not to lose our reading audience in the often dry and unfamiliar material.

We decided that a consistent chapter format would benefit the flow so that students understood what kind of material was about to be presented and where to find the information that they needed. Each chapter begins with a case study of a real patient assessed and interviewed on camera by Vicky Graham. The case studies establish a conceptual framework for the rest of the chapter.

A short Overview of Concepts introduces the basic content of the chapter and is followed by the details of the topic or system. We built up the neuroanatomical framework of the system with descriptions that are presented in language comprehensible to novices and still sophisticated enough for students familiar with the concepts. This is not always an easy synthesis, and we hope we struck the right balance.

After "building" the neurological systems, we broke them, discussing the physiologic processes of damage and clinical presentation, including observable behaviors after injury or disease. We also recognized that the often dense presentation of information could benefit from short interesting interludes, so we introduced a scattering of boxes that expand on issues relating to Neuroplasticity, Response to Injury, and Frontiers in Research, that hopefully are informative and interesting.

Chapter organization of the text begins traditionally, with an Overview chapter and a chapter on Nervous System Development. These generate an anatomical scaffold on which the rest of the book is built. Understanding fetal development helps students understand the complex structure and connectivity found in the developing, mature, and recovering brain.

We have noticed that most physical therapy students have minimal understanding of cell biology. We felt that it was important for students to understand the cytology of the components of the nervous system, especially some of the basic molecular biology. Much of neuronal function is driven by the expression of various proteins, their insertion into the cell membrane, and their release into extracellular space. This information facilitates student understanding of neurophysiological concepts presented in the following chapter. We felt that this level of detail was important in light of the way that numerous injuries and degenerative diseases alter cellular and intercellular functions. This was an expression of our underlying desire to assist students to gain a deeper understanding of the mechanisms of function, injury, and recovery that their patients will undergo.

Both of us, as well as most of our colleagues, teach the functional nervous system from the "bottom up," that is, starting with the spinal cord, ascending through the brainstem and diencephalon, up to the cerebral cortex. Many texts are organized from the top down, beginning with the cortex. We felt that our organization would be as beneficial to the professors as to the students. So we started in the spinal cord and ascended to the cortex. Of course, we still faced the challenge of integrating clinical and scientific information in a way that was manageable for students, so we inserted patient presentations from a student-centric perspective. We anticipate that after studying our chapters, students will be prepared to apply neuroscience principles during subsequent clinical application courses as well as during patient care of this population.

For our chapter on the brainstem and cranial nerves, we recruited Maryke Neiberg, a neuro-optometrist, for assistance in preparing the portions on the sensorimotor features of the visual system. We knew we'd found a kindred spirit and creative collaborator when we heard her speak eloquently at a conference, memorably describing the circle of Willis as "a little devil." She was also a major contributor to the sections in the cerebral cortex related to visual processing for perception and association. We felt this of particular interest because of the enormous diagnostic value in assessment of vision and extrinsic and intrinsic motor function of the eyes.

After each chapter, there is a discussion of the outcomes of the introductory case study. These sections are often very intimate and in some cases include discussions from the patients themselves. We feel that this personalizes the patients and leads students away from thinking about the disease or injury and toward viewing patients as the people they will spend the rest of their working lives helping.

Each chapter ends with ten Review Questions to help students think about the information in a way that prepares them for further study for board exams. Additional materials include a Glossary to collect terminology that might be difficult to remember when seen in subsequent parts of the book. We have also developed Appendices that present more detailed pathology and that lead students through a complete neurological evaluation. To make these sections more impressive on student learning, many videos are available that demonstrate these conditions in actual patients and observations on students. Videos are available by subscription to McGraw-Hill's AccessPhysiotherapy site (accessphysiotherapy.mhmedical.com).

We are optimistic that the present work will make the enormous, but critically important, subjects of neuroscience accessible, understandable, and engaging to our students. We have created it out of our fascination with the form and function of the nervous system, from development through senescence and during recovery from injury. We created it with students in mind because we love them and want only the best for the development of their individual brilliance. Finally, we hope that this book will inform students in a way that will ultimately guide their professional selves to creatively and compassionately assist people in need.

Tony Mosconi, PhD
Victoria Graham, PT, DPT, OCS, NCS

Acknowledgments

Dr. Mosconi and I want to extend a special thanks to all of the people gracious enough to share their stories. We appreciate your honesty, candor, and contribution to the training of future health care providers. Thanks also to my physical therapy colleagues who recommended these lovely people for our book.

All of neuroscience owes a debt to Phineas Gage, our opening chapter patient case demonstrating both the amazing potential of the brain to heal and the devastating cost of brain injury. We hope someday to travel to Cambridge, Massachusetts, to pay our respects; his skull and the tamping rod are both on display at Harvard University's Medical Library. A special section on neuroplasticity featured Armando Ayala, whom I first met when he was a volunteer in our campus PT clinic, and it has been a pleasure to know him since. He is featured in a photograph demonstrating mirror therapy and a video discussing his experiences with phantom limb pain after amputation.

It was inspiring to interview David for Chapter 2. This intelligent, compassionate man fights every day for his own continued recovery as well as for the rights of others. David Karchem described a life-altering journey after sustaining a severe hemorrhagic stroke, his rehabilitation and ongoing recovery, and subsequent dedication to advocacy. He signs his correspondence with several inspirational quotes regarding resilience and his experiences, but my favorite is his own: "The 'rehabilitation myth' will only hold you back if you allow it."

For Chapter 3, we were looking for someone with myasthenia gravis, and a first-year DPT student told me about a family friend, Howard Berkey. It was a short trip down to San Diego County to meet with Howard and his wife for a candid and revealing interview. I am inspired by his strength of character and passion for living a life full of travel and joy in the face of ongoing struggles with this challenging disease. Thanks to both him and his wife for sharing their journey with our future students.

Miles Campa will be turning three about the time this book will go to print; he is one of our cover models, demonstrating a critical developmental milestone and a memorable smile. His mother, Jasmine Campa, was one of my students many years ago, and now a colleague and friend. She agreed to be interviewed when pregnant, and I had the distinct pleasure of visiting the agreeable and cooperative baby Miles several times during his first year to demonstrate normal infant development for our chapter on the developing nervous system. I look forward to seeing his continued development and growth into adulthood, and hope he does not mind being teased in college about his tenure as an infant cover model for our book.

Many years ago, when I still had dark hair, Robert Rohan wheeled past me on his way to a patient room on the neurorehabilitation unit to speak with a newly injured young man. Not only was he a peer mentor at Northridge Hospital Medical Center, but he also served in this role at several Southern California hospitals. It had been a few years since the original injury, and he was active in peer mentoring, played on the wheelchair basketball team Northridge Knights, and shared his experiences with new therapy staff like me. I learned so much from Bobby, information I shared with other patients regarding the reality of living with spinal cord injury. When I began teaching, he was gracious enough to come and speak with my students about his experiences, and readers of this book are also fortunate to meet this optimistic, resourceful, and compassionate man profiled in Chapter 5. He is also one of our cover models, and I love the image of fitness and unlimited possibility in his photo.

Finding a patient who not only survived a brainstem lesion but also went to the Paralympics after completing neurorehab was incredible. Sean Boyle agreed to be interviewed for the book after being contacted by Carlos Roel, who was guest speaking in my class about his experience as a physical therapist to the 2016 Rio de Janeiro Paralympics soccer team. We were standing in line for lunch when I asked him if he knew anyone we could profile for our brainstem chapter. Carlos pulled out his phone and called Sean, who agreed to discuss his amazing triumph from a nearly fatal condition. One day I hope to meet Sean in person, cheer him on from the sidelines, and thank him for his kindness and generosity in sharing this personal story highlighted in Chapter 6.

Many thanks to our Chapter 7 cover girls, Tabitha Jacobs and her physical therapist, Jen Wong. Tabitha's brain tumor grew in response to her pregnancy hormones, unfortunately causing such subtle and slow changes that she and her sweet baby, Mali, were in serious danger by the time anyone figured out the source of her problems. An amazing health care team, combined with the love of family and a strong faith, saw them both through to a better future. It has been such a joy to spend time with Tabitha and her family. Tony and I both look forward to seeing Mali continue to thrive in their loving arms.

Interviewing the former provost Dr. Harry Hellenbrand for Chapter 8 was an honor, and more relaxed than I'd anticipated. He put me at ease with his easy, informal style when we met in his office on campus. Writing his story was daunting. I confess that I wanted to craft a story worthy of such an eminent scholar and published author. Harry, thank you for your candid interview on the struggles of living with Parkinson's disease. I admire your courage and perspective on living a full life, and hope our students will also be inspired as they pursue the difficult study of neuroscience.

Alzheimer's disease is a terrible neurodegenerative disease that impacts far too many families. Our Chapter 9 case describes the journey of my dear grandmother, Norma Bazett, who made it to age 99, surrounded by music, love, and laughter until the very end. Her daughter and son-in-law, Barbara Bazett and Al Deaton, were kind enough to describe the final years as her caregivers. Grandma Norma would have been pleased to know that her story would benefit students; she spent years as a music teacher, and education was her life's passion. Hopefully her story will inspire readers to appreciate the needs of caregivers as well as the patients, particularly in progressive, degenerative neurologic disease.

Thanks to Isabel Burrows, his physical therapist, I interviewed the remarkable Dr. Jan Tillisch for our final chapter case. Dr. Tillisch is the first person I've ever met who diagnosed *himself* with a rare and nearly fatal condition, while in the hospital recovering from a severe stroke. Meeting with him and his wife in their lovely and interesting home was such a treat. Dr. Tillisch is a renaissance man—not only a physician, scholar, and educator but also a skilled woodworker, musician, avid collector, and historian. I anticipate continued recovery due to his amazing resources, both premorbid and poststroke. I thank both of them for their warm and gracious hospitality, and for sharing their journey with our future students.

We had fun taking pictures with and of our student models for the Appendix. All of them have bright futures in health care, and we thank them for their time. Demonstrating clinical examination of cranial nerves with vision function were students Jillian Price and Sharlyn Ramirez from MCPHS School of Optometry, in Worcester, Massachusetts. For the remaining cranial nerves, we thank the students from Casa Loma College in Van Nuys, California: Garry Davis, Gabriel Gadia, Juan Garcia, Tricia Mina, Karen Quindara, and Manuel Santos.

Finally, we thank the Peeps-loving staff of the Pasadena Public Library and apologize to those who had to repeatedly shush us. We also give a shout-out to the guys at Express Yourself, who kept us caffeinated. To our long-suffering editor, Michael Weitz, whose patience we repeatedly tested over this very long journey, we say it is time again for dinner! We've waited long enough. A special thank-you to Peter Boyle, Richard Ruzycka, Vivek Khandelwal, and Guarav Prabhu for their thoughtful and incisive editing; we could not have done it without their help! To Gaby, thanks for all the delicious lunches she packed for us both, including the homemade cakes that kept our blood sugar adequately maintained. We thank our peer reviewers, Michael Biel and Debbie Lowe, for taking time to give feedback on our manuscript.

Vicky Graham and Tony Mosconi, 2017

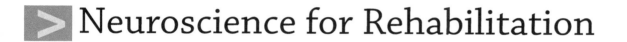
Neuroscience for Rehabilitation

CHAPTER 1

Structural and Functional Organization of the Nervous System

> **CASE 1** No Longer Phineas Gage

In 1848, a 25-year-old railroad foreman named Phineas Gage was in charge of a work crew tasked with blasting rock to lay track for the Rutland & Burlington Railroad in Vermont. As he had countless times before, Gage prepared to pack the charge into a hole in the rock, using a three-and-a-half-foot-long tamping iron. This time, however, the charge was improperly placed. As he plunged it into the hole, the rod set off a spark that detonated the charge and blew the tamping iron through Gage's left cheek and orbit, and clear through his left frontal lobe and skull, landing 80 feet away. Incredibly, some accounts tell that he never lost consciousness, spoke soon after the tragic event, and helped himself into a cart to leave the site. Dr. John Martyn Harlow became Gage's physician throughout the ordeal and for a time afterward during his recovery. He returned to his family home in New Hampshire, and after a few days in a semi-comatose state, Gage sat up and began an almost miraculous recovery. He spent several months convalescing at his family home, then returned to Vermont, where Dr. Harlow pronounced him in good health except for loss of vision in his left eye, ptosis (drooping) in his left eyelid, and a large scar and indentation in his forehead. Dr. Harlow remained Gage's physician throughout his recovery.

Over the ensuing years, Phineas Gage's personality underwent a profound change. No longer was he the quiet, competent work foreman, so he lost his job on the railroad. He performed numerous jobs afterward, including driving stagecoaches in Chile. His behavior and demeanor became increasingly erratic, prone to outburst, and inappropriate, until his friends stated that he was "no longer Gage." He died in May 1860, 12 years after his tragic accident, but his skull and the offending tamping iron currently reside in Harvard Medical School's Warren Anatomical Museum.

Both Dr. Harlow's original observation of Gage's injury, including probing the wound by inserting his finger into the hole, and subsequent modern computed tomography (CT) reconstructions based on images from Gage's actual skull, suggest that the iron destroyed Gage's left frontal lobe, largely sparing his right hemisphere and the rest of his brain. The reconstruction infers significant damage to the prefrontal cortex and the underlying white matter tracts that likely contributed to the prolonged behavior and personality changes. Because of the incomplete understanding of his brain injury and the often contradictory reports of Gage's mental deterioration, both sides of the nineteenth-century discussion of whether function is localized in specific parts of the brain were able to cite Gage's case as supporting their hypotheses.

I OVERVIEW OF KEY CONCEPTS

The brain with its central, peripheral, and autonomic components is the most complex and still least understood organ system in the human body. When it functions well, it controls bodily functions; interprets internal and external stimuli; mediates memory, emotion, and cognitive function; and remains the only organ capable of examining itself. When its function is impaired by injury, disease, or degeneration, the deficits can be permanently life altering. Combined knowledge of the morphology and circuitry of the nervous system (regional neuroanatomy) and the effects that activation or inactivation of particular structures have on behavior (functional neuroanatomy) are essential for developing an understanding of nervous system organization sufficient to allow localization of a lesion based on deduction from subjective and objective observations or prediction of deficits that will be produced by a lesion in a specific location.

Regional neuroanatomy defines the major brain divisions and details spatial relationships and connections among structures within portions of the nervous system. Functional neuroanatomy, in contrast, examines those parts of the nervous system that work together to accomplish a particular task. Nervous system functions are conducted by specific complex neural circuits within and between regions of the nervous system. Understanding specific responses to injury and recovery is essential for effective rehabilitation of function and movement.

The nervous system can be divided into two parts: the central nervous system (CNS) and the peripheral nervous system (PNS) (Figure 1.1). The PNS (Figure 1.1A), composed of nerves and collections of cells within ganglia, essentially acts as the interface between the CNS and the world in relation to the body, monitoring the condition of the body internally and externally, and affecting behavioral changes in response to those conditions. The CNS (Figure 1.1B, C), composed of the spinal cord and brain, is the overall control center, converting objective stimuli into subjective perceptions and sensations, translating the "plan" for behavioral responses, such as grasping, swimming, or smiling, into directions that drive behavioral responses and mediating those cognitive functions that confer consciousness and personality.

Within the CNS, specific locations, structures, or sets of interrelated structures carry out clearly defined functions that are predictably lost with injury (Figure 1.1C). The spinal cord is the interface between the PNS innervating the body and the CNS that responds to the needs of the individual relative to changing peripheral conditions. Ascending and descending connections (i.e., the groups of axons that travel between regions; also known as tracts, columns, fascicles, pathways, or lemnisci) pass through a region called the brainstem. The brainstem includes the medulla and pons ventrally, the cerebellum posteriorly, and the midbrain superiorly. Each region contains numerous specific cellular structures, known as nuclei, which

also have characteristic functions. Above the midbrain, the CNS is called the forebrain, and it includes the diencephalon (the thalamus and hypothalamus) and the telencephalon (basal ganglia and cerebral cortex). This region is supposed to be related to executive motor function, integration of sensory and motor function, and cognition.

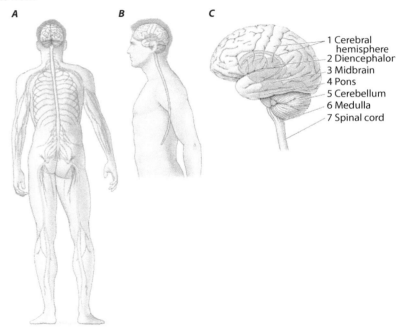

A *B* *C*

1 Cerebral hemisphere
2 Diencephalor
3 Midbrain
4 Pons
5 Cerebellum
6 Medulla
7 Spinal cord

FIGURE 1.1

CNS-PNS overview. *A.* Location of the central and peripheral nervous systems in the body. Major peripheral nerves are shown in yellow. ***B.*** The brain and spinal cord, viewed laterally. ***C.*** There are seven major divisions of the central nervous system: (1) cerebral hemispheres, (2) diencephalon, (3) midbrain, (4) pons, (5) cerebellum, (6) medulla, and (7) spinal cord. The midbrain, pons, and medulla comprise the brain stem. (Reproduced with permission from Organization of the Central Nervous System. In: Martin JH. eds. Neuroanatomy Text and Atlas, 4e New York, NY: McGraw-Hill; 2012).

❚❚ STRUCTURE OF THE NERVOUS SYSTEM

Regional Neuroanatomy

Standardized language serves as a frame of reference for students embarking on the study of the nervous system. Structures exist in precise, and often elegant, relationships with others, and unambiguous terminology is essential for clarity. The following section introduces the general (gross) relationships among the nervous tissues, in preparation for detailed functional discussions to come.

Introduction to neuroanatomical planes

The terminology of neuroanatomy is specialized for describing the brain's complex three-dimensional organization for cogent discussion of both form and function of the nervous system. The CNS is organized along the rostrocaudal, dorsoventral, and mediolateral axes of the body (Figure 1.2). These axes are most easily understood in quadrupedal animals with a more linear CNS than that of humans. In the rat (Figure 1.2A), the rostrocaudal axis runs approximately in a straight line from the nose (*rostrum*) to the tail (*cauda*). This comprises the longitudinal axis of the nervous system and is often termed the neuraxis because the CNS has a predominant longitudinal organization. The dorsoventral axis is perpendicular to the rostrocaudal axis and runs from the back to the abdomen. The terms *posterior* and *anterior* are synonymous with *dorsal* and *ventral* and are used more commonly among clinicians (Figure 1.2B). Mediolateral axes refer to relationships extending from the midline to the side and are particularly important for describing relationships within divisions along the neuraxis.

The longitudinal axis of the human nervous system is not straight as it is in the quadruped. During development, the brain, and therefore its longitudinal axis, undergoes a prominent bend, or flexure, at the midbrain. Instead of describing structures located rostral to this flexure as dorsal or ventral, we typically use the terms *superior* and *inferior*. This bend in the neuraxis reflects the persistence of the cephalic flexure (see Figure 4.3, Chapter 4).

We define three principal planes in which anatomical sections are made, relative to the longitudinal axis of the nervous system (Figure 1.3). Horizontal sections in the forebrain are cut parallel to the longitudinal axis. As one continues caudally through the neuraxis, inferior to the cephalic flexure and into the brainstem and spinal cord, the horizontal (also called *transverse*) plane is oriented perpendicular to the longitudinal axis. Sections cut through the cerebral hemisphere, roughly parallel to the coronal suture of the skull, are called coronal sections. Sagittal sections are cut in the dorsoventral plane, parallel both to the longitudinal axis of the CNS and to the midline. A midsagittal section divides the CNS into two symmetrical halves, whereas a parasagittal section is cut lateral to the midline.

Nervous system: Peripheral and central components

The nervous system is organized into two anatomically separate but functionally interdependent parts: the peripheral and central nervous systems (Figure 1.1A). The peripheral nervous system is subdivided into somatic and autonomic divisions. The somatic division contains the sensory neurons that innervate the skin, muscles, and joints that form the body wall and limbs. These neurons detect and inform the CNS of external stimuli. This division also includes the axons of motor neurons that innervate skeletal muscle, although the cell bodies of these motor neurons lie within the CNS. Motor axons transmit control signals to muscles to regulate muscle contraction. The autonomic division contains the neurons that innervate glands and smooth muscle of the body wall, viscera, and blood vessels. This division, with its separate sympathetic, parasympathetic, and enteric subdivisions, regulates body functions based, in part, on information about the body's internal state.

The CNS consists of the spinal cord and brain (Figure 1.1B). The brain is further subdivided into the medulla, pons, cerebellum, midbrain, and forebrain. Included in the forebrain are the diencephalon, containing the hypothalamus and thalamus, and cerebral hemispheres, which contain the basal ganglia, amygdala, hippocampal formations, and cerebral cortex (Figure 1.1C). Externally, the surface of the cerebral cortex is characterized by gyri (convolutions), sulci (grooves), and fissures (particularly deep grooves) (Figure 1.11A). Four lobes comprise the cerebral cortex: frontal, parietal, temporal, and occipital. The insular cortex, often referred to as a fifth lobe, lies buried beneath the frontal, parietal, and temporal lobes. The corpus callosum is a large decussating (crossing the midline) band of axons that interconnects each of the lobes with their contralateral counterparts (Figure 1.11B). Three sets of structures lie beneath the cortical surface: the hippocampal formation, the amygdala (Figure 1.4A), and the basal ganglia (Figure 1.4B). The limbic system comprises a

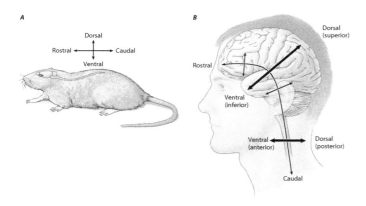

FIGURE 1.2

CNS axes. The axes of the central nervous system are illustrated for the rat (**A**), an animal whose central nervous system is organized in a linear fashion, and the human (**B**), whose central nervous system has a prominent flexure at the midbrain. (Reproduced with permission from Martin JH. Organization of the Central Nervous System. In: Martin JH. eds. *Neuroanatomy Text and Atlas*, 4e. New York, NY: McGraw-Hill; 2012).

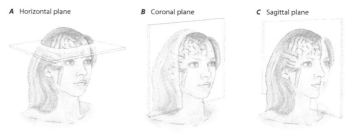

FIGURE 1.3

CNS planes. The three main anatomical planes: (**A**) horizontal, (**B**) coronal, and (**C**) sagittal. (Reproduced with permission from Organization of the Central Nervous System. In: Martin JH. eds. Neuroanatomy Text and Atlas, 4e New York, NY: McGraw-Hill; 2012).

A

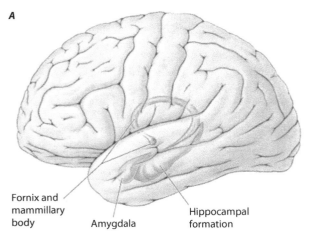

Fornix and mammillary body

Amygdala

Hippocampal formation

B

Striatum

Ventricular system

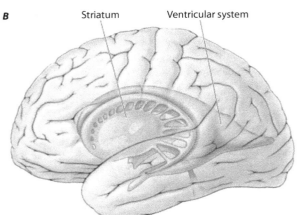

diverse set of cortical and subcortical structures. The olfactory bulbs lie on the orbital surface of the frontal lobes.

Ventricular System

Within each of the CNS divisions resides a component of the ventricular system, a labyrinth of fluid-filled cavities that serve various supportive functions (Figure 1.5). The cavities of the ventricular system are filled with cerebrospinal fluid and are located in relation to specific divisions of the CNS. One of the two lateral ventricles is located in each of the cerebral hemispheres; the third ventricle is located in the diencephalon; and the fourth ventricle is situated between the pons and medulla ventrally and the cerebellum dorsally. The interventricular foramina (of Monro) connect the two lateral ventricles with the third ventricle. The cerebral aqueduct descends through the midbrain and connects the third and fourth ventricles. Two lateral apertures (foramina of Luschka) and a single midline median aperture (foramen of Magendie) allow cerebrospinal fluid to exit the ventricles and circulate in subarachnoid space (see below).

FIGURE 1.4

Three-dimensional views of deep structures of the cerebral hemisphere. *A.* The hippocampal formation (red) and amygdala (orange). The fornix (blue) and mammillary body (purple) are structures that are anatomically and functionally related to the hippocampal formation. ***B.*** Striatum is a component of the basal ganglia with a complex three-dimensional shape. The ventricular system is also illustrated. Note the similarity in overall shapes of the striatum and the lateral ventricle. (Reproduced with permission from Organization of the Central Nervous System. In: Martin JH. eds. Neuroanatomy Text and Atlas, 4e New York, NY: McGraw-Hill; 2012).

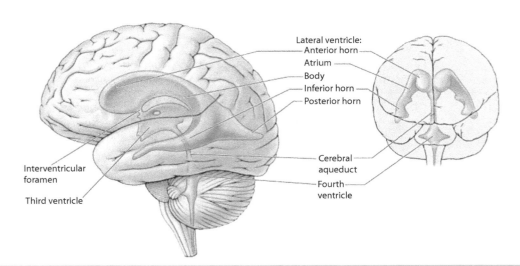

Lateral ventricle:
Anterior horn
Atrium
Body
Inferior horn
Posterior horn

Interventricular foramen

Third ventricle

Cerebral aqueduct
Fourth ventricle

FIGURE 1.5

Ventricular system. The lateral ventricles, third ventricle, cerebral aqueduct, and fourth ventricle are seen from the lateral brain surface (left) and the front (right). The lateral ventricle is divided into four main components: anterior (or frontal) horn, body, inferior (or temporal) horn, and posterior (or occipital) horn. The atrium of the lateral ventricle is the region of confluence of the body, inferior horn, and posterior horn. The interventricular foramen (of Monro) connects each lateral ventricle with the third ventricle. The cerebral aqueduct connects the third and fourth ventricles. (Reproduced with permission from Organization of the Central Nervous System. In: Martin JH. eds. Neuroanatomy Text and Atlas, 4e New York, NY: McGraw-Hill; 2012).

Meninges

The CNS is covered by three meningeal layers, from outermost to innermost: dura mater, arachnoid mater, and pia mater. Arachnoid mater and pia mater are separated by the subarachnoid space, which also contains cerebrospinal fluid. Two prominent double-folded meningeal planes separate brain structures. The falx cerebri separates left and right cerebral hemispheres, and the tentorium cerebelli separates the cerebellum from the forebrain. Also formed within the meningeal folds are the dural sinuses, low-pressure blood vessels draining venous blood and excess cerebrospinal fluid out of the cranium and into the internal jugular vein.

III   FUNCTIONAL NEUROANATOMY

Spinal Cord: Gray Matter and White Matter Regions

The spinal cord participates in processing sensory information from the limbs, trunk, and many internal organs; in controlling body movements directly; and in regulating many visceral functions (Figure 1.6A). It also provides a conduit for the transmission of both sensory information in the tracts that ascend to the brain and motor information in the descending tracts. The spinal cord is the only part of the human CNS that has an external segmental organization (Figure 1.6B).

Each spinal cord segment contains a pair of nerve roots (and associated rootlets) called the dorsal and ventral roots (Figure 1.6C). According to the Bell-Magendie Law, dorsal roots contain only afferent axons that transmit sensory information into the spinal cord, and ventral roots contain motor axons that transmit efferent motor commands to striated and smooth muscles of the body wall, limbs, and other body organs. Dorsal and ventral roots exemplify the separation of function in the nervous system, a principle that is examined further in subsequent chapters. These sensory and motor axons become intermingled in the spinal nerves en route to their peripheral targets.

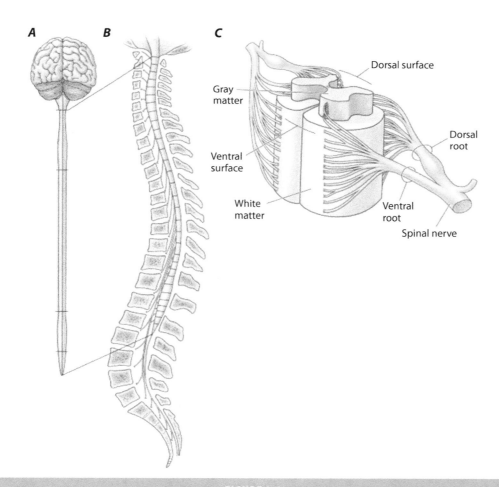

FIGURE 1.6

Spinal cord organization. A. A dorsal view of the central nervous system. The horizontal lines over the spinal cord mark the locations of the different spinal cord divisions; these are considered in more detail in later chapters. **B.** A lateral view of the spinal cord and the vertebral column. **C.** Surface topography and internal structure of the spinal cord. (Adapted from Snell RS. Clinical Neuroanatomy. 7th ed. Lippincott Williams & WIlkins, 2010).

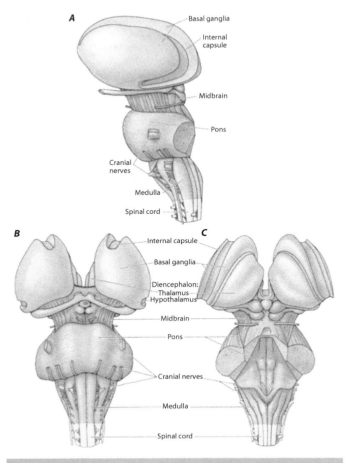

FIGURE 1.7

Thalamus. (*A*) Lateral, (*B*) ventral, and (*C*) dorsal surfaces of the brain stem. The thalamus and basal ganglia are also shown. The different divisions of the brain are shaded in different colors. (Reproduced with permission from Organization of the Central Nervous System. In: Martin JH. eds. Neuroanatomy Text and Atlas, 4e New York, NY: McGraw-Hill; 2012).

Integration of Systems
Neurological Coordination to Produce Movement
Many different integrated systems work together to produce human behavior, and with advances in technology, our appreciation of the complexity of the connections among the various regions is becoming more complete. Multiple areas of the brain become activated during even simple tasks, and even watching a task being done can cause similar areas to activate in the brain of the observer. Following chapters will explore different aspects of human behavior and current understanding of neurological coordination to produce movement.

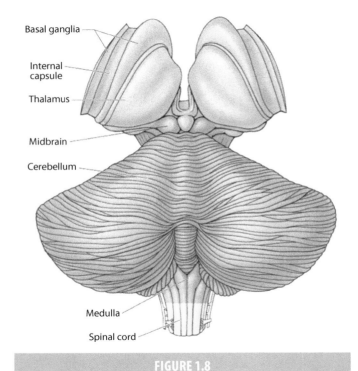

FIGURE 1.8

Dorsal view of the brain stem, thalamus, and basal ganglia, together with the cerebellum. (Reproduced with permission from Organization of the Central Nervous System. In: Martin JH. eds. Neuroanatomy Text and Atlas, 4e New York, NY: McGraw-Hill; 2012).

Brainstem and Cerebellum

The medulla, pons, and midbrain comprise the brainstem (Figure 1.7). The brainstem has three general functions. First, it receives sensory information from cranial structures and controls the muscles of the head. These functions are similar to those of the spinal cord. Cranial nerves, the sensory and motor nerve roots that enter and exit the brainstem, are parts of the peripheral nervous system and are analogous to the spinal nerves. Second, similar to the spinal cord, the brainstem is a conduit for information flow because ascending sensory and descending motor tracts travel through it between the forebrain and the spinal cord. Finally, nuclei in the brainstem integrate information from a variety of sources regulating vegetative functions, as well as arousal and other higher brain functions.

In addition to these three general functions, the various divisions of the brainstem each subserve specific sensory and motor functions. For example, portions of the medulla participate in essential blood pressure and respiratory regulatory mechanisms. Indeed, significant damage to these parts of the brain is almost always life threatening. Parts of the pons and midbrain play a key role in the control of eye movement.

The cerebellum is a major sensorimotor integration center, and its principal functions are to regulate eye and limb movements and to maintain posture and balance (Figure 1.8). Limb movements become poorly coordinated when the cerebellum is damaged. In addition, parts of the cerebellum play a role in higher brain functions, including language, cognition, and emotion.

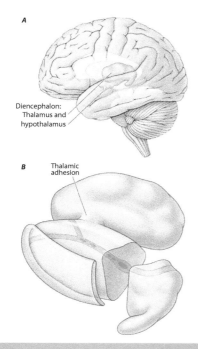

FIGURE 1.9

Diencephalon. *A.* Lateral surface of the cerebral hemispheres and brain stem, illustrating the location of the thalamus and hypothalamus. ***B.*** Three-dimensional structure of the thalamus. The separate structure lateral to the main portion of the thalamus is the thalamic reticular nucleus, which forms a lamina over the lateral sides of the thalamus. (Reproduced with permission from Organization of the Central Nervous System. In: Martin JH. eds. Neuroanatomy Text and Atlas, 4e New York, NY: McGraw-Hill; 2012).

Diencephalon: Thalamus and Hypothalamus

Two principal parts of the diencephalon, the thalamus and the hypothalamus, participate in diverse sensory, motor, and integrative functions (Figure 1.9). The thalamus (Figure 1.9B) is a key structure for transmitting information to the cerebral hemispheres. It is composed of numerous separate nuclei that transmit information to different cortical areas. In the brains of most people, a small portion of the thalamus in each half adheres at the midline, the thalamic adhesion (interthalamic adhesion, massa intermedia). The other component of the diencephalon, the hypothalamus (Figure 1.9A), controls endocrine hormone release from the pituitary gland and the overall functions of the autonomic nervous system.

Cerebral Hemispheres: Complex Topography of Gyri and Sulci

The cerebral hemispheres are the most highly developed portions of the human CNS (Figure 1.10). Each hemisphere is a distinct half, and each has four major components: cerebral cortex, hippocampal formation, amygdala, and basal ganglia. Together, these structures mediate the most sophisticated of human behaviors, and they do so through complex anatomical connections.

Four lobes of cerebral cortex: Distinct but interconnected functions

The cerebral cortex, which is located on the surface of the brain, is highly convoluted. The total area of the human cerebral cortex is approximately 2500 cm². Convolutions are an evolutionary adaptation to fit a greater surface area within the confined space of the cranial cavity. In fact, only one quarter to one third of the cerebral cortex is exposed on the surface. Gyri are elevated convolutions on the cortical surface, separated by grooves called sulci and fissures (which are particularly deep sulci). Cerebral hemispheres are separated from each other by the sagittal (or interhemispheric) fissure (Figure 1.10).

The four lobes of the cerebral cortex are named after the cranial bones that overlie them: frontal, parietal, occipital, and temporal (Figure 1.10 inset). Although intricately interconnected, the functions of the different lobes are remarkably distinct, as are the functions of individual gyri within each lobe. Below is presented a brief overview of some of the functions of each lobe. Detailed discussions will be presented in appropriate sections later in the text.

The frontal lobe serves diverse behavioral functions, from thoughts to actions, cognition, and emotions. The precentral gyrus contains the primary motor cortex, which participates in controlling components of movement, such as the direction and speed of reaching. Much of the frontal lobe is association cortex. Psychiatric disorders of thought, as in schizophrenia, and mood disorders, such as depression, are linked with abnormal functions of frontal association cortex. The basal forebrain, which is on the ventral surface of the frontal lobe, contains a special population of neurons that uses acetylcholine to regulate cortical excitability. Although the olfactory sensory organ, the olfactory bulb, is located on the ventral surface of the frontal lobe, its connections are predominantly with the temporal lobe.

The parietal lobe is separated from the frontal lobe by the central sulcus and mediates perceptions of touch, limb position, and, in part, sensations of pain. These functions are carried out by the primary somatosensory cortex located in the postcentral gyrus. Primary sensory areas are the initial cortical processing stages for sensory information. The remaining portion of the parietal lobe on the lateral brain surface consists of the superior and inferior parietal lobules, which are higher-order somatic sensory areas for further processing of information related to spatial awareness and integrating diverse sensory information for visual perception and language, mathematical reasoning, and cognition. They are essential for a complete self-image of the body, and they mediate behavioral interactions with the world around us.

The occipital lobe is separated from the parietal lobe on the medial brain surface by the parietooccipital sulcus. On the lateral and inferior surfaces, there are no distinct boundaries, only an imaginary line connecting the preoccipital notch with the parietooccipital sulcus. The occipital lobe is involved only with vision. Primary visual cortex is located in the walls and depths of the calcarine fissure on the medial brain surface extending to the occipital pole. Whereas the primary visual cortex is important in the initial stages of visual processing, the surrounding higher-order visual areas, as well as their profuse connections with parietal and temporal association areas, play roles in elaborating the sensory message that enables us to see the form and color of objects and to identify them, and to appreciate our bodies within our multi-dimensional environment.

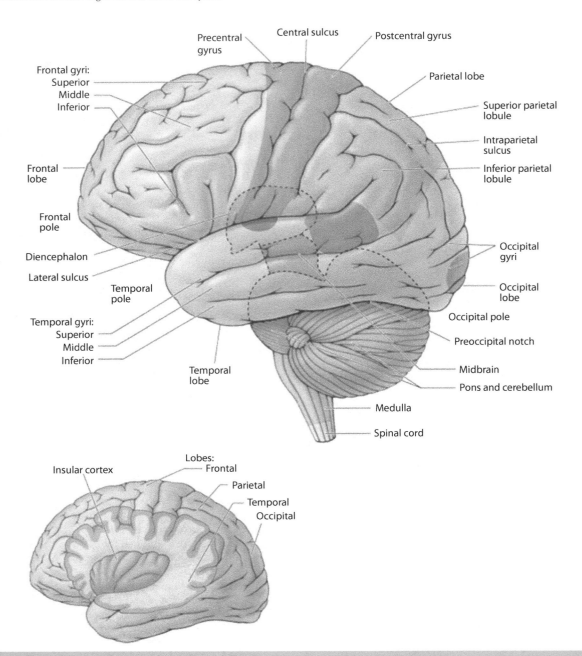

FIGURE 1.10

Brain topography. Lateral surface of cerebral hemisphere and brain stem and a portion of the spinal cord. The different colored regions correspond to distinct functional cortical areas. The primary motor and somatic sensory areas are located in the pre- and postcentral gyri, respectively. The primary auditory cortex lies in the superior temporal gyrus adjacent to the sensory and motor areas. Broca's area comprises most of the inferior frontal gyrus, and Wernicke's area is in the posterior part of the superior temporal gyrus. Boldface labeling indicates key structures. The inset shows the four lobes of the cerebral cortex and the insular cortex in relation to the four lobes. (Reproduced with permission from Organization of the Central Nervous System. In: Martin JH. eds. Neuroanatomy Text and Atlas, 4e New York, NY: McGraw-Hill; 2012).

The temporal lobe, separated from the frontal and parietal lobes by the lateral sulcus (or Sylvian fissure), mediates a variety of sensory functions and participates in memory and emotions. Primary auditory cortex, located on the superior surface of the superior temporal gyrus, works with surrounding areas for perception and localization of sounds. The posterior part of the superior temporal gyrus on the left side, Wernicke's area, is specialized for speech. Lesion of Wernicke's area impairs the understanding of speech. The middle temporal gyrus, especially the portion close to the occipital lobe, is essential for perception of visual motion, while the inferior temporal gyrus mediates the perception of visual form and color. Cortex located at the temporal pole, together with adjacent portions of the medial temporal lobe and inferior and medial frontal lobes, is important for emotions.

Deep within the lateral sulcus are portions of the frontal, parietal, and temporal lobes. This territory is called the insular cortex (Figure 1.10 inset). It becomes buried late in prenatal development. Portions of the insular cortex are important in taste, internal body senses, pain perception, and balance.

Tracts containing axons that interconnect the two sides of the brain are called commissures (containing commissural fibers), and the corpus callosum is the largest of the brain's commissures. To integrate the functions of the two halves of the cerebral cortex, axons of the corpus callosum course through each of its four principal parts: rostrum, genu, body, and splenium (Figure 1.11). Information between the occipital lobes travels through the splenium of the corpus callosum, whereas information from the other lobes travels through the rostrum, genu, and body.

Subcortical Components

The hippocampal formation is important in learning and memory, whereas the amygdala not only participates in emotions but also helps to coordinate the body's response to stressful and threatening situations, such as preparing to fight (Figure 1.4A). These two structures are part of the limbic system, which includes other parts of the cerebral hemispheres, diencephalon, and midbrain. Because parts of the limbic system play a key role in mood, it is not surprising that psychiatric disorders are often associated with limbic system dysfunction.

Basal ganglia comprise a set of collections of neurons (nuclei) located deep within the cerebral hemisphere (Figure 1.4B). The importance of the basal ganglia in the control of movement is clearly revealed when they become damaged, as in Parkinson's disease. Tremor and a slowing of movement are some of the overt signs of this disease. Basal ganglia also participate in cognition and emotions in concert with the cerebral cortex and are key brain structures involved in addiction.

Cavities within the CNS contain cerebrospinal fluid

The CNS has a tubular organization that is especially obvious early in development. Within it are cavities and channels, collectively termed the ventricular system, that contain cerebrospinal fluid (Figure 1.5). Cerebrospinal fluid is a watery fluid that cushions the CNS from physical shocks, buoys the brain to reduce pressure on its base, and is a medium for chemical communication.

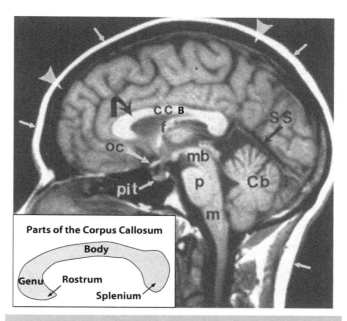

Parts of the Corpus Callosum

Body

Genu **Rostrum**

Splenium

FIGURE 1.11

Normal head MR images. Sagittal T1-weighted image. Note differences in signal between gray matter (large arrows), white matter (curved arrows), CSF (small arrowheads), fat (small arrows), and cortical bone (large arrowheads). Parts labeled on the MRI include the corpus callosum (cc), fornix (f), optic chiasm (oc), pituitary gland (pit), midbrain (mb), pons (p), medulla (m), cerebellum (Cb), straight sinus (SS), and the body of the corpus callosum (B). The inset shows parts of the corpus callosum: rostrum, genu, body, and splenium. (Reproduced with permission from Zapadka ME, Bradbury MS, Williams DW, III. Chapter 12. Brain and Its Coverings. In: Chen MM, et al. eds. Basic Radiology, 2e New York, NY: McGraw-Hill; 2011).

An intraventricular vascular structure, the choroid plexus, secretes most of the cerebrospinal fluid.

The ventricular system consists of chambers, or ventricles, where cerebrospinal fluid accumulates, and narrow channels through which the ventricles communicate. There are two lateral ventricles, each within one cerebral hemisphere, the third ventricle, between the two halves of the diencephalon, and the fourth ventricle, which is located between the brainstem and cerebellum. The interventricular foramina (of Monro) connect each of the lateral ventricles with the third ventricle, and the cerebral aqueduct (of Sylvius) in the midbrain connects the third and fourth ventricles. Three additional openings, or apertures can be seen in the fourth ventricle: a single, posterior median aperture (of Magendie) and two lateral apertures (of Luschka) that allow cerebrospinal fluid to exit the ventricular system into subarachnoid space (see below). The ventricular system extends into the spinal cord as the central canal, although its lumen typically closes off during adulthood.

Three meningeal layers in the CNS

The meninges consist of the dura mater, the arachnoid mater, and the pia mater (Figure 1.12). (Meninges are more commonly called the dura, arachnoid, and pia, without using the term *mater*.) The dura is the thickest and outermost of these membranes and serves a protective function. Ancient surgeons knew that patients could survive even severe skull fractures if bone fragments had not penetrated the dura. Two important partitions arise from the dura and separate different components of the cerebral hemispheres and brainstem (Figure 1.13). The falx cerebri separates the two cerebral hemispheres. It has a small inferior continuation, the falx cerebelli, that separates the two cerebellar hemispheres. The tentorium cerebelli separates the cerebellum from the overlying cerebral hemispheres. The dura is fused externally with the periosteum of the skull and is removed only with difficulty.

The arachnoid mater adjoins but is not tightly bound to the dura mater, thereby allowing a potential space, the subdural space, to exist between them. This space is important clinically. The innermost meningeal layer, the pia mater, is very delicate and adheres to the surface of the brain and spinal cord. Subarachnoid space is situated between the arachnoid mater and pia mater. Filaments of arachnoid mater pass through the subarachnoid space and connect to the pia mater, giving this space the appearance of a spider's web. Because the dura mater contains blood vessels, breakage of one of its vessels due to head trauma can lead to subdural bleeding and to the formation of a blood clot (a subdural hematoma). In this condition the blood clot pushes the arachnoid mater away from the dura mater, fills the subdural space, and compresses underlying neural tissue.

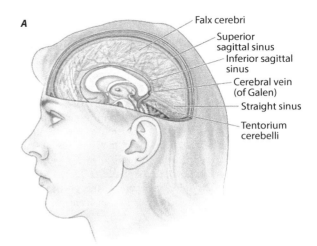

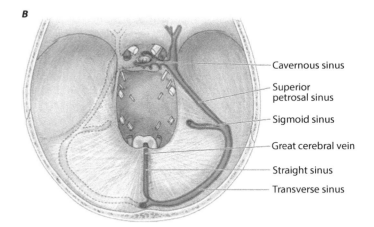

FIGURE 1.12

The dura, arachnoid, and pia maters also surround the brain and as shown here the relationships among the cranial meninges are similar to those of the spinal cord. The diagram includes arachnoid villi, which are outpocketings of arachnoid away from the brain, which penetrate the dura mater and enter blood-filled venous sinuses located within that layer. The arachnoid villi function in releasing excess CSF into the blood. Blood vessels from the arachnoid branch into smaller arteries and veins that enter brain tissue carrying oxygen and nutrients. These small vessels are initially covered with pia mater, but as capillaries they are covered only by the perivascular feet of astrocytes. (Reproduced with permission from Nerve Tissue & the Nervous System. In: Mescher AL. eds. Junqueira's Basic Histology, 14e New York, NY: McGraw-Hill; 2016).

FIGURE 1.13

Falx cerebri, tentorium cerebelli, and superior sagittal sinus. *A.* From a lateral perspective. ***B.*** View of cranial cavity with the brain removed, showing the return of blood from the sinuses to the venous system. (Reproduced with permission from Vasculature of the Central Nervous System and the Cerebrospinal Fluid. In: Martin JH. eds. Neuroanatomy Text and Atlas, 4e New York, NY: McGraw-Hill, 2012).

IV RESPONSE TO INJURY

Tissue-Specific Response to Injury

Nervous system tissue responds to injury differently than other tissues in the body. A basic overview of phases of tissue healing is necessary to provide context for future discussion. Any injury or disruption to tissue is treated as a wound by the body, with emergent needs for survival of the system. There are three phases of wound healing: (1) inflammation, (2) proliferation, and (3) maturation (Figure 1.14). The inflammation phase occurs in all tissue types immediately after injury with a hemostatic response that includes vasoconstriction of any injured local blood vessels to stop bleeding and prepare the wound for healing (Figure 1.15). Liberated platelets attach to exposed collagen fibers on the vessel walls to form a platelet plug. The plug is strengthened by coagulation, in which fibrin strands trap red blood cells and platelets. Clot size is limited by coagulation inhibitors and fibrinolysis. Next, mast cells release histamine and serotonin, causing capillaries to dilate and increase permeability, leading to heat, redness, swelling, pain, and loss of function. Blood plasma leaks into the local tissues as a result of the dilation, and white blood cells are free to migrate into the wound. These white blood cells clean the wound in preparation for the next phase of tissue healing. Neutrophils digest breakdown products and contaminants, then die after a few days. Monocytes migrate in to continue the process, maturing into macrophages. Macrophages are now the key cells for phagocytosis of injury-related debris, with their activity mediated by cytokines. The inflammation phase is necessary for healing; however, it can become inappropriate, such as in autoimmune diseases, causing damage and excessive scarring. The discovery of cytokines and recognition of the profound role of inflammation in disease is changing health delivery. Inflammatory cytokines are linked to major depressive disorder, Alzheimer's disease, cancer, heart disease, auto-immune diseases, Type II diabetes mellitus, non-alcoholic fatty liver disease, and obesity. Their expression is modified by drug therapy, diet, movement, and exercise.

The proliferation phase of tissue healing permanently closes the wound and rebuilds the tissue. Macrophages release chemicals that degrade the clot, promote wound closure, and build a base for new tissue. Angiogenesis provides oxygenation to the healing wound and removes waste products. Fibroblasts lay down new collagen, and granulation tissue spreads to create a new extracellular matrix for the final phases of epithelialization that close the wound.

The last phase of tissue healing is the maturation phase. This long term process lasts up to a year and involves a balance of synthesis (production) and lysis (destruction) of collagen in the scar tissue. During this phase, mobile type III collagen is replaced with stronger, realigned, more organized type I collagen.

Response to injury in the central and peripheral nervous system is an area of great interest to biomedical researchers, health care providers, and patients. The ability of nervous tissue to heal and resume function significantly impacts long term recovery and prognosis; these tissue properties and responses are discussed more fully in Chapter 3.

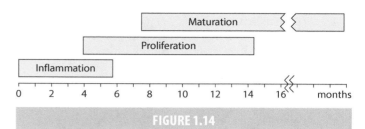

Phases of healing

FIGURE 1.14

The cellular, biochemical, and mechanical phases of wound healing. (Reproduced with permission from Barbul A, et al. Chapter 9. Wound Healing. In: Brunicardi F, et al., eds. *Schwartz's Principles of Surgery*, 9e. New York, NY: McGraw-Hill; 2010).

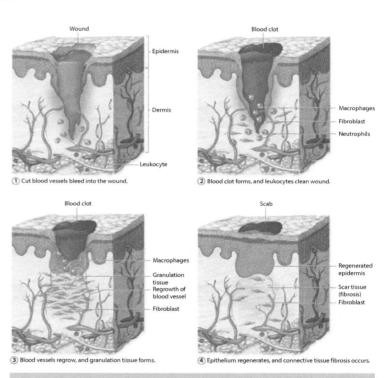

FIGURE 1.15

Stages of wound healing. Skin repair occurs in overlapping stages, shown here schematically. (1) The process begins with blood quickly clotting at the wound site, releasing platelet-derived growth factors and other substances. (2) Macrophages and neutrophils enter the wound as inflammation begins, and epithelial cells from the cut edges of the stratum basale begin to migrate beneath and through the blood clot. (3) Under the influence of growth factors and hydrolytic enzymes released in part from macrophages, fibroblasts proliferate and produce much new collagen to form "granulation tissue" containing many new, growing capillaries. (4) The epidermis gradually reestablishes continuity over the wound site, but excessive collagen usually remains in the dermis as scar tissue. (Adapted from Brunicardi F, et al., eds. *Schwartz's Principles of Surgery*, 9e. New York, NY: McGraw-Hill; 2010).

> Neuroplasticity

Application to Rehabilitation

The nervous system is shaped by environmental demands throughout our lifetime. *Neuroplasticity* describes changes in neural pathways and synapses in response to injury, disease, environmental demands, and changing behavior. This ability to change is a relatively new discovery that fundamentally altered our perception of human potential after nervous system injury or disease. Since the 1940s, researchers have detailed the process of neuroplasticity with elegant studies of non-human animals and, more recently, human beings.

Neuroplasticity occurs extensively within the nervous system,

affecting such diverse functions as gene expression, neuronal morphological and biochemical differentiation, and reorganization of cortical maps. Synaptic pruning is a significant process affecting both developmental and post-traumatic plasticity in the nervous system, notably in organization (or reorganization) of cerebral cortical representations. Environmental deprivation during a developmental critical period results in permanent changes to functional neural substrates. Subsequently, the brain is unable to activate the deprived system, even if the rest of the pathway is intact. Amputation studies in animals have demonstrated that the central representation of adjacent uninjured territories expands into the cortical area vacated by the missing structure.

Synaptic pruning not only occurs during critical periods, but it plays a significant role in maladaptive or "negative" plasticity. As many as 90% of humans experience phantom limb pain after amputation that appear to be related to maladaptive remapping of the somatosensory cortex. Ramachandran and his coworkers have developed behavioral interventions using mirrors to manipulate patient perception and redirect cortical remapping. During mirror therapy, the subject places the amputated limb behind a mirror and the intact limb in front of the mirror in a position that creates the illusion that the amputated limb is actually present. The subject then simulates bilateral tasks while looking at the illusion in the mirror. With practice, the technique

drives neuroplastic changes that "convince" the brain that the limb is truly gone, eliminating any residual phantom sensations.

Rehabilitation extensively uses the brain's capacity for neuroplastic change, and an effective health care practitioner must be expert in applying appropriate therapies that promote functional recovery. Ideal experiences should be meaningful to the patient, with adequate intensity and repetition to enhance positive neurological outcomes. Interventions that begin too soon after injury may actually induce maladaptive changes. Even simple exercise such as walking is now recognized as beneficial to the nervous system.

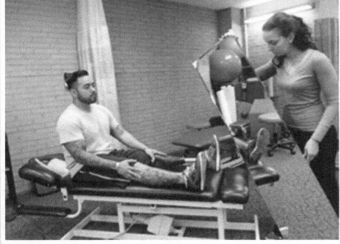
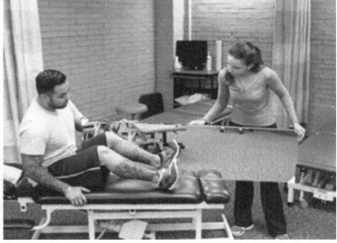

> CASE 1   DISCUSSION: No Longer Phineas Gage

The destruction of Phineas Gage's prefrontal cortex stimulated excitement in two competing schools of thought among neuroscience researchers of the time. The first group espoused a theory of modularity originally proposed by phrenologists, stating that each region of the brain has a specific

and unique function. They cited additional observations, such as the localization of speech functions to the left cerebral hemisphere, and the fusiform face area, in the temporal lobe, specialized for face recognition. Many of the predictions of the modularity group have been supported by modern functional MRI studies. In contrast, the distributive

processing group limits the focal specificity mainly to motor and sensory functions, but proposes an extensive interconnectedness for cognitive functions. Recently, groups have suggested that a combination of modular and distributed circuitry is most likely. Phineas Gage became the first traumatic brain injury case study.

REFERENCES

Allen NJ, Barres BA. Glia: more than just brain glue. *Nature*. 2009; 457:675–677.

Chapman SB, Aslan S, Spence JS, Defina LF, Keebler MW, Didehbani N, Lu H. Shorter term aerobic exercise improves brain, cognition, and cardiovascular fitness in aging. *Front Aging Neurosci*. 2013 Nov 12;5:75.

Duvernoy HM. *The Human Hippocampus*. Munich, Germany: J.F. Bergmann Verlag; 1988.

Filippi M, Charil A, Rovaris M, Absinta M, Rocca M. Insights from magnetic resonance imaging. *Handb Clin Neurol*. 2014;122:115–149.

Haas L. Phineas Gage and the science of brain localisation. *J Neurol Neurosurg Psychiatry*. 2001;71:761.

Hötting K, Röder B. Beneficial effects of physical exercise on neuroplasticity and cognition. *Neurosci Biobehav Rev*. 2013 Nov;37(9 Pt B): 2243–2257.

Lee PR, Fields R. Regulation of myelin genes implicated in psychiatric disorders by functional activity in axons. *Front Neuroanat*. 2009;3:4.

Lee SK, Wolfe SW. Peripheral nerve injury and repair. *J Am Acad Orthop Surg*. 2000;8(4):243–252.

Macmillan M, Lena M. Rehabilitating Phineas Gage. *Neuropsychol Rehabil*. 2010 Oct;20(5):641–658.

O'Driscoll K, Leach JP. "No longer Gage": an iron bar through the head. Early observation of personality change after injury to the prefrontal cortex. *BMJ*. 1998;317:1673–1674.

Paxinos G, Mai JK, eds. *The Human Nervous System*. London: Elsevier, 2004.

Raichle ME. A brief history of human brain mapping. *Trends Neurosci*. 2009;32(2):118–126.

Ramachandran VS, Rogers-Ramachandran D. Phantom limbs and neuroplasticity. *Arch Neurol*. 2000;57:317–320.

Ratiu P, Talos I-F. The tale of Phineas Gage, digitally remastered. *N Engl J Med*. 2004;351:23. www.nejm.org.

Sherman DL, Brophy PJ. Mechanisms of axon ensheathment and myelin growth. *Nat Rev Neurosci*. 2005;6(9):683–690.

Van Horn JD, Irimia A, Torgerson CM, Chambers MC, Kikinis R, et al. Mapping connectivity damage in the case of Phineas Gage. *PLoS ONE*. 2012;7(5):e37454.

Volterra A, Meldolesi J. Astrocytes, from brain glue to communication elements: the revolution continues. *Nat Rev Neurosci*. 2005;6(8): 626–640.

Zigmond MJ, Smeyne RJ. Exercise: is it a neuroprotective and if so, how does it work? *Parkinsonism Relat Disord*. 2014 Jan;20(Suppl 1):S123–S127.

REVIEW QUESTIONS

1. Functional neuroanatomy is defined as:
   A. knowledge of the morphology and circuitry of the nervous system.
   B. effects activation or inactivation of particular structures have on behavior.
   C. interaction of physiology and anatomy of particular central nervous system structures.
   D. chemical transmission of information via neurotransmitters.

2. The ability to change neural pathways in response to lifetime demands is called:
   A. phagocytosis.
   B. neuroplasticity.
   C. neurotransmission.
   D. synaptic transmission.

3. A person sustains a connective tissue injury. There is bleeding and inflammation at the injury site. Which of the following cell types plays a phagocytic role in eliminating blood and tissue debris?
   A. Schwann cells
   B. Mast cells
   C. Macrophages
   D. Neurons

4. Which of the following is *not* part of the peripheral nervous system?
   A. Motor neuron cell body
   B. Sympathetic ganglia
   C. Dorsal root
   D. Ventral root

5. Which of the following best describes sulci and gyri?
   A. Functional regions of the brain are located on gyri.
   B. Sulci separate the lobes of the brain.
   C. Gyri are the bumps, and sulci are the grooves that separate the gyri.
   D. Sulci are the bumps, and gyri are the grooves that separate the sulci.

6. Which of the following best describes the location of major brain regions?
   A. The thalamus is located rostral to the midbrain.
   B. The basal ganglia are located ventral to the cerebellum.
   C. The midbrain is located caudal to the medulla.
   D. The cerebellum is located ventral to the pons.

7. A patient has a tumor in the region of the insular cortex. Which of the following choices best describes the location of the tumor?
   A. It is buried beneath the brain surface, under the frontal lobe.
   B. It is buried beneath the frontal and parietal lobes.
   C. It is buried beneath the frontal, parietal, and temporal lobes.
   D. It is buried beneath the frontal, parietal, temporal, and occipital lobes.

8. A pitcher was hit in the head with a baseball. The impact of the ball hitting his head caused a skull fracture over his left orbit. Which of the following brain structures is located closest to the site of fracture?
   A. Inferior frontal lobe
   B. Postcentral gyrus
   C. Calcarine fissure
   D. Anterior horn of lateral ventricle

9. The falx cerebri separates:
   A. the occipital lobes and the cerebellum.
   B. the cerebellum and the medulla.
   C. the two cerebral hemispheres.
   D. the two halves of the diencephalon.

10. The atrium of the lateral ventricle is located within which major central nervous system division?
    A. Pons
    B. Cerebellum
    C. Cerebral cortex
    D. Diencephalon

CHAPTER 2

Vascular Supply of the Central Nervous System

CASE 2 Atrioventricular Malformation

David K was driving through a busy southern California intersection when his left arm and leg stopped working. He glided to the side of the road, partially blocking traffic. Realizing something was wrong, he called 911 and reported, "I'm at Plummer and Reseda," but the operator kept asking him to repeat himself. His memories of the event fade in and out; he unlocked his car and put a note on his windshield to call for help. When the paramedics arrived, they found him slumped over the steering wheel and asked his name, but he was only able to point to his wallet in response to their questions. His speech returned during the ambulance ride; he spent the entire time trying to convince them to stop for hamburgers. Once at the local hospital, he was transported to CT scan to determine the cause of his acute neurologic decline. Clinical findings were consistent with a cerebral vascular accident. Test results were positive for ischemic rather than hemorrhagic onset, qualifying him for the drug t-PA (tissue plasmin activator).

David K was an active man in his early 50s, working as a software engineer. His true passion, however, was his volunteer work. Thirty years of running around soccer fields as a referee gave him strong legs and excellent cardiovascular fitness. This high level of fitness may be the reason his physician neglected to follow up with a cardiology consultation when he found an abnormal heart rate (arrhythmia) during a routine check-up six months prior. Atrial fibrillation causes inefficient blood circulation, subsequent pooling, and increased risk of clot development. Released clots impede circulation

and cause tissue damage through ischemia. David had several large clots (thrombi), which settled in his right middle and posterior cerebral arteries. The t-PA is most effective when delivered during the first few hours after ischemic stroke, and probably saved David's life. However, the neurologic damage was severe, and he remained unable to control motion of his left side. Four days later, David developed a thrombus in his right calf, underwent vascular surgery, and was placed on temporary bed rest.

A dislodged thrombus (thromboembolism) can travel up to the heart or brain and cause serious damage, including death. This prolonged period of inactivity cost him dearly, as he developed severe tightness in his knee, which delayed his recovery and ability to participate in therapy. David remembers fighting for every week of rehabilitation, constantly being told that there was little chance of improving. His course of care was typical, even better than the average, as he had insurance and spent six weeks in an acute care hospital with several weeks in a CARF (Commission on Accreditation of Rehabilitation Facilities)–accredited interprofessional inpatient rehabilitation unit. This unit provided hours of daily intensive rehabilitation therapy, with coordination by a physiatrist (physician specializing in physical medicine and rehabilitation). The program included occupational, physical, speech, and recreation therapy; neuropsychiatric evaluation; social work; and consistent nursing services emphasizing family training, emotional coping, and self-care. He was discharged to home health

and subsequently outpatient care for continued physical, occupational, and speech therapy.

One year after his stroke, David remained severely impaired, with no use of his left hand. He developed spasticity in the finger and wrist flexors and required a splint to maintain his hand position. He learned to walk with a cane, finding ways to cope with his continued imbalance and slow gait by avoiding uneven ground, curbs, and sidewalks pushed up by tree roots. Loss of smell and taste, and poor saliva production, made eating difficult and less enjoyable. Although he used chin-positioning strategies the speech-language pathologist taught, different textures such as carrots with a sandwich or a salad with a runny dressing remained challenging. His speech returned, but he noticed weakness after talking a long time. He worked with a specialist to manage his visual agnosia (difficulty naming items) and compensate for left lower quadrant field loss. He learned to identify the container lids by organizing them by size, shape, and color. David's happiest accomplishment was resuming driving. The local hospital had a driving rehabilitation program that included behind-the-wheel sessions. He bought a new car with automatic transmission, installing a spinner knob and crossover bar for one-handed steering and vehicle manipulation. His instructor was an occupational therapist who taught him individual strategies for visual scanning and safety, use of adaptive equipment, and prepared him for the Department of Motor Vehicles examination, which he passed on the first try!

I OVERVIEW OF KEY CONCEPTS

Brain vasculature disorders constitute a major class of nervous system disease. The principal source of nourishment for the CNS is glucose, and oxygen is necessary for cell function. Neither glucose nor oxygen is stored in appreciable amounts, so brain functions become severely disrupted when the blood supply of the CNS is interrupted, even briefly.

Much of what is known about the arterial supply to the CNS derives from three observational approaches. First, classical anatomical studies in normal postmortem tissue use colored dye injected into a blood vessel to identify the areas it supplies. Second, in postmortem tissue or on radiological examination, the portion of the CNS supplied by a particular artery can be inferred by observing the extent of damage that occurred after the artery became occluded. Third, radiological techniques, such as cerebral angiography and magnetic resonance angiography, make it possible to view the arterial and venous circulation in the living brain (Appendix 1). These important clinical tools also permit localization of a vascular obstruction or other pathology.

Brain vasculature is closely related to the ventricular system and the watery fluid contained within it, the CSF. This is because most CSF is produced continually by the choroid plexus via active secretion of ions from blood plasma. Therefore, to maintain a constant brain volume, CSF is returned to the blood through valves between the subarachnoid space and the dural sinuses.

II ARTERIAL SUPPLY

The principal blood supply for the brain comes from two arterial systems, each of which receives blood from different systemic arteries (Figure 2.1A). Anterior circulation is fed by the internal carotid arteries, and posterior circulation receives blood from the vertebral arteries (Figure 2.1C right inset). Anterior circulation is also called *carotid circulation*, and posterior circulation is referred to as *vertebral-basilar*. Anterior and posterior circulations are not independent, but are connected by anastomotic (interconnected) networks of arteries on the ventral surface of the diencephalon and midbrain and on the cortical surface (Figure 2.2). Anastomosis with extracranial arteries is minimal.

The brainstem, in contrast, receives blood only from posterior circulation. The arterial supply for the spinal cord is provided by vertebral arteries along with systemic circulation, which also supplies muscle, skin, and bones. Spinal arteries are part of the general systemic circulation, draining into veins that return blood directly to the heart. In contrast, many cerebral arteries connect with cerebral veins that drain first into dural sinuses, a set of large venous collection channels in the dura mater (Figure 2.7), and from there into the internal jugular vein to return to systemic circulation.

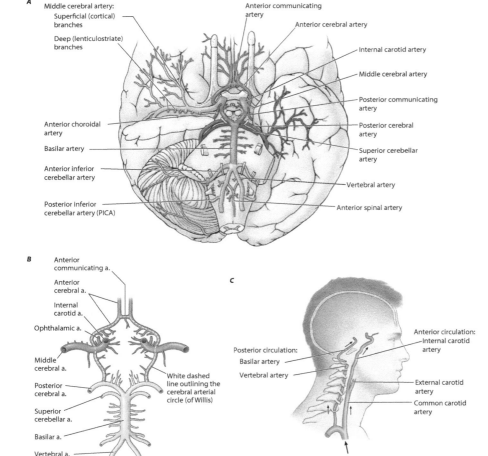

FIGURE 2.1

Diagram of the ventral surface of the brain stem and cerebral hemispheres, illustrating the key components of the anterior (carotid) circulation and the posterior (vertebral-basilar) circulation. *A.* The anterior portion of the temporal lobe of the right hemisphere is removed to illustrate the course of the middle cerebral artery through the lateral (Sylvian) fissure and the penetrating branches (lenticulostriate arteries). ***B.*** The circle of Willis is formed by the anterior communicating artery, the two posterior communicating arteries, and the three cerebral arteries. ***C.*** The extracranial and cranial courses of the vertebral, basilar, and carotid arteries. Arrows indicate normal direction of blood flow. (***A-C***, Reproduced with permission from Vasculature of the Central Nervous System and the Cerebrospinal Fluid. In: Martin JH. eds. Neuroanatomy Text and Atlas, 4e New York, NY: McGraw-Hill; 2012; ***B***, Reproduced with permission from Chapter 16. Brain. In: Morton DA, Foreman K, Albertine KH. eds. The Big Picture: Gross Anatomy New York, NY: McGraw-Hill; 2011).

Internal Carotid Arteries

The internal carotid artery consists of four segments (Figure 2.3A): (1) The cervical segment ascends from the bifurcation of the common carotid into the external and internal carotid arteries (Figure 2.2) to enter the cranium through the carotid canal; (2) the intrapetrosal segment courses through the petrous portion of the temporal bone; (3) the intracavernous segment enters at the cavernous sinus, a venous structure overlying the sphenoid bone; and (4) the cerebral segment extends to the bifurcation of the internal carotid artery into anterior and middle cerebral arteries. The intracavernous and cerebral portions together form the carotid siphon, an important radiological landmark (Figure 2.3A).

The internal carotid artery divides near the basal surface of the cerebral hemisphere to form the anterior cerebral and middle cerebral arteries (Figure 2.3A, B). Thus, the anterior and middle cerebral arteries receive their blood from anterior circulation and, as described above, the posterior cerebral artery receives blood from posterior circulation. The cerebral cortex is supplied by the distal, or cortical, branches of the anterior, middle, and posterior cerebral arteries. Knowledge of the approximate boundaries of the cortical regions supplied by the different cerebral arteries helps explain the functional disturbances that follow vascular obstruction, or other pathology, of the cerebral vessels.

Like many parts of the cerebral hemisphere, the anterior cerebral artery is C-shaped (Figure 2.3B). It originates where the internal carotid artery bifurcates and courses within the sagittal fissure around the genu of the corpus callosum (Chapter 1, Figure 1.6). The anterior cerebral artery supplies the dorsal and medial portions of the frontal and parietal lobes. It supplies sensory representation and motor control to the lower extremity in the primary somatosensory and primary motor cortices.

The middle cerebral artery (MCA) supplies blood to most of the lateral convexity of the cortex (Figure 2.3A). It begins at the bifurcation of the internal carotid artery, taking an indirect course through the lateral sulcus and over the inner surfaces of the frontal, temporal, and parietal lobes along the surface of the insular cortex. Distal branches finally emerge onto the lateral convexity. This complex configuration can be seen on radiological images of brain vasculature (Appendix 1). There are deep and cortical branches of the three cerebral arteries (Figure 2.4). The deep branches come off

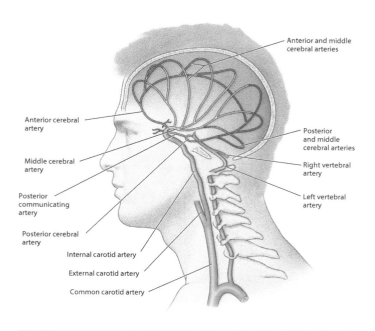

FIGURE 2.2

Paths for collateral blood supply and the course of the major cerebral arteries over the lateral and medial cortical surfaces. Anastomotic channels between the middle and anterior cerebral arteries, and the middle and posterior cerebral arteries are depicted. The left side of the circle of Willis is shown: anterior communicating artery (purple; unlabeled), posterior communicating artery, and posterior cerebral artery. (Reproduced with permission from Vasculature of the Central Nervous System and the Cerebrospinal Fluid. In: Martin JH. eds. *Neuroanatomy Text and Atlas,* 4e New York, NY: McGraw-Hill; 2012).

the arteries proximally and supply deep brain gray matter and white matter regions. The cortical branches at the terminal endings of the cerebral arteries supply the various neuronal laminae of the cerebral cortex. Areas supplied by the MCAs bilaterally include remaining body representation in primary somatosensory and primary motor cortices, and in the left hemisphere only, the speech centers.

> ### > Neuroplasticity
> **Cerebral angiogenesis**

Every year, people gather to watch the magnificent horses of the Kentucky Derby race. The animals have large, hypertrophic muscles rippled with new capillaries, grown in direct response to the intensive metabolic demands of running. This outward sign in our equine athletes of vascular response to tissue demand, called angiogenesis, is also present in humans. Angiogenesis occurs to support nervous system function as well. Brain activity increases metabolic demand, met with increased blood flow to the specific region, which can be detected with functional magnetic resonance imaging (fMRI).

Angiogenesis occurs naturally during the intensive period of brain development in utero. Later, and throughout life, learning takes place through synaptogenesis, the formation of interneuronal connections. This process increases metabolic demands, mainly in the hippocampus, which requires adequate oxygen perfusion through increased blood flow. Aerobic exercise stimulates blood flow, not just in muscles, but also in the brain, to improve tissue perfusion, and promote angiogenesis and synaptogenesis in nervous system structures associated with learning and memory. So, to achieve maximal cognitive performance, such acing a neuroscience exam, in addition to studying, regular exercise will support the metabolic demands required for learning and mastery of the new material.

In contrast to the rather manageable demands placed on a healthy brain during learning, nervous system disease or injury often produces (or is produced by) impaired blood supply. Through the process of angiogenesis, new capillaries infiltrate the damaged areas, replenishing an adequate blood supply necessary to support the high metabolic demands for tissue repair, neuroplastic synaptogenesis, and return of neurological activity for recovery. Scientists are developing treatments to promote and direct early angiogenesis that may one day hasten neurologic recovery and optimize function after damage.

Vertebral Arteries

The vertebral arteries join at the junction of the medulla and pons (pontomedullary junction) on the ventral surface of the brainstem to form the basilar artery, which lies unpaired along the pontine midline, establishing vertebral-basilar circulation (Figure 2.1). The posterior cerebral artery (PCA) originates where the basilar artery bifurcates near the midbrain (Figure 2.3B) and courses around the lateral margin of the midbrain. The PCA supplies the occipital lobe and the medial and inferior portions of the temporal lobes. Functional territories supplied by the posterior cerebral artery include the visual cortex and the hippocampal formation. Both the

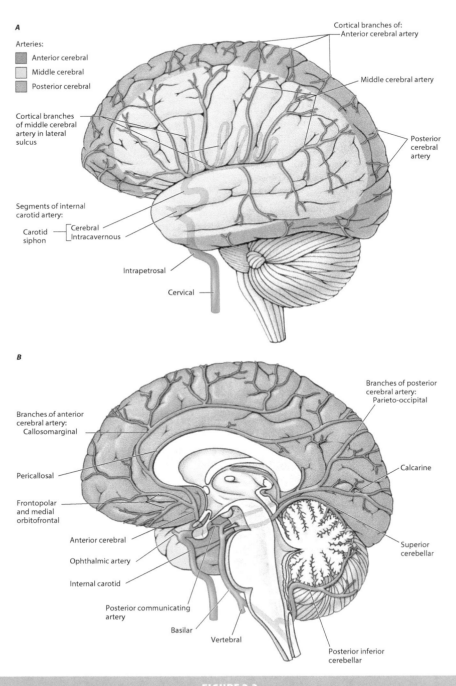

FIGURE 2.3

The courses of the three cerebral arteries are illustrated in views of the lateral (*A*) and midsagittal (*B*) surfaces of the cerebral hemisphere. The territories supplied by each cerebral artery are shown in different colors. Note that the anterior cerebral artery (*B*) courses around the genu of the corpus callosum. (Reproduced with permission from Vasculature of the Central Nervous System and the Cerebrospinal Fluid. In: Martin JH. eds. *Neuroanatomy Text and Atlas*, 4e New York, NY: McGraw-Hill; 2012).

brainstem and cerebellum receive their arterial supply from posterior circulation (Figure 2.5). Arteries supplying most of the brainstem arise from the ventral surface only, in contrast to the spinal arteries, which are located both ventrally and dorsally. Branches emerge from these ventral arteries and either penetrate directly (penetrating or paramedian branches) or run around the circumference (circumferential branches) of the brainstem to supply dorsal brainstem structures and the cerebellum.

Near their entry into the cranium through the foramen magnum, a highly variable series of circumferential and penetrating branches extend from the vertebral arteries (Figures 2.1 and 2.5).

Usually, the first pair of small branches joins at the ventral midline of the medulla, descending as the unpaired anterior spinal artery into the cervical spinal cord. Dorsally, a pair of posterior spinal arteries emerges from the vertebral arteries and descends into the rostral spinal cord. Both the anterior spinal artery and the posterior spinal arteries supply the caudal medulla as they descend into the cervical spinal cord. Spinal arteries lie close to the dorsal and ventral medullary midline, and penetrating branches nourish the deepest areas (Figure 2.5). The anterior spinal artery supplies axons of the corticospinal tract (descending motor pathway) and the medial lemniscus (ascending discriminative touch pathway) in the ventral medulla.

A major laterally emerging branch from the vertebral artery, the posterior inferior cerebellar artery (PICA), nourishes the most dorsolateral region of the medulla. Because this region of the medulla receives blood from no other artery, any occlusion to the PICA typically results in significant medullary tissue damage and functional disruption. This area contains neurons that mediate a wide variety of functions, such as motor neurons to the face, and vital cell groups that regulate cardiovascular function.

The two vertebral arteries join near the pontomedullary junction to form the basilar artery, which supplies the pons via two different sets of branches. Short branches supply the base, where corticospinal fibers are located. A long circumferential branch, the anterior inferior cerebellar artery (AICA) supplies the caudal pons. The basilar artery continues rostrally and emits the superior cerebellar artery, another long circumferential branch arising just proximal to the bifurcation of the basilar artery into the posterior cerebral arteries (Figure 2.5). The cerebellum is supplied by the PICA and AICA caudally and the superior cerebellar artery rostrally, with the long circumferential branches of the vertebral and basilar arteries supplying the rest (Figures 2.1 and 2.5).

The basilar artery splits at the pons-midbrain junction into the two posterior cerebral arteries. The posterior cerebral artery nourishes most of the midbrain (Figures 2.1, 2.3B, and 2.5), visual cortex, and hippocampal formation. Short branches supply the base and tegmentum of the midbrain, whereas long circumferential branches supply the tectum dorsally. The superior and inferior colliculi, the principal portion of the tectum, also receive a small supply by the superior cerebellar artery.

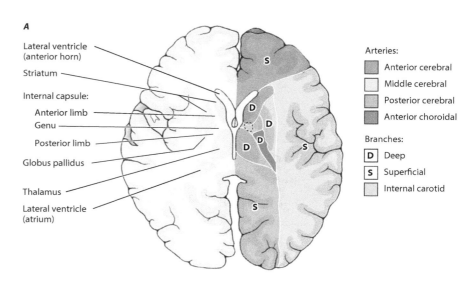

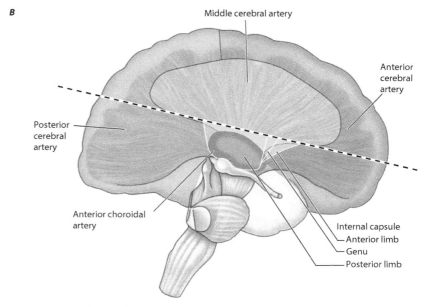

FIGURE 2.4

The arterial circulation of deep cerebral structures and cerebral white matter. A. Distributions of deep and superficial branches of the cerebral arteries are shown. **B.** Arterial supply of the subcortical white matter and internal capsule. Different dorsoventral levels of the internal capsule and limbs receive their arterial supply from different cerebral arteries. The dashed line indicates the plane of the horizontal section in **A.** The territories supplied by each cerebral artery are shown. (Reproduced with permission from Vasculature of the Central Nervous System and the Cerebrospinal Fluid. In: Martin JH. eds. *Neuroanatomy Text and Atlas,* 4e New York, NY: McGraw-Hill; 2012).

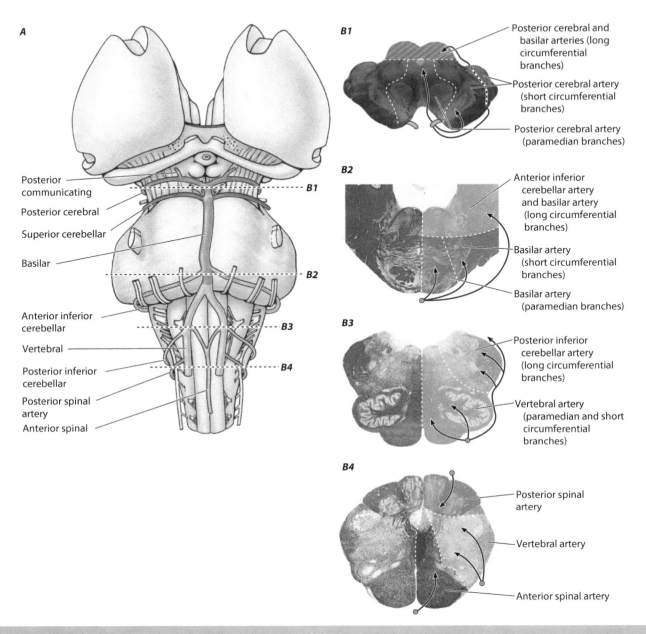

FIGURE 2.5

Brainstem arterial distribution A. Arterial circulation of the brain stem is schematically illustrated on a view of the ventral surface of the brain stem. **B.** Four transverse sections through the brain stem are shown, illustrating the distribution of arterial supply. In the upper medulla (**B3**), pons (**B2**), and midbrain (**B1**), portions of tissue from medial to dorsolateral are supplied by paramedian, short circumferential, and long circumferential branches. The caudal medulla receives its arterial supply from the vertebral and spinal arteries (**B4**). The dashed lines in **A** indicate the planes of section in **B**. (Reproduced with permission from Vasculature of the Central Nervous System and the Cerebrospinal Fluid. In: Martin JH. eds. *Neuroanatomy Text and Atlas*, 4e New York, NY: McGraw-Hill; 2012; Photo used with permission from Howard J Radzyner).

The arterial supply of the diencephalon, basal ganglia, and internal capsule derives from both the anterior and posterior circulations (Figure 2.6). This supply is complex, with many individual variations. Branches supplying these structures emerge from the proximal portions of the cerebral arteries or directly from the internal carotid artery. Many of the small proximal branches of the anterior and middle cerebral arteries are also termed the lenticulostriate arteries. The superior half of the internal capsule is supplied primarily by lenticulostriate branches of the middle cerebral artery. The inferior half of the internal capsule's anterior limb is supplied primarily by the anterior cerebral artery. The posterior limb and genu are supplied by the lenticulostriate branches of the middle cerebral artery, with contribution from the anterior choroidal artery (Figure 2.1). The basal ganglia receive their arterial blood supply from the anterior and middle cerebral arteries and the anterior choroidal artery (Figures 2.1 and 2.6). The thalamus is nourished by branches of the posterior cerebral and posterior communicating arteries. The hypothalamus is fed by branches of the anterior and posterior cerebral arteries and the two communicating arteries.

Circle of Willis

On the ventral surface of the brain, proximal portions of the cerebral and communicating arteries form the circle of Willis (Figure 2.1B). The circle of Willis is an example of a network of interconnected arteries, or an anastomosis. Communication between anterior and posterior circulations is valuable because decreased flow in one system can be compensated by increased flow in the other. The

two posterior communicating arteries allow blood to flow between the middle and posterior cerebral arteries on each side, and the anterior communicating artery allows blood to flow between the anterior cerebral arteries. When either the posterior or the anterior arterial circulation becomes occluded, collateral circulation may occur through the circle of Willis to rescue the region deprived of blood. Many individuals, however, lack one of the components of the circle of Willis, resulting in incomplete cerebral perfusion by the surviving system.

Another site for anterior-posterior circulation communication is the dorsal convexity of the cerebral hemisphere, where the terminal ends of the cerebral arteries anastomose (Figure 2.2). These interconnections occur between branches only when they are located on the cortical surface in the grey matter, not after the artery has penetrated into the white matter. When a major artery becomes compromised, these anastomoses limit the extent of cortical damage. For example, if a branch of the posterior cerebral artery becomes occluded, the occipital lobe may be rescued by collateral circulation from the middle cerebral artery. In contrast, little collateral circulation exists in the deeper white matter.

Although collateral circulation provides the cerebral cortex with a safety margin during arterial occlusion, the dorsal anastomotic network that provides such insurance is vulnerable to ischemia. When systemic blood pressure is reduced, the region served by this network is particularly susceptible to ischemia because such anastomoses occur at the terminal ends of the arteries, regions where perfusion is lowest. The peripheral borders of the territory supplied by major vessels are termed *border zones*, and an infarction occurring in these regions is termed a *border zone infarct*.

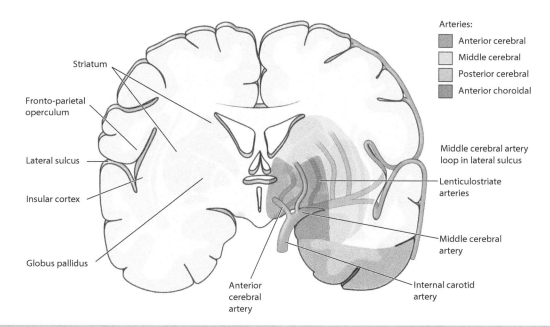

Arteries:
- Anterior cerebral
- Middle cerebral
- Posterior cerebral
- Anterior choroidal

Striatum
Fronto-parietal operculum
Lateral sulcus
Insular cortex
Globus pallidus
Anterior cerebral artery

Middle cerebral artery loop in lateral sulcus
Lenticulostriate arteries
Middle cerebral artery
Internal carotid artery

FIGURE 2.6

Middle cerebral artery and vascular supply of the diencephalon. The course of the middle cerebral artery through the lateral sulcus and along the insular and opercular surfaces of the cerebral cortex is shown in a schematic coronal section. Deep structures of the diencephalon and basal ganglia have a complex blood supply. In this representation, different arterial territories are shaded different colors. (Adapted from DeArmond SJ, Fusco MM, Dewey MM. *Structure of the Human Brain*, 3rd ed. Oxford University Press; 1989).

III VENOUS DRAINAGE

Drainage of blood from the CNS into the major vessels emptying into the heart—systemic circulation—is achieved through either a direct or an indirect path. Spinal cord and caudal medullary veins drain directly through a network of veins and plexuses, into the systemic circulation. By contrast, the rest of the CNS drains indirectly; veins first empty into dural sinuses before returning blood to the systemic circulation (Figure 2.7).

Venous drainage of the cerebral hemispheres is provided by superficial and deep cerebral veins. Superficial veins vary in distribution, arising from the cerebral cortex and underlying white matter. The deep cerebral veins, such as the internal cerebral vein (Figure 2.7, inset), drain the more interior portions of the white matter as well as the basal ganglia and parts of the diencephalon. Many deep cerebral veins drain into the great cerebral vein of Galen.

Major dural sinuses located within layers of the dura include the superior sagittal, inferior sagittal, straight, transverse, sigmoid, superior, and inferior petrosal. Dural sinuses function as low-pressure channels for venous blood flow back to the systemic circulation, mainly through the internal jugular vein (Figure 2.7 and Chapter 1, Figure 1.14).

Superficial cerebral veins drain into the superior and inferior sagittal sinuses. The superior sagittal sinus runs along the midline at the superior margin of the falx cerebri. The inferior sagittal sinus courses along the inferior margin of the falx cerebri just above the corpus callosum. The inferior sagittal sinus, together with the great cerebral vein of Galen, returns venous blood to the straight (sometimes called *rectus*) sinus.

Veins of the midbrain drain into the great cerebral vein, which empties into the straight sinus, whereas the pons and rostral medulla drain into the superior petrosal sinus (Chapter 1, Figure 1.14). Cerebellar veins drain into the great cerebral vein and the superior petrosal sinus.

At the occipital pole, the superior sagittal sinus and the straight sinus join to form the two transverse sinuses. Finally, these sinuses drain into the sigmoid sinuses, which return blood to the internal jugular veins. The cavernous sinus, into which drain the ophthalmic and facial veins, is also illustrated in Chapter 1, Figure 1.14. It provides an area of communication between intra- and extracranial circulation and may allow infection to enter the brain. If infection is transmitted into the cavernous sinus, venous blood in the infected sinus clots, producing a thrombus (a solid blood clot) that can compress multiple cranial nerves, particularly those that affect eye movements and face sensation. Patients can quickly develop sepsis with fever and nuchal rigidity consistent with meningitis. Cavernous sinus infection is an emergent condition, and if left untreated, can be fatal.

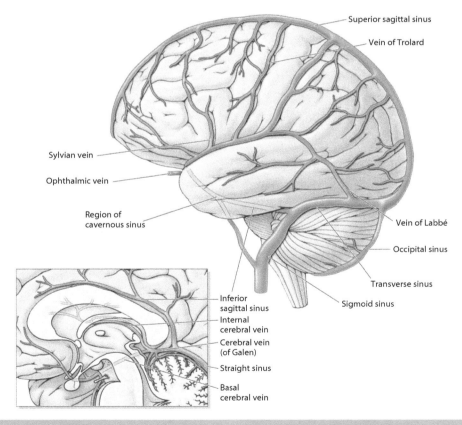

FIGURE 2.7

Cerebral veins and sinuses. Lateral view of the brain, showing major superficial veins and the dural sinuses. Inset shows veins on midline. (Reproduced with permission from Vasculature of the Central Nervous System and the Cerebrospinal Fluid. In: Martin JH. eds. *Neuroanatomy Text and Atlas,* 4e New York, NY: McGraw-Hill; 2012).

Blood–Brain Barrier

The intravascular compartment is isolated from the extracellular compartment of the CNS. This feature, the blood–brain barrier (Figure 2.8), was discovered when intravenous dye injection stained most tissues and organs of the body, but not the brain. This permeability barrier protects the brain from neuroactive compounds and rapid changes in the ionic constituents of the blood that can affect neuronal excitability.

Unique characteristics of endothelial cells in the capillaries of the brain and spinal cord create the blood–brain barrier (Figure 2.8A1, A2). Peripheral capillary endothelial cells have fenestrations (pores) between adjacent cells that allow large molecules to flow into the extracellular space, with additional nonselective transport by pinocytosis (internalization of liquid). In contrast, CNS capillaries restrict motion for several reasons. First, adjacent tightly joined endothelial cells in CNS capillaries prevent movement of compounds both in and out of the extracellular compartment. Additionally, transcellular movement of compounds from intravascular to extracellular compartments is limited because the endothelial cells lack the required transport mechanisms, and pinocytosis does not occur in

the CNS. Further, astrocytes (support cells in the CNS) emit processes that terminate as flattened endfeet/foot processes that are intimately applied to the outer surfaces of the capillary endothelial cells. Astrocytic endfeet form a scale-like or lace-like network of lamellar (flattened) processes that enclose the capillary, reinforcing the barrier. Finally, astrocytes may release substances that promote formation of tight junctions and regulate capillary permeability.

Although most of the CNS is protected by the blood–brain barrier, eight brain structures lack a blood–brain barrier. These structures are close to the midline, and because they are closely associated with the ventricular system, they are collectively termed *circumventricular organs* (Figure 2.8B). Circumventricular organs include the (1) area postrema in the medulla, (2) subcommissural organ, (3) subfornical organ, (4) vascular organ of the lamina terminalis, (5) median eminence, (6) neurohypophysis (part of the pituitary gland), (7) choroid plexus, and (8) pineal gland. At each organ, neurosecretory products secreted into the blood or local neurons detect blood-borne compounds as part of a mechanism for regulating the body's internal environment. One circumventricular organ, the area postrema, triggers vomiting in response to circulating blood-borne chemicals.

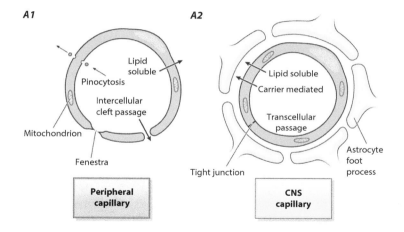

A1 *A2*

Lipid soluble
Pinocytosis
Intercellular cleft passage
Mitochondrion
Fenestra

Peripheral capillary

Lipid soluble
Carrier mediated
Transcellular passage
Tight junction
Astrocyte foot process

CNS capillary

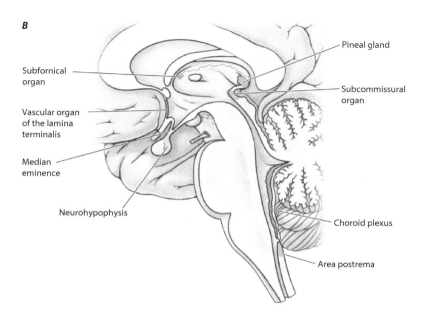

B

Subfornical organ
Vascular organ of the lamina terminalis
Median eminence
Neurohypophysis

Pineal gland
Subcommissural organ
Choroid plexus
Area postrema

FIGURE 2.8

Blood–brain barrier and circumventricular organs. **A.** Schematic illustration of a section through a peripheral (*A1*) and central nervous system (*A2*) capillary. There is less restricted transport across the endothelium of the peripheral than central capillary. **B.** Circumventricular organs are brain regions that do not have a blood–brain barrier. The locations of the eight circumventricular organs are shown on a view of the midsagittal brain: neurohypophysis (also termed posterior lobe of pituitary gland), median eminence, vascular organ of the lamina terminalis, subfornical organ, pineal gland, subcommissural organ, choroid plexus, and area postrema. Note that all circumventricular organs are located centrally, in close association with the components of the ventricular system. (Reproduced with permission from Vasculature of the Central Nervous System and the Cerebrospinal Fluid. In: Martin JH. eds. *Neuroanatomy Text and Atlas*, 4e New York, NY: McGraw-Hill; 2012).

Ventricular System and Cerebrospinal Fluid

CSF fills the ventricles (Figure 2.9). It also fills the subarachnoid space and thus bathes the external brain surface. Together, the ventricles and subarachnoid space contain approximately 140 mL of CSF, of which 25 mL are in the ventricles and the remaining in the subarachnoid space. Intraventricular pressure is normally around 10–15 mm Hg. Total CSF production by both sources is approximately 500 mL per day, and excess fluid is eliminated through communication with venous drainage in dural sinuses (see below).

CSF serves at least three essential functions. First, CSF buoys the brain, reducing pressure on delicate tissue of the ventral brain surface and cushioning the brain from physical shocks. Second, it serves an excretory function and regulates the chemical environment of the CNS. Because the brain has no lymphatic system, diffusion into the CSF is the method of removing waste. Although the production of CSF by the choroid plexus has been discussed, it also serves to remove waste and excess neurotransmitters from the CNS via the blood–CSF barrier. Tight junctions between epithelial cells in the choroid plexus form a barrier to movement of water-soluble molecules between the choroid plexus and adjacent capillaries. A variety of transport channels in the choroid epithelial cells provide a means whereby waste products are actively removed from the CSF into the capillaries for elimination from the brain tissues. Third, it acts as a channel for chemical communication within the CNS. Neurochemicals released by neurons can enter the CSF and be taken up by cells on the ventricular floor and walls. Once in the CSF, these compounds have relatively free access to neural tissue adjacent to the ventricles because much of the ventricular lining presents no barrier between the CSF compartment and the extracellular compartment of the brain.

Cerebrospinal fluid circulation

Pia and blood vessels form the core of the choroid plexus and the choroid epithelium which secretes CSF (Figure 2.9A). The choroid plexus is present only in the ventricles: in the roof of the third and fourth ventricles and in the ventricular roof and floor of the lateral ventricles. A barrier imposed by the choroidal epithelium prevents the transport of materials from blood into the CSF. This is the blood–CSF barrier, analogous to the blood–brain barrier. The choroidal epithelium is innervated by autonomic fibers, which serve a regulatory function. For example, denervation of the sympathetic fibers produces hydrocephalus in animals.

The rest of the CSF is secreted by brain capillaries. This extrachoroidal source of CSF enters the ventricular system through ependymal cells, ciliated cuboidal epithelial cells that line the ventricles. Although the principal function of the choroid plexus is CSF secretion, the plexus also has a reabsorptive function. The choroid plexus can eliminate from the CSF a variety of compounds introduced into the ventricles.

Cerebrospinal fluid circulation through the ventricles and subarachnoid space.

The lateral ventricle is a C-shaped structure, as are many deep neuronal regions of the cerebral hemispheres. CSF produced by the choroid plexus in the lateral ventricles (Figure 2.9A) flows through the interventricular foramina (of Monro) and mixes with CSF produced in the third ventricle. From the third ventricle, CSF flows through the cerebral aqueduct (of Sylvius) and into the fourth ventricle. Three apertures in the roof of the fourth ventricle drain CSF from the ventricular system into the subarachnoid space: the median aperture, or foramen of Magendie, located on the midline, and the two lateral apertures, or foramina of Luschka, located at the lateral margins of the fourth ventricle (Figure 2.9A inset).

Subarachnoid space is dilated in certain locations, called *cisterns* (CSF pools here). Five prominent cisterns are located on the midline: (1) the interpeduncular cistern, between the basis pedunculi on the ventral midbrain surface, (2) the quadrigeminal cistern, dorsal to the superior and inferior colliculi (which are also called the *quadrigeminal bodies*, or *corpora quadrigemina*), (3) the pontine cistern, ventral to the pontomedullary junction, (4) the cisterna magna, dorsal to the medulla, and (5) the lumbar cistern, in the caudal vertebral canal. The subarachnoid space also contains the blood vessels of the CNS (Figure 2.9B). Blood vessels penetrate the brain together with

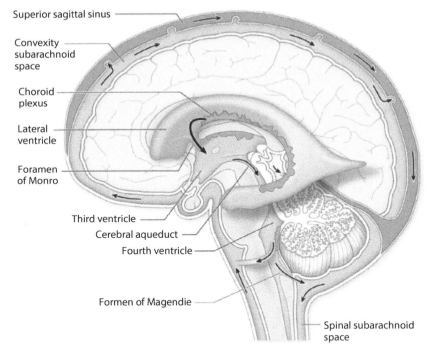

Superior sagittal sinus

Convexity subarachnoid space

Choroid plexus

Lateral ventricle

Foramen of Monro

Third ventricle

Cerebral aqueduct

Fourth ventricle

Formen of Magendie

Spinal subarachnoid space

FIGURE 2.9

Schematic representation of the bulk flow of CSF from the lateral ventricles, through the third and fourth ventricles, outward from the basal foramina (Luschka and Magendie), upward around the brainstem and basal cisterns to both the convexities of the hemispheres and downward to spinal subarachnoid space. Most absorption is presumed to occur over the cerebral convexities, abutting the sagittal sinus. (Reproduced with permission from Disturbances of Cerebrospinal Fluid, Including Hydrocephalus, Pseudotumor Cerebri, and Low-Pressure Syndromes. In: Ropper AH, et al., eds. *Adams and Victor's Principles of Neurology*, 11e New York, NY: McGraw-Hill; 2019).

the pia, creating a perivascular space between the vessels and pia for a short distance, and a path for CSF flow from the subarachnoid space to interstitial spaces within the brain and spinal cord.

Lumbar puncture. CSF can be safely withdrawn from the lumbar cistern without risking spinal cord damage (Figure 2.10). This can be understood by considering how the caudal vertebral column and spinal cord develop. Throughout the first three months of development, the spinal cord grows at about the same rate as the vertebral column (Figure 2.10A). During this period, the spinal cord occupies the entire vertebral canal within the vertebral column. The dorsal and ventral roots associated with each segment pass directly through the intervertebral foramina to reach their target structures. Later, the growth of the vertebral column exceeds that

of the spinal cord. In the adult, the most caudal spinal cord segment is located at the level of the first lumbar vertebra. This differential growth produces the lumbar cistern, an enlargement of the subarachnoid space in the caudal portion of the spinal canal. The dorsal and ventral roots from the lumbar and sacral segments, which subserve sensation and movement of the legs, travel within the lumbar cistern before exiting the vertebral canal. In dissection these roots resemble a horse's tail; hence the name *cauda equina*. CSF can be withdrawn from the lumbar cistern without risk of damaging the spinal cord, by inserting a needle through the intervertebral space between either the third and fourth or fourth and fifth vertebrae (Figure 2.10B). The roots are displaced by the needle rather than being pierced. This procedure is known as a spinal or lumbar tap.

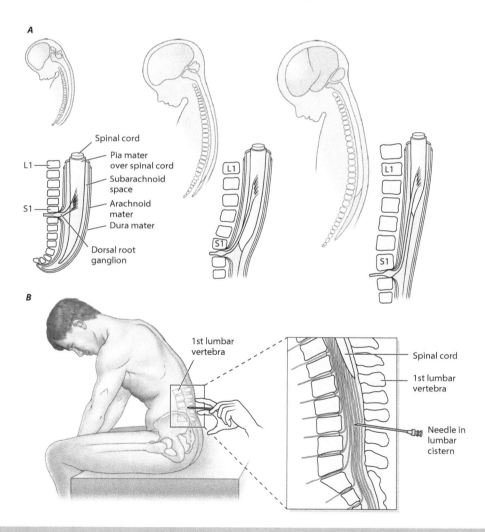

FIGURE 2.10

The lumbar cistern and the lumbar puncture. The lumbar cistern forms because the vertebral column grows in length more than the spinal cord. **A.** Side view of the lumbosacral spinal cord and vertebral column at three developmental stages: 3 months, 5 months, and in the newborn. The insets show the fetus at these stages. **B.** Schematic showing principle of withdrawal of cerebrospinal fluid from the lumbar cistern (lumbar puncture). The needle is inserted into the subarachnoid space of the lumbar cistern. The view on the right shows the relationship between the needle and the roots in the cistern. Note that the lumbar puncture is performed with the patient lying on his or her side. In this figure, the patient is sitting upright to simplify visualization of the procedure and comparison with the anatomy of the vertebrae. (**A-B**, Adapted from House EL, Pansky B, and Siegel A. *A Systematic Approach to Neuroscience*, 3rd ed. New York, NY: McGraw-Hill; 1979).

CSF return through dural sinuses. CSF passes from the subarachnoid space to the venous blood through specialized structures called *arachnoid villi* (Figure 2.11 and Chapter 1, Figure 1.13). Arachnoid villi are microscopic evaginations (outpocketings) of the arachnoid mater that protrude into the dural sinuses as well as directly into certain veins. CSF flows through a system of large vacuoles in the arachnoid cells of the villi and through an extracellular path between cells of the villi. Numerous clusters of arachnoid villi are present over the dorsal (superior) convexity of the cerebral hemispheres in the superior sagittal sinus, where they form a macroscopic structure called the arachnoid granulations. The arachnoid granulations can be imaged on MRI (Figure 2.9C). The arachnoid villi are also present where the spinal nerves exit the spinal dural sac. These villi direct the flow of CSF into the radicular veins.

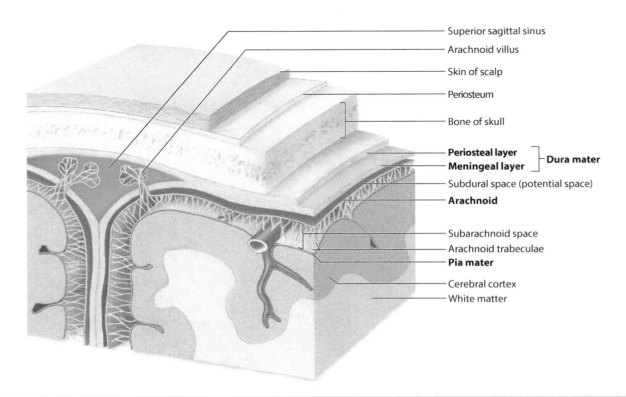

Superior sagittal sinus
Arachnoid villus
Skin of scalp
Periosteum
Bone of skull
Periosteal layer
Meningeal layer ⎱ **Dura mater**
Subdural space (potential space)
Arachnoid
Subarachnoid space
Arachnoid trabeculae
Pia mater
Cerebral cortex
White matter

FIGURE 2.11

Meninges around the brain. The dura, arachnoid, and pia maters also surround the brain, and as shown here, the relationships among the cranial meninges are similar to those of the spinal cord. The diagram includes arachnoid villi, which are outpocketings of arachnoid away from the brain, which penetrate the dura mater and enter blood-filled venous sinuses located within that layer. The arachnoid villi function in releasing excess CSF into the blood. Blood vessels from the arachnoid branch into smaller arteries and veins that enter brain tissue, carrying oxygen and nutrients. These small vessels are initially covered with pia mater, but as capillaries they are covered only by the perivascular feet of astrocytes. (Reproduced with permission from Mescher AL. Chapter 9. Nerve Tissue & the Nervous System. In: Mescher AL. eds. *Junqueira's Basic Histology: Text & Atlas*, 13e. New York, NY: McGraw-Hill; 2013).

IV RESPONSE TO INJURY

Cerebrovascular Injury

Local regions of the CNS receive blood from small sets of penetrating arteries that receive their blood from the major arteries. Disruption in the blood supply can be devastating to local tissue. Decreased blood supply typically occurs when an artery becomes occluded or when systemic blood pressure drops substantially, such as during a heart attack. Occlusion commonly occurs because of an acute blockage (Figure 2.12B), such as from an embolus, or the gradual narrowing of the arterial lumen (stenosis), as in atherosclerosis. Interruption or reduction of arterial supply to an area results in decreased delivery of oxygenated blood to the tissue, a condition termed *ischemia*. A brief reduction in blood flow produces transient neurological signs, attributable to lost functions of the oxygen-deprived area. This transient (temporary) ischemic attack is defined by the lack of infarction on subsequent imaging studies, and increases risk of future vascular events. Ischemia that persists, or other types of brain injury, can produce an infarct, a region of dead and necrotic tissues (Figure 2.12A).

Clinical presentation of ischemic stroke (cerebral vascular accident) is based on anatomic distribution of tissue damage. The most common type is termed *subclinical* or *silent*, with subtle disruption of higher brain function such as critical thinking, motivation, and self-control. Many strokes follow the entire arterial supply of a cerebral vessel (Figure 2.12B) creating predictable clinical manifestations such as loss of contralateral sensory and motor function. Another common type of ischemic stroke is termed *lacunar* (Latin for "empty space"), with tissue damage often localized to the deep nuclei or pons (Figure 2.13).

Lacunar stroke carries a higher 30-day survival rate than other types, possibly due to the localized, less diffuse pattern of damage.

In contrast to ischemic stroke, hemorrhage produces diffuse and extensive damage to brain tissue. Hemorrhagic stroke can occur when an artery ruptures, releasing blood into the surrounding tissue (Figure 2.14). This not only interrupts downstream flow but also can damage brain tissue at the rupture site due to pressure on tissues from uncontrolled bleeding. A common cause of hemorrhagic stroke is an aneurysm (ballooning of an artery due to weakening of the muscular wall) that ruptures. Hemorrhagic stroke generally leads to more diffuse damage and extensive clinical impairments due to increased size and permanence of tissue damage. It is common to see a combination of ischemic and hemorrhagic damage. This clinical presentation may be termed *mixed cerebrovascular disease*.

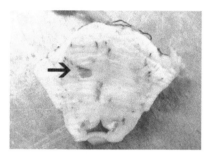

FIGURE 2.13

Lacunar infarct of the pons. The arrow indicates a lacunar infarct. Lacunar infarcts are small (<1.0 cm) and can be the result of hypertensive cardiovascular disease. Because of their small size, most lacunar infarcts are asymptomatic. (Reproduced with permission from Chapter 11. Neuropathology. In: Kemp WL, Burns DK, Brown TG. eds. *Pathology: The Big Picture* New York, NY: McGraw-Hill; 2008).

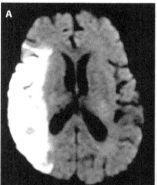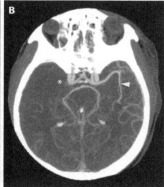

FIGURE 2.12

Neuroradiological imaging after stroke. A. Diffusion weighted image (DWI) showing large right middle cerebral artery infarction. The white region corresponds to the infarcted territory of the middle cerebral artery (clinical representation has left side of the picture representing the right side of the brain). **B.** Magnetic resonance angiogram (MRA) showing normal perfusion in the left artery (arrowhead) and a complete lack of perfusion of the right middle cerebral artery (asterisk). This demonstrates occlusion at its proximal portion. (Reproduced with permission from Ropper AH et al. *Adams & Victor's Principles of Neurology*, 9th ed. New York: AccessMedicine, 2009.)

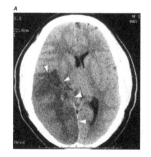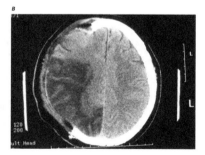

FIGURE 2.14

CTs of hemorrhagic atroke pre- and post-surgery. A. Head computed tomography scan of a patient with a 4-day-old stroke that occluded the right middle cerebral and posterior cerebral arteries. The infarcted tissue is the hypodense (dark) area indicated by the arrowheads. The patient presented with left-sided weakness and left visual field loss but then became less responsive, prompting this head computed tomography. Note the right-to-left midline shift. **B.** Same patient status post decompressive right hemicraniectomy. Note the free expansion of swollen brain outside the normal confines of the skull. (Reproduced with permission from Chapter 11. Neuropathology. In: Kemp WL, Burns DK, Brown TG. eds. *Pathology: The Big Picture* New York, NY: McGraw-Hill; 2008).

Increased Intracranial Pressure

The cranial vault acts as a closed chamber containing brain, blood, and CSF. Maintenance of intracranial pressure is essential because the brain, especially the gray matter, is delicate, and elevated pressure can distort and damage soft tissue. The Monro-Kellie doctrine states that intracranial pressure is related to the sum of the volumes of these three elements so that intracranial pressure remains relatively constant. An increase in one element is equalized by decreases in one or both of the other elements (Figure 2.15). In a normal person, increases in systolic blood pressure are common during exercise, without accompanying damaging increases in intracranial pressure.

Increases in brain volume by space-occupying lesions (intracranial bleeding, hydrocephalus, tumors) stimulate accommodative responses most easily in the venous and CSF circulatory systems. If the pressure increase exceeds the compensation effects of the blood and ventricular mechanisms, the soft brain tissue can herniate (be forced across rigid structures in the cranium), damaging the tissue and producing severe injury that can even result in death. Because of this, intracranial pressure is closely watched, using a variety of monitors in the Intensive Care Unit (Figure 2.16).

Two types of herniation are recognized and described in relation to the tentorium cerebelli: supratentorial and infratentorial (Figure 2.17). Three locations are prone to herniation: crossing the midline below the inferior margin of the falx cerebri (subfalcine); across the sharp border of the tentorium cerebelli (uncal and central); and through the foramen magnum (tonsillar). With a subfalcine herniation, the most common type of supratentorial cerebral herniation, forebrain tissue is forced across the midline, compressing the anterior cerebral artery and producing frontal and parietal lobe infarcts. Often, a subfalcine herniation is a prelude to more severe infratentorial herniations. Although less frequent, tissue can also be extruded upward through the tentorium cerebelli. Infratentorial

Integration of Systems
The Risks of Stroke

Stroke, or cerebral vascular accident, was once considered untreatable and unpreventable. Considerable gains in prevention and treatment have been made over the past 50 years. However, stroke incidence remains high due to imperfect public awareness, adherence to unhealthy lifestyles, and variable access to quality health care.

Stroke risk factors are generally well known. Authors of an international case-control study identified the top 10 risk factors: (1) hypertension, (2) diabetes, (3) cardiac causes, (4) current smoking, (5) abdominal obesity, (6) hyperlipidemia, (7) physical inactivity, (8) alcohol consumption, (9) diet, and (10) psychosocial stress and depression. A brief review of this list indicates that most risk factors are modifiable, and therein lies another challenge: how to inspire broad behavioral change in a population. Considering the large number of risk factors for stroke, and the fact that stroke symptoms are not uniform between people or populations, preventing stroke remains an urgent challenge.

Stroke commonly causes death, dementia, or disability, with clinical presentation depending on location and severity of tissue damage. These effects take severe physical, emotional, and financial tolls on both the individual and society. Brain mapping studies in animal models have allowed rigorous study of response to localized brain injury, and response to rehabilitation has exceeded expectations. Translational research is demonstrating benefit from behavioral interventions after stroke to reduce edema and promote neuroplastic changes. Rapid treatment in quality stroke centers and rehabilitation improve recovery after cerebral vascular accident. Multimodal therapy after stroke has been shown to be efficacious, leading to improved function and health outcomes. However, because it remains impossible to specifically predict the amount and timeline for individual recovery after stroke, care dosing remains uncertain.

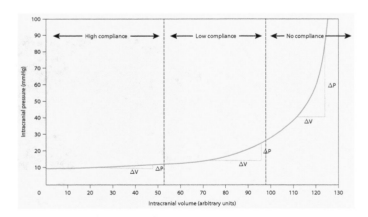

FIGURE 2.15

Pressure-volume curve demonstrating the effect of changing the volume of intracranial contents on intracranial pressure. Note the compensated zone, with little change of pressure with change of volume, and the uncompensated zone, with significant change of pressure with change of volume. (Adapted with permission from Morton R, Ellenbogen RG: Intracranial consciousness, in Ellenbogen RG et al (eds): *Principles of Neurosurgery*, 3rd ed. Philadelphia: Elsevier Saunders, 2012, p 313. Copyright Elsevier).

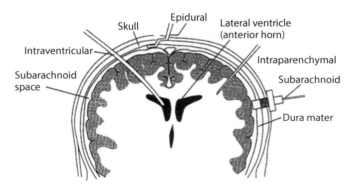

FIGURE 2.16

Various anatomic sites to monitor intracranial pressure. (Reproduced with permission from Frank JI, Rosengart AJ. Chapter 65. Intracranial Pressure: Monitoring and Management. In: Hall JB, Schmidt GA, Wood LH. eds. *Principles of Critical Care*, 3e. New York, NY: McGraw-Hill; 2005).

herniations often produce more severe effects on patients because the structures at and below the tentorium include critical motor and sensory structures and vital function control centers.

The uncus is a medial protrusion of tissue on the inferomedial surface of the inferior temporal lobe. With increased supratentorial pressure, the uncus can be forced through the tentorial notch and compress underlying structures, beginning with the oculomotor nerve. Thus the first symptom of an uncal herniation is fixed pupillary dilation and loss of ipsilateral eye movement. If the uncal herniation is larger, it can compress the posterior cerebral artery and produce an infarct in the visual cortex, producing loss of vision in the contralateral visual hemisphere. With a central herniation, more of the temporal lobes bilaterally, and portions of the diencephalon, are forced through the tentorial notch, damaging the midbrain and possibly extending farther caudally along the brainstem. This type of infratentorial herniation is extremely dangerous and requires immediate intervention. Frequently the patient will become comatose and display abnormal posturing related to interruption of descending motor pathways. Also diagnostic of a central infratentorial herniation from increased intracranial pressure is the appearance of Cushing's reflex (Cushing's triad). Patients with this level of injury present increased blood pressure, bradycardia (decreased heart rate), and irregular respiration; cardiovascular and respiratory centers are located in the caudal brainstem. Cushing's reflex frequently presages death, so immediate treatment is imperative.

Tonsillar herniation (also called a *Chiari malformation*) involves the inferomedial portion of the cerebellum, called the tonsil, being forced through the foramen magnum, primarily due to a space-occupying mass in the posterior cranial fossa (where the caudal brainstem and cerebellum are located). It can be caused by, or it can produce, hydrocephalus due to interrupted CSF flow. Patients present with symptoms reflecting hydrocephalus, nausea, irritability, and headaches, as well as other signs of impaired caudal cranial nerves, such as weakness in facial muscles, dysphagia (difficulty

swallowing), vertigo, and nystagmus (rhythmic horizontal eye oscillation). Severe cases may produce paralysis, coma, or death, but mild cases may be asymptomatic.

Although thrombolytic drug therapy represents a significant advance in treating ischemic stroke, reperfusion of the microvasculature in the ischemic area can lead to intracerebral stroke and expansion of tissue damage due to two factors: (1) collapse of microvasculature destroying membranes; and (2) increasing permeability across the walls of capillaries and arterioles. Effects of increasing permeability include influx of Ca^{++} and Na^+, leading to release of bioactive molecules, including large amounts of glutamate, which can poison connecting cells by overexciting them (excitotoxicity). These molecules can lead to necrosis or programmed cell death and production of an infarct (Figure 2.18).

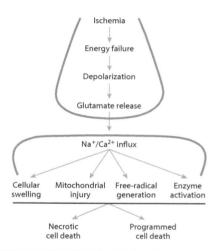

FIGURE 2.18

Pathogenesis of the ischemic cascade. Ischemia deprives the brain of metabolic substrates, especially oxygen and glucose, making it impossible for cells to carry out energy-dependent functions such as the maintenance of transmembrane ion gradients. Loss of these gradients depolarizes cell membranes, leading to the influx of calcium through voltage-gated calcium channels and triggering the release of neurotransmitters such as glutamate from presynaptic nerve terminals. Glutamate binds to receptors on the postsynaptic neuronal membrane to activate the influx of sodium and calcium. This sets in motion a cascade of biochemical events that causes cellular swelling; injures mitochondria; generates toxic free radicals; and activates proteases, nucleases, and other enzymes. Depending on the severity and duration of ischemia, neurons may die rapidly from necrosis or more gradually from programmed cell death or apoptosis. Necrotic cell death is characterized by shrinkage of the nucleus (pyknosis), early loss of membrane integrity, structural changes in mitochondria, and eventually cellular lysis. Programmed cell death (PCD) depends on the synthesis of new proteins. Apoptosis, one form of PCD, is associated with margination of nuclear chromatin, relative preservation of cell membrane and mitochondrial integrity, and the formation of membrane-bound extracellular blebs (apoptotic bodies). Necrosis and PCD can coexist in different regions of an ischemic lesion. (Reproduced with permission from Aminoff MJ, Greenberg D, Simon RR: *Clinical Neurology*, 6th ed. New York, McGraw-Hill Companies; 2005).

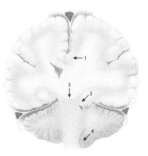

FIGURE 2.17

Schematic drawing of brain herniation patterns. (1) Subfalcine herniation. The cingulate gyrus shifts across midline under the falx cerebri. (2) Uncal herniation. The uncus (medial temporal lobe gyrus) shifts medially and compresses the midbrain and cerebral peduncle. (3) Central transtentorial herniation. The diencephalon and midbrain shift caudally through the tentorial notch. (4) Tonsillar herniation. The cerebellar tonsil shifts caudally through the foramen magnum. (Reproduced with permission from Cohen DS, Quest DO: Increased intracranial pressure, brain herniation and their control. In: Wilkins RH, Rengachary SS [eds]: *Neurosurgery*, 2nd ed. New York: McGraw Hill, 1996).

Drugs to Minimize Stroke Effects

As drug treatments and angioplasty were developed to treat heart attacks, some scientists recognized similarities between heart attack and stroke, both events caused by arterial clotting. They administered similar treatments to combat the effects of ischemic stroke; however, the treatments were not effective, and that line of research was abandoned. The development of thrombolytic drugs and their use to treat ischemic stroke is a relatively new emergence in stroke care. Recognizing a critical three-hour window for preventing permanent ischemic damage, timely delivery of thrombolytic therapy is now understood to be essential. One drug used today is tissue plasmin activator (t-PA), first found during cancer research. It is activated by cancer cells to destroy extracellular matrix (Figure 2.19). In fact, the first cell line of t-PA was derived from a human with malignant melanoma. Currently the human t-PA gene is cloned and grown for drug delivery in a lab. As described in Chapter 1, during the inflammatory response to injury, a clot is formed by platelets and strengthened by a fibrin mesh. Tissue plasmin activator generates plasminogen, which degrades the fibrin found in a clot. This treatment of arterial blockage reduces permanent nervous tissue damage and death. When people are properly diagnosed with a thrombotic stroke (as administering thrombolytic drug therapy to a patient with hemorrhagic stroke could be catastrophic) and receive t-PA within a three-hour window, clinical signs of stroke are prevented or reduced dramatically. Because this requires public awareness of stroke signs and early access to appropriate healthcare, public health campaigns regarding stroke risk factors, signs, and urgent care needs are becoming more common globally.

Frontiers in Research
Genetic Markers for Ischemic Stroke

The cause of ischemic stroke remains uncertain, or cryptogenic, in over a third of all cases. This makes prevention difficult. Researchers are combining genetic marking with brain imaging to identify probable causes of ischemic stroke. In time, a gene expression profile could be used commonly to more specifically identify and target treatment to prevent stroke. Other scientists have discovered that, when ischemia disrupts neuronal function, damaged tissues release specific peptides into the bloodstream through the compromised blood–brain barrier. They found among these peptides fragments of N-methyl-D-aspartate (NMDA), the receptor for one of the key excitatory neurotransmitters, glutamate. Antibodies to the NMDA fragments develop and can be measured in the bloodstream, allowing differentiation of hemorrhagic versus ischemic stroke, providing earlier, less costly detection of silent stroke and TIA, which both carry increased risk of future cardiovascular events.

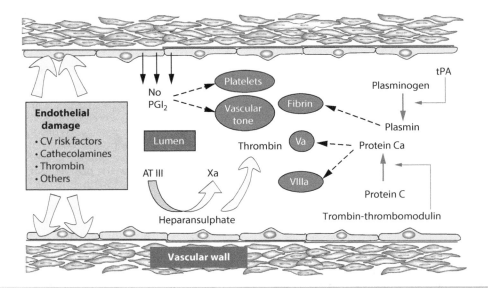

FIGURE 2.19

Simplified diagram of the physiologic anticoagulation system. AT, antithrombin; CV, cardiovascular; NO, nitrous oxide; t-PA, tissue plasminogen activator. (Reproduced with permission from Badimon J, Ibanez B, Fuster V, Badimon L. Chapter 53. Coronary Thrombosis: Local and Systemic Factors. In: Fuster V, Walsh RA, Harrington RA. eds. *Hurst's The Heart*, 13e. New York, NY: McGraw-Hill; 2011).

CASE 2 DISCUSSION: Atrioventricular Malformation

Seven years after David's stroke, he continues his fight for full recovery. He spent a good deal of time in the early years reading and researching, searching for his purpose. He began volunteering as a patient model, allowing students to practice new skills while they were training to become occupational or physical therapists at several local universities. He enrolled in a master's program and graduated with a degree in assistive technology while expanding his volunteer service at local hospitals to include support groups and case management as well as peer mentorship in a robotic technology program.

Last year he attended a New Year's Eve party and took a bite of chicken satay, cooked over an open flame and covered in a creamy, sweet peanut sauce, noticing that not only did it taste delicious, but he could smell it as well! He had a wonderful evening sampling every type of food served, including a dessert buffet. Not long after that, he dreamed of moving his paralyzed left hand, waking to see his fingers opening and closing for the first time under his control. Progress is slow, but he remains motivated and committed to helping not only himself but others through this journey. He signs his emails, "The rehab myth will only hold you back if you let it." During his long recovery David was told many times that progress was only possible early after injury, a statement he considers "the rehab myth." He is currently continuing his training as a doctoral candidate, so he can help even more people with his blend of personal experience, determination, and knowledge.

REFERENCES

Abbott NJ, Ronnback L, Hansson E. Astrocyte-endothelial interactions at the blood–brain barrier. *Nat Rev Neurosci*. 2006;7(1):41–53.

Adams HP, et al. Guidelines for Thrombolytic Therapy for Acute Stroke: A Supplement to the Guidelines for the Management of Patients with Acute Ischemic Stroke. Stroke Council, American Heart Association, 1996.

Ayling J. Managing head injuries. *Emerg Med Serv*. 2002;31:42.

Ballabh P, Braun A, Nedergaard M. The blood–brain barrier: an overview. Structure, regulation, and clinical implications. *Neurobiol Dis*. 2004;16:1–13.

Bourque CW. Central mechanisms of osmosensation and systemic osmoregulation. *Nat Rev Neurosci*. 2008;9(7):519–531.

Brodbelt A, Stoodley M. CSF pathways: a review. *Br J Neurosurg*. 2007;21(5):510–520.

Choi JH, Mohr JP. Brain arteriovenous malformations in adults. *Lancet Neurol*. 2005;4:299.

Davson H, Keasley W, Segal MB. *Physiology and Pathophysiology of the Cerebrospinal Fluid*. New York: Churchill Livingstone; 1987.

Delude C. Clot busters! *Discovery of Thrombolytic Therapy for Heart Attack and Stroke*. Bethesda, MD: Federation of American Societies for Experimental Biology; 2004.

Dunn LT. Raised intracranial pressure. *J Neurol Neurosurg Psychiatry*. 2002;73(Suppl I):i23–i27.

Duvernoy HM. *The Superficial Veins of the Human Brain*. Heidelberg, Germany: Springer-Verlag; 1975.

Duvernoy HM. *The Human Brain Stem and Cerebellum: Surface, Structure, Vascularization, and Three-dimensional Sectional Anatomy with MRI*. Vienna, Austria: Springer-Verlag; 1995.

Duvernoy HM. *Human Brain Stem Vessels: Including the Pineal Gland and Information on Brain Stem Infarction*. New York: Springer; 1999.

Fisher CM. Modern concepts of cerebrovascular disease. In: Meyer JS, ed. *The Anatomy and Pathology of the Cerebral Vasculature*. Wooster and Cambridge, OH: Spectrum Publications; 1975:1–41.

Fishman RT. *Cerebrospinal Fluid in Diseases of the Nervous System*, 2nd ed. Philadelphia: Saunders; 1992.

Fodstad H, Kelly PJ, Buchfelder M. History of the Cushing reflex. *Neurosurgery*. 2006;59:1132–1137.

Gao L, et al. What stroke symptoms tell us: association of risk factors and individual stroke symptoms in the REasons for Geographic and Racial Differences in Stroke (REGARDS) study. *Stroke Cerebrovasc Dis*. 2012 July;21(5):411–416.

Gross PM. Morphology and physiology of capillary systems in subregions of the subfornical organ and area postrema. *Can J Physiol Pharmacol*. 1991;69(7):1010–1025.

Hachinche V. Stroke: Working toward a prioritized world agenda. *Stroke*. 2010 June;41(6):1084–1099.

Karibe H, Shimizu H, Tominaga T, Koshu K, Yoshimoto T. Diffusion-weighted magnetic resonance imaging in the early evaluation of corticospinal tract injury to predict functional motor outcome in patients with deep intra-cerebral hemorrhage. *J Neurosurg*. 2000; 92:58–63.

Laterra J, Goldstein GW. The blood–brain barrier, choroid plexus, and cerebrospinal fluid. In: Kandel ER, Schwartz JH, Jessell TM, Siegelbaum SA, Hudspeth AJ, eds. *Principles of Neural Science*, 5th ed. New York, NY: McGraw-Hill; 2012.

McKinley MJ, Clarke IJ, Oldfield BJ. Circumventricular organs. In: Paxinos G, ed. *The Human Nervous System*. London: Elsevier; 2004:563–591.

McKinley MJ, McAllen RM, Davern P, et al. The sensory circumventricular organs of the mammalian brain. *Adv Anat Embryol Cell Biol*. 2003;172:III–XII, 1–122.

Noda M. The subfornical organ, a specialized sodium channel, and the sensing of sodium levels in the brain. *Neuroscientist*. 2006;12(1):80–91.

O'Connor WT, Smyth A, Gilchrist MD. Animal models of traumatic brain injury: a critical evaluation. *Pharmacol Ther*. 2011;130:106–113.

Osborn AG. *Handbook of Neuroradiology: Brain and Skull*. Maryland Heights, MO: Mosby; 1996.

Ovbiagele B, Nguyen-Huynh MN. Stroke epidemiology: advancing our understanding of disease mechanism and therapy. *Neurotherapeutics*. 2011;8:319–329.

Price CJ, Hoyda TD, Ferguson AV. The area postrema: a brain monitor and integrator of systemic autonomic state. *Neuroscientist*. 2008;14(2):182–194.

Riley J. Anatomy of stroke injury predicts gains from therapy. *Stroke*. 2011 February;42(2):421–426.

Ropper AH, Samuels MA. Cerebrovascular diseases. In: Ropper AH, Samuels MA, eds. *Adams & Victor's Principles of Neurology*, 9th ed. New York: McGraw-Hill; 2009.

Sanchez-Covarrubias L, Slosky LM, Thompson BJ, Davis TP, Ronaldson PT. Transporters at CNS barrier sites: obstacles or opportunities for drug delivery? *Curr Pharm Des*. 2014;20(10):1422–1449.

Savitz SI, Caplan LR. Vertebrobasilar disease. *N Engl J Med.* 2005;352: 2618.

Scremin OU. Cerebral vascular system. In: Paxinos G, Mai JK, eds. *The Human Nervous System.* London: Elsevier; 2004:1326–1348.

Segal MB. The choroid plexuses and the barriers between the blood and the cerebrospinal fluid. *Cell Mol Neurobiol.* 2000;20:183–196.

Smith WS, English JD, Johnston SC. Cerebrovascular diseases. In: Fauci AS, Braunwald E, Kasper D, et al., eds. *Harrison's Principles of Internal Medicine.* New York: McGraw-Hill; 2008.

Zipser BD, Johanson CE, Gonzalez L, et al. Microvascular injury and blood–brain barrier leakage in Alzheimer's disease. *Neurobiol Aging.* 2007;(28): 977–986.

REVIEW QUESTIONS

1. The primary visual cortex is supplied primarily by the:
   A. middle cerebral artery.
   B. anterior cerebral artery.
   C. posterior cerebral artery.
   D. lenticulostriate branches of the MCA.
   E. basilar artery.

2. The ventricular system:
   A. contains the interventricular foramina that allow CSF to pass directly into the fourth ventricle.
   B. has arachnoid granulations that empty directly into the subarachnoid space.
   C. circulation can be blocked without usually causing significant problems.
   D. has a cerebral aqueduct that is the defining ventricular structure of the midbrain.
   E. has foramina of Luschka connecting the lateral ventricles with the third ventricle.

3. Which of the following arteries is not part of the circle of Willis?
   A. Posterior cerebral artery
   B. Anterior communicating artery
   C. Superior cerebellar artery
   D. Anterior cerebral artery
   E. Posterior communicating artery

4. The course of the anterior cerebral artery is best shown with an arteriogram that provides a:
   A. frontal view of the brain.
   B. medial or lateral view of the brain.
   C. frontal-inferior view of the brain.
   D. posterior view of the brain.

5. A 38-year-old male suspected of having Guillian-Barré syndrome will have a lumbar tap to sample protein content in CSF. Which of the following best explains why CSF sampling is by lumbar tap?
   A. CSF pools within the subarachnoid space located at the most inferior portion of the CNS.
   B. CSF exits from the ventricular system at the caudal terminus of the vertebral column.
   C. The lumbar cistern is the only part of the subarachnoid space in which there is sufficient CSF for sampling.
   D. It is safe to sample CSF from the lumbar cistern because it contains only nerve roots since the caudal termination of the spinal cord is rostral to the lumbar cistern.

6. Which of the following arteries supplies part of the posterior limb of the internal capsule?
   A. Anterior choroidal artery
   B. Posterior cerebral artery
   C. Posterior choroidal artery
   D. Ophthalmic artery

7. Which description of brain stem arterial distributions is most accurate?
   A. Arterial branches supply pie-shaped wedges of tissue, beginning at dorsal midline and extending circumferentially.
   B. Short circumferential branches supply the dorsal brain stem; long circumferential branches supply the ventral brain stem.
   C. Arteries course on the ventral surface and send branches dorsally.
   D. The basilar artery supplies the midline; the vertebral arteries, the next lateral territory; and the cerebellar arteries supply most laterally.

8. Which arterial interfaces are not locations of collateral circulation?
   A. Anterior cerebral artery and middle cerebral artery
   B. Middle cerebral artery and posterior cerebral artery
   C. Anterior cerebral artery and posterior cerebral artery
   D. Posterior inferior cerebellar artery and vertebral arteries

9. A patient has a subdural hematoma. Which of the following best describes the space within which blood accumulates?
   A. The space between the dura and the arachnoid
   B. The space between the dura and the pia
   C. The space between the dura and the cortex surface
   D. Any space within a part of the CNS covered by the dura

10. CSF exits the ventricles through the _____ and then from the subarachnoid space to the venous sinuses through the _____.
    A. foramen of Luschka; foramen of Magendie
    B. foramen of Magendie; foramen of Luschka
    C. foramina of Luschka and Magendie; arachnoid villi
    D. arachnoid villi; foramina of Luschka and Magendie

CHAPTER 3

Cellular Organization of the Nervous System

> ## CASE 3 Myasthenia Gravis

HB was a career navy man, working as a civilian in the area of logistics management ever since he retired 22 years ago as a chief petty officer. One day two years ago, he noticed his eyes kept drooping as he drove to the navy base. He didn't think about it again until lunch, when he had to hold his eyes open to see enough to drive home. Concerned, HB went to Urgent Care, where they referred him to a neurologist.

The neurologist ordered blood tests specifically looking for antibodies against acetylcholine receptors and changes in the amount of thymus hormones. Results were positive for the antibodies, confirming a diagnosis of myasthenia gravis, an autoimmune

disease. Myasthenia gravis causes the body to attack the receptors for acetylcholine, the main neurotransmitter for motor (muscle) function, causing muscle weakness.

The neurologist treated him with pyridostigmine (Mestinon), a drug that promotes neurotransmitter function by blocking the enzyme acetyl cholinesterase that degrades acetylcholine in the motor end plate. His symptoms resolved quickly, allowing HB to return to work. His neurologist also managed his symptoms with medications that decreased the autoimmune response. His wife searched the Internet and found discussion boards and websites with information on this rare disease, including prognosis and how to cope with the uncertainty. HB was a strong,

self-determined man who took these challenges as a sign to live his life to the fullest, so he and his wife began traveling in earnest.

Over the next two years, HB managed his condition with the help of a supportive wife and attentive neurologist. He survived mild episodes of recurrent weakness, each time a little different: discoordinated nasal speech, difficulty swallowing, poor balance. Two months ago, he had to take a break from work due to neck weakness and pronounced difficulty swallowing; he started a course of steroids and hoped the symptoms would resolve. After discussing things with his wife, they cancelled a trip to Machu Picchu so he could rest and try to return to work.

> Neuroplasticity
BRAIN Initiative

Understanding the process of neuroplastic change after central nervous system damage allows clinicians to determine the ideal timing and approach for treatment. It is long established that delayed care results in poorer outcomes. However, by identifying the cellular recovery mechanisms, we now understand neuroplastic changes following injury. The damaged system must first reestablish the cell membrane resting potential, and it uses a great deal of energy to restore ionic gradients and repair injured organelles. Any new demands on the healing synapse can potentially hinder recovery. The

ideal timing for rehabilitation and activity after stroke remains unanswered. In animal models, introducing exercise too soon after brain injury is shown to hinder hippocampal function, an area essential for learning and memory. Extrapolating these findings to the human brain is an area that should be explored in the near future, due in large part to the efforts of current collaboration between bench and clinical science fostered by the BRAIN Initiative.

Acceleration in our understanding of the human brain began in earnest with the 2013 BRAIN (Brain Research through Advancing Innovative Neurotechnologies) Initiative. Launched at the request of US

President Obama in 2013 to map the human brain, it challenged researchers from diverse fields to collaborate and coordinate, using innovative new discoveries and technologies. These advances include mapping of the human genome, advances in animal models used in biomedical research, and new technologies for imaging the live human brain. New developments fostered by this project will transform many fields of study, inform biomedical science, and potentially save many lives from the devastation of neurological disease and injury.

To guide the process, the BRAIN Initiative Working Group convened. They recommended neuronal activity as key to begin

the process, stating in their 2014 Preliminary Report:

The working group identified the analysis of circuits of interacting neurons as being particularly rich in opportunity, with potential for revolutionary advances. Truly understanding a circuit requires identifying and characterizing the component cells, defining their synaptic connections with one another, observing their dynamic patterns of activity in vivo during behavior, and perturbing these patterns to test their significance. It also requires an understanding of the algorithms that govern information processing within a circuit, and between interacting circuits in the brain as a whole.

I OVERVIEW OF KEY CONCEPTS

Neurons comprise the functional units of the nervous system. Although most of the organelles in the neuron are similar to those of other cells in the body, the phenotypes of neurons vary widely in their form and function. Understanding subcellular components and vital processes occurring both within and between neurons creates a more thorough understanding of nervous system function. Impairment of cellular function underlies many of the pathologies seen by health care providers.

Neurons have specialized regions for specific functions: axons transmit signals; dendrites receive signals; and the cell body receives a large number of inputs directly. The synapse is the mechanism of electrochemical communication in the nervous system. It is a highly organized system composed of elements from the presynaptic (transmitting) axon terminal and the postsynaptic (receiving) cell membrane. An electrical impulse initiates the release of neurotransmitter molecules that cross the thin cleft between the two elements. Special receptors line the postsynaptic membrane, which bind to the neurotransmitter molecules and produce an electrical response in the target cell.

In addition to neurons, there are cells in both the CNS and PNS that support neuronal metabolic and physiological function. In the CNS, support cells are known collectively as glia. There are two main types of glial cells: astrocytes and oligodendrocytes. Astrocytes provide metabolic support and create a blood–brain barrier against movement of material into brain tissue. Oligodendrocytes invest CNS axons with myelin, an insulating sheath around the axon, which greatly increases the velocity of impulse transmission along the axon. In the PNS, axonal support cells are called Schwann cells. These axons are invested either with a thin layer of cytoplasm and extracellular matrix proteins or with a thicker layer of myelin.

Central and peripheral axons are thin, delicate processes, and damage can produce deficits of movement, sensation, and cognition in an individual. After injury, the axon distal to the injury and its myelin sheath are degraded and cleared away in a process known as Wallerian degeneration. In the PNS, this is followed by sprouting of neurites (thin axonal processes) from the proximal segment and regenerative elongation until the target tissue is reinnervated. In the CNS, the process of regeneration is inhibited by physical and chemical barriers produced, in part, by glia. Circumventing this inhibition is a fundamental goal of researchers investigating CNS repair.

II NERVOUS SYSTEM CYTOLOGY

CNS Support Cells: Glia

Glial cells support neural function (Figure 3.1), outnumbering neurons by about 10 to 1 in the human brain.

The two major classes of glia, microglia and macroglia, provide structural and metabolic support for neurons during development and in maturity. Microglia serve in a phagocytic or scavenger role, responding to nervous system infection or damage. They are rapidly

CNS Glial Cells

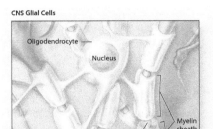

A Oligodendrocyte

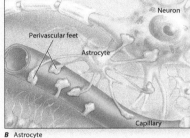

B Astrocyte

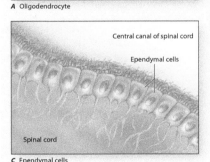

C Ependymal cells

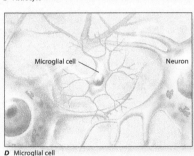

D Microglial cell

PNS Glial Cells

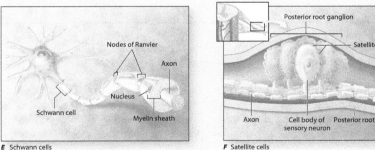

E Schwann cells

F Satellite cells

FIGURE 3.1

Glial cells of the CNS and PNS. There are four major types of glia in the CNS. **A.** Oligodendrocytes myelinate parts of several axons. **B.** Astrocytes have multiple processes and form perivascular endfeet that completely enclose all capillaries (only a few such feet are shown here, to allow their morphology to be seen). **C.** Ependymal cells are epithelial-like cells that line the ventricles and central canal. **D.** Microglial cells have protective, phagocytic, immune-related functions. Two glial cell types occur in the PNS. **E.** Schwann cells form a cuff of myelin ensheathing axons. **F.** Satellite cells are restricted to ganglia, where they cover and support the large neuronal cell bodies. (Reproduced with permission from Chapter 9. Nerve Tissue & the Nervous System. In: Mescher AL. eds. *Junqueira's Basic Histology: Text & Atlas*, 13e New York, NY: McGraw-Hill; 2013).

mobilized in response to different patho-physiological conditions and trauma. Activated microglia can destroy invading microorganisms, remove debris, and promote tissue repair. Activated microglia also mediate changes in neuronal properties. These actions, helpful in early healing, later hinder recovery. For example, neurons often become hyperexcitable after nervous system damage, and microglia can be involved in this process. This chronic hyperexcitability can lead to conditions such as central neuropathic pain and neuronal death through cytotoxicity.

Macroglia, of which there are four separate types—oligodendrocytes, Schwann cells, astrocytes, and ependymal cells—have a variety of support and nutritive functions. Oligodendrocytes and Schwann cells form the myelin sheaths around central and peripheral axons. Myelin is a fatty substance composed of many different myelin proteins. Along with providing metabolic support to the axon, the myelin sheath increases the velocity of action potential conduction. In the PNS, Schwann cells proliferate after injury, stimulating axon elongation and regeneration. A single CNS oligodendrocyte can myelinate dozens of axons.

Damage to oligodendrocytes creates myelin debris adjacent to the injury and also stimulates proliferation of oligodendrocyte precursor cells. Both the debris and molecules released by the precursor cells contribute to inhibition of CNS axon regeneration.

Astrocytes have important structural and metabolic functions. In the developing nervous system, they act as scaffolds for growing axons and guide migrating immature neurons. Many synapses have astrocyte processes that may monitor synaptic actions and provide chemical feedback. Astrocytes also contribute to the blood–brain barrier, a specialized feature of brain circulation not seen in other capillary systems (Figure 3.2).

Endothelial cells forming the walls of brain capillaries are joined by tight junctions creating a semipermeable membrane restricting the movement of large molecules while permitting passage of small molecules such as water, oxygen, or hormones. Larger molecules, such as glucose, required for cellular function, must be actively transported across the barrier. The endothelial cells are covered by the endfeet of astrocytes, which support those cells physically and metabolically. Breakdown of the blood–brain barrier has been implicated in such diseases as meningitis, multiple sclerosis, and Alzheimer's disease. The last class of macroglia includes ependymal cells, which line fluid-filled cavities in the central nervous system. They play an important role in regulating the flow of chemicals from these cavities into the brain.

PNS Support Cells: Schwann Cells and Satellite Glial Cells

Schwann cells support peripheral axons. There are two types: myelinating and non-myelinating. A myelinating Schwann cell supplies only one axon, whereas a non-myelinating Schwann cell provides a thin layer of cytoplasm around many fine caliber axons (Figure 3.3).

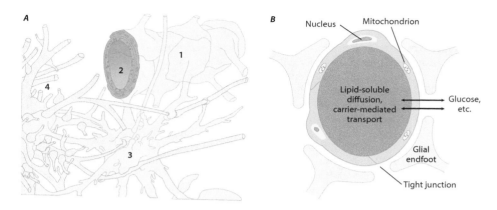

FIGURE 3.2

Astrocytes and the blood–brain barrier. *A.* Relation of fibrous astrocyte (3) to a capillary (2) and neuron (4) in the brain. The endfeet of the astrocyte processes form a discontinuous membrane around the capillary (1). Astrocyte processes also envelop the neuron. (Adapted with permission from Krstic RV. *Die Gewebe des Menschen und der Säugetiere.* New York: Springer, 1978.) ***B.*** Transport across cerebral capillaries. Only free lipid-soluble substances can move passively across the endothelial cells. Water-soluble solutes, such as glucose, require active transport mechanisms. Proteins and protein-bound lipids are excluded. (Reproduced with permission from Circulation Through Special Regions. In: Barrett KE, Barman SM, Boitano S, Brooks HL. eds. *Ganong's Review of Medical Physiology,* 25e New York, NY: McGraw-Hill; 2016).

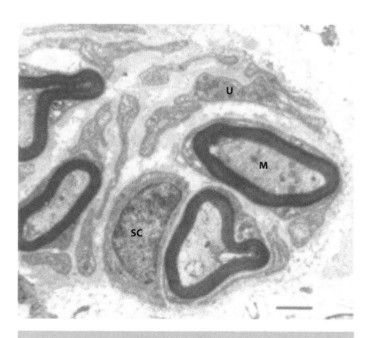

FIGURE 3.3

Transmission electron micrograph of a peripheral nerve in cross section. Electron micrograph of myelinated (M) and unmyelinated (U) axons of a peripheral nerve. Schwann cells (SC) may surround one myelinated or several unmyelinated axons. ×16,000. (Reproduced with permission from Sevilla T, Cuesta A, Chumillas MJ, et al. Clinical, electrophysiological and morphological findings of Charcot–Marie–Tooth neuropathy with vocal cord palsy and mutations in the GDAP1 gene. *Brain.* 2003;126(Pt 9):2023–2033).

The primary role of the myelin enclosing axons is to increase conduction rate of the electrical signal, the action potential. Myelinating Schwann cells also assist in organizing formation of connective tissue sheaths surrounding peripheral nerves during normal development and also in maturity during axon regeneration following damage.

Satellite glial cells are found in sensory, sympathetic, and parasympathetic ganglia. They serve similar supportive roles to those performed by CNS glia. An array of satellite cells encloses individual neurons in the ganglia. They are in close chemical communication with the neurons through exocytosis (local secretion) of neurotransmitters such as ATP, bradykinin, GABA, and glutamate. Satellite glial cells also communicate with the environment surrounding the neurons, with adjacent satellite glial cells, and with sensory and autonomic neurons on which they might exert a modulatory effect. More recent research implicates glial cells in chronic pain conditions due to phenotypic changes in injured peripheral glia extending proximally through the entire central nociceptive pathway.

Wallerian Degeneration and Axon Regeneration

Nerve injury that produces discontinuity between proximal and distal regions of the axon also damages myelin-producing cells in the vicinity. These injuries initiate a cascade of cellular events, primarily distal to the injury, called Wallerian degeneration (Figure 3.4).

Wallerian degeneration occurs distal to an injury in myelinated axons in both the PNS and CNS. Macrophages first infiltrate the trauma site and begin to remove the segment of damaged myelin proximal to the site of injury. This degeneration only extends proximally to the next healthy myelin segment. The proximal stump of the severed axon recedes in preparation for the signal to regenerate. Changes also occur in the cell body of the injured neuron in a process called chromatolysis. Within the cell body, the Nissl substance (collections of ribosomes and rough endoplasmic reticulum normally dispersed throughout the cytoplasm) dissolve; the nucleus is displaced toward the periphery of the cell body; and the entire cell body hypertrophies. With successful regeneration, chromatologic changes reverse, and cell function returns. If regeneration fails, the cell can die; this is more common in the CNS.

Distal to the site of injury, macrophages remove myelin and axon debris, leaving only a thin basement membrane, a layer of extracellular matrix proteins laid down by the Schwann cells. Macrophages and Schwann cells phagocytize myelin debris along the distal axon segment to the terminal. Schwann cells then enter a phase of rapid proliferation. The new Schwann cells use the basement membrane as a scaffold to form a cellular tube that directs the regenerating axon from the proximal stump to its original target cell. Schwann cells release neuroactive molecules into the basement membrane and extracellular matrix to promote axon elongation and facilitate regeneration. When the axon reinnervates its target, the Schwann cells begin to form new, shorter myelin sheath segments. Although the reinnervation provides virtually full functional recovery, the shortened myelin segments permanently reduce axonal conduction velocities.

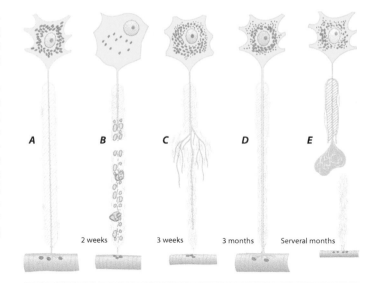

FIGURE 3.4

Wallerian degeneration and neuronal chromatolysis. Main changes that take place in an injured nerve fiber. **A.** Normal nerve fiber, with its perikaryon and the target cell (striated skeletal muscle). Notice the central position of the neuron nucleus and the amount and distribution of Nissl bodies. **B.** When the fiber is injured, the neuronal nucleus moves to the cell periphery, Nissl bodies become greatly reduced in number (chromatolysis), and the nerve fiber distal to the injury degenerates along with its myelin sheath. Debris is phagocytized by macrophages. **C.** The muscle fiber shows pronounced disuse atrophy. Schwann cells proliferate, forming a compact channel that is penetrated by the growing axon. The axon grows at a rate of ~1 to 10 mm/d. **D.** In this example, the nerve fiber regeneration was successful, and the muscle fiber was also regenerated after receiving nerve stimuli. **E.** When the axon does not penetrate the cord of Schwann cells, its growth is not organized and successful regeneration does not occur; formation of a painful neuroma is common. (Used with permission from Willis RA and Willis AT. *The Principles of Pathology and Bacteriology*, 3rd ed. Oxford: Butterworth-Heinemann, 1972.)

In some cases, the distance between the proximal and distal axon segments after injury is too great to retain continuity in the basement membrane, and the scaffold for creating the Schwann cell tube is interrupted. This complicates reinnervation as acquiring the distal segment becomes problematic. Additionally, if the gap between proximal and distal segments is excessive, or if alignment of proximal and distal segments is impaired, axon elongation can create a neuroma, a painful tangle of exposed neurites embedded in connective tissue.

Common Morphological Plan for All Neurons

There are estimated to be 80-100 billion neurons in the adult human brain. Neurons express a broad range of morphological and biochemical phenotypes related to their function and connections (Figure 3.5). Axons from projection neurons can be quite long; for example, the axon from a motor neuron descending from the cerebral cortex to the sacral spinal cord can extend beyond one meter. The energy requirement and manufacturing potential of a neuron are prodigious. The Purkinje cell in the cerebellar cortex has an elaborate dendritic arbor that is nearly two-dimensional.

Although neurons come in different shapes and sizes, they all have four morphologically and biochemically specialized regions with particular functions: cell body, dendrites, axon, and axon terminals. The cell body, or soma (*pl.* somata or somas), encloses the machinery for cell function and maintenance, receives information (synapses) from other neurons, and serves important integrative functions. Dendrites and axons are fine processes (neurites) extending from the cell body. Dendrites receive information from other neurons. The axon conducts information (encoded in the form of action potentials) to the axon terminals. Two neurons in a neural circuit communicate through synapses between the axon terminal of the presynaptic neuron and the receptive membrane of the postsynaptic neuron. Synapses can be located on the dendrites and dendritic spines, the cell body, or presynaptically on the axon terminal. (Figure 3.6)

Despite a wide range of morphology, we can distinguish three classes of neuron based on the configuration of their dendrites and axons: unipolar, bipolar, and multipolar. Unipolar neurons are the simplest in shape. They have no true dendrites; the cell body of unipolar neurons receives and integrates incoming information. A single axon, which originates from the cell body, gives rise to multiple terminal processes. In the human nervous system, unipolar neurons are the least common. They control exocrine gland secretions and smooth muscle contractility.

Bipolar neurons have two processes that arise from opposite poles of the cell body. The flow of information in bipolar neurons is from one of the processes, which functions like a dendrite, across the cell body to the other process, which functions like an axon. Bipolar cells are common in the retina. One subtype of bipolar neurons is the pseudounipolar

neuron. During development the two processes of the embryonic bipolar neuron fuse into a single process in the pseudounipolar neuron, which bifurcates at a distance from the cell body. Many somatic (located in the body) sensory neurons, such as those that transmit information to the brain about odors or touch, are bipolar and pseudounipolar neurons.

Multipolar neurons feature a complex array of dendrites on the cell body and a single axon that branches extensively. Most of the neurons in the brain and spinal cord are multipolar. Multipolar neurons with long axons that terminate in distant sites are called projection neurons. Projection neurons mediate communication between regions of the nervous system, and between the nervous system and peripheral targets, such as striated muscle cells and skin. Other multipolar neurons, commonly called interneurons, have short axons that remain in the same region of the nervous system in which the cell body is located. Interneurons help to process neuronal information within a local brain region.

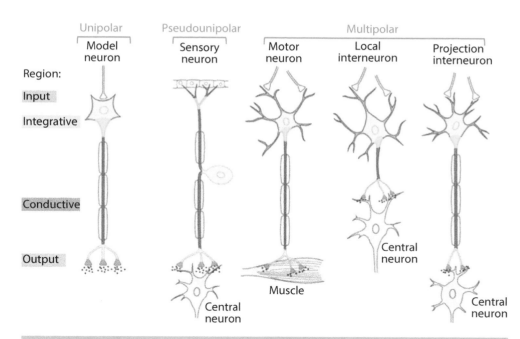

FIGURE 3.5

Some of the types of neurons in the mammalian nervous system. A. Unipolar neurons have one process, with different segments serving as receptive surfaces and releasing terminals. **B.** Bipolar neurons have two specialized processes: a dendrite that carries information to the cell and an axon that transmits information from the cell. **C.** Some sensory neurons are in a subclass of bipolar cells called pseudo-unipolar cells. As the cell develops, a single process splits into two, both of which function as axons—one going to skin or muscle and another to the spinal cord. **D.** Multipolar cells have one axon and many dendrites. Examples include motor neurons, hippocampal pyramidal cells with dendrites in the apex and base, and cerebellar Purkinje cells with an extensive dendritic tree in a single plane. (Reproduced, with permission, from Kandel ER, Schwartz JH, Jessell TM, Siegelbaum SA, Hudspeth AJ, eds. *Principles of Neural Science*. 5th ed. New York: McGraw-Hill; 2013.)

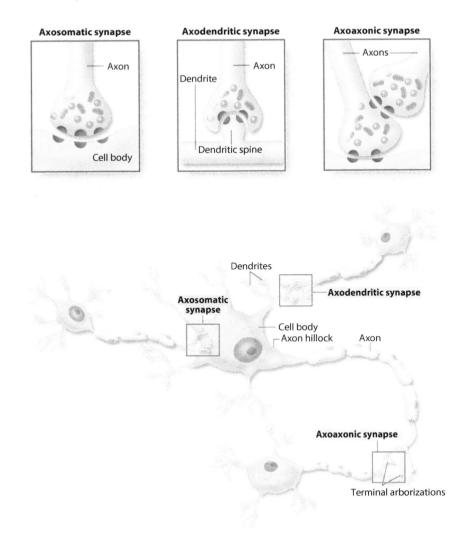

Types of synapses. Axon terminals usually transmit the nerve impulse to another neuron's cell body (soma) or to its dendrites (or a dendritic spine). Less frequently, axon terminals form synapses with another axon terminal, an arrangement that helps modulate synaptic activity. Features of these three common morphologic types of synapses are shown at the top of the figure. (Reproduced with permisson from Chapter 9. Nerve Tissue & the Nervous System. In: Mescher AL. eds. *Junqueira's Basic Histology: Text & Atlas*, 13e New York, NY: McGraw-Hill; 2013).

Neurocytology

Subcellular components of neurons are, in great part, the same as those found in most somatic cell types; a few will be discussed here (Figure 3.7). Centrally located within the neuronal cytoplasm (neuroplasm) is a large nucleus, the repository of DNA. The nucleus is involved in cellular processes such as protein synthesis, mitosis (cell division), and cell growth. The nucleus contains one, sometimes two, smaller nucleoli. One main responsibility of the nucleolus is to transcribe ribosomal RNA and combine it with proteins to create functional ribosomes which are transported into the neuroplasm of the cell body, dendrites, and axons. When cells reproduce, their nucleolus disappears, there is a reduction in active protein synthesis, and they construct the mitotic apparatus

necessary for mitosis. Recent studies of adult neurogenesis have demonstrated neuronal mitosis in the adult human brain. Adult mitosis may replenish cerebral cortical neurons and help maintain cognition. Interruption of this ongoing process is proposed to underlie some forms of dementia. The vast majority of mature neurons, however, appear not to reproduce, thus a loss of cells in most of the brain is permanent. Neurons contain a protein cytoskeletal scaffold that serves as mechanical support for axons and dendrites and provides an internal transport system between the axons and dendrites and the cell body. The principle fibrillar component of the cytoskeleton is the microtubule. Their main purpose is structural, but they also bind to the transport molecules, kinesin and dynein, which move vesicles in the anterograde (away from the soma) or retrograde (toward the soma) direction, respectively. Neurofilaments, or intermediate filaments, are specifically neuronal cytoskeletal fibrils providing longitudinal support and regulating axonal diameter. Microfilaments, or actin filaments, are the thinnest of the neuronal cytoskeletal proteins. They form a thin network underlying the cell membrane. Receptor proteins, ion channels, and presynaptic apparatus for cell-cell signaling are anchored in place by binding to actin fibrils.

Ribosomes translate the code for building proteins. They are either membrane bound on the rough endoplasmic reticulum (ER) or floating free in the neuroplasm. Free floating ribosomes produce water soluble proteins that are not associated with the membranes of the cell or the organelles; these may include large protein complexes and enzymes.

The endomembranous system is an interconnecting system of stacked flattened cisternae (membrane-bound, fluid filled chambers) that communicate with each other directly or through pinching off ("budding") and fusion of vesicles at the perimeters of the cisternae (Figure 3.8). It is also a protein trafficking pathway through which proteins, especially trans- or intramembranous

proteins and secretory proteins, are constructed, processed, and packaged for insertion into the membrane or release from the axon terminal. The system includes the nuclear envelope, the smooth ER, the rough ER, the Golgi apparatus (a.k.a., Golgi body, Golgi), the small vesicular organelles such as lysosomes and vacuoles, and the plasmalemma. The surface of the rough ER is studded with ribosomes. Ribosomes translate messenger RNA, which carries the code for the appropriate sequence of amino acids that make up a protein. As the newly formed protein elongates, it extends into the lumen of the rough ER. Small vesicles bud off the perimeter of the rough ER and pass onward to merge with the membrane of the Golgi apparatus and empty their contents into its lumen. Smooth ER is involved with steroid metabolism, drug detoxification, and carbohydrate metabolism, and is most abundant in gonadal and liver cells.

In the Golgi apparatus, proteins and protein complexes are packaged into vesicles destined for use elsewhere in the cell. Vesicles containing secretory proteins, such as neurotransmitters, bud off the periphery of the Golgi to be shipped to the axon terminal and await the signal for release into extracellular space.

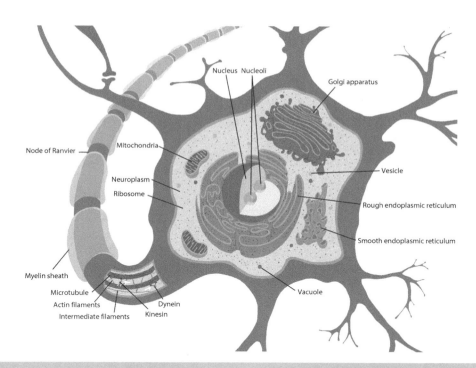

FIGURE 3.7

Diagram of the subcellular organization of a neuron. Much of the subcellular apparatus in the neuronal soma is involved in manufacture and transport of proteins. The nucleus, containing one or two nucleoli, produces ribosomal proteins and mRNA, which are transported into the neuroplasm. Ribosomes, either free floating in the neuroplasm or bound to the membrane of the rER, translate the mRNA message into a specific protein. Proteins formed inside the rER cisternae are destined for delivery to remote parts of the neuron, such as the axon terminal. Vesicles containing nascent proteins (green circles) separate from the rER and fuse with the membrane of the Golgi apparatus for posttranslational modification. As the vesicles bud off the Golgi, they bind to the motive protein, kinesin (inside the axon cutout), and are transported along microtubules to their terminal targets within the cell. Vesicles of endocytosed material (red circles) are transported in the retrograde direction by dynein molecules, also along microtubules. Fine intermediate filaments provide structural support to the neuron and its processes, and actin filaments serve to anchor subcellular structures. Smooth ER is present in the neuronal soma and contributes to some posttranslational protein and lipid processing; however, they also sequester Ca^{++} for use by the cell. As in other cells, mitochondria make ATP for cellular metabolism. A series of myelin segments, separated by nodes of Ranvier, insulate the axon and greatly increase action potential propagation. (Image provided by Jamie Graham © 2014)

Integration of Systems
Drug Therapy

Understanding the complexities of cellular behavior is fundamental in developing drug therapies for many neurological conditions. Drugs acting on the CNS primarily impact the synapse (see figure), increasing or decreasing neurotransmitter release to impact disease. For example, one of the most prevalent and best-studied degradative enzymes is acetylcholinesterase, which hydrolyzes acetylcholine into its choline and acetate components. Malfunction of acetylcholine synaptic transmission creates pathological conditions, such as Alzheimer's disease, where cholinergic cells die. Acetylcholinesterase-blocking drugs are used to prevent degradation of acetylcholine, extending its time in the synaptic cleft and prolonging its effects on the postsynaptic cell.

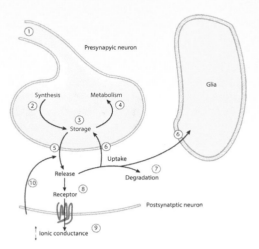

Sites of drug action. Schematic drawing of steps at which drugs can alter synaptic transmission: (1) action potential in presynaptic fiber, (2) synthesis of transmitter, (3) storage, (4) metabolism, (5) release, (6) reuptake into the nerve ending or uptake into a glial cell, (7) degradation, (8) receptor for the transmitter, (9) receptor-induced increase or decrease in ionic conductance, and (10) retrograde signaling. (Reproduced with permission from Nicoll RA. Chapter 21. Introduction to the Pharmacology of CNS Drugs. In: Katzung BG, Masters SB, Trevor AJ. eds. *Basic & Clinical Pharmacology*, 12e New York, NY: McGraw-Hill; 2012).

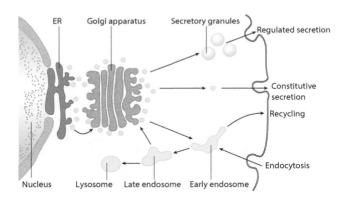

FIGURE 3.8

The endomembranous system: subcellular structures involved in protein processing. Proteins are constructed from translated DNA-to-mRNA segments that pass through the nuclear envelope into the cytoplasm. In the cytoplasm, mRNA binds to either free-floating or rER-bound ribosomes and are translated. Vesicles bud off the distal face (surface) of the rER containing newly formed proteins. Vesicles (yellow circles) merge with the membrane of the proximal face of the Golgi apparatus for posttranslational modification. Secretory granules merge with the membrane of the terminal and release their contents into extracellular space. Endocytosis engulfs extracellular materials and transports them back to the cell body; some are hydrolyzed in lysosomes. (Reproduced with permission from Overview of Cellular Physiology in Medical Physiology. In: Barrett KE, Barman SM, Boitano S, Brooks HL. eds. *Ganong's Review of Medical Physiology*, 25e New York, NY: McGraw-Hill; 2016).

Membrane Proteins: Ion Channels and Receptors

All of the elements comprising the endomembrane system are constructed from the unit membrane, a fluid phospholipid bilayer with hydrophilic inner and outer surfaces sandwiching a hydrophobic core. Although flip-flopping (exchanging inner and outer portions of the protein) is impossible, integral proteins can move within the plane of the membrane (Figure 3.9), permitting redistribution of the proteins within membrane as required for cell function, such as clustering of sodium channels at nodes of Ranvier on myelinated axons.

The nuclear DNA contains the code for synthesizing proteins required for cellular function. This process engages the endomembrane system to create cytoplasmic, secretory, and membrane bound proteins. A discussion of protein synthesis in neurons is necessary to understand construction of the highly dynamic neuronal membrane. The nucleolus contains ribosomal RNA, that forms a complex with nuclear proteins to create functional ribosomes that are shuttled into the neuroplasm through the nuclear pores. DNA contains the genes, the regions that code for specific proteins.

In a process called transcription (Figure 3.10), the double helical DNA molecule opens to expose a single strand of DNA, the template. The DNA template is read by an enzyme that moves along the DNA to form a messenger RNA (mRNA). The mRNA transcript is also transported into the cytoplasm where it will be bound to a ribosome for protein construction. In the cytoplasm, numerous ribosomes bind simultaneously with the mRNA and "read" the code in a process called translation. Another type of RNA, transfer RNA (tRNA), also binds to the mRNA strand. The tRNA molecules have one end that binds to the mRNA, and another end that binds to only one amino acid. Appropriate amino acids are bound together to form an elongating polypeptide chain that will become a protein molecule.

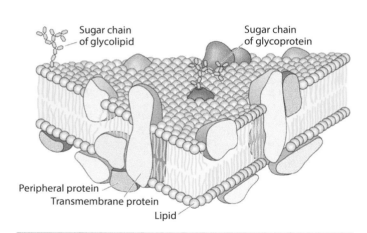

FIGURE 3.9

Proteins associated with the membrane lipid bilayer. The fluid mosaic model of membrane structure emphasizes that the phospholipid bilayer of a membrane also contains inserted or peripheral proteins; many move within the fluid lipid phase. Integral proteins are firmly embedded in the lipid layers; those that completely span the bilayer are called transmembrane proteins. Uncharged portions of these proteins interact with the hydrophobic fatty acid portions of the membrane lipids. (Reproduced with permission from Chapter 2. The Cytoplasm. In: Mescher AL. eds. *Junqueira's Basic Histology: Text & Atlas*, 13e New York, NY: McGraw-Hill; 2013).

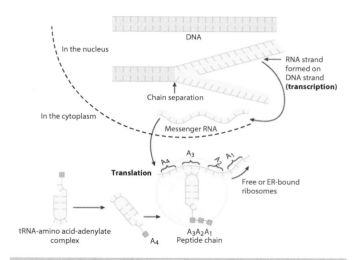

FIGURE 3.10

Major steps in the control of gene expression. Transcription from the DNA strand to the construction of messenger RNA (mRNA) takes place in the nucleus. The mRNA strands are shuttled into the cytoplasm, where they are translated by ribosomes into proteins. Transfer RNA (tRNA) brings specific amino acids to bind onto the growing polypeptide chain (i.e., the elongating protein molecule). (Reproduced with permission from General Principles & Energy Production in Medical Physiology. In: Barrett KE, Barman SM, Boitano S, Brooks HL. eds. *Ganong's Review of Medical Physiology*, 25e New York, NY: McGraw-Hill; 2016).

There are two pathways through which proteins are formed depending on the location of the ribosomes in the neuronal cytoplasm (Figure 3.11). Some ribosomes float freely in the cytoplasm, and others are bound to the membrane of the rough ER (rER). Proteins formed on free ribosomes include those that are soluble in the cytoplasm or packaged into mitochondria and peroxisomes, or transported back into the nucleus. Proteins produced by rER-bound ribosomes are released inside the lumen of the rER. Protein-filled vesicles bud off the rER and are shuttled into the Golgi for posttranslational processing and sorting. From the Golgi, proteins have three possible fates: they can be packaged into lysosomes for use within the cell; packaged into secretory vesicles for extracellular release, such as neurotransmitters and neurotrophic factors for support and maintenance of target tissues; or inserted into the vesicle membrane as transmembrane proteins (Figure 3.12).

Because it is extremely difficult and metabolically expensive to insert proteins into the lipid bilayer, they can be built directly into the rER membrane as integral membrane proteins. As amino acids are added to the lengthening polypeptide chain, translocons, specialized protein complexes in the lipid bilayer of the rER membrane, insert the elongating proteins into the membrane so that the transmembranous, intracellular (C-terminus), and extracellular portions (N-terminus) are in the proper orientation. The walls of the vesicles now contain the intramembranous proteins destined to be inserted into the axon terminal, dendrites, and the soma. The walls of the vesicle incorporate into the neuronal membrane and replenish the lipid bilayer as they insert new membrane proteins.

Misfolding of proteins during posttranslational processing can produce infectious prions that propagate by disrupting the protein structure in the host. Among the best-known prion diseases in humans is Creutzfeldt–Jakob disease, a condition similar to bovine spongiform encephalopathy (mad cow disease), in which neurodegeneration leaves the brain riddled with holes, giving a spongelike appearance.

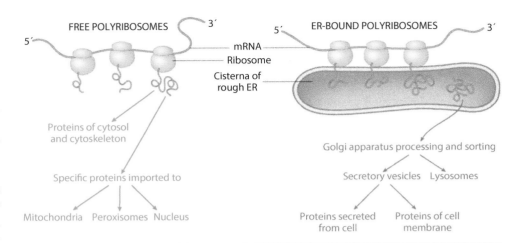

FIGURE 3.11

Polyribosomes: free or bound to the endoplasmic reticulum. Free polyribosomes (not attached to the ER) synthesize cytoplasmic and cytoskeletal proteins and proteins for import into the nucleus, mitochondria, and peroxisomes. Proteins that are to be incorporated into membranes, stored in lysosomes, or eventually secreted from the cell are made by polysomes attached to the membranes of rER. The proteins produced by bound ribosomes are segregated during translation into the interior of the ER's membrane cisternae. Secretory vesicles contain both molecules to be secreted into extracellular space and proteins that will be inserted into the terminal membrane. (Reproduced with permission from Chapter 2. The Cytoplasm. In: Mescher AL. eds. *Junqueira's Basic Histology: Text & Atlas*, 13e New York, NY: McGraw-Hill; 2013).

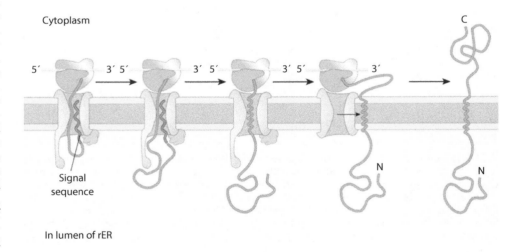

FIGURE 3.12

The translocon: Insertion of a membrane protein. The mRNA binds to a ribosome that is associated with the translocon, a protein complex attached to the cell membrane. The signal sequence forms a hydrophobic channel through which the transmembrane portion of a transmembrane protein forms. The signal sequence is cleaved off, leaving the polypeptide chain to cross the membrane with the amino (N) terminus (extracellular domain) of the polypeptide chain exposed in the ER lumen. The protein exits the channel laterally and becomes anchored in the ER membrane. Continued translation generates a membrane-spanning protein with its carboxy (C) terminus (intracellular domain) on the cytoplasmic side. (Reproduced with permission from Cooper GM and Hausman RE. *The Cell: A Molecular Approach*. Sunderland, MA: Sinauer, 2009.)

Axon Transport

Vesicles containing more mature forms of transmembrane and secretory proteins bud off the distal face of the Golgi apparatus. These vesicles are targeted for attachment to microtubules through kinesin molecules, which provide mechanical force to propel the vesicle distally in a process called anterograde axoplasmic transport (Figure 3.13). Anterograde axoplasmic transport is an ongoing process that replenishes the membrane and membrane proteins. It is involved in initial axon elongation during development and is an integral part of axon regeneration. Different forms of kinesin molecules conduct their cargo at different rates. Construction of the cytoskeletal scaffold is the rate-limiting step in axon regeneration (and return of neural function), and slow anterograde axoplasmic transport occurs on average at approximately 1–10 mm per day.

Fast anterograde axoplasmic transport moves at 50–400 mm per day, carrying vesicles and organelles to the axon terminal.

Retrograde axoplasmic transport uses a motive molecule called dynein to transport vesicles from the axon terminal toward the cell body. Extracellular material, such as neurotrophic factors and neuroactive chemicals near the terminal, is transported proximally at a rate of approximately 100–200 mm per day. Impaired axoplasmic transport, both anterograde and retrograde, appears to be related to a number of pathological neurodegenerative diseases such as Parkinson's disease or Alzheimer's disease. Certain cancer medications disrupt microtubule structure and impair axoplasmic transport and mitosis in malignant cells. In neurons, disruption of axoplasmic transport leads to Wallerian degeneration distally along the axon.

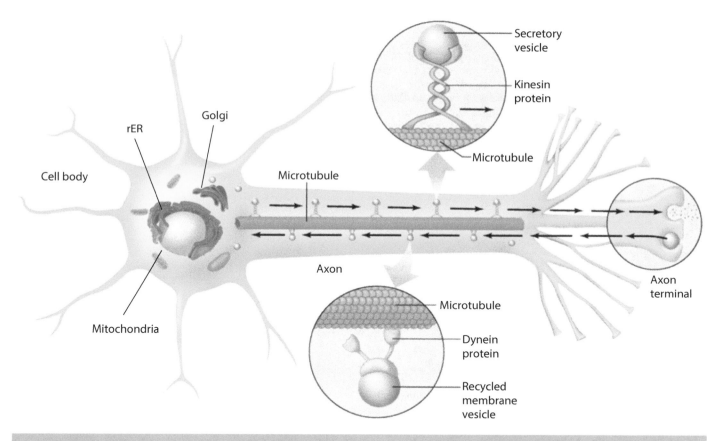

FIGURE 3.13

Axonal transport along microtubules by kinesin and dynein. Fast (400 mm/day) and slow (1–10 mm/day) anterograde axonal transport occurs along microtubules that run the length of the axon from the cell body to the terminal. Retrograde transport (~200 mm/day) occurs from the terminal to the cell body. Kinesin is the motive protein of anterograde axoplasmic transport, and dynein is used in retrograde transport. (Reproduced with permission from Widmaier EP, Raff H, and Strang KT. *Vander's Human Physiology.* New York: McGraw-Hill, 2008.)

III NEURONAL SIGNALING

Information flow along a neuron is polarized. The dendrites and cell body receive and integrate incoming information, which is transmitted along the axon to the terminals as electrical signals called action potentials. Communication of information from one neuron to another also is polarized and occurs at specialized sites called synapses. The neuron that sends information is the presynaptic neuron, and the one that receives the information is the postsynaptic neuron. An action potential is transmitted along the presynaptic axon to its synaptic terminal. At the terminal, the electrical signal elicits a release of a chemical signal, the neurotransmitter, which elicits a new electrical signal in the postsynaptic cell. Understanding the production and transmission of the action potential along an axon and across the synaptic gap requires a brief discussion of the physiological properties of the excitable membrane.

Neuronal Cell Membrane: Separation of Charges, Excitability, and the Membrane Potential

The neuronal membrane maintains an ionic concentration gradient of certain ions, such as Na^+, K^+, Cl^-, and Ca^{2+} (Table 3.1), and establishes a separation of charges across the membrane with negative intracellular and positive extracellular charges (Figure 3.14). This gradient is maintained by simple or facilitated diffusion through specific ion channels, and by active transport at a metabolic cost to the cell. For example, the Na^+/K^+ ATPase pump expends cellular energy to move two K^+ ions into the cell while pumping three Na^+ ions out. Charge separation across the membrane produces an electrical potential. Each ion has its own unique electrical potential, its ionic equilibrium potential, at which point ionic influx and efflux are in equilibrium. Each excitable cell has its own membrane potential, which is the voltage at which influx and efflux of all of the permeable ions are in equilibrium. Mammalian neurons typically have a resting membrane potential around −65 mV. On application of a stimulus, the membrane permeability to certain ions is changed with concomitant changes in membrane potential. Membrane potential approaches, but never reaches, the ionic potential of the most permeable ion.

Ions cross the membrane through channels that form a conduit through which specific ions enter or exit the cell. There are several types of ion channels that are opened in response to different types of stimuli (Figure 3.15). Perhaps the simplest of these is activated by mechanical distortion of the membrane. This type of ion channel can be found on the terminals of sensory axons. Indentation of the skin stretches the membrane of the sensory ending, opening the ion channels and initiating a change in membrane potential.

Table 3.1 Ionic Potentials. Ionic potentials for ions related to the action potential and synaptic transmission.

Ion	Concentration Gradient	Ionic Potential (mV)
Na^+	Out > In	62
K^+	Out < In	−80
Cl^-	Out > In	−65
Ca^{++}	Out > In	123

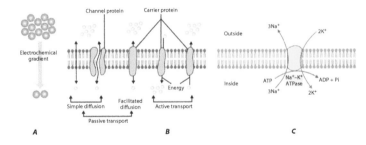

FIGURE 3.14

Movement of ions across the neurolemma. A. Illustration of membrane transport proteins. (Used with permission from Alberts B et al: *Molecular Biology of the Cell*. Garland, 1983.) **B.** Used diffusion through lipid bilayer or simple channel. Facilitated diffusion via a channel, and active transport either into or out of the cell. **C.** Na^+–K^+ ATPase membrane channel. (B., C. Used with permission from Naik P: *Biochemistry*, 3rd edition, Jaypee Broth Used publishers (P) Ltd., 2009.)

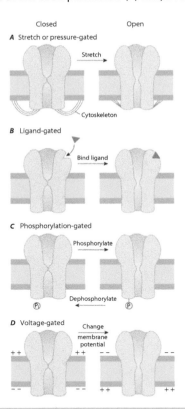

FIGURE 3.15

Regulation of gating in ion channels. Several types of gating are shown for ion channels. **A.** Mechanical stretch of the membrane results in channel opening. **B.** Ligand-gated channels open in response to ligand binding. **C.** Protein phosphorylation or dephosphorylation (often through a second messenger) regulate opening and closing of some ion channels. **D.** Changes in membrane potential alter channel openings (voltage-gated channels). (Adapted from Ion Channels. In: Kandel ER, et al., eds. *Principles of Neural Science,* Fifth Edition New York, NY: McGraw-Hill; 2012).

Other ion channels are activated by the binding of a protein ligand (a chemical messenger such as neurotransmitters) onto a specific region of the ion channel complex; neurotransmitter receptors can be ligand-gated ion channels or can lead indirectly to opening of ion channels (e.g., through intracellular enzyme-mediated phosphorylation/dephosphorylation or through G-protein coupled receptors; see below). Of particular significance to the generation and propagation of action potentials are voltage-gated ion channels. Stimulation changes membrane permeability and perturbs the membrane potential from its resting state. When the membrane potential reaches its action potential threshold, usually around −50 mV to −55 mV, voltage-gated ion channels open and initiate the sequence of membrane potential changes that make up the action potential "spike."

Some ligand-gated channels indirectly open ion channels through a transmembrane signaling system employing G-protein coupled receptors and a second messenger (Figure 3.16). G-proteins are bound to the intracellular portion of the transmembrane receptor protein. As the ligand binds to the receptor, a conformational change exposes and releases a part of the G-protein, which binds to an intramembranous effector protein on the intracellular surface

of the membrane, releasing a second messenger (an intracellular signal molecule). Depending on the type of second messenger molecule, the second messenger can open a transmembrane ion channel, open channels on the nuclear membrane, or activate intracellular organelles. Thus the G-protein-coupled second messenger system can prolong or intensify the effects of ligand binding and can produce significant changes in gene expression. A wide variety of second messenger systems exist in neurons, and malfunction is implicated in many pathological conditions, including depression, migraine, diabetes, and osteoporosis.

The Action Potential

When a stimulus is applied to a neuron, Na^+ channels open, allowing influx of that ion and a rapid positive change in the membrane potential, or depolarization (Figure 3.17). Depolarization that exceeds the action potential threshold produces a full action potential spike. The term *spike* derives from the appearance of the electrophysiological tracing made from a stimulated neuron. This is an all-or-none process: if depolarization exceeds threshold, there must

Ligand-gated ion channel

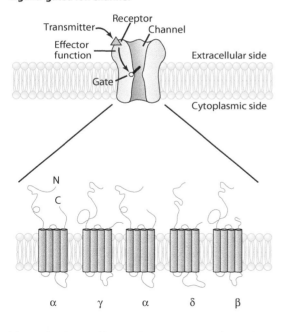

G protein-coupled receptor

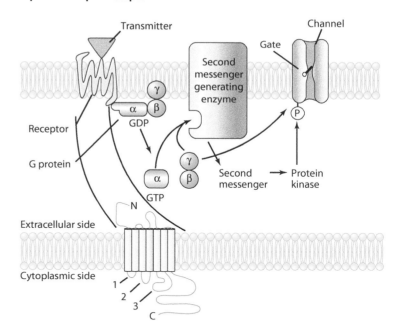

FIGURE 3.16

Ligand-gated channels and G protein–coupled receptors. Ligand-gated ion channels, which mediate fast synaptic transmission, are composed of one or more subunits (eg, α β γ δ) embedded in the plasma membrane that form a central, gated pore. In response to the binding of transmitter, this type of receptor undergoes a conformational change, opening the gate and allowing ions to diffuse passively along concentration gradients through a hydrophilic opening in an otherwise hydrophobic bilayer. G protein–coupled receptors, which mediate slow synaptic transmission, transduce neurotransmitter signals through a different mechanism. These proteins do not form gated pores in the membrane; rather, the binding of transmitter induces a conformational change that allows the receptor to activate a heterotrimeric G protein (Chapter 4). The activated G protein dissociates into a free α subunit bound to GTP and a free βγ subunit dimer. Both can activate enzymes that synthesize second messengers; in addition, βγ dimers directly regulate certain ion channels. Second messengers also regulate ion channels, most often by activating protein kinases, which subsequently phosphorylate such channels (P). 1, 2, 3, cytoplasmic domains of G protein–coupled receptor; C, C-terminal tail of the receptor. (Reproduced with permission from Overview of Synaptic Transmission. In: Kandel ER, et al, eds. Principles of Neural Science, Fifth Editon New York, NY: McGraw-Hill; 2012).

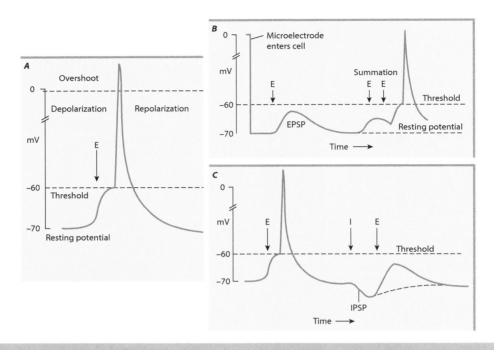

FIGURE 3.17

Action potential ("spike potential") recorded with one electrode inside cell. *A.* In the resting state, the membrane potential (resting potential) is about −70 mV. When the axon is stimulated, there is a small depolarization. If this depolarization reaches the firing level (threshold), there is an all-or-none depolarization (action potential). The action potential approaches ENa and overshoots the 0-mV level. The action potential ends when the axon repolarizes, again settling at resting potential. E = excitation stimulus. ***B.*** Subthreshold depolarization produces an EPSP. Consecutive subthreshold stimuli can summate if the later stimuli are presented before the membrane potential can degrade to resting potential. ***C.*** Inhibitory synapses hyperpolarize the membrane, driving membrane potential farther away from threshold (IPSP). Excitatory and inhibitory inputs summate; if the change in overall membrane potential meets or exceeds threshold, an action potential will be formed. (Reproduced with permission from Gray JA, Nicoll RA. Introduction to the Pharmacology of CNS Drugs. In: Katzung BG, Trevor AJ. eds. *Basic & Clinical Pharmacology*, 13e New York, NY: McGraw-Hill; 2015.)

be an action potential spike; if the depolarization does not reach threshold, membrane potential degrades back to its resting voltage. Subthreshold depolarization does not produce a postsynaptic action potential in the target cell. Instead, it produces an excitatory postsynaptic potential (EPSP) that will degenerate back to resting potential over time. Several subthreshold EPSP changes in membrane potential can be added together (summated) to reach threshold, thus initiating the action potential. Two types of summation are recognized: temporal and spatial. Temporal summation occurs when the number of EPSPs per unit of time carried on a single axon is increased so that the cumulative change in membrane voltage exceeds the threshold voltage. Spatial summation occurs when additional axons input EPSPs to the same target cell. Inhibitory postsynaptic potentials (IPSPs) occur when postsynaptic Cl⁻ channels open instead of Na^+ channels, making Cl⁻ the most permeable ion. IPSPs hyperpolarize the membrane and drive it further away from threshold. A neuron's response to synaptic inputs is determined by the sum of all of the EPSPs and IPSPs that converge on it;

if threshold is reached, the action potential ensues; otherwise, the membrane returns to resting potential.

During the depolarization phase of the action potential (Figure 3.18), Na^+ is the most permeable ion, and the membrane potential rises rapidly toward the ion potential for Na^+, which is around +60 mV. During the depolarization phase, continuing through most of the repolarization phase, no amount of additional stimulus can elicit another action potential; this is referred to as the absolute refractory period, and summation is not in effect during this time. As the membrane potential ascends past 0 mV (overshoot phase), it nears the apex of the action potential spike. At this point, voltage-gated Na^+ channels change their conformation so that they are inactivated. As the membrane potential nears its apex, K^+ channels begin to open, and that ion begins to flow out of the cell. During the repolarization phase of the action potential spike, membrane potential is driven negatively toward the K^+ ionic potential, $\sim{-}80$ mV. As the membrane repolarizes, there is a brief period, called the afterpotential phase, during which the K^+

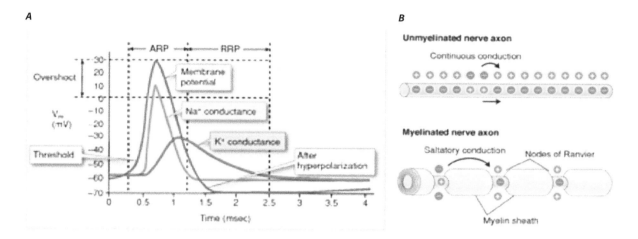

FIGURE 3.18

Nerve action potential. A. The upstroke of the action potential results from increased Na⁺ conductance. Repolarization results from a declining Na⁺ conductance combined with an increasing K⁺ conductance; afterhyperpolarization is due to sustained high K⁺ conductance. **B.** Action potential propagation. Local current flow causes the threshold potential to be exceeded in adjacent areas of the neuron membrane. Because the upstream region is refractory, an action potential is only propagated downstream. In myelinated axons, action potentials propagate faster by "jumping" from one node of Ranvier to the next node by saltatory conduction. ARP, absolute refractory period; RRP, relative refractory period. (Reproduced with permission from General Physiology. In: Kibble JD, Halsey CR. eds. Medical Physiology: The Big Picture New York, NY: McGraw-Hill; 2009).

channels have not yet closed and Na⁺ channels have not yet been reactivated, and the membrane potential drops below the −80 mV ionic potential of K⁺. During the afterpotential phase, a period known as the relative refractory period occurs, during which a suprathreshold stimulus can elicit a new action potential. At the end of the afterpotential phase, the membrane potential returns to its resting voltage, and all ion movement across the membrane returns to equilibrium.

Axon Conduction

Once produced, the action potential must travel along the axon to its terminal to initiate electrochemical transmission. A single stimulus creates a local depolarization across the axon membrane. The region of local depolarization spreads passively from the site of initiation, diminishing with increasing distance from the initiation site. At some point, the membrane potential decreases until it is below threshold; the action potential becomes an EPSP and eventually degrades to resting potential.

The distance that action potential can travel before the membrane potential drops below threshold is related to two anatomical factors, axon diameter and myelination. The electrophysiological features of axon conductance are analogous to electrical conduction along a wire. An action potential conducted along a very thin axon (some can be as small as ~0.2 μm in diameter) travels only a short distance before its charge falls below threshold.

Resistance in the thin axon is due to the small number of ion channels, reducing the rate of voltage change (membrane potential change) with distance from the initiation site. The result of high resistance and short distance of passive spread of charge is that thin axons conduct slowly, ~0.5–2.0 m/sec (Table 3.2). Noxious (nociceptive, damaging), thermal, and chemical stimuli are carried on thin, often unmyelinated axons, as are peripheral autonomic fibers. Large caliber axons, like thick wires, conduct rapidly because they have less resistance to ion flow. Large caliber axons, especially those covered with a thick layer of myelin, may conduct at ~120 m/sec. The thickest fibers serve as somatic motor axons and as proprioceptive sensory axons. Intermediate thickness axons supply the majority of sensitive mechanoreceptors.

The second factor increasing the rate of axon conduction is the presence and amount of myelination on the axon (Figure 3.19). Recall that in the CNS, myelinating cells are called oligodendrocytes, and in the periphery they are called Schwann cells. Both types of myelinating cells enclose the axon like a cuff in densely packed spiraling layers of compressed axoplasmic membrane. At any single level along an axon, each myelin segment is formed by a single Schwann cell or oligodendrocyte. Consecutive cuffs of myelin lie adjacent to each other along the length of the axon. Small gaps, known as nodes of Ranvier, exist between myelin segments. Only at the nodes is the axon membrane exposed. The exposed membrane at the nodes of Ranvier contains dense clusters of Na⁺ channels, so it is relatively easier for depolarization to

Table 3.2 Functional Classifications of Axons

	Aα/Type I	Aβ/Type II	Aγ	Aδ/Type III	C/Type IV
Sensory modality	Proprioception	Mechanoreceptors		Pain, temperature	Pain, temperature
Motor function	Somatic motor		Intrafusal motor		Postganglionic autonomic
Myelin	Very thick	Thick	Thick	Thin	Unmyelinated
Diameter (μ)	13–20	6–12	5–8	1–5	0.2–1.5
Conduction velocity (m/sec)	80–120	35–75	4–24	5–30	0.5–2

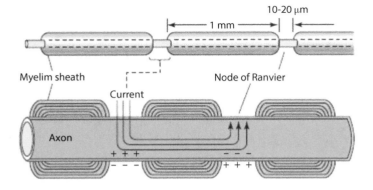

FIGURE 3.19

Myelin and saltatory conduction along axons. Nodes of Ranvier contain a high density of Na$^+$ channels. Depolarizing current enters a myelinated axon at one node and exits at the next node, effectively "jumping" node-to-node. Unlike the continuous exit of current that occurs in unmyelinated axons the myelin sheath decreases the passive spread and decrement of charge and greatly increases conduction velocity. (Reproduced with permission from Cellular Basis of Communication. In: Nestler EJ, et al., eds. *Molecular Neuropharmacology: A Foundation for Clinical Neuroscience.* 3rd ed. New York, NY: McGraw-Hill; 2015).

reach threshold there than in other sites along the axon. Passive degeneration of action potential with increasing distance from spike initiation is substantially reduced by the myelin. In this way, the suprathreshold membrane potential is maintained for a great distance under the insulating myelin sheath until it reaches the next node of Ranvier and its cluster of Na$^+$ channels; a new action potential is then initiated. This process of "jumping" from node to node is called saltatory conduction. Sites where Na$^+$ channels are clustered are referred to as spike initiation centers, and they are locations where it is relatively easy to initiate an action potential. Spike initiation centers are found at predictable sites, such as the nodes of Ranvier, dendritic spines, the soma, and the axon hillock (initial segment), the part of the axon extending from the cell body and the first myelin segment. Also, some stretch receptor endings

on sensory axons in the skin have a concentration of mechanically activated Na$^+$ channels.

Synapses: Sites of Electrochemical Signal Transmission

Synapses are points of communication between presynaptic neuronal axons and the postsynaptic cell body (axosomatic), the dendrites (axodendritic), or another axon (axoaxonic) (Figure 3.20). The synapse consists of three distinct elements: (1) presynaptic terminal, the axon terminal of the presynaptic neuron; (2) synaptic cleft, the narrow intercellular space between the presynaptic and postsynaptic neurons; and (3) receptive membrane of the postsynaptic neuron. Synapses located on different sites can serve different functions.

Arrival of the action potential at the axon terminal initiates a cascade of events culminating in target cell response: depolarization (postsynaptic EPSP), hyperpolarization (postsynaptic IPSP), or muscle contraction. As the action potential reaches the terminal bouton, voltage activated Ca^{++} channels open, allowing influx of Ca^{++}. The entry of Ca^{++} activates vesicle binding proteins that bring the vesicle membrane into contact with the active zone membrane of the terminal. Fusion of these membranes inserts any trans- or intramembranous proteins that were constructed within the vesicle membrane, and allows exocytosis (extracellular release) of the contents of the vesicles, neurotransmitters, into the synaptic cleft.

Neurotransmitter molecules diffuse across the synaptic cleft and bind to receptors on the postsynaptic membrane. This binding changes the permeability of particular ions across the neuronal membrane. A neurotransmitter can either excite the postsynaptic neuron by depolarizing it (i.e., increasing the flow of sodium ions into the neuron) or inhibit the neuron by hyperpolarizing it (i.e., increasing the flow of chloride ions into the neuron).

To prevent prolonged excitation/inhibition in the postsynaptic cell, neurotransmitter molecules must be removed from the synaptic cleft. This is accomplished by the hydrolytic actions of a degradative enzyme in the postsynaptic membrane. Simple diffusion clears away degradative products from the synaptic cleft into interstitial fluids ultimately to be removed by the liver and kidneys. Some metabolically expensive components of the degraded neurotransmitter are recycled back into the presynaptic terminal through re-uptake receptors. Once back in the presynaptic terminal, the recycled components are used to resynthesize the neurotransmitter, which is then packaged into new synaptic vesicles to await the arrival of the next action potential.

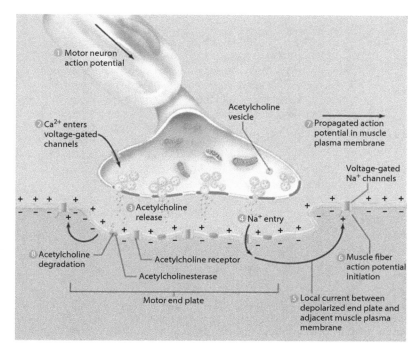

FIGURE 3.20

Diagram of the stereotypical synapse: the neuromuscular junction. Events at the neuromuscular junction that lead to an action potential in the muscle fiber plasma membrane. The impulse arriving in the end of the motor neuron (1) increases the permeability of its endings to Ca^{++} (2) which enters the endings and triggers exocytosis of the acetylcholine (ACh)-containing synaptic vesicles (3). ACh diffuses and binds to nicotinic cholinergic (NM) receptors in the motor end plate, which increases Na^+ (4) and K^+ conductance. The resultant influx of Na+ produces the end plate potential (5). The current sink created by this local potential depolarizes the adjacent muscle membrane to its firing level (6). Action potentials are generated on either side of the end plate and are conducted away from the end plate in both directions along the muscle fiber and the muscle contracts (7). ACh is then removed from the synaptic cleft by acetylcholinesterase (8). (Reproduced with permission from Chapter 6. Synaptic & Junctional Transmission. In: Barrett KE, Boitano S, Barman SM, Brooks HL. eds. Ganong's Review of Medical Physiology, 24e New York, NY: McGraw-Hill; 2012).

IV · RESPONSE TO INJURY

PNS Response to Injury

In the PNS, nerve injury can produce profound motor and sensory deficits, such as flaccid paralysis, loss of sensation, and abolished reflexes. Partial injury, such as nerve compression, is often extremely painful. Still, with proper care and rehabilitation, a person usually can recover fully from a PNS nerve injury. Compression of a peripheral nerve without dividing the nerve and all of its connective tissue coverings into proximal and distal segments can interrupt action potential conduction, producing temporary paresis or paralysis and sensory abnormalities; this situation is called neurapraxia. There is no Wallerian degeneration distal to the site of nerve injury, and full recovery is certain within days to weeks. Axonotmesis is a more emergent condition seen after a severe compression injury that breaks continuity between proximal and distal axon segments, but leaves the basement membrane and connective tissue sheaths intact. Wallerian degeneration of the axons in the distal nerve section occurs, and nerve conduction distal to the injury is abolished, eliminating sensory and motor functions. When incomplete, axonotmesis can be extremely painful, as seen in patients with herniated intervertebral discs. Recovery is likely, although the rate is limited to ~1–10 mm per day. Neurotmesis is the most severe nerve injury under this classification scheme, and it involves separation of the axon, its basement membrane, and its connective tissue sheaths. Neurotmetic injuries, such as laceration or nerve root avulsion, require surgical intervention to reattach proximal and distal nerve segments as precisely as possible. Wallerian degeneration occurs distally, but with the loss of continuity of the basement membrane, sprouting axons are no longer channeled directly to their targets, and mismatches between proximal and distal segments occur. In some cases, these mismatches are minor and cause no significant impediment to recovery, whereas in others they develop into painful neuromas.

When a peripheral nerve is injured, a process known as collateral sprouting begins. Damaged tissue and neurons change their phenotypes, converting from maintenance and normal function to survival and regeneration modes. Tissues support regeneration by increasing expression of neurotrophic molecules (neurotrophins) to attract and nourish extending regenerative neurites. Wallerian degeneration provides a rich extracellular matrix that is both permissive and facilitative to the elongating neurites, and neuronal gene expression promotes the production of neurotrophin receptor proteins. Axon sprouts emerge from adjacent uninjured, unmyelinated axons; myelinated axons in adults do not exhibit collateral sprouting. Collateral sprouting from intact axons is supported by expression of nerve growth factor in the denervated tissue. The injured axons then begin to regenerate in a process that is independent of nerve growth factor. When the original axons reinnervate their targets, the collateral sprouts withdraw. Other neurotrophic factors appear to be related to regenerative sprouting, and exogenous application may provide a therapeutic approach to facilitating recovery of the peripheral end of injured axons. Motor neurons have somewhat delayed regeneration and functional recovery, owing partially to the more extensive cellular changes (chromatolysis) in the cell bodies. These motor neurons regain function while the cellular changes slowly resolve.

CNS Response to Injury

CNS response to injury is different and less successful than seen in the PNS (Figure 3.21), although, in both, Wallerian degeneration occurs in the amputated distal segment. A traumatic injury in the CNS initiates a cascade of events that establishes a physical and chemical barrier to regenerative axon sprouting. Nerve injury damages CNS tissue, allowing molecules and non-neural cell infiltration across the ruptured blood–brain barrier. After blood clots to close the injury site, microglia clear the breakdown products of the damaged tissue. Next, reactive astrocytes form a glial scar to separate damaged tissue from adjacent healthy tissue and reestablish the blood–brain barrier. During the proliferation phase, astrocytes impose a physical barrier to axon sprouting from the proximal stump, and they secrete molecules into the extracellular matrix that prevent axon elongation.

Processes occurring normally to maintain order in the developing nervous system can become detrimental during healing after injury. For example, oligodendrocytes secrete the protein Nogo to prevent axon collaterals from sprouting, which maintains order during CNS tract development. However after injury, Nogo expression limits sprouting and prevents reestablishment of synapses in the injured CNS.

The intrinsic ability of the nervous system to reorganize in response to changing conditions during development, with learning, and in reaction to injury is called neuroplasticity. Medical professionals exploit this faculty to rehabilitate patients after central and peripheral injury or disease. In some instances, such as the development of chronic neuropathic pain after peripheral nerve injury, neuroplastic alterations are maladaptive, and the goal of rehabilitation is to reverse or prevent these changes. Neuroplasticity occurs at multiple levels: at the molecular level, with changes in gene expression; at the synaptic level, altering the effectiveness or efficiency of pre- and postsynaptic elements; at the morphological level, with changes in the dendritic arbor and axonal distribution; and at the system level, with changes in the central distribution of synaptic area. In addition to morphological plasticity, the nervous system also exhibits synaptic plasticity.

As discussed above, recovery from long CNS tract damage is hindered by glial scar development combined with the release of

Frontiers in Research
Promoting CNS Axon Elongation
Researchers have demonstrated in animal models that CNS axons are capable of elongation after transection. In experimental preparations using rats, a peripheral nerve segment was attached to a nick in the medulla, extending down to a similar nick in the spinal cord. Medullary axons extended sprouts into the PNS nerve segment for a distance of 30 μm, thus demonstrating that it is the morphological and biochemical characteristics of the environment around the site of injury that is inhibitory to CNS axon outgrowth and not an intrinsic incapacity of the axons. Recognition of this feature has opened several lines of research that aim to modify the environment at the site of injury in ways that permit and promote CNS axon elongation.

substances inhibitory to axon elongation and regeneration. Still, the CNS has a robust capacity to remodel itself morphologically and biochemically to limit functional loss and promote recovery. Uninjured axon collaterals and dendrites extend into adjacent denervated territories and increase the density of the dendritic spines in an example of morphological plasticity. Expanded dendritic territory increases the area available for synaptic input. The area in the cortex that contained the lost body representation is filled by the expanded representation of the surrounding regions.

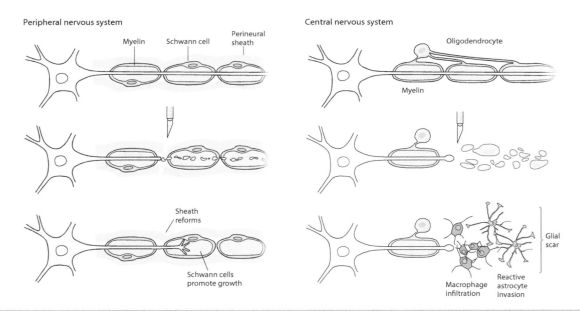

Peripheral nervous system

Central nervous system

FIGURE 3.21

Axons in the periphery regenerate better than those in the central nervous system. After sectioning of a peripheral nerve, the perineural sheath reforms rapidly and Schwann cells in the distal stump promote axonal growth by producing trophic and attractant factors and expressing high levels of adhesive proteins. After sectioning of axonal tracts in the central nervous system, the distal segment disintegrates and myelin fragments, exposing elongation-inhibiting Nogo proteins. In addition, reactive astrocytes and macrophages are attracted to the lesion site. This complex cellular milieu, termed a glial scar, inhibits axonal regeneration. (Reproduced with permission from Repairing the Damaged Brain. In: Kandel ER, Schwartz JH, Jessell TM, Siegelbaum SA, Hudspeth AJ, Mack S. eds. Principles of Neural Science, Fifth Editon New York, NY: McGraw-Hill; 2012).

> **CASE 3** DISCUSSION: Myasthenia Gravis

In the case of myasthenia gravis, the body attacks the main neurotransmitter for motor (muscle) function, acetylcholine. This causes rapid onset of profound muscle weakness, first noticeable in the small muscles of the face, where any weakness is obvious. Pharmacological management includes cholinesterase inhibitors and immunosuppressive drugs to reduce production of antibodies that block acetylcholine receptors. At the start of this chapter, our patient HB was recently recovering from a new onset of weakness, choosing to cancel an upcoming trip to Machu Picchu. He and his wife subsequently traveled to Amsterdam with a tour group, where his symptoms worsened, producing difficulty swallowing. HB realized at that time that stress was the primary trigger for his myasthenia gravis symptoms, so he slowed his travel pace and used a wheelchair to navigate the large Schiphol Airport. He returned from this trip humbled by the experience, deciding to leave his consulting job. His job placed physical demands on his body, with extensive walking, long hours of speaking that taxed his voice, and the additional challenge of frequent travel. HB was frustrated by the paucity of resources or support available socially, which was mediated by a local support group. There is currently no cure for myasthenia gravis; however, due to advances in drug therapy, people can reduce symptoms and learn to modify behavior to minimize stress. With the help of a strong support system, people can continue to lead satisfying and healthy lives, like our patient HB.

 REFERENCES

Abbott NJ, Patabendige AAK, Dolman DEM, Yusof SR, Begley DJ. Structure and function of the blood–brain barrier. *Neurobiol Dis*. 2010;37:13–25.

Allen NJ, Barres BA. Glia: more than just brain glue. *Nature*. 2009; 457:675–677.

Anand P, Singh B. A review on cholinesterase inhibitors for Alzheimer's disease. *Arch Pharm Res*. 2013;36:375–399.

Barnett MW, Larkman PM. The action potential. *Pract Neurol*. 2007;7:192–197.

Bean BP. The action potential in mammalian central neurons. *Nature Reviews Neuroscience*. 2007;8:451–465.

Chen ZJ, Ughrin Y, Levine JM. Inhibition of axon growth by oligodendrocyte precursor cells. *Mol Cell Neurosci*. 2002;20:125–139.

Duvernoy HM. *The Human Hippocampus*. Munich, Germany: J.F. Bergmann Verlag, 1988.

Gardiner NJ. Integrins and the extracellular matrix: key mediators of development and regeneration of the sensory nervous system. *Develop Neurobiol*. 2011;71:1054–1072.

Henry DE, Chiodo AE, Yang W. Central nervous system reorganization in a variety of chronic pain states: a review. *PM&R*. 2011 Dec;3(12):1116–1125.

Herculano-Houzel S, Lent R. Isotropic fractionator: a simple, rapid method for the quantification of total cell and neuron numbers in the brain. *J Neuroscience*. 2005, March 9;25:2518–2521.

Hitoshi Kawano H, Kimura-Kuroda J, Komuta Y, et al. Role of the lesion scar in the response to damage and repair in the central nervous system. *Cell Tissue Res*. 2012;349:169–180.

Insel TR, Landis SC, Collins FS. Research priorities: the NIH BRAIN initiative. *Science*. 2013;340(6133):687–688.

Johnson AE, van Waes MA. The translocon: a dynamic gateway at the ER membrane. *Annu Rev Cell Dev Biol*. 1999;15:799–842.

Kawano H, Kimura-Kuroda J, Komuta Y, Yoshioka N, Li HP, Kawamura K, Li Y, Raisman G. Role of the lesion scar in the response to damage and repair of the central nervous system. *Cell Tissue Res*. 2012;349:169–180.

Lee PR, Fields RD. Regulation of myelin genes implicated in psychiatric disorders by functional activity in axons. *Front Neuroanat*. 2009;3:4. doi:10.3389/neuro.05.004.2009.

McGleenon BM, Dynan KB, Passmore AP. Acetylcholinesterase inhibitors in Alzheimer's disease. *Br J Clin Pharmacol*. 1999;48:471–480.

Nash M, Pribiag H, Fournier AE, Jacobson C. Central nervous system regeneration inhibitors and their intracellular substrates. *Mol Neurobiol*. 2009;40:224–235.

Navarro X, Vivo M, Valero-Cabré A. Neural plasticity after peripheral nerve injury and regeneration. *Prog Neurobiol*. 2007;82:163–201.

Paxinos G, Mai JK, eds. *The Human Nervous System*. London: Elsevier, 2004.

Praveen Ballabh P, Braun A, Nedergaard M. The blood–brain barrier: an overview. Structure, regulation, and clinical implications. *Neurobiol Dis*. 2004;16:1–13.

Purves D, Augustine GJ, Fitzpatrick D, et al., eds. *Neuroscience*, 2nd ed. Sunderland, MA: Sinauer, 2001.

Raichle ME. A brief history of human brain mapping. *TINS*. 2009; 32(2):118–126.

Roux BT, Cottrell GS. G protein-coupled receptors: what a difference a 'partner' makes. *Int J Mol Sci*. 2014;15:1112–1142.

Samuel DS, Aguayo AJ. Axonal elongation into peripheral nervous system "bridges" after central nervous system injury in adult rats. *Science*. 1981;214:931–933.

Sherman DL, Brophy PJ. Mechanisms of axon ensheathment and myelin growth. *Nat Rev Neurosci*. 2005;6(9):683–690.

Stein DG, Hoffman SW. Concepts of CNS plasticity in the context of brain damage and repair. *J Head Trauma Rehabil*. 2003 Jul–Aug;18(4): 317–341.

Volterra A, Meldolesi J. Astrocytes, from brain glue to communication elements: the revolution continues. *Nat Rev Neurosci*. 2005;6(8):626–640.

Ward NS. Neural plasticity and recovery of function. *Prog Brain Res*. 2005;150:527–535.

Wettschureck N, Offermanns S. Mammalian G proteins and their cell type specific functions. *Physiol Rev*. 2005;85:1159–1204.

Young JA, Tolentino M. Neuroplasticity and its applications for rehabilitation. *American Journal of Therapeutics*. 2011;18:70–80.

> REVIEW QUESTIONS

1. In the CNS, astrocytes:
   A. buffer Na+ in the CNS neuropil.
   B. promote axonal elongation.
   C. create the blood–brain barrier.
   D. form myelin around CNS axons.
   E. emit inhibitory axons to pain endings.

2. Concerning the generation and propagation of action potentials, which of the following is *correct*?
   A. Subthreshold excitatory stimuli do not summate; either they produce an action potential or they do not.
   B. Demyelination produces "bare" areas on axons and allows faster saltatory conduction.
   C. "Cable properties" of axons indicate that axons with a small cross-section area have less resistance to ion flow and therefore conduct action potentials faster than large axons.
   D. Myelinated axons conduct impulses rapidly because the myelin is contractile and squeezes the charged ions forward.
   E. If a stimulus exceeds the threshold of the action potential, a spike will be produced; if not, the cell will return to its resting membrane potential (all-or-none principle).

3. Concerning protein synthesis and transportation in neurons, which of the following statements is *correct*?
   A. Membranes of the Golgi apparatus are studded with ribosomes.
   B. Kinesin is the most important transport molecule related to retrograde axon transport.
   C. Free ribosomes package newly formed proteins into vesicles.
   D. RNA polymerase converts ribosomal RNA into messenger RN.
   E. Translation is the process that ends with a new protein being formed.

4. Comparing axons and dendrites:
   A. only axons contain microtubules.
   B. both can be sites of synapses.
   C. most dendrites are thinly myelinated.
   D. axons are the main input sites and dendrites the main output sites.
   E. both participate in the neuromuscular junction.

5. Which of the following statements is *false*?
   A. Healing after injury is more difficult in the CNS.
   B. Astrocytes are a type of macroglia that contribute to the blood–brain barrier in the CNS.
   C. Satellite glial cells in the PNS perform similar tasks as glial cells in the CNS.
   D. All Schwann cells are myelinating, enclosing the neuron in myelin for conduction.
   E. Oligodendrocytes produce myelin in the CNS.

6. Ribosomes are organelles that translate messenger RNA to:
   A. properly code the sequence of amino acids for protein synthesis.
   B. ensure mitochondrial function occurs for cell function.
   C. maintain appropriate ion gradient for resting cell membrane.
   D. convert endoplasmic reticulum for ion transport.
   E. support cell metabolism via Golgi apparatus merger.

7. Why are some proteins built directly into the lipid bilayer of the endoplasmic reticulum?
   A. To create prions
   B. For metabolic efficiency
   C. To avoid transcription errors
   D. For transport via ribosomes across the lipid bilayer
   E. To attach to the Golgi apparatus

8. Which item below is *not* a type of ion channel?
   A. Voltage gated
   B. Ligand gated
   C. Synapse gated
   D. Pressure gated
   E. Phosphorylation gated

9. Saltatory conduction is described as:
   A. active transport to open Ca++ channels.
   B. passive depolarization in unmyelinated axons.
   C. Na+ channel potentiation at the synaptic cleft.
   D. depolarization at spaces between myelin in the axon sheath.
   E. active transport to remove neurotransmitters from the synaptic cleft.

10. Wallerian degeneration is best described as a process that:
    A. closes the blood–brain barrier.
    B. occurs both proximal and distal to the injured axon.
    C. can occur in both myelinated and non-myelinated axons.
    D. can occur in both PNS and CNS.
    E. is irreversible, resulting in cell death.

CHAPTER 4

Development of the Central Nervous System

> **CASE 4** Normal Infant Development

Jasmine and Richard had mixed emotions when the pregnancy test came back positive. Their previous pregnancy was not successful because of chromosomal abnormalities. This had been devastating for them both, and they planted a tree in the backyard in honor of that child not meant to be. A human karyotype consists of 22 pairs of autosomal chromosomes and one pair of allosomes for gender. Fetal development often ends prior to the first trimester of a pregnancy, primarily due to karyotype deficiencies such as an extra chromosome, XXY, or a missing chromosome, X only. They were relieved when the chorionic villi sampling (CVS) test in the first trimester was negative for chromosomal abnormalities. CVS is a common prenatal test performed in high-risk pregnancies; the physician extracts tissue from the placenta for fetal genetic testing.

Jasmine was careful with her diet, eating healthy foods and taking prenatal vitamins. She was very fit, and her physician supported her decision to remain active, with modifications as needed, as long as she felt good and the baby was doing well. She worked as a physical therapist at the hospital until her 39th week of pregnancy. Additionally, visitors to the local health club were surprised to meet a vibrant and very pregnant woman teaching both Zumba and spinning up until her ninth month!

Jasmine worked Friday and went into labor over the weekend, giving birth to Miles on a Monday evening in October, after 39 weeks of gestation. At 8 pounds 5 ounces, Miles was full term; however, a complication developed during delivery when the umbilical cord wrapped around his neck. The obstetrician asked Jasmine to hold off on pushing while he unwound the cord, and Miles was delivered. He was a little blue, with a hearty cry and an Apgar score of 9/10 (he lost one point for color), which increased to a 10/10 at five minutes. Infant health is assessed at one minute and five minutes after delivery, using the Apgar scale, which evaluates infant status for cardiovascular and neurologic function, indicating need for resuscitation support to thrive. The one-minute score offers a glimpse of how the infant tolerated delivery, and the five-minute score relates to postpartum tolerance. It does not correlate to long-term infant health, nor can it predict morbidity or mortality. Miles' Apgar reflected the minimal amount of time he had the cord wrapped around his neck, thus saving him from potentially damaging events such as anoxia.

Miles is a very fortunate baby, with many loving caregivers in his life, offering a supportive and varied environment. From day one, Miles enjoyed multisensory enrichments including sound, touch, and varied postures. His parents sang to him daily, and he would listen as they read to Fiona, his older sister. Each bath ended with infant massage, and he came to appreciate daily "tummy time," to promote head extension and development of motor milestones. His grandparents were bilingual and spoke to him in Spanish as well as English to promote neurologic pathways for language and avoid synaptic pruning. This type of early enrichment promotes positive neuroplastic changes during the critical period of synaptic pruning.

I OVERVIEW OF KEY CONCEPTS

The nervous system is one of the earliest organ systems to develop. Its general layout is established during the first trimester; maturation continues through the first 20 years of life; and fundamental changes continue at cellular and subcellular levels according to life demands. Failure in the development of the nervous system is responsible for the high rate of spontaneous loss of pregnancies during the first trimester.

Developmentally, the body and all its structures arise from three embryonic tissue layers, the endoderm, mesoderm, and ectoderm. The nervous system develops from a specialized portion of the ectoderm, the neural plate. Originally a flattened sheet of cells, the neural plate forms a tubelike structure—termed the *neural tube*—from which the neurons and glial cells derive. These early neural progenitors undergo prodigious mitosis, followed by migration to their final destinations where they will make connections and develop functional circuits. Neural tube walls form the central nervous system, and the cavity forms the ventricular system containing cerebrospinal fluid produced mainly by the choroid plexus. Cerebrospinal fluid normally exits from the ventricular system into the space overlying the central nervous system's surface through foramina in the fourth ventricle.

Differential rates of rapid cell proliferation within the limited volume of the cranial vault forces the developing neural tube to fold, producing a series of flexures that delineate the major portions of the CNS. The cerebral cortex is folded into an array of ridges and grooves, gyri and sulci, that greatly increase the surface area within the confined space of the cranium. Complexities in the distribution of cell clusters (nuclei), nerves, and tracts (axon pathways in the CNS) arise in part because connections are made before the cells migrate to their mature positions. These early connections are possible because the embryo is tiny, with small distances between cell bodies and target tissues. Differential rates of growth between nervous and somatic tissues draw axons sometimes great distances from their cell bodies at maturity. Thus the familiar configuration of the mature brain is the result of a complex interplay among physical interactions between adjacent tissues, highly regulated spatiotemporal expression of a sequence of reproductive and growth-promoting proteins, and programmed cell death (apoptosis).

II STRUCTURE OF THE BRAIN DURING NORMAL DEVELOPMENT

During the first week of embryonic life, the embryo consists of a flattened three-layered structure. Mesenchymal tissue differentiates during the third week, in a process called induction, into the notochord, releasing chemical agents that stimulate early differentiation of the overlying ectoderm into a flattened disc called the neural plate. Neural plate cells are still pluripotent, capable of differentiating into neurons and glia. With induction, the development of the nervous system begins.

Neurulation

Differential rates of mitosis lead to alterations in the embryonic nervous system that create the neural tube, the source of all neurons and glia that form the CNS (Figure 4.1). During the fourth week, cell reproduction in the neural plate is greatest at its margins, which forms a shallow groove on the dorsum of the plate called the

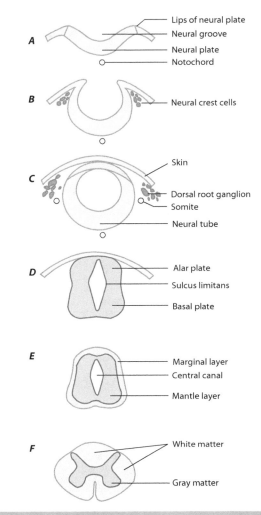

FIGURE 4.1

Schematic cross sections showing the development of the spinal cord. A. The appearance of the notochord stimulates formation of a midline disc (neural plate). Along the midline of the neural plate, differential rates of mitosis generate a shallow furrow, the neural groove. The lips of the neural plate extend toward each other. **B.** As the neural groove deepens, a specialized set of neurons in the lips of the neural groove differentiates into the neural crest cells, which will generate the neurons of the PNS. **C.** The neural groove has closed forming the neural tube, the lumen of which will form the ventricular system of the CNS. Neural crest cells have further differentiated into sensory cells of the dorsal root ganglia. Tissues around the dorsal root ganglia form the somites, which will differentiate into locally appropriate muscles and bones. **D.** Spinal cord differentiation of the neural tube creates a dorsal, sensory region, the alar plate; and a ventral, motor region, the basal plate, separated by a longitudinal groove, the sulcus limitans, which extends bilaterally within the wall of the neural tube. **E.** Cells in the mantle differentiate into gray matter; the marginal layer is composed of axons that comprise white matter tracts. **F.** A mature spinal cord has a central gray matter region surrounded by white matter. The central canal in adults is largely obliterated. (Reproduced with permission from Waxman SG. Chapter 5. The Spinal Cord. In: Waxman SG. eds. Clinical Neuroanatomy, 27e. New York, NY: McGraw-Hill; 2013).

neural groove. This initial differentiation of cells is called primary neurulation and establishes cell lines that become the epidermis, neural tube, and neural crest. Neurulation continues as the lips of the neural groove grow together and merge on the dorsal midline, seal the roof, and construct the patent neural tube along the rostral-caudal axis of the embryo. Secondary neurulation occurs as the cells of the neural tube begin to differentiate into neurons and glia. Cells in the dorsal part of the tube differentiate into the roof plate, which establishes the dorsum and dorsal midline of the embryo and influences neural crest cell differentiation and migration.

As the neural tube closes, bilaterally a small collection of cells, the neural crest, differentiates from cells in the lips of the neural groove. Neural crest cells migrate ventrolaterally and develop into the neurons and support cells of the PNS as well as several non-neural structures such as facial cartilage and cells in the adrenal medulla.

Three- and Five-Vesicle Stages

The neural tube at first is open rostrally and caudally, presenting the anterior and posterior neuropores. Proper development of the rest of the CNS requires closure at both ends of the tube, which occurs under a strictly regulated spatiotemporal schedule. Premature closure of the anterior neuropore results in severe dysraphic cranial deformities including incomplete brain development (microcephaly; "small brain") as well as malformation of the boney and muscular

structures of the head (microcephaly; "small head"). Anencephaly combines the worst of both microencephaly and microcephaly and is often incompatible with life (Figure 4.2). Rostral dysraphic defects can involve extrusion of meninges, CSF, and brain tissue into a sac usually protruding from the back of the head.

Caudally, failure of posterior neuropore closure presents as spina bifida, and myeloschisis is the severest form of spina bifida. Like rostral dysraphic defects, spina bifida can present as a dorsal protrusion of a fluid-filled sac, which can contain meninges and spinal cord tissue. Spina bifida occulta is a mild form of the condition and may appear as a tuft of coarse hair on the back. The degree of impairment experienced by patients with neural tube defects is dependent on how much CNS tissue is extruded into the sac, and the impairments can be severe.

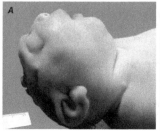 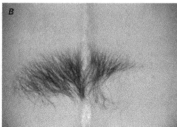

FIGURE 4.2

Failure of closure of the neuropores. A. Anencephaly represents one of the most extreme forms of neural tube defect, resulting in the nearly complete absence of the cranial vault and brain above the level of the ears and eyes. (Reproduced with permission from Kemp WL, Burns DK, Brown TG. Chapter 11. Neuropathology. In: Kemp WL, Burns DK, Brown TG. eds. Pathology: The Big Picture. New York, NY: McGraw-Hill; 2008). **B.** A large, wide tuft of thick terminal hair on the lumbosacral spine noted at birth. This woman had underlying tethered cord (note midline scar due to surgical repair). (Reproduced with permission from Chang M. Chapter 107. Neonatal, Pediatric, and Adolescent Dermatology. In: Goldsmith LA, et al., eds. Fitzpatrick's Dermatology in General Medicine, 8e. New York, NY: McGraw-Hill; 2012).

Integration of Systems
Primitive Reflexes and Motor Development; and the Role of the Environment in Neural Plasticity

Due to the large brain size of humans, infants are born prematurely to allow the infant head to travel safely through the birth canal. This premature neurological state causes humans to be born without significant volitional motor control. Instead, infants are born with "primitive" reflexes that direct motion. One example is the rooting reflex, which is triggered by a touch on the cheek. This stimulus produces a motor (movement) response in the muscles that turn the head toward the touch. This encourages a nursing infant to turn her head toward her mother's nipple. The sucking reflex then produces a strong contraction of the orbicularis oris muscle that encircles the mouth, along with other muscles involved in sucking. With time, the infant develops volitional control and sufficient strength for head control and nursing and no longer needs the rooting reflex. Many of these primitive reflexes create an adequately stimulating environment to give an infant experiences that mold future behavior. A touch on the cheek from a random stimulus is rewarded with joyous images, including a parent's smiling face.

Absence of pleasing and rewarding experiences can also have a profound impact upon human development. A tragic example of neurologic damage caused by neglect was the overcrowded and poorly run Romanian orphanage system. After the Romanian leader Nicolae Ceausescu was executed in 1989, the world discovered horrific conditions within their large, state-run orphanages. This included severe sensory and social deprivation, with children left unattended all day on their backs, tied to their beds. Nearly half of these children became physically developmentally delayed, for example teenagers the size of six-year-olds, with pronounced neurological impairments such as speech loss and permanent cognitive damage due to the lack of social and physical stimulation.

With closure of the neuropores, the rostral end of the tube dilates, forming vesicles that establish different regions of the CNS (Figure 4.3). During the fourth embryonic week, three vesicles differentiate. The most rostral, the prosencephalon will develop into forebrain structures. The middle vesicle is the mesencephalon, which develops into the midbrain, and the caudal vesicle is the rhombencephalon, progenitor of the hindbrain. The caudal portion of the neural tube becomes the spinal cord. During the second gestational month, continued mitosis leads to the formation of five vesicles from the original three. The prosencephalon forms the telencephalon and the diencephalon. The telencephalon appears as bilateral bulges that will become the two cerebral hemispheres and the underlying basal ganglia. The diencephalon is the embryonic origin of the thalamus and hypothalamus. Eye cups emerge from the diencephalon to develop into the eyes. The mesencephalon (midbrain) lies caudal to the diencephalon, and most caudally, the rhombencephalon develops into the metencephalon (pons and cerebellum) and myelencephalon (medulla).

Ventricle Development

As discussed in Chapter 1, the ventricles form a system of CSF-filled chambers communicating through narrow channels. Each of the brain regions correlates with a specific and predictable portion of the ventricular system (Figure 4.3). The central canal continues rostrally into the developing brainstem, merging with the fourth ventricle; the spinal cord central canal is largely obliterated in adulthood. Ascending through the brainstem, the central canal opens into the fourth ventricle. It is narrow at the spinal cord–medulla junction (the "closed medulla"), broadest near the pons–medulla junction ventral to the cerebellum (the "open medulla"), and tapers as it ascends toward the midbrain, where its lumen narrows again to create the cerebral aqueduct providing communication with the third ventricle at the level of the diencephalon. The lumina of the two vesicles of the telencephalon (developing cerebral hemispheres) form the lateral ventricles. Continuity between the third ventricle and the lateral ventricles is maintained through the interventricular foramina (of Monro).

Cephalic, Cervical, and Pontine Flexures

Evolution has given humans brains of approximately 1200 cc, extraordinarily large in proportion to our body size. Developing bipedalism and a large brain simultaneously evolved so that the head of a newborn is relatively large, and the size and shape of the female pelvis puts constraints on the size of the fetal head. Humans have developed two strategies to accommodate these features: remarkable convolution of the brain within a pliable infant skull and altricial birth (meaning that infants are born underdeveloped and needing extensive

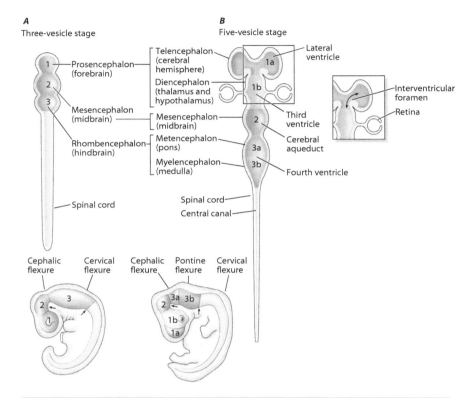

A Three-vesicle stage

B Five-vesicle stage

FIGURE 4.3

Schematic illustration of the three- and five-vesicle stages of the neural tube. The top portion of the figure shows dorsal views of the neural tube drawn without flexures. The bottom portion of the figure presents lateral views. **A.** Three-vesicle stage. **B.** Five-vesicle stage. The lineage of each vesicle at the five-vesicle stage is indicated by the colored shading. The two secondary vesicles from the forebrain have different green shades, and the two vesicles that derived from the hindbrain have different blue shades. The inset shows the location of the interventricular foramen on one side in the five-vesicle stage. (Reproduced with permission from Kandel ER, Schwartz JH, and Jessell TM, eds. *Principles of Neural Science*, 3rd ed. McGraw-Hill, 1991)

maternal care). Much of the anatomical and functional development of the brain occurs postnatally, even extending into young adulthood.

During the third and fourth embryonic weeks, the relatively straight neural tube develops a series of bends, called flexures, which initiate the folding of the brain required to fit within the confined cranium. The cephalic flexure appears at the developing mesencephalon, delineating midbrain and forebrain structures from the more caudal parts of the brain. Appearing around the same time as the cephalic flexure is the cervical flexure, marking the division between the brain and spinal cord at the caudal margin of the medulla. The pontine flexure appears around the seventh gestational week, distinguishing pons rostrally from medulla caudally. The end of the eighth week marks the end of the embryonic period of human development and configuration of most of the structures of the brain. Failure of folding in the embryo can result in incomplete or abnormal brain development, with accompanying cognitive difficulties, and visible craniofacial malformations.

Development of Segmentation

Induction produces tissue changes to establish order among the neural and non-neural structures in the embryo and set up basic body organization. The mesoderm, ectoderm, and endoderm differentiate simultaneously as the embryo develops. Soon after the closure of the neural tube, tissues that develop into muscular, skeletal, and nervous system elements group together in a series of segmented blocks of partially differentiated mesodermal tissues. Rostrally the segments form in relation to pairs of mesenchymal condensations called branchial (pharyngeal) arches (Figure 4.4), which appear as the embryo enters its fourth week. Contained within these structures are neural tube and neural crest cells that will differentiate into separate clusters of neurons related by location, connectivity, and function. These neuron clusters are called nuclei in the CNS and ganglia in the PNS. Branchial arches form features in the head and neck, including such diverse structures as the muscles of mastication along with the mandible, muscles of facial expression, and the skeletal and muscular structures associated with the palate, pharynx, and larynx. Timed changes in gene expression along the rostral neuraxis coincide with differentiation of a transient series of cellular condensations called neuromeres. Little mixing of cells from adjacent neuromeres occurs; thus each neuromere develops into a particular set of genetically isolated structures and a single cranial nerve nucleus. Continued cellular migration and tissue development obscure the segmentation of the brain, but the connections made persist, contributing to the often tortuous pathways seen in the mature CNS.

Caudal to the developing brain, a series of segmental blocks of tissue, called somites, differentiates. Somites form a striking array of modules along the dorsum of the embryo, and embryonic age can be determined based on the number of somites. Consecutive somitic segments further differentiate to form sclerotomes, myotomes, and dermatomes. Sclerotomes differentiate into the vertebrae and rib cartilage; myotomes form muscles of the back; and dermatomes form the skin on the back. Failure of differentiation of somites can delay or repress development of cartilage forming limb buds. Clusters of neural crest neurons within the somites form the dorsal root ganglia (DRG), and their peripheral axons elongate into spinal nerves and seek target tissues in the body.

Spinal Cord Development

Caudal to the cervical flexure, the neural tube forms the spinal cord. The roof plate has established the dorsal-ventral relationships in the embryo. Within the walls inside the lumen of the neural tube, bilateral longitudinal furrows (sulcus limitans) appear, which delineate the dorsal (posterior) and ventral (anterior) portions of the spinal cord. Proliferation of cells in the dorsal half of the neural tube forms the alar plate, creating a column of neurons extending the length of the spinal cord; this region will become the dorsal horn, the sensory region of the spinal cord gray matter. Ventrally, cells of the basal plate differentiate into spinal somatic and visceral motor neurons populating the ventral and lateral horns. Axons from first-order (primary) sensory neurons in the DRG penetrate the dorsal horn and innervate second-order neurons there, becoming the first synapses in the ascending pathway for processing sensation from the body. Cells in the spinal cord gray matter begin to emit axons that form the marginal zone comprising the earliest white matter tracts (axon bundles). Axons from the somatic and visceral motor neurons emerge from the ventral horn and extend distally as ventral roots. Just distal to the DRG, ventral roots merge with the peripheral axons of the sensory neurons in the ganglia to form spinal nerves that distribute to peripheral targets.

Distances between the spinal nerves and their peripheral targets are quite short when axons first arise from the developing spinal cord. Emerging nerves from all spinal segments take nearly straight trajectories to their targets. Growth of the vertebral column soon outstrips that of the spinal cord; thus in the adult, the caudal terminus of the cord (conus medullaris) extends only to about the level of the first or second lumbar vertebra. The roots are drawn out caudally, forming the cauda equina ("horse's tail"), as they descend to the level of the appropriate intervertebral foramina and exit from the spinal column (Figure 4.5).

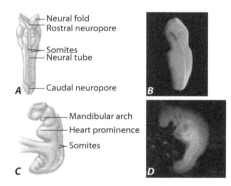

FIGURE 4.4

Development of somites. A. Dorsal view of an embryo during 22 to 23 days of development showing a series of somites. **B.** Lateral views of embryo at 24 days. **C.** Dorsal view of embryo at 24 days. The mandibular arch is the first branchial arch, and the heart prominence accommodates the rapidly growing heart. **D.** Lateral view of embryo at about 28 days. (**A, C,** (Reproduced with permission from Embryogenesis and Fetal Morphological Development. In: Cunningham F, et al, eds. Williams Obstetrics, Twenty-Fourth Edition New York, NY: McGraw-Hill; 2013). **B, D,** From Embryogenesis and Fetal Morphological Development. In: Cunningham F, et al., eds. *Williams Obstetrics*, Twenty-Fourth Edition New York, NY: McGraw-Hill; 2013.)

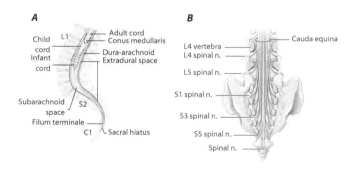

FIGURE 4.5

Development of the cauda equina. A. Sagittal view through the lumbar vertebrae and sacrum. Note the end of the spinal cord rises with development from approximately L3 to L1. The dural sac (dura-arachnoid) normally ends at S2. The filum terminale tethers the conus medullaris to the coccyx. (Reproduced with permission from Butterworth JF, IV, et al. Chapter 45. Spinal, Epidural, & Caudal Blocks. In: Butterworth JF, IV, et al., eds. Morgan & Mikhail's Clinical Anesthesiology, 5e. New York, NY: McGraw-Hill; 2013). **B.** Caudal end of the vertebral canal revealing spinal roots forming the cauda equina before exiting the vertebral canal through the intervertebral and sacral foramina. (Reproduced with permission from Morton DA, et al. Chapter 1. Back. In: Morton DA, et al, eds. The Big Picture: Gross Anatomy. New York, NY: McGraw-Hill; 2011).

Brainstem Development

Established early in development, brainstem organization persists throughout life, and appreciating the functional regionalization of the brainstem facilitates mental three-dimensional construction of CNS anatomy for precise localization of injuries.

The brainstem consists of the medulla most caudally, and the pons and the midbrain most rostrally. The fourth ventricle separates the brainstem anteriorly from the cerebellum posteriorly. As the central canal ascends into the brainstem, it merges with the fourth ventricle. The fourth ventricle spreads widely at the level of the pontomedullary junction, diverging along the roof plate. As the ventricular lumen widens, the bilateral remnants of the roof plate differentiate into the cerebellum.

Within the brainstem numerous nuclei are derived from the rostral neuromeres. Among the most prominent nuclei are those of the cranial nerves, which provide sensory and motor functions in the head and neck as well as in more distant structures such as the thoracic and abdominal viscera. In the brainstem, the sulcus limitans roughly distinguishes columns of cranial nerve sensory nuclei dorsolaterally and columns of motor nuclei ventromedially (Figure 4.6). The cranial nerves are numbered I–XII, from rostral to caudal, within the cranium.

The first two cranial nerves, the olfactory and optic nerves, are derivatives of the prosencephalon (CNS) and have no brainstem nuclei. The nuclei of cranial nerves III–XII, however, are aligned by function and position within the brainstem. For example, four different cranial nerve somatic motor nuclei, one each in the medulla and pons, and two in the midbrain, which supply muscles that control voluntary eye and tongue movements, comprise a discontinuous cellular column located near the midline ventromedial to the sulcus limitans (Figure 4.7).

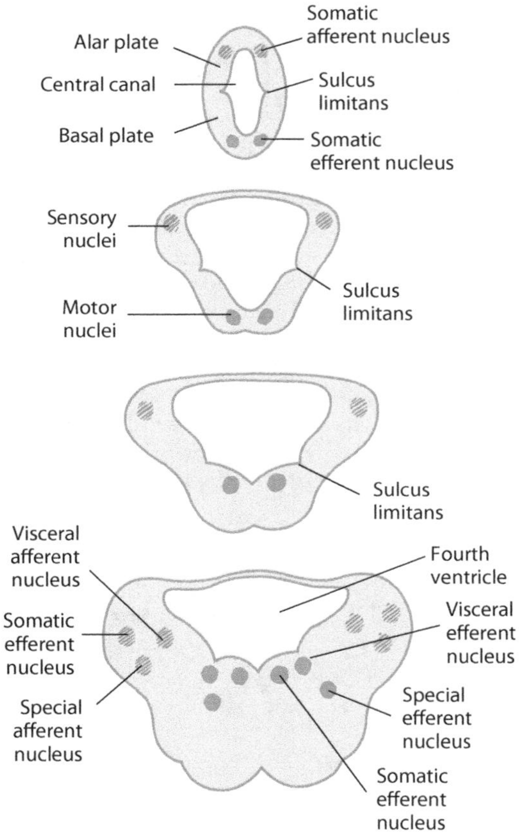

FIGURE 4.6

Schematic illustration of widening of the central cavity in the lower brain stem. The alar plate generates sensory cells and nuclei, and the basal plate forms motor cells. The sulcus limitans extends rostrally within the lumen of the neural tube and fourth ventricle. Clusters of neurons migrate dorsolaterally and form visceral, somatic, and special sensory nuclei. Other clusters migrate ventromedially to form corresponding motor nuclei. (Reproduced with permission from Waxman SG. Chapter 7. The Brain Stem and Cerebellum. In: Waxman SG. eds. Clinical Neuroanatomy, 27e. New York, NY: McGraw-Hill; 2013).

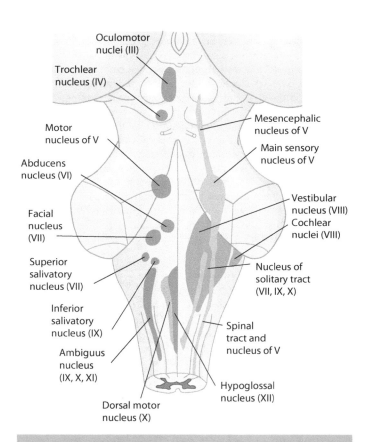

FIGURE 4.7

Cranial nerve nuclei. Dorsal view of the human brain stem with the positions of the cranial nerve nuclei projected on the surface. Motor nuclei are on the left; sensory nuclei are on the right. The oculomotor, trochlear, abducens, and hypoglossal nuclei form a discontinuous column of cells with somatic motor functions (see text). (Reproduced with permission from Waxman SG. Chapter 7. The Brain Stem and Cerebellum. In: Waxman SG. eds. Clinical Neuroanatomy, 27e. New York, NY: McGraw-Hill; 2013).

Other cranial nerve nuclei are similarly grouped in columns in different regions within the brainstem. Cranial nerves make their earliest peripheral target contacts after about three weeks of gestation. At this time, not all of the neurons comprising the nuclei have migrated to their mature locations. Once again, this contributes to the irregular pathways taken by some cranial nerves in adults, such as the looping genu of the facial nerve and the elongated axons of the portion of the vagus nerve that supplies thoracic and abdominal viscera.

Forebrain Development

In mature cerebral cortical organization, specific functions (motor, sensory, and mixed—e.g., somatosensory) are localized to highly predictable cortical areas. This functional parcellation begins during the embryonic period with the interactions of differential and opposing concentration gradients of a pair of gene products in the early neocortex that direct differentiation and migration of newly born cortical neurons. Emx2 and Pax6, transcription factor protein products of the *Emx2* and *Pax6* genes, respectively, are expressed so that high concentrations of Emx2 and low concentrations of Pax6 result in the differentiation of sensory cortices (such as the visual cortex), and the reverse gradient generates motor cortices; intermediate ratios of these proteins stimulate differentiation of cortices that integrate sensory and motor connections. This process not only divides the CNS into dorsal and ventral portions, but it also has significant influence on the development of dorsal and ventral compartments within the PNS. This is a single, extremely simplified example of the complex interaction of factors affecting the earliest separation of cortical function, and new genes and interactions are being discovered continually.

The early fetal period of human gestation (eighth week through mid-gestation) is a critical time in the development of the neocortex; most of the cortical neurons are born and early connections made during this period. All mammal species possess a six-layered cerebral cortex. Cortical neurons and glia derive from cells lining the ventricles and migrate superficially to their appropriate layers. As embryogenesis continues, different nervous system regions undergo mitosis at different rates. Rostrally in the telencephalon, exuberant neuronal mitosis results in the formation of folds, gyri, separated by grooves, sulci, in a process called gyrification. Gyrification proceeds rapidly during the third trimester and creates the familiar, extensively convoluted cortical surface, substantially increasing cerebral surface area. Major sulci form early; the lateral fissures, for example, appear during the second trimester, although they are not complete until after birth. Abnormal gyrification has ramifications postnatally. Normal maternal intrauterine growth restrictions limit prenatal formation of gyri and, if extreme, may be correlated with ADHD and schizophrenia in postnatal life. Conversely, excessive formation of undersized gyri (polymicrogyria) also causes numerous postnatal developmental disorders.

Synaptogenesis (formation of interneuronal connections) begins during the first trimester and continues into young adulthood. As the synapses form and early connectivity is stabilized, oligodendrocytes begin to myelinate the axons and build white matter tracts. By week 16, the corpus callosum, the largest CNS fiber bundle, can be identified by ultrasound. Elaboration and growth of fiber tracts continues postnatally; this has been shown by tensor diffusion imaging, which analyzes diffusion of water molecules in tissues including fiber bundles. Postnatal maturation of tracts is extremely active in the first decade of life and, for some systems, throughout much of the second postnatal decade. During the second trimester and continuing into early postnatal life, coinciding with a period of rapid synaptogenesis, many neurons undergo apoptosis (programmed cell death), during which more than half of the neurons in the brain are eliminated. As synapses are strengthened, axons that are unable to compete for growth factors are pruned (eliminated) with subsequent neuronal death. This is a normal process that results in survival for only those neurons making the most stable connections.

Synaptogenesis continues throughout life as individuals learn, experience novel situations, and recover from injury. Synapse formation is prolific during early stages of these events, and pruning of the excess refines the precision of cortical connectivity. The classical example of the influence of synaptic pruning and cortical sculpting is the creation of ocular dominance columns in the mammalian visual cortex. Neurons within a mature ocular dominance column are responsive only to inputs from one eye, and adjacent columns respond to alternate optic input. In tangential sections through the visual cortex, the alternating inputs generate a striking pattern (Figure 4.8). Typically, the earliest projections to visual cortex are profuse, and inputs from both eyes are mixed and do not yet respect the boundaries of the eye-specific columns. In 1963, eventual Nobel laureates Hubel and Wiesel demonstrated that removing light stimulus to one eye during a kitten's first three months of life resulted in permanent loss of vision, even after the eye was reopened. When one eye is blinded, inputs from the closed eye fail to make functional synapses and are eliminated, with the concomitant maladaptive expansion of inputs from the intact eye across the entire cortex and loss of ocular dominance columns. These results attest to the importance of light stimulation during the pruning period; it strengthens appropriate synapses and promotes withdrawal of inappropriate ones.

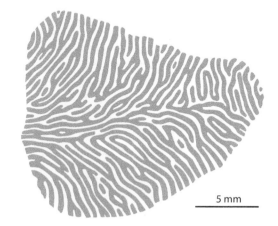

5 mm

FIGURE 4.8

Reconstruction of ocular dominance columns in the right visual cortex of a rhesus monkey. Dark stripes represent one eye; light stripes represent the other. (Reproduced, with permission, from LeVay S, Hubel DH, and Wiesel TN. The pattern of ocular dominance columns in macaque visual cortex revealed by a reduced silver stain. *J Comp Neurol* 1975;159:559.)

Frontiers in Research
Animal Models: The Mighty Mouse

For both practical and ethical reasons, the use of humans in genetic research is necessarily limited. Animal models, particularly mouse models, have proven to be invaluable for this line of study because of their short lifespan and gestation, as well as more amenable legal and ethical considerations. Further, humans and mice share many genes, so data are relevant to human studies. In 2007, the Nobel Prize in Physiology or Medicine was awarded for the discovery of a method of altering the genetic code in mice. Researchers injected a specific gene into a fertilized oocyte (single cell embryo). This embryo was then transferred into a host mother. Once born, mouse pups were screened to confirm that the alien gene was integrated. Transgenic mice produce a protein that is foreign to that mouse strain, and the altered expression can be passed down to later generations. Introduction of this gene produces phenotypic or behavioral changes that can be attributed to the new genetic conditions. In subsequent models, expression of a particular protein was eliminated by "knocking out" the gene encoding a particular protein. Knockout technology was further developed into conditional versions, with activation (or inactivation) of the gene of interest by administering a drug or other exogenous biochemical. Altering gene expression by eliminating the action of an important gene product often produces other unintended effects, such as cytotoxicity or developmental disruption that can easily confound interpretation of the findings. Conditional transgenic mouse manipulations are tissue specific, targeting genes in only one organ system and reducing or eliminating inadvertent systemic consequences of gene alteration. The knockout mouse model is named after the replaced gene, such as Park2 knockout mice created to study the neurological disease Parkinson's.

Transgenic mouse technology. DNA is microinjected into a pronucleus of a fertilized egg, which is then transplanted into a foster mother. The microinjected egg develops offspring mice. Incorporation of the injected DNA into offspring is indicated by the different coat color of offspring mice.

Although a one-to-one correlation between gene function and disease is not always possible, the relative specificity with which transgenic technology can assess particular gene function has revolutionized medical research. It has opened the way to development of the new field of genomics, with which the actions of select genes or combinations of genes and their relation to diseases are being discovered, and new diagnostic and therapeutic strategies tailored to the individual patient are being developed. (Reproduced with permission from Feng X, et al. Molecular and Genomic Surgery. In: Brunicardi F, et al, eds. *Schwartz's Principles of Surgery*, 10e. New York, NY: McGraw-Hill; 2014.)

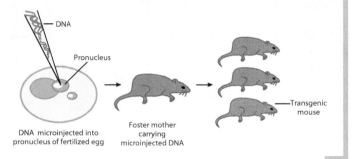

The efficacy of this process is diminished, however, when there is paucity of stimulation during the critical period under both developmental and regenerative conditions. Limited stimulus and reduced activation during the critical period produces neuronal atrophy and dendritic retraction that can severely impair functional development, learning, and posttraumatic recovery.

III   RESPONSE TO INJURY

Rehabilitation after CNS damage promotes neuroplasticity and provides better long-term functional outcomes in both human and animal studies. This is due to enhanced dendritic sprouting, synaptogenesis, and neurochemical production. In animal models, early initiation of rehabilitation creates a GABA-induced excitotoxicity counterproductive to recovery. Thus rehabilitation in animals is ideally initiated several days post injury. Ideal timing is yet to be determined for humans, although in the days following an injury, the same GABA-mediated inhibition is activated, this time aimed at minimizing damage and restoring homeostasis. This activation, however, temporarily prevents acquisition of new learning early in the recovery. Evolving technology will soon allow clinicians to determine when the damaged nervous system is metabolically prepared for rehabilitation. Wahl and Schwab proposed a three-step model for timing of rehabilitation after stroke or spinal cord injury that includes: (1) neuroimaging and assessment of biomarkers to determine metabolic readiness; (2) therapies that enhance neuroplasticity, such as using customized antibodies to block post-injury expression of inhibitory proteins; and (3) selection and stabilization of neural pathways through behavioral interventions.

> Neuroplasticity
Neurological Readiness

A young brain has tremendous capacity for new learning and post-injury relearning. There is a time frame, called the critical period, during which the brain is especially receptive to modification. Different systems have different critical periods. For example, a baby will make all of the sounds that are used in any language and can learn to communicate even in sign language. Eventually, after the critical period for language development ends, this expansive capacity is significantly reduced so that it becomes more difficult for adults to learn new languages. A critical period was also found for hearing and for vestibular function, but they occur under different temporal controls. Although experts now

agree that the critical period is a time of enhanced neuroplasticity and capacity for learning, controversy persists regarding the concept of an absolute window for acquisition of new learning. Recent research shows that critical periods are mediated by cortical inhibitory neurons. Researchers identified a protein, Lynx1 (which is chemically similar to snake venom), which impaired visual neuroplasticity; by eliminating the gene for Lynx1, adult mice were able to regain vision, even after prolonged sensory deprivation initiated in infancy. Dubbed the "molecular brakes," these proteins gradually increase over a lifetime, reducing neuroplasticity and limiting the capacity for new learning.

The adage "You can't teach an old dog new tricks" has been

challenged in recent years. The long-held belief that new learning diminishes with increasing age is no longer dogma. In fact, exposure to new tasks and new challenges appears to keep the nervous system healthy and is considered neuroprotective against diseases such as Alzheimer's. A study of cab drivers in London demonstrates the intrinsic ability of adult brains to alter in response to novel demands. As the cabbies developed their internal three-dimensional map of London, their hippocampal areas associated with spatial relationships expanded.

The axiom "If you don't use it, you'll lose it" remains salient today. We now know that exercise and exposure to novel and complex physical and cognitive tasks promote

long-term molecular changes and formation of new synapses. Conversely, the plastic and highly adaptive brain also down-regulates protein synthesis and reduces or removes neurons and synapses with inactivity and stress throughout our lifetimes. Leading a life with high stress or low demand can both promote loss of cognition. A sedentary lifestyle and failure to comply with therapeutic exercise protocols after trauma present significant impediments to recovery. Neuronal projections into areas in the cortex that once received input related to the injured structure are lost, and adjacent intact projections encroach into the denervated cortex, resulting in long-lasting functional loss.

Neuroplasticity is, as the saying goes, "a double-edged sword."

> CASE 4   DISCUSSION: Normal Infant Development

Jasmine had a three-month maternity leave, and the day she went back to work, Miles rolled from prone to supine for the first time. He stayed at home another six weeks during his father's paternity leave. Miles started at a local day care with his older sister when he was five months old, just as he became able to sit unsupported. Twelve months later, Miles is on track, reaching all of his cognitive, sensory,

and motor function milestones and within age-normal values for height and weight. Miles's story exemplifies the value of genetic health and proactive prenatal care, combined with rich postnatal stimulation to support healthy neurological development. Lacking this combination of resources puts many of our patients at a disadvantage. Because neurologic injury in adulthood disinhibits primitive reflexes, understanding normal

infant development is essential for rehabilitation in both infancy and throughout the lifespan. Following the normal developmental sequence is a time-honored approach to neurologic rehabilitation. Before he can learn to walk, an infant must develop strong trunk muscles through sitting unsupported and overcome reflexes that may disrupt postural control, and the same principles can be applied to adult neurologic rehabilitation.

REFERENCES

Achiron R, Achiron A. Development of the human fetal corpus callosum: a high-resolution, cross-sectional sonographic study. *Ultrasound Obstet Gynecol.* 2001;18:343–347.

Andersen SL. Trajectories of brain development: point of vulnerability or window of opportunity? *Neurosci Biobehav Rev.* 2003 Jan–Mar;27(1–2):3–18.

Baker RE, Schnell S, Maini PK. A clock and wavefront mechanism for somite formation. *Developmental Biology.* 2006;293:116–126.

Bockamp E, Maringer M, Spangenberg C, et al. *Physiol Genomics.* 2002;11:115–132.

Chen Y, Wang G, Ma ZL, et al. Adverse effects of high glucose levels on somite and limb development in avian embryos. *Food Chem Toxicol.* 2014 Sep;71:1–9.

Chizhikov V, Millen KJ. Roof plate-dependent patterning of the vertebrate dorsal central nervous system. *Dev Biol.* 2005;277:287–295.

Colson SD, Meek JH, Hawdon JM. Optimal positions for the release of primitive neonatal reflexes stimulating breastfeeding. *Early Hum Dev.* 2008 Jul;84(7):441–449.

Dubois J, Benders M, Borradori-Tolsa C, et al. Primary cortical folding in the human newborn: an early marker of later functional development. *Brain.* 2008;131:2028–2041.

Duce IR, Keen P. Can neuronal smooth endoplasmic reticulum function as a calcium reservoir? *Neuroscience.* 1978;3(9):837–848.

Eluvathingal TJ, Chugani HT, Behen ME, et al. Abnormal brain connectivity in children after early severe socioemotional deprivation: a diffusion tensor imaging study. *Pediatrics.* 2006;117:2093–2100.

Giza C, Prins M. Is being plastic fantastic? Mechanisms of altered plasticity after developmental traumatic brain injury. *Dev Neurosci.* 2006;28:364–379.

Hevner R, Haydar T. The (not necessarily) convoluted role of basal radial glia in cortical neurogenesis. *Cerebral Cortex.* 2012;22:465–468.

Hötting K, Röder B. Beneficial effects of physical exercise on neuroplasticity and cognition. *Neurosci Biobehav Rev.* 2013 Nov;37(9 Pt B):2243–2257.

Huang H, Zhang J, Wakana S, et al. White and gray matter development in human fetal, newborn and pediatric brains. *NeuroImage.* 2006;33:27–38.

Huang X, Saint-Jeannet JP. Induction of the neural crest and the opportunities of life on the edge. *Dev Biol.* 2004;275:1–11.

Hubel DH, Wiesel TN. Receptive fields, binocular interaction and functional architecture in the cat's visual cortex. *J Physiol.* 1962;160:106–154.

Jacobson S, Marcus EM. *Neuroanatomy for the Neuroscientist,* 2nd ed. New York: Springer, 2011. p. 147.

Jin Y, Fischer I, Tessler A, Houle J. Transplants of fibroblasts genetically modified to express BDNF promote axonal regeneration from supraspinal neurons following chronic spinal cord injury. *Exp Neurol.* 2002;177(1):265–275.

Levelt CN, Hübener M. Critical-period plasticity in the visual cortex. *Annu Rev Neurosci.* 2012 July;35:309–330.

Levi DM, Li RW. Perceptual learning as a potential treatment for amblyopia: a mini-review. *Vision Res.* 2009 October; 49(21):2535–2549.

Levin AR, Zeanah CH, Fox NA, Nelson CA. Motor outcomes in children exposed to early psychosocial deprivation. *J Pediatr.* 2014 Jan;164(1):123–129.

Liu Y, Himes BT, Murray M, Tessler A, Fischer I. Grafts of BDNF-producing fibroblasts rescue axotomized rubrospinal neurons and prevent their atrophy. *Exp Neurol.* 2002;150:164.

Lodygensky G, Vasung L, Sizonenk S, Huppi P. Neuroimaging of cortical development and brain connectivity in human newborns and animal models. *J Anat.* 2010;217:418–428.

Maguire EA, Woollett K, Spiers HJ. London taxi drivers and bus drivers: a structural MRI and neuropsychological analysis. *Hippocampus.* 2006;16(12):1091–1101.

Maulden SA, Gassaway J, Horn SD, Smout RJ, DeJong G. Timing of initiation of rehabilitation after stroke. *Arch Phys Med Rehabil.* 2005 Dec;86(12 Suppl 2):S34–S40.

Monteagudo A, Timor-Tritsch IE. Development of fetal gyri, sulci and fissures: a transvaginal sonographic study. *Ultrasound Obstet Gynecol.* 1997 Apr;9(4):222–228.

Morishita H, Miwa JM, Heintz N, Hensch TK. Lynx1, a cholinergic brake limits plasticity in adult visual cortex: a cure for amblyopia through nicotinic receptor signaling. *Science.* 2010, November 26;330(6008):1238–1240.

Müller F, O'Rahilly R. Occipitocervical segmentation in staged human embryos. *J Anat.* 1994;185:251–258.

Pourquié O. Segmentation of the vertebrate spine: from clock to scoliosis. *Cell.* 2011, May 27;145(5):650–663.

Rakic P. Specification of cerebral cortical areas. *Science.* 1988;241 (4862):170–176.

Ramırez O, Couve A. The endoplasmic reticulum and protein trafficking in dendrites and axons. *Trends Cell Biol.* 2011;21(4):219–227.

Rash BG, Rakic P. Neuroscience. Genetic resolutions of brain convolutions. *Science.* 2014;343(6172):744–745.

Resende T, Andrade R, Palmeirim I. Timing embryo segmentation: dynamics and regulatory mechanisms of the vertebrate segmentation clock. *Biomed Res Int.* 2014;2014:718683.

Scholz J, Klein MC, Behrens TEJ, Johansen-Berg H. Training induces changes in white-matter architecture. *Nature Neurosci.* 2009;12:1370–1371.

Smart I, McSherry OM. Gyrus formation in the cerebral cortex of the ferret: description of the internal histological changes. *J Anat.* 1986;147:27–43.

Stephenson SEM, Taylor JM, Lockhart PJ. Parkinson's Disease and Parkin. Insights from Park2 Knockout Mice, Mechanisms in Parkinson's Disease—Models and Treatments. Dushanova J, ed. InTech. DOI: 10.5772/18148. http://www.intechopen.com/books/mechanisms-in-parkinson-s-disease-models-and-treatments/parkinson-s-disease-and-parkin-insights-from-park2-knockout-mice.

Stiles J, Jernigan TJ. The basics of brain development. *Neuropsychol Rev.* 2010;20:327–348.

Takesian AE, Hensch TK. Balancing plasticity/stability across brain development. *Prog Brain Res.* 2013;207:3–34.

Tau GS, Peterson BS. Normal development of brain circuits. *Neuropsychopharmacology Reviews.* 2010;35:147–168.

Urban JPG, Roberts S, Ralphs JR. The nucleus of the intervertebral disc from development to degeneration. *Amer Zool.* 2000;40:53–61.

Van Essen DC. A tension-based theory of morphogenesis and compact wiring in the central nervous system. *Nature.* 1997, Jan 23;385(6614):313–318.

Vasung L, Fischi-Gomez E, Hüppi PS. Multimodality evaluation of the pediatric brain: DTI and its competitors. *Pediatr Radiol.* 2013 Jan;43(1):60–68.

Wahl A, Schwab M. Finding an optimal rehabilitation paradigm after stroke: enhancing fiber growth and training of the brain at the right moment. *Front Human Neurosci.* 2014 June;8(38):1–13.

Walker HK. The suck, snout, palmomental, and grasp reflexes. In: Walker HK, Hall WD, Hurst JW, eds. *Clinical Methods: The History, Physical, and Laboratory Examinations,* 3rd ed. Boston: Butterworths, 1990. Ch 71.

Weisel T, Hubel D. Extent of recovery from the effects of visual deprivation in kittens. *J Neurophysiol.* 1965 Nov;28(6):1060–1072.

Wilson DB. Embryonic development of the head and neck: part 5, the brain and cranium. *Head Neck Surg.* 1980 Mar–Apr;2(4):312–320.

Wittman AB, Wall LL. The evolutionary origins of obstructed labor: bipedalism, encephalization, and the human obstetric dilemma. *Obstet Gynecol Surv.* 2007 Nov;62(11):739–748.

Woollett K, Maguire EA. Acquiring "the knowledge" of London's layout drives structural brain changes. *Curr Biol.* 2011;21:2109–2114.

Zhou J, Thompson B, Hess RF. A new form of rapid binocular plasticity in adults with amblyopia. *Scientific Reports.* 2013;3:2638.

Zilles K, Palomero-Gallagher N, Amunts K. Development of cortical folding during evolution and ontogeny. *Trends Neurosci.* 2013 May;36(5):275–284.

REVIEW QUESTIONS

1. Which embryonic layer develops into the nervous system?
   A. Endoderm
   B. Ectoderm
   C. Mesoderm
   D. Induction

2. What are the functional consequences of gyrification?
   A. It allows normal brain growth in limited space during early fetal period.
   B. Inadequate gyrification may cause CNS dysfunction after birth such as schizophrenia.
   C. Excess gyrification may lead to undersized gyri and postnatal complications.
   D. All of the above

3. What do the vesicles develop into later?
   A. Forebrain, midbrain, spinal cord
   B. Forebrain, midbrain, cranium
   C. Spinal cord, midbrain, progenitor of hindbrain
   D. Forebrain, midbrain, progenitor of hindbrain

4. Consequences of improper neuropore closure include all of the following *except*:
   A. anencephaly.
   B. spina bifida.
   C. polymicrogyria.
   D. microencephaly.

5. What process creates the cauda equina?
   A. Growth of somites delays spinal cord development.
   B. Growth of the vertebral column occurs more quickly than the spinal cord.
   C. Growth of the spinal nerves is delayed due to neurulation.
   D. Growth of the medulla oblongata delays spinal cord development.

6. In the brainstem, the sulcus limitans separates motor nuclei, located_____, from sensory nuclei, which are located_____.
   A. medially, dorsally
   B. ventromedially, dorsolaterally
   C. dorsally, medially
   D. dorsolaterally, ventromedially

7. Which statement regarding synaptogenesis and neural pruning is false?
   A. It ensures only the most stable neurological connections survive.
   B. The process only occurs in early childhood during the critical period.
   C. It occurs in adulthood after injury or with new learning.
   D. Pruning destroys more than 50% of neurons during the perinatal period.

8. What limits neuroplasticity in the adult?
   A. The end of the critical period permanently restricts synaptogenesis.
   B. Inhibitory neurons that close the critical window gradually increase over time.
   C. Synaptogenesis only occurs in childhood during the critical period.
   D. Neural pruning is most active in the perinatal period.

9. What are the potential consequences of somite failure?
   A. Inadequate development of cranial nerves
   B. Myeloschisis, the most severe form of spina bifida
   C. Inadequate limb development
   D. All of the above

10. Which of the following factors has the least impact on long-term success of rehabilitation after stroke or SCI?
    A. Timing of rehabilitation after injury
    B. Noncompliance with exercise and rehabilitation program
    C. Metabolic readiness of cortex after injury
    D. High levels of stress after injury

CHAPTER 5

The Spinal Cord

> **CASE 5** Spinal Cord Injury

Bobby was a fearless child; his mother told stories of him riding his big wheel down the stairs outside his Colorado home. He preferred individual sports, so he took up racket ball and swimming when his family later moved to California. In high school he became a triathlete, joining a group of dedicated older athletes who met regularly to swim, ride, and run. Sunday mornings they swam 3 miles in the ocean, and after a rest finished the day with a 13-mile run. Cycling through 56 miles of Southern California mountains and canyons completed the weekly training. It was a disciplined, active life he shared with his best friend.

Everything changed on a beautiful March day when he was 17. It was too pretty to be inside at the gym, so he decided to go for an easy ride, from his parents' house, past the high school and back a few laps. A car darted toward him from the side, and as he swerved to avoid that collision, he ran into the back of a bus that was illegally parked in front of a fire hydrant. The accident fractured his spine, permanently damaging his spinal cord at the fifth cervical level.

In the hospital, reality came slowly as he gradually became aware of his new limitations. He was placed in traction initially while they ran tests to determine the severity of the injury. He heard words like *quadriplegic*, and struggled to move his arms as he lay in bed. Once, he was able to wiggle his shoulders and flex his arm in front of his body, only to have it get stuck against his face, unable to extend his elbow due to paralyzed triceps brachii. A few days after the accident, he lay there while a physician told him he would never walk again, news he did not fully accept at that point. Far more immediate was the plan to place him in a halo for the next few months. A halo-stabilizing device immobilizes the cervical spine with a metal band encircling the skull, fixed by four screws. Long metal rods extend downward from the halo and attach to a vest worn around the torso. Bobby's father had worn a halo a few years before due to a cervical fracture, and he remembered his father's pain and discomfort very well, fearing the next few months living in the halo more than anyone on the rehabilitation team imagined.

Once he was transferred to the rehabilitation unit, Bobby found comfort and familiarity in the routine. He focused on learning new skills in occupational and physical therapy, and mentally planned to complete a race in a few months, once he recovered. The positive, focused nature of the rehab team made each day easier, along with a tremendous support network of family and friends, who filled the hallways each day until the staff had to request a limit on the number of visitors. His training partners were mostly older, mature individuals providing social and emotional support to young Bobby throughout the early months of his recovery.

A few weeks after the injury, Bobby had a moment of clarity and acceptance. He realized that he would not return to racing or even walking again. He cried for the loss of his old life, mourning future accomplishments that were no longer possible. He found rehabilitation much easier after that point, and he could now fully embrace his new life in a wheelchair. The day he was discharged from the hospital, he boarded a plane to watch the Hawaii Ironman Triathlon, in a trip funded by his friends and family.

> ## > Neuroplasticity
> ### Stem Cell Therapies
> A great deal of research and hope has been directed toward finding effective treatments for spinal cord injury. The peripheral nervous system has great capacity for neuroplasticity, yet functional central plasticity is minimal. Stem cells are unlike most cells because they can differentiate into other types of tissue. Transplantation after tissue damage has the potential to be highly effective because, if properly stimulated, stem cells can differentiate into the desired target tissue. Mouse stem cells were first isolated in the early 1980s, followed by human stem cells nearly 20 years later. Years of research demonstrate that these stem cells have tremendous value in tissue repair, with applications after heart and other organ damage. However, the use of stem cell–based transplantation to restore function after spinal cord injury has yet to be realized. Scientists are still working to uncover the mechanisms of repair after spinal cord trauma and overcome obstacles, such as glial scarring (see Chapter 3), that block axonal regeneration. Additionally, stem cell properties are not fully understood, including their mechanism of differentiation, needed to fully integrate stem cell therapy. A recent meta-analysis of human studies using bone marrow stem cells demonstrated some benefit, with minor reduction in sensory and motor loss for participants. How this translates into improved quality of life remains undetermined, as few studies reported subjects' perceived benefit. At this time, researchers know that stem cell–based transplantation therapy after spinal cord injury requires a combination of phenotype replacement for the damaged neural tissue and ongoing support of neural growth to be successful.

I   OVERVIEW OF KEY CONCEPTS

The spinal cord is the interface between the CNS and the PNS connectivity with the body; it is the first site of somatosensory input from the limbs and body, and the source of somatic and autonomic motor output. Ascending and descending white matter fiber pathways form the outer portion, surrounding the cellular gray matter core. The massive volume of information passing through and processed within the spinal cord demands an unparalleled degree of order and organization that is established from its first embryonic appearance and maintained throughout life.

White matter fibers comprise ascending afferent (sensory) and descending efferent (motor) pathways. A variety of end organs, specifically designed to extract different features from a single stimulus, communicate sensory information to modulate behavior. Axons in these pathways have a precise somatotopy, maintaining point-to-point relationships that precisely reflect peripheral sensory and motor topography. Functionally specific axonal fiber bundles (fasciculi, tracts) are spatially segregated within the spinal cord. This organization means that small focal lesions of white matter can impair some functions while sparing others, and neurologic localization of spinal cord lesions can be quite precise based on the spectrum of resulting deficits.

It is common knowledge that, for much of the CNS, the left side of the brain controls the right side of the body, and vice versa. This relationship implies that at some point along the pathways, the fibers must cross the midline on their ascent (for sensory axons) or descent (for motor axons) to their targets. The decussations for each of the long systems occur at different locations along the pathway. Recalling locations of these decussations is essential when determining the level and laterality of a lesion.

Because of the anatomical and functional precision in the long pathways (projection neurons) and the local circuits (interneurons), injuries to the spinal cord produce predictable behavioral difficulties, such as spasticity or paresthesia. Also, because the spinal cord receives both incoming information about noxious (potentially damaging, pain-producing) stimuli and descending central suppression of those inputs, the role of the spinal cord in the perception and response to pain is a major topic of research.

II   STRUCTURE OF THE SPINAL CORD

Because of the complexity and the volume of information carried in the spinal cord, order in the arrangement of gray and white matter is essential. Groups of cells and collections of axons are arranged somatotopically so that their peripheral target tissues are represented in precise point-to-point order centrally. This somatotopic organization is a fundamental feature of development and establishes a representation of the body at different levels within the gray matter columns and along the white matter pathways. Because the majority of spinal cord injuries are incomplete, damage to the gray and white matter typically involves only part of the structure. An understanding of the internal arrangement of body representation is essential to making accurate diagnoses of the location as well as the extent of a spinal cord injury.

Surface Features

The spinal cord is an elongated tubelike structure extending from the medulla in the brainstem to the level of the first lumbar vertebra (LV1); it does not extend the entire length of the vertebral column because of differential rates and duration of growth during development (Chapter 4). It is a remarkably small structure given the enormous amount of information it carries. From its inferior end, an extension of the pia mater, the filum terminale, loosely anchors the cord to the coccyx. The filum terminale is a non-neural structure that descends among the spinal root fibers that compose the cauda equina (Figure 5.1). Dorsal and ventral rootlets emerge from the dorsal and ventral surfaces of the cord (Figure 5.2). The rostrocaudal extent of the roots indicates the borders of the corresponding spinal segment. Root fibers join just distal to the dorsal root ganglion (DRG), which occupies space in the intervertebral foramen to form spinal nerves. Spinal cord meninges terminate as the spinal nerve commences, becoming continuous with the connective tissue sheath enclosing peripheral nerves.

Segmental Anatomy

Differences in the gross appearance of the cord can be related to differences in the density of sensory and motor innervation to the peripheral regions supplied. The cervical and lumbar enlargements represent dense sensory and motor axon innervation to upper and lower extremities, particularly the hands and feet. Conversely, the sparse motor and sensory innervation distributed to the chest and back relates to the relatively small cross-sectional area of the thoracic spinal cord. The shape of the cord and the proportions of white and gray matter at each spinal level are characteristics that identify the level, allowing for easy identification visually in a transverse image such as MRI.

Internal Organization of the Spinal Cord: Gray Matter

Developmental processes described in Chapter 4 establish a central gray matter cellular region surrounded by white matter axon tracts. Very early during development, the dorsal half of the gray matter becomes the dorsal horn, which serves sensory functions, and the ventral half becomes the ventral horn, which performs motor functions. Motor neurons are located in the ventral horn; they project their axons to the periphery via the ventral roots. Because the spinal cord has a longitudinal organization, the dorsal and ventral horns form columns of neurons that run rostrocaudally.

Between the dorsal and ventral horns is an overlapping region, the intermediate zone. From the level of first thoracic vertebra (TV1) through the second lumbar vertebra (LV2), lateral to the intermediate zone gray matter, there is a lateral protrusion, the lateral horn (Figure 5.1). It contains a column of preganglionic sympathetic neurons. Their axons exit with the ventral roots to join a spinal nerve; thus all of the axons in the ventral roots are motor efferents (and all the dorsal roots are sensory afferents). Myelinated preganglionic axons peel off each spinal nerve and enter the sympathetic chain ganglia, a string of interconnected sympathetic chain ganglia (Figure 5.2) ascending on the posterior wall of the thoracic cavity between TV1 and LV2. Preganglionic axons enter the sympathetic chain as a small fascicle called the white ramus communicans. After synapsing, unmyelinated postganglionic axons also form small fascicles, the gray rami communicantes, that rejoin and distribute with the spinal nerves.

Also in the thoracolumbar gray matter, the dorsal nucleus of Clarke, or the dorsal (posterior) thoracic nucleus, extends from about CV7–TV1 down to LV3–4. In stained spinal cord sections, the nucleus presents a conspicuous oval of cells in the medial part

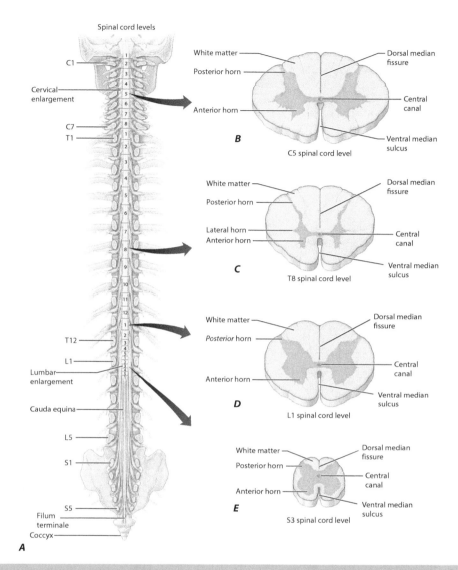

FIGURE 5.1

Diagram of (A) spinal cord in situ and (B–E) sections at four different levels. **A.** Dorsal view of the spinal cord within the vertebral canal. Observe the divergence between the spinal cord, spinal nerve, and vertebral levels. Note the caudal position of the filum terminale. **B–E.** C5, T8, L1, and S3 cross sections of the spinal cord, respectively. Compare the shape and volume of gray and white matter at the various levels. (Reproduced with permission from Morton DA, et al. Chapter 1. Back. In: Morton DA, et al,. eds. The Big Picture: Gross Anatomy. New York, NY: McGraw-Hill; 2011).

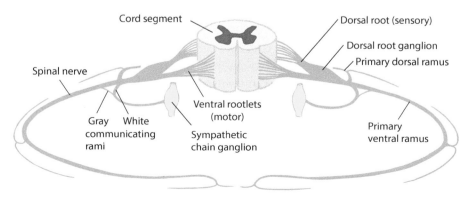

FIGURE 5.2

Illustration of a spinal cord segment with its roots, ganglia, and branches. Dorsal roots contain central axons of sensory neurons in the dorsal root ganglia. Ventral roots contain motor fibers exiting motor and sympathetic cells in the ventral and lateral horns, respectively. Sympathetic fibers connect to the sympathetic chain ganglia through white and gray rami communicantes. (Reproduced with permission from Waxman SG. Chapter 5. The Spinal Cord. In: Waxman SG. eds. Clinical Neuroanatomy, 27e. New York, NY: McGraw-Hill; 2013.)

of lamina VII of the intermediate zone (see below). Inputs to the dorsal nucleus of Clarke include collaterals of annulospiral endings, muscle proprioceptors, which have some of the thickest Aα axons in the PNS. Axons that emerge from neurons in Clarke's nucleus dorsalis decussate and ascend in the contralateral dorsal (posterior) spinothalamic tract to the cerebellum for sensorimotor processing at the unconscious level.

In the intermediate zone extending from SV2 through SV4 are preganglionic parasympathetic neurons. Their axons contribute to the pelvic splanchnic nerves that supply the pelvic viscera.

The spinal gray matter has a laminar organization (I–X); this system designates regions of sensory and motor function (Figure 5.3). Generally, laminae I–VI serve sensory functions. Lamina I is Lissauer's tract, mostly thinly myelinated Aδ and unmyelinated C fibers carrying information relating to potentially damaging peripheral stimuli (nociception). Lamina II comprises the substantia gelatinosa, which contains second-order neurons of the anterolateral system. Second-order axons from this cell column decussate in the anterior white commissure to form the contralateral spinothalamic tract (see Figure 5.6).

Laminae III–VI form the nucleus proprius. Its neurons receive synapses from primary low-threshold mechanoreceptor axons and from some primary nociceptive axons. Axons emerging from nucleus proprius cells can participate in local circuitry or ascend to brainstem or diencephalic structures.

Lamina VII, along with lamina X, form the intermediate zone. Cells are sparser in this region, except in the more medial dorsal nucleus of Clarke and the more lateral intermediolateral cell column.

Laminae VIII and IX are motor neuron columns containing large alpha-motor (α-motor) neurons. The column of motor neurons innervating limb muscles, lamina IX, is located in the lateral part of ventral horn. In contrast, motor neurons innervating axial and girdle muscles (i.e., neck and shoulder muscles) are located in the medial part of the ventral horn (Figure 5.4). Neurons in the medial part of the ventral horn supply axial and proximal limb muscles; those supplying the distal limb muscles are in the lateral part. Further, the flexor muscles (preaxial muscles) are represented more dorsally within the ventral horn and the extensor muscles (postaxial muscles) more ventrally.

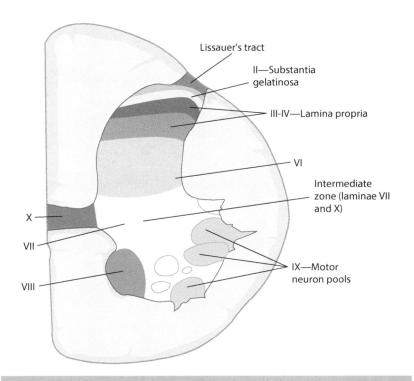

FIGURE 5.3

Gray matter laminae in the spinal hemicord. The dorsal horn is related to processing of sensory information; the ventral horn, to motor efferent function. (Reproduced with permission from Waxman SG. Chapter 5. The Spinal Cord. In: Waxman SG. eds. Clinical Neuroanatomy, 27e. New York, NY: McGraw-Hill; 2013.)

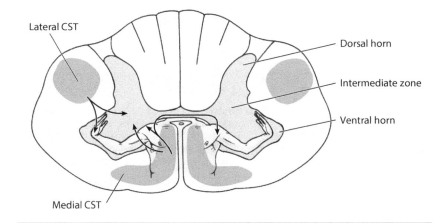

FIGURE 5.4

Somatotopic organization of the ventral horn. Diagram of the spinal cord shows the somatotopic organization of the ventral horn. In general, motor neurons innervating the proximal limb and axial muscles are located medially in the ventral horn and distal muscles laterally. Flexor muscles are represented dorsally and extensors, ventrally. A partial homunculus is superimposed on the ventral horns. (From Descending Motor Pathways and the Motor Function of the Spinal Cord. In: Martin JH. eds. Neuroanatomy Text and Atlas, 4e New York, NY: McGraw-Hill, 2012).

Internal Organization of the Spinal Cord: White Matter

Spinal cord white matter includes both descending (motor) and ascending (sensory) pathways (Figure 5.5). Three spinal pathways of special functional significance discussed in detail include the corticospinal tract (Figure 5.5A), controlling activation of motor neurons in the ventral horn; the dorsal columns (Figure 5.5B), carrying fine tactile inputs, including two-point discrimination, vibration, and proprioception; and the anterolateral system (spinothalamic tract) (Figure 5.5C), which mediates mechanical and thermal nociceptive inputs, as well as crude (nondiscriminative) touch. Each of these pathways occupies a predictable region in spinal cord white matter, and each conforms to strict somatotopic organization (Figure 5.6).

The other descending pathways are called extrapyramidal tracts, activating muscles responsible for more automatic functions such as postural adjustment and movement of the head and neck in response to outside cues. Extrapyramidal pathways include the rubrospinal tract, the reticulospinal tracts, the tectospinal tract, and the vestibulospinal tracts (Figure 5.7). These are discussed below.

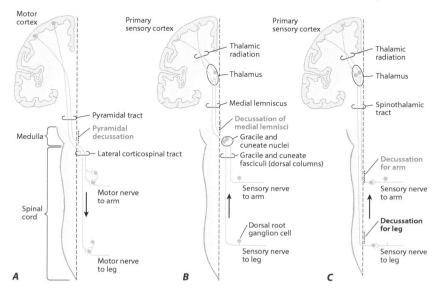

FIGURE 5.5

The three major long pathways between the spinal cord and the cerebral cortex. *A.* Corticospinal (pyramidal) tract. ***B.*** Dorsal column-medial lemniscus system. ***C.*** Spinothalamic (anterolateral) system. (Reproduced with permission from Waxman SG. Chapter 4. The Relationship Between Neuroanatomy and Neurology. In: Waxman SG. eds. Clinical Neuroanatomy, 27e. New York, NY: McGraw-Hill; 2013).

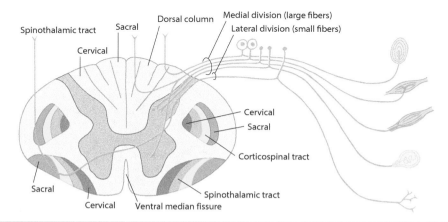

FIGURE 5.6

Illustration of a spinal cord segment with associated peripheral structures. A variety of sensory endings is represented on the left side; small fibers within the lateral division of the dorsal root supply primarily nociceptor endings. Somatotopy is represented in the dorsal columns with sacral body situated medially and cervical levels laterally. In the CST and spinothalamic tracts, cervical representation is in green; thoracic, in yellow; lumbar, in brown; and sacral, in pink. (Reproduced with permission from Waxman SG. Chapter 14. Somatosensory Systems. In: Waxman SG. eds. Clinical Neuroanatomy, 27e. New York, NY: McGraw-Hill; 2013).

III   MOTOR PATHWAYS

The cerebral cortex and brain stem contribute descending motor axons to the muscles of our limbs and trunk or face. The brain stem motor pathways engage in relatively automatic control, such as rapid postural adjustments and in-flight correction of misdirected movements. By contrast, the cortical motor pathways participate in more refined, flexible, and adaptive control, such as reaching for objects, grasping, and tool use.

Seven major descending motor control pathways terminate in motor centers of the brain stem and spinal cord (Figure 5.7). Three of these pathways originate in layer V of the cerebral cortex, primarily in the frontal lobe: (1) the lateral corticospinal tract; (2) the medial corticospinal tract; and (3) the corticobulbar tract. The corticobulbar tract terminates primarily in cranial motor nuclei in the pons and medulla, producing neck and facial motor function; it is the cranial equivalent of the two corticospinal tracts. Collectively, these cortical pathways participate in controlling the most adaptive and flexible movements, such as finger control during tool use, regulating posture during limb movements, and speech. The remaining four pathways originate from brain stem nuclei and are considered extrapyramidal tracts: (4) the rubrospinal tract, involved in automatic upper limb control; (5) the reticulospinal tracts, which participate in automatic control of proximal muscles and locomotion; (6) the tectospinal tract, involved in coordinating head movements with eye movements; and (7) the vestibulospinal tracts, critical for maintaining balance.

Medial and Lateral Corticospinal (Pyramidal) Tracts

The corticospinal tracts (CST) control spinal circuits through their direct spinal projections (Figure 5.7). In addition, the cortical motor regions project to brain stem nuclei that give rise to motor pathways: the red nucleus, superior colliculus, reticular formation, and vestibular nuclei. The lateral CST is the principal motor control pathway in humans, originating from the primary motor cortex as well as premotor cortical regions (supplementary motor area, cingulate motor area, and premotor cortex) and the somatic sensory cortical areas. The lateral CST occupies much of the lateral funiculus, and the medial CST is in the anterior funiculus, situated near the ventral median fissure on the midline medial to the ventral horns. The lateral CST controls more distal limb muscles. In contrast, the medial CST fibers control axial and limb girdle muscles.

The lateral CST descends from the primary motor cortex through the crus cerebri in the ventral part of the midbrain basis pedunculi (cerebral peduncle). Its descent continues through the basilar pons, where it is broken into smaller fascicles because of the presence of the pontine nuclei. The fiber bundle coalesces in the medulla, forming a ventral protrusion called the pyramid (thus the name *pyramidal tract* for the lateral CST). At the inferior border of the pyramid, about 90% of the axons cross the midline at the pyramidal decussation. From there downward, lateral CST axons descend ipsilaterally to the ventral horn motor neurons that they will innervate. This innervation supplies muscles that perform the finest, most dexterous movements.

In the internal somatotopy of the lateral CST, the fascicle has a body representation with the neck medial and the sacrum lateral.

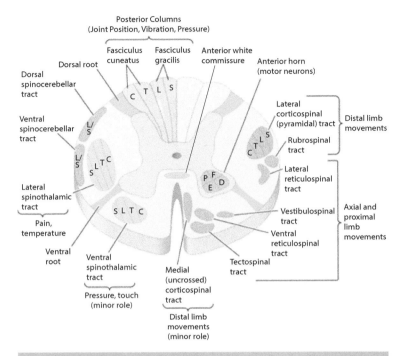

FIGURE 5.7

Transverse section through the spinal cord; principal ascending sensory pathways shown on the left and descending motor pathways right. A brief statement of the function of each pathway is included. C, cervical; D, distal; E, extensors; F, flexors; L, lumbar; P, proximal; S, sacral; T, thoracic. (From Kirkland TN, Fierer J. Coccidioidomycosis: A Reemerging Infectious Disease. Emerging Infectious Diseases. 1996;2(3):192-199. doi:10.3201/eid0203.960305).

The lateral CST has its greatest volume in the cervical cord, carrying axons down to all of the spinal segments. Within the fascicle, axons that supply neck muscles, and those that participate in the brachial plexus supplying the upper extremity, occupy the portion nearest the ventral horn motor neurons. The medial most axons exit the CST fascicle and innervate (synapse on) segmental motor neurons and interneurons while the remainder continue to descend. As the lateral CST descends, axons continually exit the medial side of the fascicle, and it becomes progressively smaller until it ends at the sacral level.

The medial CST originates from the primary motor cortex and the various premotor areas and descends to the medulla along with the lateral CST. It contains the remaining uncrossed 10% of the descending motor axons. Many of these decussate segmentally within the spinal cord; thus the medial CST provides bilateral supply of the postural muscles. They synapse on motor neurons in the medial ventral horn and on interneurons in the intermediate zone. This fiber pathway extends caudally to about the lower thoracic level, below which the lateral CST provides innervation to the distal leg muscles.

Cortical efferents descend in the spinal cord pathways described above to synapse on and activate motor neurons in the ventral horn. These motor neurons emit axons that distribute with spinal nerves. The different functions of these two sets of neurons become even more apparent when they are injured. Damage to the cortical neurons or their axons produces an array of behavioral changes in motor activity, including spasticity, hyperreflexia, hypertonicity, and clonus, collectively referred to as an upper motor neuron syndrome. If ventral horn motor neurons or their peripheral axons are injured, the resultant behavioral changes contrast sharply with those after an upper motor neuron injury: flaccid paralysis, abolition of reflexes, and hypotonicity, altogether referred to as a lower motor neuron syndrome.

Corticobulbar Tract

The corticobulbar tract arises from the primary motor cortex, the supplementary motor area, the premotor cortex, and the cingulate motor area. These are the same cortical regions that control limb and trunk muscles as noted above; however, the corticobulbar tract projects to various brain stem motor nuclei within the somatic skeletal and branchiomeric motor columns to innervate facial, tongue, jaw, laryngeal, and pharyngeal muscles. This tract is considered in detail in Chapter 6.

Extrapyramidal Tracts

The four descending tracts that originate outside the cortex and do not travel through the pyramids are the rubrospinal, reticulospinal, vestibulospinal, and tectospinal tracts. The rubrospinal tract, which has fewer axons overall than the CST, originates from neurons in the red nucleus, primarily from the caudal part. This portion is termed the magnocellular division because many rubrospinal tract neurons are large. The rubrospinal tract decussates in the midbrain and descends in the dorsolateral portion of the brain stem. Similar to the lateral CST, the rubrospinal tract is found in the dorsal portion of the lateral column and terminates primarily in the lateral portions of the intermediate zone and ventral horn of the cervical cord. In humans, the rubrospinal tract does not descend into the lumbosacral cord, suggesting that it functions in arm, but not leg, control.

The reticulospinal tracts originate from different regions of the pontine and medullary reticular formation. The pontine reticulospinal tract descends in the ventral column of the spinal cord, whereas the medullary reticulospinal tract descends in the ventrolateral quadrant of the lateral column. The reticulospinal tracts descend predominantly in the ipsilateral spinal cord but exert bilateral motor control effects. Laboratory animal studies show that the reticulospinal tracts control relatively automatic movements, such as maintaining posture or walking over even terrain. Because simultaneous contraction of muscles on opposing sides of a joint results in an isometric contraction, antagonist supression makes movement possible by inhibiting the contraction of opposing muscles (e.g., elbow flexors suppressed to allow the elbow extensors to straighten the arm).

The vestibulospinal tracts are essential for maintaining balance. They receive their principal input from the vestibular organs, discussed in more detail in Chapter 6. Originating in the vestibular nuclei of the medulla and pons, the vestibulospinal tracts descend in the ventromedial spinal white matter. There are separate medial and lateral vestibulospinal tracts. The medial vestibulospinal tract only projects to the upper cervical spinal cord and is important in coordinating head movements with eye movements. By contrast, the lateral vestibulospinal tract projects throughout the full length of the spinal cord to control all axial and proximal muscles. Note that despite its name, the lateral vestibulospinal tract is a medial descending motor pathway.

The tectospinal tract originates primarily from neurons located in the deeper layers of the superior colliculus, which comprises a large part of the tectum, the portion of the midbrain dorsal to the cerebral aqueduct. The tectospinal tract also has a limited rostrocaudal distribution, projecting only to the cervical spinal segments. It therefore participates primarily in the control of neck, shoulder, and upper trunk muscles. Because the superior colliculus also plays a key role in controlling eye movements, the tectospinal tract contributes to coordinating head and eye movements.

Integration of Systems
Movement Synergies (Normal and Abnormal)

Normal human movement begins in utero, and may be determined by fetal position as well as anatomy and neurophysiology. Early postnatal movement is produced by a series of primitive reflexes. These reflexes typically become suppressed as infant experiences drive the development of volitional movement. These reflexes become incorporated into normal human movement and may be seen under fatigue, stress, or unskilled movement patterns. Persistence of these reflexes beyond the normal time frame indicates certain medical conditions or diseases, such as cerebral palsy. In adults, neurologic injury or disease may lift the central suppression of these primitive reflexes so that they are seen again, as in amyotrophic lateral sclerosis (ALS).

The study of human movement incorporates many fields, ranging from cellular and neurophysiological assessment to direct observation of human behavior. The neural substrates of human motor control are relatively well defined, with additional value in new technologies to study in vivo conditions. The discovery of spinal or central pattern generators (CPGs) in mammals has generated a new area of study into the role of the spinal cord to coordinate and produce movement. After observing that many complex motions were still possible in animal models even after spinal cord dissection, scientists sought to understand the mechanism. They discovered that spinal burst generators that activate lumbosacral motor neuron pools, with very specific activation patterns that generate complex, rhythmic, repetitive motions requiring muscle activation across joints, coordinated temporally in a specific sequence. Afferent input from the periphery, primarily muscle spindles, modulates the motion. This discovery impacted rehabilitation after spinal injury or stroke, as studies showed benefit of promoting use of CPGs to generate locomotion. In fact, the results were so compelling that clinics began to use treadmills with overhead harness support to unload the demands of body weight, thus allowing patients with weak limbs to begin practicing walking motions despite paresis.

IV SOMATOSENSORY PATHWAYS

The somatic sensory systems mediate our bodily sensations, including mechanical sensations, protective senses, and a wide range of visceral sensory experiences. Apart from our basic sensory capabilities, like discriminating textures and shapes of grasped objects, or ensuring that we are not hurt when we hold something too hot, somatic sensations are also critical for many integrative functions. Consider the capacity of touch to quiet the cry of a newborn baby or awaken us from a deep sleep. Somatic sensory information is essential for controlling movements, from the simplest reflexes, such as the stretch or withdrawal reflexes, to the finest voluntary movements.

There are two main somatosensory pathways in the spinal cord: the dorsal columns carrying fine, highly detailed, precisely localized mechanical information interpreted as discriminative touch; and the spinothalamic tract (anterolateral system) transmitting noxious inputs interpreted as painful. Additionally, the trigeminal system, which is discussed in Chapter 6, carries touch and pain information from the face. In all of the major somatosensory systems, the pathways comprise a three-neuron chain. Primary afferent neurons are sequestered in peripheral ganglia, specifically the dorsal root ganglia for the spinal sensory systems, and the trigeminal ganglion for the majority of facial sensation. Primary afferent axons project to second-order target neurons located at different locations for the different systems. Second-order axons decussate and construct a fascicle that ascends to synapse on third-order neurons in the thalamus. The main thalamic nucleus receiving sensory inputs from the body is the ventroposterolateral nucleus, and from the face, the ventroposteromedial nucleus. Thalamic output proceeds to the primary somatosensory cortex in the postcentral gyrus.

Because afferent information ascends through the CNS, injury to the pathway before the decussation produces ipsilateral deficits below the level of the lesion. After the fibers decussate, an injury will produce a contralateral sensory deficit. It is essential to know the level of the decussation to be able to make an accurate differential diagnosis.

Sensory Modalities

A brief description of sensory modalities and their receptors is helpful before describing their complex neurologic pathways. Basic sensations in the periphery include touch, vibration, proprioception, pain, itch, and differentiating heat versus cold. Touch is a complex sensory modality encompassing many different aspects of mechanical stimuli. Fine, discriminative touch is detected by several different receptors, most of which are supplied by medium-sized myelinated Aβ fibers. Fine touch receptors, which contribute axons to the dorsal columns, allow us to sense smooth and rough textures and the shapes of objects produced by low-energy, low-force deformations of the skin. Touch also includes perception of pressure exerted by objects pressed onto the skin over muscle (deep pressure). Vibration sensitivity is carried on dorsal column axons. Single sensory receptors (notably Pacinian corpuscles) encode the rate and force of repeated fine stimuli, which the cortex interprets as vibration of varying frequency and amplitude. Clinicians routinely use vibration, not only for sensory testing but also as stimuli to enhance activity in specific muscle groups to increase strength and stability. People with impairments in these modalities

experience clumsiness and incoordination. Proprioception is our sense of static limb position; kinesthesia is the sensation of limb movement. Both of these sensory modalities are detected by different ending types within the muscle spindle apparatus. Sensory endings in muscle spindles detect joint position (proprioception) and small changes in limb position and direction, force, and speed of joint movement (kinesthesia). Thermal senses separate warmth and cold, provide critical information about the safety and comfort of our environment, and enable us to maintain our body temperature within narrow limits. Pain alerts the individual of tissue damage, present or impending. Pain is mediated by specific nociceptors. It comprises sharp pricking pain and a dull burning pain. Itch is triggered selectively by chemical irritation of the skin, especially in response to particular tissue inflammatory agents. Itch provokes the urge to scratch, thereby tending to remove the offending substance. Visceral sensation provides not only awareness of the internal state of our body but also the information for regulating many bodily functions, such as blood pressure and breathing. Many aspects of visceral sensation are never conscious, such as arterial pressure, and others are only so under special circumstances, such as nausea and fullness.

Dorsal Column–Medial Lemniscus

Low-threshold (extremely sensitive) mechanoreceptors are specialized types of dorsal root ganglion neurons that provide the major sensory input to the dorsal column–medial lemniscal system. The central axons of mechanoreceptors emit collateral branches. Some branches synapse in the spinal cord, which is primarily important for bringing information to spinal motor circuits for reflex function. Others ascend to synapse on second-order cells in the medulla. The ascending branches are the principal ones for perception. They travel in the dorsal columns that occupy the spaces between the dorsal horns and the dorsal median septum (Figure 5.8). Each dorsal column transmits somatic sensory information from the ipsilateral side of the body to second-order target cells located in the dorsal column nuclei in the ipsilateral caudal medulla. As the sensory roots enter the cord, precise somatotopy is established as each new layer of axons from progressively higher spinal levels builds from medial to lateral; thus the dorsal columns become increasingly broader as they ascend. Axons transmitting information from the lower limb ascend in the gracile fasciculus, the more medial portion of the dorsal column. Axons from the lower trunk ascend lateral to those from the lower limb, but still within the gracile fascicle. Axons from the upper trunk, upper limb, neck, and occiput ascend within the cuneate fascicle, a structure that begins approximately at the level of the sixth thoracic segment. The dorsal intermediate septum separates the gracile and cuneate fascicles, with the dorsal columns of the two halves of the spinal cord separated by the dorsal median septum. Spinal cord injury can interrupt the dorsal column axons, resulting in an ipsilateral mechanosensory loss below the level of the injury.

The synapse in the dorsal column nuclei in the medulla is the first major relay in the dorsal column–medial lemniscal system. Here, the first-order axons in the pathway synapse on the second-order neurons in the central nervous system. The second-order axons decussate in the medulla and travel in the medial lemniscus, which transmits information primarily to the ventral posterior lateral nucleus of the thalamus. Thalamic neurons in this nucleus project their axons to the primary somatic sensory cortex in the

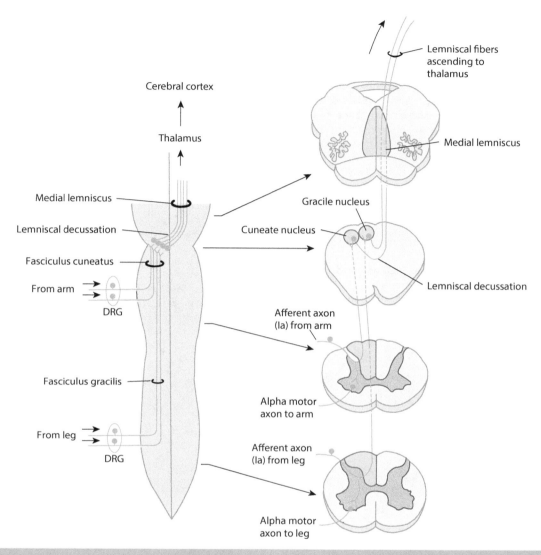

Cerebral cortex

Thalamus

Medial lemniscus

Lemniscal decussation

Fasciculus cuneatus

From arm

DRG

Fasciculus gracilis

From leg

DRG

Lemniscal fibers ascending to thalamus

Medial lemniscus

Gracile nucleus

Cuneate nucleus

Lemniscal decussation

Afferent axon (Ia) from arm

Alpha motor axon to arm

Afferent axon (Ia) from leg

Alpha motor axon to leg

FIGURE 5.8

The dorsal column system in the spinal cord. Primary afferent neurons in the DRG emit axons that enter the dorsal roots and ascend in the ipsilateral dorsal column, sacral representations medially in the gracile fasciculus and cervical laterally in the cuneate fasciculus. Primary axons synapse on secondary neurons in the ipsilateral gracile and cuneate nuclei in caudal medulla. Second-order axons decussate and construct the medial lemniscus, which ascends to the thalamus. (Reproduced with permission from Waxman SG. Chapter 5. The Spinal Cord. In: Waxman SG. eds. Clinical Neuroanatomy, 27e. New York, NY: McGraw-Hill; 2013.)

postcentral gyrus. This cortical area is important in localization of mechanical stimuli and in identifying the quality of such stimuli.

From the primary somatic sensory cortex, information is transmitted to higher-order cortical areas, located posteriorly, that play a role in more complex aspects of touch and position sense. Cortical areas that are located ventrally, including the secondary somatic sensory cortex, are important for recognizing objects by touch and grasp alone—that is, "what" something is. Dorsal areas, including area 5, are important in spatial localization, or "where" something is located. The dorsal areas are also important in using mechanosensory information for guiding hand and arm movements. We will

learn that the visual and auditory cortical areas also have dorsal, or "where," and ventral, "what," areas.

Whereas the majority of axons in the dorsal column are the central branches of mechanoreceptors, a small number of dorsal horn nociceptive neurons project their axons into the dorsal columns, comprising approximately 10%–15% of the axons in the path. These axons are important for visceral pain sensation. The branching patterns of the pain, temperature, and itch fibers, which all have a small-diameter axons, are different from those of the mechanosensory fibers, terminating within the more dorsal portion of the dorsal horn.

Spinocerebellar Tracts

The dorsal column–medial lemniscus and the anterolateral system carry information to the ventroposterolateral nucleus of the thalamus. These inputs are consciously recognized as specific sensations localized precisely on the body. The dorsal column–medial lemniscus even carries proprioceptive information so that we can appreciate our body position in space. This is necessary so that meaningful goal-oriented movements can proceed with coordination and control. Consider what it would do to our ability to move smoothly if we were required to consciously monitor our every movement. If we had to consider our body, leg, and foot positions during every step, we would never get anywhere! Because constant sensory feedback is necessary for coordinated movement, there must be a mechanism that continually monitors our changing position without rising to a conscious level. Unconscious proprioception, therefore, is a function of spinal cord inputs to the cerebellum through two spinocerebellar tracts (Figure 5.9).

In the thoracic spinal cord, generally coextensive with the location of the lateral horn, is a pair of nuclei situated in lamina VII called Clarke's nucleus dorsalis (dorsal nucleus of Clarke). Another cluster of neurons is found in the lateral margin of the ventral horn; these are the spinal border cells. Primary proprioceptive afferent axons enter the cord and give off at least three sets of collateral branches. The first branch ascends in the ipsilateral dorsal column to the dorsal column nucleus and to the contralateral ventroposterolateral thalamic nucleus for conscious interpretation of joint position. The other two sets of primary afferent terminals will synapse either onto cells in Clarke's nucleus dorsalis or spinal border cells. Outputs from both of these cell types ascend to the cerebellum for sensorimotor integration at an unconscious level. Axons from cells in Clarke's nucleus ascend in the ipsilateral spinal cord lateral to the CST in the lateral funiculus, comprising the uncrossed dorsal spinocerebellar tract. These fibers ascend through the inferior cerebellar peduncle into the cerebellum. Axons arising from spinal border cells decussate and ascend in the crossed ventral spinocerebellar tract. These axons ascend to enter the cerebellum through the superior cerebellar peduncle. Both the dorsal and ventral spinocerebellar tracts contribute to ongoing proprioceptive feedback from the lower extremity and trunk. Rostrally in the cervical spinal cord, the cuneate fasciculus contains fibers carrying unconscious proprioceptive inputs to the cerebellum from the upper limb. Collectively, these

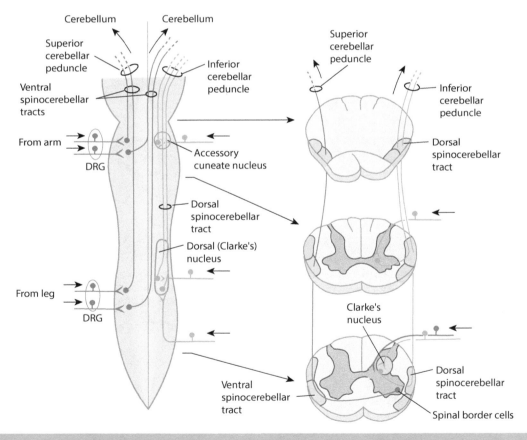

FIGURE 5.9

The spinocerebellar pathways in the spinal cord. Proprioceptor inputs project collaterals to three places: ipsilateral dorsal column, Clarke's nucleus dorsalis, and the spinal border cells. Outputs from Clarke's nucleus dorsalis emit uncrossed axons to form the dorsal spinocerebellar tract. Axons emerging from the spinal border cells decussate and ascend as the crossed ventral spinocerebellar tract. Ascending fibers from the accessory cuneate nucleus comprise the cuneocerebellar tract to the ipsilateral cerebellum. (Reproduced from Waxman SG. Chapter 14. Somatosensory Systems. In: Waxman SG. eds. Clinical Neuroanatomy, 27e. New York, NY: McGraw-Hill; 2013.)

three pathways provide the cerebellum with continuous inputs related to changing joint positions in the entire body necessary for making minute modifications to the motor plan as we carry out goal-oriented behaviors.

Anterolateral System (Spinothalamic Tract)

Potentially damaging mechanical (noxious), thermal, and chemical stimuli are transmitted in the anterolateral system (Figure 5.10), which ascends in the anterior portion of the lateral column of the spinal cord and synapses in different brain regions. The spinothalamic tract ascends in the anterolateral spinal cord contralateral to their primary nociceptive neurons. The pathway continues to the thalamus, where the axons synapse onto third-order neurons in the

ventroposterolateral nucleus as well as other thalamic relay centers. From the thalamic nuclei, noxious information is distributed to several different subcortical and cortical centers for interpretation of the sensation and the processing of the emotional and cognitive effects of the pain.

Because of the lateral location of the spinothalamic tract in the spinal cord and its distance from the dorsal columns, it is possible to produce a surgical lesion that affects only transmission of pain inputs: a lateral cordotomy. A small transverse slice is made into the anterolateral aspect of the spinal cord contralateral and one or two segments rostral to the painful segment. Significantly, although most axons in the dorsal columns, approximately 85%, are the central branches of mechanoreceptors, the remaining 15% carry nociceptive information. Persistence of this complement of nociceptors

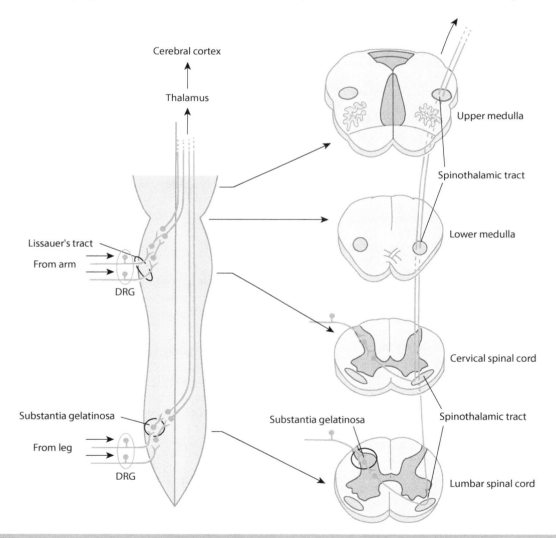

FIGURE 5.10

The spinothalamic (anterolateral) system in the spinal cord. One significant difference between the spinothalamic tract and the dorsal column-medial lemniscus pathway is the location of the second-order neurons and the decussation. Second-order cells for the anterolateral system lie in the substantia gelatinosa (and the nucleus proprius) one or two segments above the entry point of the primary axons into the spinal cord. Axons from these neurons decussate and construct the spinothalamic tracts that ascend in the anterolateral column contralateral to the primary afferent neuron cell bodies. (Reproduced with permission from Waxman SG. Chapter 5. The Spinal Cord. In: Waxman SG. eds. Clinical Neuroanatomy, 27e. New York, NY: McGraw-Hill; 2013).

after lateral cordotomy aimed at severing the pain-transmitting spinothalamic tract may contribute to the refractory nature of surgical pain relief.

The anterolateral system comprises multiple pathways for several distinctive functions. In subsequent chapters we focus on the role of these pathways in three aspects of pain: (1) sensory-discriminative aspects of pain, (2) emotional aspects of pain, and (3) arousal and feedback control of pain transmission. Here we examine the sensory-discriminative aspects of pain. The lateral spinothalamic tract carries discriminative aspects of pain, including information about the location, intensity, and quality of noxious stimuli; this projection is somatotopically organized. Neurophysiological studies have shown that this projection encodes the physical intensity of the stimulus, not the person's subjective impression of intensity. The ventral spinothalamic tract carries a sensory modality referred to as crude (poorly localized and indiscriminate) touch, as well as more emotional information that contributes to anxiety-producing aspects of pain.

Small DRG neurons with thinly myelinated $A\delta$ and unmyelinated C-fiber axons sensitive to noxious (i.e., painful) mechanical, thermal, and pruritic (i.e., itch-provoking) stimuli provide the major sensory inputs to the anterolateral system. Nociceptive primary afferents enter the Lissauer's tract on entry into the spinal cord, then branch to ascend and descend one or two segments before penetrating to synapse on second-order neurons in the nucleus proprius and substantia gelatinosa in the dorsal horn. This divergence of inputs contributes to the reduced precision of localization of pain compared to the high degree of acuity produced by activation of the low-threshold mechanoreceptors contributing to the dorsal columns. Nociceptive primary afferent axons synapse on second-order projection neurons in the ipsilateral dorsal horn. Axons emitted by second-order neurons decussate in the anterior white commissure, which is located just ventral to the central canal, and ascend in the contralateral spinal cord and brainstem to the thalamus.

As the anterolateral system ascends through the brainstem, it includes additional components that comprise smaller brainstem tracts to several additional locations en route to the thalamus. These include the spinoreticular tract, the spinomesencephalic tract, and the spinohypothalamic tract. Each can be distinguished by its targets and by the effects that those connections produce.

The spinoreticular tract engages a subcortical emotional pathway. This pathway synapses in the medullary and pontine reticular formations. Many of these reticular formation neurons project to the intralaminar thalamic nuclei that have broad projections to the basal ganglia and cerebral cortex for arousal.

The spinomesencephalic tract terminates primarily in the periaqueductal gray and the midbrain tectum. The projection to the tectum integrates somatic sensory information with vision and hearing for orienting the head and body to salient, notably noxious, stimuli. Projections to the periaqueductal gray matter play a role in the feedback regulation of pain transmission in the spinal cord. Spinomesencephalic fibers ascend in the dorsal part of the *lateral funiculus*, which is possibly why an anterolateral cordotomy is only partially effective in relieving chronic pain. Other projections form the spinohypothalamic tract, which innervates the hypothalamus and influences the autonomic effects of pain, such as increased heart rate, sweating, and general anxiety. Pathways from the hypothalamus are also related to descending pain modulation, discussed below.

Visceral Sensation

There is a special pathway for pain from caudal visceral structures, such as in the pelvic region and parts of the lower gut, that is different from that of pain originating from other body parts. Rather than synapse on dorsal horn neurons that send their axons into the anterolateral white matter, dorsal horn visceral pain neurons send their axons into the medial portion of the dorsal columns, the gracile column. Surprisingly, the visceral pain pathway follows a course similar to the mechanosensory pathway rather than the nociceptive pathway, synapsing in the dorsal column nuclei, decussating in the medulla, ascending in the brain stem in the medial lemniscus, and synapsing within the thalamus. The main difference is that the visceral pain pathway synapses in different portions of the dorsal column nuclei and thalamus than the mechanosensory pathway. Much less is known of this potentially very important pathway than the anterolateral pathways.

Vascular Supply of the Spinal Cord

Blood supply to the spinal cord derives from the subclavian artery through the vertebral arteries, and from segmental branches from the aorta (Figure 5.11). A small artery, the anterior spinal artery, arises within the cranium by the fusion of descending branches from the vertebral arteries just inside the foramen magnum. It descends on the ventral midline of the cord all the way to the conus medullaris. It supplies the ventrolateral white matter as well as most of the gray matter, including the dorsal horn, accounting for the blood supply of about two-thirds of the spinal cord area. Also arising from the vertebral arteries near the point where the posterior inferior cerebellar arteries branch off, the posterior spinal arteries descend on the dorsal surface of the spinal cord bilaterally, anastomosing bilaterally with the posterior spinal branches off the aorta. The spinal cord can be divided into two related halves called hemicords. Each hemicord deals primarily, but not exclusively, with inputs and outputs from the ipsilateral side of the body. A number of spinal cord surface features are directly related to functional differences. As stated above, the diameter of the cord at cervical and lumbar levels is larger than that seen in the thoracic and sacral levels.

V NEUROPHYSIOLOGY OF THE PERIPHERAL NERVOUS SYSTEM

Chapter 4 provided basic information on cellular neurophysiology, as these features influence grosser level nervous system functions. The initial part of this section describes spinal cord motor circuitry, the internal local and projection synaptic complexes; motor endplate neurophysiology was discussed in detail in Chapter 3. Neurophysiological characteristics, as well as circuitry, influence the way peripheral stimuli are encoded and carried rostrally, and therefore influence sensory perception.

Spinal Motor Circuitry

The descending pyramidal tract pathways target the alpha-motor neurons (α-motor neurons) in the ventral horn (Figure 5.12). Alpha-motor neurons provide motor signals to muscle fibers. A single α-motor neuron connects to a limited set of fibers within one muscle, termed the motor unit. There is a direct relationship between the size of the motor unit and the precision of movement.

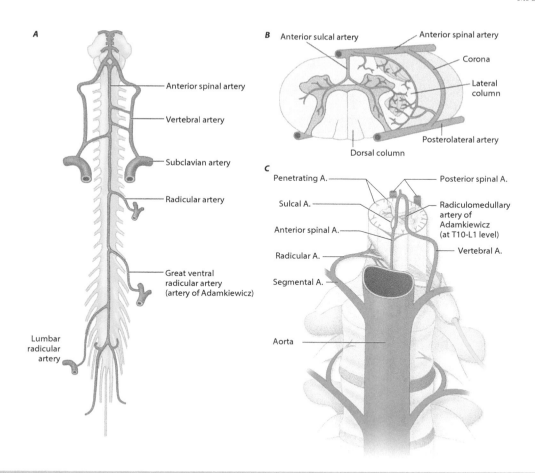

A. Anterior spinal artery
Vertebral artery
Subclavian artery
Radicular artery
Great ventral
radicular artery
(artery of Adamkiewicz)
Lumbar
radicular
artery

B. Anterior sulcal artery
Anterior spinal artery
Corona
Lateral
column
Posterolateral artery
Dorsal column

C. Penetrating A.
Sulcal A.
Anterior spinal A.
Radicular A.
Segmental A.
Aorta
Posterior spinal A.
Radiculomedullary
artery of
Adamkiewicz
(at T10-L1 level)
Vertebral A.

FIGURE 5.11

Arterial supply to the spinal cord. *A.* Anterior view showing principal sources of blood supply: the anterior spinal artery from the vertebral arteries, and radicular branches farther caudally. (Reproduced with permission from Chapter 45. Spinal, Epidural, & Caudal Blocks. In: Butterworth JF, IV, Mackey DC, Wasnick JD. eds. Morgan & Mikhail's Clinical Anesthesiology, 5e New York, NY: McGraw-Hill; 2013). ***B.*** Cross-sectional view through the spinal cord showing paired posterior spinal arteries and a single anterior spinal artery. Note that the anterior spinal artery supplies approximately two-thirds of the cord ventrally. (Reproduced with permission from Chapter 6. The Vertebral Column and Other Structures Surrounding the Spinal Cord. In: Waxman SG. eds. Clinical Neuroanatomy, 27e New York, NY: McGraw-Hill; 2013.) ***C.*** Cross section of the arteries in the cervical spinal cord. There are numerous variations in the vascular supply. (Used with permission from Prasad S, Price RS, Kranick SM et al: Clinical reasoning: A 59-year-old woman with acute paraplegia. Neurology 69:E41, 2007).

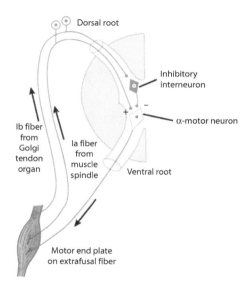

Dorsal root
Inhibitory
interneuron
α-motor neuron
Ib fiber
from
Golgi
tendon
organ
Ia fiber
from
muscle
spindle
Ventral root
Motor end plate
on extrafusal fiber

FIGURE 5.12

Illustration of the pathways responsible for the monosynaptic knee jerk (stretch) reflex and the polysynaptic inverse stretch reflex. Stretch stimulates the muscle spindle annulospiral endings, and impulses pass up the Ia fiber to excite (+) the α-motor neuron. The stretch also stimulates the Golgi tendon organ, and impulses passing up the Ib fiber activate an inhibitory interneuron to suppress (−) α-motor neuron activity. (Reproduced with permission from Reflex & Voluntary Control of Posture & Movement. In: Barrett KE, Barman SM, Boitano S, Brooks HL. eds. Ganong's Review of Medical Physiology, 25e New York, NY: McGraw-Hill; 2016).

Small motor units, such as those in the digits and extraocular eye muscles, provide exquisite control, allowing us to make watches or track rabbits while hunting in the wild; large motor units, such as those in the gluteal muscles, provide coarser movements.

As the motor pathways descend from the cortex, about 90% of the lateral CST fibers cross the midline at the pyramidal decussation in the caudal medulla, and the remaining 10% remain uncrossed, forming the medial CST (Figure 5.13). The decussation of the lateral CST brings the axons to synapse directly on the α-motor neurons on the ipsilateral (same) side as the muscles they activate. Axons of these cortical efferent "upper" motor neurons synapse onto "lower" α-motor neurons in the ventral horn, whose axons extend into the ventral roots and continue into peripheral nerves that provide motor innervation to individual muscles or muscle groups. Injury to CST neurons or their axons produces an upper motor neuron syndrome including spasticity, hypertonicity, and clonus. Injury to lower motor neurons produces flaccidity, abolition or reduction of reflexes, and rapid atrophy.

The CSTs directly control volitional movements; however, that is not the only way α-motor neurons can be activated. They function relatively independently at the spinal segmental level, requiring no cortical direction, to produce reflexive movements. Descending CST axons also synapse onto ventral horn interneurons. For muscles of the limbs and trunk, motor neurons and most interneurons are found in the ventral horn and intermediate zone of the spinal cord. The intermediate zone corresponds primarily to the spinal gray matter lateral to the central canal; it is sometimes included within the ventral horn. For muscles of the head, including facial muscles, the motor neurons and interneurons are located in the cranial nerve motor nuclei and the reticular formation. Interneurons can be excitatory or inhibitory, depending on the circuitry in which they participate. For example, an inhibitory interneuron activated by descending CST projections can suppress activation of an α-motor neuron. Excitatory interneurons function differently, promoting or facilitating α-motor neuron activation. Other interneurons receive input from somatic sensory receptors for the reflex control of movement. For example, particular interneurons that receive input from nociceptors excite motor neurons to produce limb withdrawal reflexes in response to painful stimuli, such as when you jerk your hand away from a hot stove. Other interneurons coordinate the left–right limb motor actions during walking, and still others are important for upper limb–lower limb coordination.

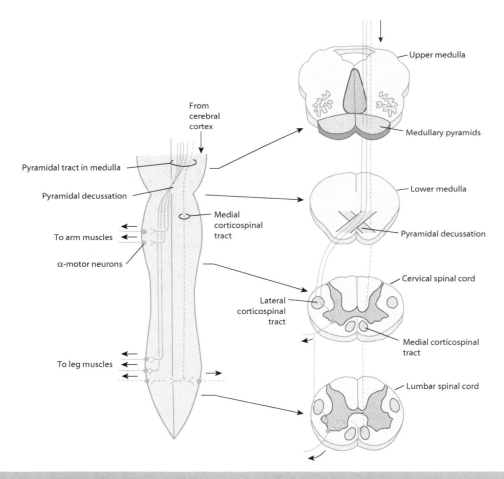

FIGURE 5.13

The corticospinal tract fibers in the spinal cord with cross sections at representative levels. CST fibers descend through the caudal medulla where ~90% cross at the pyramidal decussation forming the lateral CST. The remaining ~10% descend uncrossed into the cord to form the medial CST. Note that the volume of the lateral CST decreases caudally as axons exit the fascicle segmentally. (Reproduced with permission from Waxman SG. Chapter 5. The Spinal Cord. In: Waxman SG. eds. Clinical Neuroanatomy, 27e. New York, NY: McGraw-Hill; 2013).

Neurophysiology of Sensory Receptors

Somatic sensation is a CNS interpretation of the features of an object based on information generated by activation of sensory endings in the PNS. The somatic senses consist of many distinct components, or modalities. This diversity adds to the richness of somatic sensations. The peripheral axon terminal is the receptive portion of the PNS neuron. Here, stimulus energy is transduced into neural signals by membrane receptor-channel complexes that respond to a particular stimulus energy (e.g., mechanical or thermal). Mechanoreceptors are activated when the energy produces skin deformation that opens stretch-activated channels in the receptor membrane that produces a burst of action potentials that is carried centrally (Chapter 3). A different type of sensory receptor mediates each sensory modality (Figure 5.14). Common activities require integration of different senses for controlled function. For example, in picking up a cup of coffee, you use proprioception in

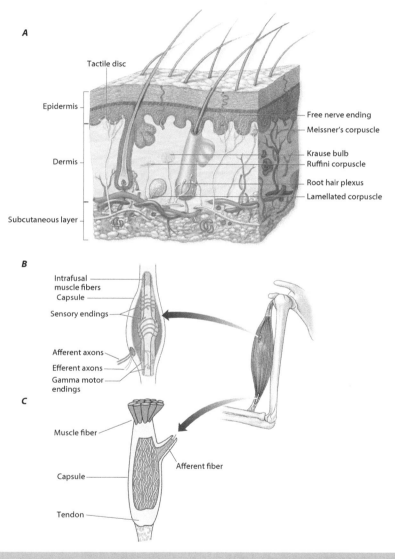

FIGURE 5.14

Diagram of different types of sensory receptors. *A.* Block of skin containing several types of simple and encapsulated sensory receptors. Free nerve endings and tactile discs of nerve fibers associated with Merkel cells are seen in the basal layer of the epidermis. More complex, encapsulated tactile receptors are located in the dermis and hypodermis. These include Meissner corpuscles for light touch, Pacinian corpuscles detecting pressure and high-frequency vibration, and Ruffini corpuscles detecting tissue distortion (stretch). (Krause end bulbs for low-frequency vibrations/movements are distributed relatively sparsely.) (Reproduced with permission from Chapter 18. Skin. In: Mescher AL. eds. Junqueira's Basic Histology: Text & Atlas, 13e New York, NY: McGraw-Hill; 2013). ***B.*** The muscle spindle organ (top inset) is a stretch receptor located within the extrafusal muscle. Its intrafusal muscle fibers receive efferent innervation from specialized γ-motor neurons the spinal cord that maintain receptor sensitivity during muscle contraction. ***C.*** Located within tendons, Golgi tendon organs respond to force generated by muscle contraction. ***B, C,*** (From Chapter 4, The Physiology of Small Groups of Neurons; Reflexes. In: Schmidt RF. Fundamentals of Neurophysiology, 3rd ed. Berlin, Heidelberg, New York: Springer; 1985. With permission from Springer).

Table 5.1 Functional Classifications of Axons

	Aα/Type I	Aβ/Type II	Aγ	Aδ/Type III	C/Type IV
Sensory modality	Proprioception	Mechanoreceptors		Pain, temperature	Pain, temperature
Motor function	Somatic motor		Intrafusal Motor		Postganglionic autonomic
Myelin	Very thick	Thick	Thick	Thin	Unmyelinated
Diameter (μ)	13–20	6–12	5–8	1–5	0.2–1.5
Conduction velocity (m/sec)	80–120	35–75	4–24	5–30	0.5–2

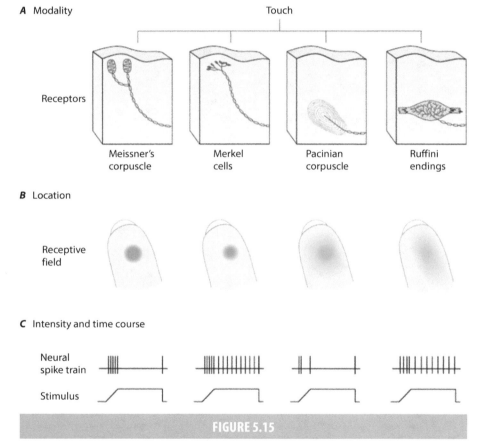

FIGURE 5.15

Modality, location (receptive field), intensity, and duration (timing) encoded by sensory endings. A. Four types of low-threshold mechanoreceptors in skin; their combined activation produces the sensation of contact with an object. Selective activation of Merkel cells and Ruffini endings causes sensation of steady pressure; selective activation of Meissner's and Pacinian corpuscles causes tingling and vibratory sensation. **B.** Mechanoreceptors are only activated by distortions of the skin near their terminals. These receptive fields, corresponding to the mechanoreceptors presented in (**A**) (shown as red areas on fingertips), differ in size. Merkel cells and Meissner's corpuscles have the smallest receptive fields and provide the most precise localization as they are most sensitive to pressure applied by a small probe. **C.** Stimulus intensity is signaled by action potential firing rates in response to skin distortion; duration of stimulus is signaled by time course of firing. Meissner's and Pacinian corpuscles are rapidly adapting, the others are slowly adapting. (Adapted from Johansson RS, Vallbo ÅB. 1983. Tactile sensory coding in the glabrous skin of the human hand. *Trends Neurosci* 6:27–32. Copyright 1983 Elsevier.)

identifying the location of your hand as you reach to grasp the handle; contact with the cup is detected by touch. If the cup is warm, your temperature sense is recruited, and if it is too hot, you experience pain. After consuming caffeine in the coffee, your heart may beat faster, which is sensed by both visceral sensory receptors and mechanoreceptors in the chest.

The stimulus sensitivity of a sensory neuron is also related to the diameter of its axon and the patterns of connections it makes in the central nervous system. Most mechanoreceptors have a large-diameter axon covered by a thick myelin sheath. The larger the diameter of the axon, the faster it conducts action potentials (Chapter 3). The mechanoreceptors are the fastest conducting sensory receptor neurons in the somatic sensory system. The dorsal column–medial lemniscal system carries sensory input principally through these fast conducting mechanoreceptors with large-diameter axons. By contrast, dorsal root ganglion neurons that are sensitive to noxious stimuli (nociceptors), temperature (thermoreceptors), and itch (pruriceptors) have small-diameter axons that are either thinly myelinated or unmyelinated. Table 5.1 lists the functional categories of primary sensory fibers, including the two fiber nomenclatures based on axonal diameter: Aα (group 1), Aβ (group 2), Aδ (group 3), and C (group 4).

Neural adaptation, the pattern and timing of the action potentials produced by contact, is different among the various receptor types; thus the cerebral cortex receives subtly different information from each type and can extract even very fine detail about the stimulus. The different types of endings correspond to different modalities of sensation. Rapidly adapting endings deliver a phasic response, changing its pattern of firing during the application of the stimulus. Slowly adapting receptors' tonic response changes little over time (Figure 5.15).

A somatic sensory modality is thought to be mediated by a single type of sensory receptor. Low-threshold mechanoreceptors encode the energy of the stimulus that will be interpreted as light touch, pressure, vibration, stretch, and proprioception. Low-activation thresholds give tissues a high degree of sensitivity to low-energy, low-force deformation. Five major types of encapsulated mechanoreceptor neurons are located in the skin and underlying deep tissue that mediate mechanical sensations: Ruffini corpuscles, Merkel receptors, Meissner's corpuscles, Pacinian corpuscles, and hair receptors. Merkel receptors and Meissner's corpuscles are located at the epidermis–dermis border. These receptors are sensitive to stimulation within a very small region of overlying skin; hence they have very small receptive fields. A smaller receptive field provides more precise localization of a stimulus. These receptors participate in fine tactile discrimination, such as reading Braille. Ruffini and Pacinian corpuscles are both located in the dermis. Ruffini endings are sensitive to skin stretch and are important in discriminating the shape of grasped objects. Pacinian corpuscles, the most sensitive mechanoreceptor, respond to subtle skin displacement as small as 500 nm, allowing you to feel the weight of an insect. Merkel's receptors and Pacinian corpuscles are rapidly adapting, responding to changes in the stimulus, such as when it begins or ends. Meissner's corpuscles and Ruffini endings are slowly adapting, firing action potentials for the duration of the stimulus. Hair receptors may be either slowly or rapidly adapting. Each primary sensory fiber has multiple terminal branches and, therefore, multiple receptive endings.

VI SENSORY-MOTOR INTERACTION

Sensory and motor pathways have been considered separately in this chapter, due to distinct anatomical pathways and structures. Normal movement, however, requires constant integration of sensory and motor information. In later chapters, this centrally mediated communication is discussed in detail, with emphasis on cerebellar and cortical interaction. The complex interaction between ascending and descending pathways begins locally in the spinal cord. A simple reflex involves sensory input that generates a motor response. Resting muscle tone is constantly adapting to sensory input to the muscle spindle, to maintain a constant ready state of appropriate muscle length and tension to produce an effective contraction.

Motor Control

Motor control research strives to define the necessary neuromotor interactions for producing and modulating movement. Despite significant progress toward deeper understanding of neural pathways, there is also dissent, as disparate theories attempt to explain the many unanswered questions. The extensive field of motor control theory is beyond the scope of this text; however, a brief overview will provide context for students of human motion. Two concepts specific to sensory and motor interaction are feedforward and feedback control. Consider the task of drinking a beverage, which includes creating a motor program to reach forward, place your hand in the proper shape, and then exert the appropriate force while grasping the beverage container to drink. This task varies greatly depending on many factors, including the container's contents, shape, and fragility. Feedforward sensory control includes visually inspecting the object, accessing cortical pathways for prior knowledge about the object's behavior, and even touching the object lightly to determine weight or temperature. Grasping a hot cup of coffee filled to

the brim in a flimsy Styrofoam container requires significantly different motor control from lifting an antique porcelain teacup. The feedback control provides information for rapid adjustment of the motor pattern during the task.

The role of the spinal cord in sharing sensory-motor information to create movement is demonstrated clearly in the simple reflex loop (Figure 5.16). Rehabilitation professionals have employed sensory input to generate specific motor responses for many years, supported by these early theories of stimulus-response, reflex-driven motor control. New evidence points to a more subtle, yet direct, role in modulating motion for the spinal cord. Development of manual dexterity is associated with expansion of both the cerebral cortical hand representation and corticomotoneural projections. In addition to these motor pathways, sensory feedback and feedforward inhibition of propriospinal neurons develop to provide real-time motor control at the spinal level. Recent studies on the control of grasp and reach in humans demonstrate coordination of sensory and motor signals at the midcervical level to modify grip pressure and precision during the task. Cervical propriospinal neurons receive peripheral inputs from joints, skin, and muscle, as well as efferent corticospinal inputs. Rather than relying solely on central coordination of the motor plan based on proprioceptive and visual feedback, this local information allows efficient and effective adjustments in subtle behavior. Successful beverage management requires a complex, constant interaction between ascending and descending pathways at multiple cortical and subcortical levels.

Muscle Tone and Reflexes

When relaxed, muscles retain a state of tension, called resting tone, which creates resistance to stretch. This is regulated by a special kind

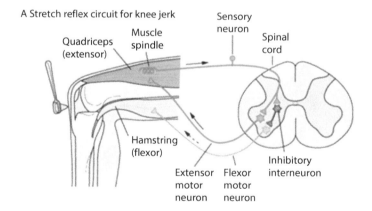

A Stretch reflex circuit for knee jerk

Quadriceps (extensor) · Muscle spindle · Sensory neuron · Spinal cord · Hamstring (flexor) · Extensor motor neuron · Flexor motor neuron · Inhibitory interneuron

FIGURE 5.16

Components of typical patellar tendon and inverse stretch reflex arcs. Patellar tendon tap stretches the extrafusal quadriceps muscle and its intrafusal muscle spindles, activating annulospiral endings. Their central axons project directly (monosynaptically) to α-motor neurons supplying the extensor muscle. A collateral from the annulospiral ending also innervates an inhibitory interneuron in the ventral horn. The interneurons inhibit contraction of the antagonistic hamstring muscles (polysynaptic antagonist inhibition). (Reproduced with permission from Nerve Cells, Neural Circuitry, and Behavior. In: Kandel ER, et al., eds. *Principles of Neural Science*, Fifth Editon New York, NY: McGraw-Hill; 2012.)

of sensory receptor known as the muscle spindle, which constantly monitors muscle tension to maintain the length–tension relationship function while conserving energy at rest. The length–tension relationship refers to the ability of connective tissue to generate tension. It involves length of the entire muscle and its associated connective tissue, including both contractile and noncontractile tissue. Contractile tissue is most effective only in the midranges. In contrast, noncontractile tissue generates tension as it is stretched. The protein titin is the molecular spring that gives stretched muscles their property of passive elasticity. Figure 5.17 shows

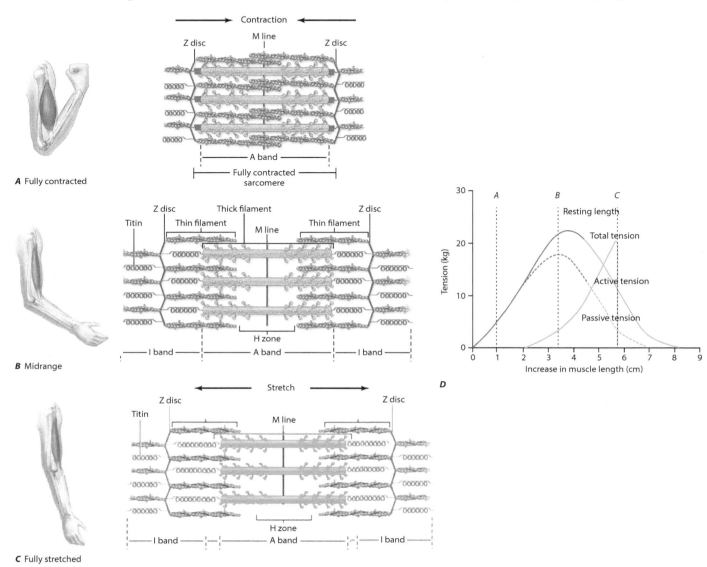

FIGURE 5.17

Length-tension relationship during skeletal muscle contraction in three different states. *A.* Fully contracted. Muscle contraction draws the Z discs closer together as they move toward the ends of thick filaments in the A band. Titin molecules, the molecular springs, are compressed during contraction and generate little to no tension passively at this length. ***B.* Midrange.** At midrange the sarcomere, I band, and H zone are at their expanded length. The springlike action of titin molecules, which span the I band, helps pull thin and thick filaments past one another in relaxed muscle, increasing the ability to produce tension passively. ***C.* Fully stretched.** In this position, Z discs are far from each other, and the thin filaments only minimally overlap the thick filaments. Titin molecules are stretched to their limits, producing the maximum amount of passive tension in this position. ***D.*** Length–tension relationship for the human triceps muscle. The passive tension curve measures the tension exerted by this skeletal muscle at each length, generated by either active muscle contraction or passive stretch. The total tension curve represents the tension developed from both active muscle contraction and passive elongation. *A, B,* and *C* correlate with the fully contracted, midrange, and fully stretched stated depicted. (*A, B,* Reproduced with permission from Chapter 10. Muscle Tissue. In: Mescher AL. eds. Junqueira's Basic Histology: Text & Atlas, 13e New York, NY: McGraw-Hill; 2013; *C* Adapted from Chapter 10. Muscle Tissue. In: Mescher AL. eds. Junqueira's Basic Histology: Text & Atlas, 13e New York, NY: McGraw-Hill; 2013; *D,* Reproduced with permission from Chapter 5. Excitable Tissue: Muscle. In: Barrett KE, Boitano S, Barman SM, Brooks HL. eds. Ganong's Review of Medical Physiology, 24e New York, NY: McGraw-Hill; 2012).

the relationship between joint position, tissue length, and tensile strength. Contraction results as the overlapping thin and thick filaments of each sarcomere slide past one another. Contraction is induced when an action potential arrives at a synapse, the neuromuscular junction (NMJ), and is transmitted along the T tubules to the sarcoplasmic reticulum to trigger Ca^{2+} release. The proper distance between Z discs is essential to produce a muscle contraction. If the motor unit is in a shortened position prior to contraction, the myosin has insufficient actin for cross bridges (Figure 5.17A). With excessive motor unit elongation (Figure 5.17C), the ability to produce strong cross-links for muscle contraction is reduced, as less myosin is available to bond with the actin. The optimum resting muscle length will produce the strongest contraction (Figure 5.17B). This is also seen with reflex testing, as little to no response is produced at either end of the joint's available range of motion. Reflex testing is therefore done in specific midjoint range positions to produce the best response.

Muscle tone is achieved via normal stretch reflexes, which represent a muscle's tendency to maintain its original length whenever it is stretched. Sustained muscle tone facilitates quick, unsustained skilled muscle movement, such as that used in speech.

Resting muscle tone is easily changed in the intact nervous system by altering sympathetic nervous system output; reduced with deep relaxation (e.g., massage) or increased with anxiety or a state of alertness. Resting muscle tone can also be altered by strength training, producing musculoskeletal hypertrophy. Pathological nervous system conditions commonly alter both resting muscle tone as well as contractile ability of the muscle through disruption of the afferent and efferent pathways.

Muscle spindles serve as sensory receptors within the extrafusal (gross) muscles (Figure 5.18). They provide information on the status of the normal stretch mechanisms in muscle. The nonneural portion of the muscle spindle apparatus includes several thin muscle fibers, called intrafusal fibers, enclosed within a connective tissue capsule. The entire complex is arranged in parallel with the extrafusal muscle fibers. Two types of sensory endings are associated with the muscle spindle. First, annulospiral endings, supplied by thick, heavily myelinated $A\alpha$ axons, are wrapped around the center of the intrafusal fibers. They are dynamic (phasic) receptors encoding the velocity of muscle stretch. Second, flower spray endings, so called because of their appearance, are supplied by $A\beta$ axons and are slower conducting than the annulospiral endings. Flower

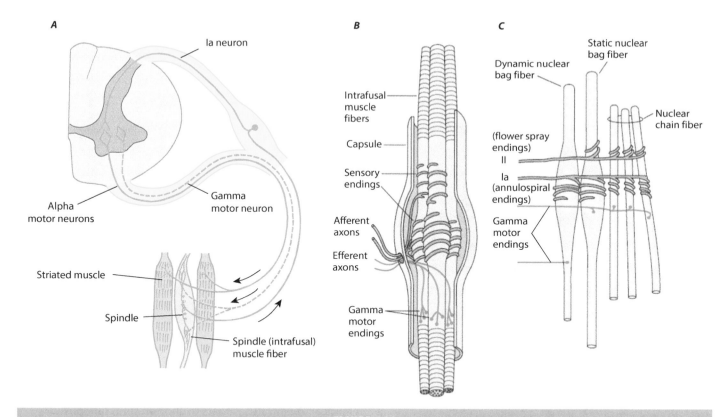

FIGURE 5.18

Connections and innervation of the muscle spindle apparatus. A. Innervation of extrafusal and intrafusal fibers and the muscle spindle. Extrafusal (striated muscle) fibers are innervated by α-motor neurons, and intrafusal fibers within muscle spindles are supplied by γ-motor neurons. Sensory annulospiral endings also distribute within the muscle spindle. (Reproduced with permission from Chapter 5. The Spinal Cord. In: Waxman SG. eds. Clinical Neuroanatomy, 27e New York, NY: McGraw-Hill; 2013). **B.** Muscle spindle apparatus within its collagenous capsule. Motor innervation is distributed to intrafusal muscle fibers at the contractile ends. Sensory innervation is distributed in the dilated, noncontractile central portion. **C.** A single Ia afferent fiber innervates all multiple fibers types to form a primary sensory ending (annulospiral endings). A group II sensory fiber innervates nuclear chain and static bag fibers to form a secondary sensory ending (flower spray endings). (**B, C**, From Chapter 12. Reflex and Voluntary Control of Posture & Movement. In: Barrett KE, et al, eds. Ganong's Review of Medical Physiology, 24e New York, NY: McGraw-Hill; 2012).

spray endings are static (tonic) receptors encoding moment-to-moment muscle length.

Muscle spindle intrafusal fibers possess motor innervation supplied by gamma-motor neurons (γ-motor neurons) (Figure 5.19). When a γ-motor neuron fires, it causes the muscle spindle fiber to contract. The shortening of the muscle spindle fiber is detected by the annulospiral endings in the muscle spindle. This results in sensory feedback to the spinal cord, where the sensory axons synapse on α-motor neurons. The α-motor neurons, in turn, send impulses back to extrafusal muscle fibers, stimulating them to contract simultaneously and proportionally with the contraction of the muscle spindle fibers. Once this parallel contraction takes place, the sensory receptor no longer detects shortening (i.e., the ending returns to its baseline rate of action potential firing); the loop is inactivated; and muscle tone is established. The muscle spindle is more complicated than the other encapsulated mechanoreceptors because it contains intrafusal muscle fibers, controlled by the central nervous system, that regulate the receptor neuron's sensitivity.

There is another deep mechanoreceptor, the Golgi tendon organ (Figure 5.14), which is entwined within the collagen fibers of tendon and is sensitive to the force generated by contracting muscle. Its rate of action potential firing increases with increasing force of muscular contraction. If the force exceeds its threshold, the Golgi tendon organ's central projections synapsing onto inhibitory interneurons inhibit α-motor neurons and halt muscle contraction (Figure 5.12). The Golgi tendon organ may also have a role in an individual's sense of how much effort it takes to produce a particular motor act. The muscle spindle and Golgi tendon organs play key roles in the reflex control of muscle contraction. The joints are innervated by mechanoreceptors, but those receptors play a greater role in sensing joint pressure and the extremes of joint motion than in proprioception.

Cortical direction does not directly participate in producing reflex movements; rather, a reflex is directed by local segmental circuitry. Motor neurons and DRG cells are the primary constituents of reflex arc, and loss of either component will abolish the reflex. Sensory inputs not only participate in the reflex loop but also send ascending collaterals toward the sensory cortex. In this way, reflex motor behaviors are separated from cortical direction, but the cortex remains aware of the sensory stimuli and directs complex, but delayed, subsequent behaviors. Thus the initial withdrawal from a hot plate is reflexive, and becoming aware of danger and moving away from it occur after recruiting cortical involvement.

Reflexes are categorized as superficial, deep, visceral, or primitive. Table 5.2 summarizes reflexes, the stimulus that activates them, and the behavior elicited by the stimulus. Although reflexes support movement and integrate it into normal function, they can also be impacted by nervous system damage. Careful testing can reveal damage to specific structures, as an intact reflex requires both normal afferent and efferent pathways. Reflexes can also be used to generate movement after conditions that impact volitional control.

Deep reflexes, also known as deep tendon reflexes, can be elicited with stretch to the muscle, resulting in a tendon distraction. They are commonly tested as part of a basic screening examination, as they provide measures of the competence of the CST and peripheral nerve performance. The best-known deep tendon reflex is the patellar (or myotatic) reflex elicited by using a reflex hammer to briskly tap the patellar tendon. The corresponding kick response is generated by a monosynaptic circuit involving the annulospiral

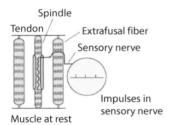

Spindle
Tendon — Extrafusal fiber
Sensory nerve
Impulses in sensory nerve
Muscle at rest

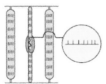

Muscle stretched

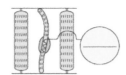

Muscle contracted

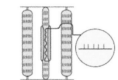

Increased γ efferent discharge

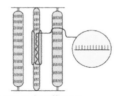

Increased γ efferent discharge—muscle stretched

FIGURE 5.19

Muscle spindle annulospiral ending discharge. Stretch of the muscle simultaneously stretches the spindle fibers and activates its sensory endings at a frequency proportional to the degree of stretching ("loading the spindle"). Without activation of γ-motor neurons, the intrafusal muscles would become flaccid, and spindle afferents would stop firing when the muscle contracts ("unloading the spindle"). Stimulation of γ-motor neurons causes the contractile ends of the intrafusal fibers to shorten simultaneously and proportionally with extrafusal muscle contraction. This stretches the intrafusal muscles, initiating impulses in sensory fibers. If the whole muscle is stretched during stimulation of the γ-motor neurons, the rate of discharge in sensory fibers is further increased. (Reproduced with permission from Barrett KE, et al. Chapter 12. Reflex and Voluntary Control of Posture & Movement. In: Barrett KE, et al., eds. Ganong's Review of Medical Physiology, 24e. New York, NY: McGraw-Hill; 2012).

Table 5.2 Reflexes

Type of Reflex	Stimulus	Motor Response	Typically Present from:
Primitive: Oral			
Rooting	Touch on either side of cheek, corner of mouth, center of upper lip	Turns head in direction of stimulus Mouth opens, seeking the stimulus	28 weeks–4 months
Sucking	Place nipple, finger, or object in mouth, centered on tongue	Divided into 3 steps: (1) Front of tongue laps on nipple (2) Back of tongue massages center of nipple (3) Esophagus pulls on tip of nipple	28 weeks–12 months
Swallowing	Liquid on back of mouth	Swallow	Persists
Gag	Touch back of throat	Esophagus tightens	19 weeks–persists
Cry	Discomfort	Nonspecific response to show discomfort	21 weeks–persists
Primitive: Facial			
Blink	Bright light, puff of air, loud noise	Eyes close	Birth–persists
Oculocephalic	Passively turn head	Eye movements lag behind head motion for seconds Seen with horizontal head turns, pull to sit	Birth–2 weeks
Nasal	Water in nose	Apnea to protect blood flow to heart and brain; other areas are shunted off	Birth–persists
Primitive: Startle			
Moro	In supine Gently drop in backward direction	Throws arms out in extension, then grimaces or cries	Birth–6 months
Startle	Noxious stimulus such as loud noise	Like the Moro, but elicit with Elbows remain flexed and hands fisted	Birth–persists
Primitive: General Body			
Palmar grasp	Place finger in open palm	Hand will close over finger; with attempted removal grip will strengthen	Birth–3 months
Plantar grasp	Stroke inner sole	Toes curl around ("grasp") examiner's finger	Birth–9 months
Babinski	Stroke outer sole	Toes spread, great toe dorsiflexion	Birth–2 years
Palmomental	Press palm	Mouth opens	Birth–6 months
Babkin	In supine Apply deep pressure to both palms	Mouth opens, eyes close, neck flexes May bring fist to mouth and suck a finger	Birth–4 months
Protective	Soft cloth is placed over the eyes and nose	Arches head and turns head side to side Brings both hands to face to swipe cloth away	Birth–4 months
Asymmetrical tonic neck (ATNR)	Head rotation	Ipsilateral UE extension, contralateral UE flexion	Birth–6 months

Symmetrical tonic neck (STNR)	Place in prone
	
	Passively extend or flex neck to produce bilateral symmetrical motor response of arms and legs
		With cervical extension:
		  UE extension, LE flexion
		With cervical flexion:
		  UE flexion, LE extension
			6 months–1 year

Crawling	Prone Stroke spine along side	Head extends, legs flex and begins reciprocal LE motion of crawling	Birth–4 months
Crossed adduction	Hold one leg in extension Rub sole of foot	The other leg will first flex, then extend/adduct with toe extension	Birth–8 months

(continued)

Table 5.2 Reflexes (*continued*)

Type of Reflex	Stimulus	Motor Response	Typically Present from:
Galant	In prone, stroke along one side of spine	Flexes whole body toward the stroked side	Birth–9 months
Head righting	In supine	Eyes open on coming to sitting (like a doll's) Head initially lags	Birth–3 months
	Grasp hands or arms and pull to sit up	Baby uses shoulders to right head position	
Placing	Hold upright Touch anterior tibia to edge of table	Knee and hip will flex to place foot on table	Birth–2 months
Standing	Hold upright Weight bearing evenly on both feet	Full lower extremity extension	Birth–4 months
Stepping	Hold upright	Alternate flexion and extension of lower extremities, as in walking	Birth (or by 2 months)–1 year
	Weight bearing evenly on both feet Lean forward, alternate pressure on sole of foot		
Later Emerging			
Auditory orienting	Sound	Turn head toward sound	Persists
Landau	Place prone	Arms and legs extend	5 months–1 year
Protective extension	Prone, head down	Arms reach out toward floor	5 months–persists
Tonic labyrinthine	Cervical extension Cervical flexion	Produces full body flexion Produces full body extension	Birth–4 years
Deep Tendon (myotactic): most commonly tested			
Biceps	Tap tendon with elbow at 90° flexion	Elbow flexes	Persists entire lifetime
Triceps	Tap tendon with elbow at 90° flexion	Elbow extends	Persists entire lifetime
Patellar	Tap tendon with knee flexed 90°	Knee extends	Persists entire lifetime
Ankle Jerk (Gastrocnemius/Soleus)	Tap tendon with ankle dorsiflexed to 5°	Ankle plantar flexes	Persists entire lifetime
Cutaneous			
Abdominal	Lightly stroke peri-abdominal region	Umbilicus deviates toward stimulus	Persists entire lifetime
Cremaster	Lightly stroke medial thigh	Contraction of ipsilateral cremaster muscle raises testis	Persists entire lifetime
Visceral Reflex			
Micturition	Urinary bladder stretched	Afferent firing increases, causing sensation of bladder fullness; reflexively relaxes urethra, contracts bladder to void	Birth to 3 years
Emesis	Mulitple stimuli possible, including: – Noxious smells – Vertigo – Touch to back of throat	Vomiting occurs	Persists entire lifetime

Table 5.3 Deep Tendon Reflex Scale

Scale	Response
0	No response
1+	Present but depressed; low normal
2+	Average; normal
3+	Increased, brisker than average; possibly, but not necessarily, abnormal
4+	Very brisk, hyperactive, clonus present; abnormal

sensory ending synapsing directly onto the α-motor neuron. The inverse stretch reflex provides for smooth, coordinated quadriceps contraction and leg extension by inhibiting antagonistic hamstring contraction. Without this inhibition, the patellar tendon tap would produce only isometric contraction and therefore no motion. Quality movement is only accomplished using inhibitory ventral horn interneurons, innervated by collaterals from the annulospiral endings, which suppress activation of neurons that drive antagonistic muscle contraction. It is important to note, however, that testing is done with joint position–specific standardized protocols based on measurements of motor responses over the range of the joint arc of motion.

A deep tendon reflex requires functioning sensory and motor innervation to that muscle segment, along with intact supraspinal inhibition to limit the reflex response. Deep tendon reflex responses are graded on a scale of 0, with no response, to 4+, indicating clonus, an uncontrollable repetition of the motor response. It is interesting to note that there are three categories of normal, ranging from low normal 1+ to normal 2+, to high normal 3+ (Table 5.3). This accounts for the normal variation in muscle tone between individuals, as well as changes throughout the day. Abnormal deep tendon reflex findings and their significance are described in the Spinal Cord Injury section.

Superficial reflexes produce motor responses to noxious cutaneous stimuli of either skin or mucous membranes. They are polysynaptic reflex loops with noxious information coded by the nociceptor carried into the dorsal horn, and a motor response generated locally to produce rapid movements, such as flexor withdrawal (and antagonistic extensor inhibition) in response to pain. Touching a hot stove activates thermal receptors in the hand, which activate a local reflex arc that produces a motor response to withdraw the hand. Thermal receptors also send collateral axons up the spinothalamic tract for cortical recognition and processing. The hand is withdrawn even before the cortex can elicit a response.

Another example of a protective reflex arc is the crossed extensor response associated with the flexor withdrawal after stepping on a piece of broken glass. The limb is withdrawn from the damage from the broken glass, but to avoid falling, the extensors in the opposite leg are activated to remain weight bearing. Collateral input from the initial nociceptor excites interneurons whose axons decussate and project to the contralateral ventral horn to activate the extensor motor neuron pool. Both flexor withdrawal and crossed extension are enduring primitive reflexes that contribute to early acquisition of reciprocal limb motion in the infant. The reflex is later integrated into normal function and typically suppressed except when called on in emergent situations, such as stepping on a painful object.

Visceral reflexes are essential for normal visceral function and also play a role in visceral pain during acute injury. A clinical test for appendicitis, called the rebound test, involves deep pressure exerted over the right lower quadrant at a point about halfway between the umbilicus and the anterior superior iliac spine (McBurney's point). Acute inflammation of the viscera will produce reflexive muscle spasm when the pressure is quickly removed, felt as exquisite tenderness and rigidity in the abdominal wall.

VII PRIMARY AND SECONDARY HYPERALGESIA

Nociception involves the transduction of damaging, or potentially damaging, stimuli to the CNS. Mechanical nociceptors respond to damaging tissue distortion and to the chemicals released from the traumatized tissue. Thermoreceptors are sensitive to cold below 5°C (41°F) and warmth greater than 45°C (113°F). Polymodal nociceptors are activated by noxious thermal or mechanical stimuli. Itch-sensitive receptors, or pruriceptors, respond to histamine. The morphology of these three classes of receptor endings is simple: they are free nerve endings only covered with a thin basal lamina produced by Schwann cells (Figure 5.14). In contrast to mechanoreceptors, with large-diameter, thickly myelinated axons (Aα and Aβ), nociceptors, thermoreceptors, and pruriceptors have small-diameter, thinly myelinated Aδ or unmyelinated C-fiber axons. A brief noxious stimulus initially evokes a sharp, pricking pain, sometimes termed "fast" pain, mediated by Aδ nociceptors, followed by a dull burning pain, termed "slow" pain, mediated by C-fiber nociceptors. Thermoreceptor axons also conduct action potentials in the Aδ and C-fiber ranges. Pruriceptors sensitive to irritants in the skin, thus triggering itch, use only C fibers. Visceral nociceptors, also called silent nociceptors, are activated by inflammation and chemical stimuli in the organ systems.

There has been much research on the mechanisms of transduction of noxious stimuli into depolarizing sensory potentials. Functional differences among the various nociceptor types are conferred, in part, by different receptor proteins inserted into the terminal membrane. Among these, the transient receptor potential vanilloid 1 (TRPV1) is the capsaicin (hot pepper) receptor. It is chemically and thermally heat-activated and mediates pain related to thermal stimuli as well as breakdown products found at the site of peripheral injury, such as H^+. Another nociceptive membrane receptor protein is the voltage-gated sodium channel Na(V)1.7, a major contributor in humans to pain signaling activated by noxious pressure. Mutations of the gene coding for Na(V)1.7 can result in patients who are congenitally insensitive to pain but still sensitive to other forms of touch. Congenital analgesia (congenital indifference to pain) results in children who are unaware of damage, often leading to more severe injury or life-threatening infection. The Mas-related G-protein-coupled receptor (Mrg) is activated by neuropeptide (e.g., substance P, calcitonin gene–related peptide [CGRP]) binding, as at an injury site. These are only a few possible nociceptive membrane receptors, but there are many more that are currently being examined for potential analgesic therapeutic use.

As anyone with a paper cut knows, there is an immediate sharp pain emanating from the exact location of the offending cut, followed a little while later by a duller, throbbing, burning pain from somewhere in the region of the cut. This demonstrates the dual nociceptive systems, one initially activated by the acute trauma, primary hyperalgesia; and the other, secondary hyperalgesia, activated later through neurogenic inflammation. There is anatomical and neurophysiological evidence that these two phases of pain perception are mediated in great part by two types of axons: Aδ; and C fibers. Aδ axons carry the fast, well-localized, pricking pain of primary hyperalgesia. Aδ axons are around 0.5–2.5 μm in diameter and only thinly myelinated. Their conduction velocity is relatively slow compared to larger, more heavily myelinated axons, but it is still more than five times faster than that of the unmyelinated C fibers carrying the signals that produce the longer lasting, poorly localized burning sensation that characterizes secondary hyperalgesia. Figure 5.20 is a simple illustration of the complex interactions that occur at an injury site, including tissue changes and activation of the innervation. At the site of tissue damage, a wide variety of tissue breakdown products and other neuroactive molecules is released. Among these are prostaglandins, proteases (enzymes), ATP, H+ (activating TRPV receptors), bradykinin, substance P, and CGRP (peptides activating Mrg-positive neurons).

Release and binding of the injury-related substances activate first the Aδ fibers, which rapidly carry the inputs centrally. Those inputs are transmitted to the second-order dorsal horn neurons, and the second-order axons decussate and build the spinothalamic tract. This wave of nociceptive input ascends to the ventroposterolateral (or ventroposteromedial for facial nociception) thalamic nucleus. This early pain perception is sharp and well localized and comprises primary hyperalgesia. The presence of those molecules in the damaged tissue causes a widespread subthreshold depolarization of endings in the area; tonic subthreshold depolarization means even innocuous stimuli activate high-threshold mechanoreceptors and cause pain. Activation of Aδ fibers and the tissue changes associated with the initial insult are often referred to as the primary flare, which includes inflammation, redness, heat, swelling, and decreased threshold to stimuli.

Secondary hyperalgesia is associated with longer-term changes in the tissue that are produced by efferent release of peptides from C fibers innervating the area immediately surrounding the primary flare in the area initial of damage. Incoming impulses from noxious stimuli activate some small DRG neurons with C-fiber axons in order to send impulses down the peripheral axon toward the injury site. Once there, neuropeptides such as substance P and CGRP are released from the nerve endings. Substance P causes mast cells to degranulate their histamine. Also, substance P and CGRP act as potent vasodilators and cause capillary walls to become "leaky." Tissue fluid is extravasated into the area, causing swelling, and increased blood flow also causes tissue to redden and become warm. Collectively, these neurogenic inflammatory changes make

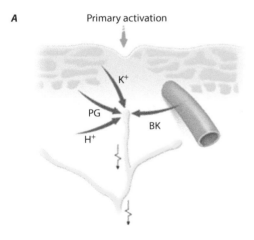

A Primary activation

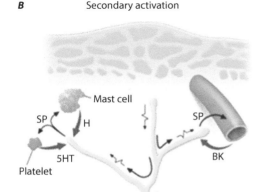

B Secondary activation

FIGURE 5.20

Events leading to activation, sensitization, and spread of sensitization of primary afferent nociceptor terminals. *A.* Primary activation. Tissue damage releases a variety of neuroactive chemicals at the injury site, including bradykinin and prostaglandins, which activate or sensitize nociceptors and produce the primary flare. Cell damage induces lower pH (H+) and leads to release of potassium (K+) and to synthesis of prostaglandins (PG) and bradykinin (BK). Prostaglandins increase the sensitivity of the terminal to bradykinin and other pain-producing substances. *B.* Secondary activation. Impulses generated in the stimulated terminal propagate not only to the spinal cord but also into other terminal branches, where they induce the release of peptides, including substance P (SP). Substance P causes vasodilation and neurogenic edema with further accumulation of bradykinin (BK). Substance P also causes the release of histamine (H) from mast cells and serotonin (5HT) from platelets. (From Somatosensory Neurotransmission: Touch, Pain, & Temperature. In: Barrett KE, et al., eds. Ganong's Review of Medical Physiology, 25e New York, NY: McGraw-Hill; 2016).

Table 5.4 Referred Pain Patterns

Affected Organ	Referred Site
Heart	Left shoulder and arm, neck, jaws
Liver	Right shoulder and neck, back, tip of scapula
Gall bladder	Upper right abdominal quadrant, right shoulder and neck, back, tip of scapula
Kidney	Back and abdomen below umbilicus down to pubis, and medial and lateral proximal thigh
Stomach	Back between scapulae
Urinary bladder	Coccyx, proximal medial thighs
Lung and diaphragm	Left neck

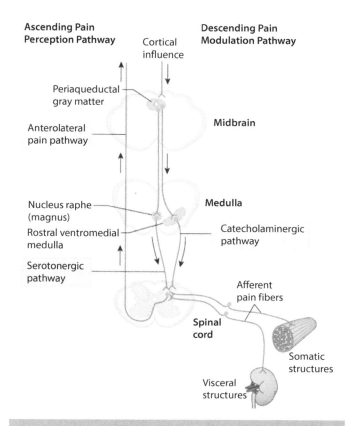

FIGURE 5.21

Illustration of the convergence-projection theory for referred pain and descending pathways involved in pain control. One hypothesis of the mechanism for referred pain involves convergence of somatic and visceral pain fibers on the same second-order neurons in the dorsal horn of the spinal cord. Rostral targets seldom receive noxious stimuli from viscera, therefore interpret the pain as arising from the somatic target. The periaqueductal gray (PAG) is a part of a descending pathway that includes serotonergic neurons in the nucleus raphé magnus and catecholaminergic neurons in the rostral ventromedial medulla to modulate pain transmission by inhibition of primary afferent transmission in the dorsal horn. (Reproduced with permission from Somatosensory Neurotransmission: Touch, Pain, & Temperature. In: Barrett KE, et al., eds. Ganong's Review of Medical Physiology, 25e New York, NY: McGraw-Hill; 2016.)

the secondary flare, also known as the axon reflex. These tissue changes maintain the nociceptors partially depolarized and sensitized so that even innocuous stimuli produce pain.

Acute pain results from tissue damage. It involves activation of nociceptive endings, nociceptive pathways peripherally and centrally, release of tissue breakdown products, anterograde (back to the site of injury) axon conduction, and rapid, reversible changes in the sensitivity of the nociceptors (hyperalgesia) as well as non-nociceptive A-fiber endings (allodynia) by alterations in gene expression. Although acute pain is related to damage to nociceptive endings and usually reverts to normal with time, if treated, chronic neuropathic pain persists well after the initial lesion is healed and involves changes in the CNS. These chronic pain states can be debilitating. They have both peripheral and CNS components, including maladaptive plasticity in the dorsal horn (see next section) and abnormal modulatory signals from the brain.

Referred Pain

Pain in the neck and left shoulder are well-known signs for myocardial infarction. Pain in a site remote from the site of actual damage is called referred pain. Referred pain is often observed in injuries or diseases producing visceral pain (Table 5.4), but it can also be present with muscle injury referring to other sites, such as tibialis anterior muscle pain referring to the ankle. The mechanism underlying this phenomenon remains elusive; however, the convergence-projection hypothesis is among the leading proposals (Figure 5.21). Afferent neurons supplying the affected organ and the nociceptor neurons innervating the referral area synapse on common dorsal horn neurons. The brain rarely encounters pain from the organ, so it interprets pain to arise from the referral area from which noxious inputs are more common.

VIII SPINAL CORD INJURY

Injury to the spinal cord may produce sensory, motor, and autonomic dysfunction. Levels and locations of spinal cord lesions can be identified based on clinical findings. Because of the degree of order in the long pathways, including somatotopic organization, injuries often produce predictable responses, or deficits. Spinal cord injury can be caused by either direct trauma or vascular insufficiency. With vascular insufficiency, hypoxia and edema follow and result in further tissue damage. Early intervention is key, with axonal transport compromised within a few hours and cord necrosis at 24 hours. Post-injury management with stabilizing body boards, spinal precautions that preclude any flexion or rotation, along with corticosteroid use to minimize edema, have improved post-traumatic outcomes.

Spinal shock, a temporary loss of all reflexes below the level of injury, is an early clinical finding after spinal injury. It consists of four distinct phases corresponding to neurological response to the injury. The initial phase of spinal shock lasts up to 24 hours and produces temporary loss of all reflexes (areflexia) below the level of injury. This initial reflex depression is due to a variety of factors such as dendrite and synapse retraction after injury, and metabolic changes reducing excitation and promoting inhibition. This phase ends with the return of polysynaptic reflexes, such as the bulbocavernosus reflex. During the brief second phase, injured neurons become more responsive to neurotransmitter release into the synapse, a condition known as denervation hypersensitivity. This promotes the return of monosynaptic cutaneous reflexes. During phase 3, which can last up to four weeks, new synapses begin to grow in the damaged areas, with local interneurons dominating. In the final phase, spinal shock resolves into a classic upper motor neuron presentation as newly developed local circuits are accompanied by loss of cortical inhibition.

Clinical examination during the early hours and days of recovery provides prognostic value, as return of reflexes and sensory function typically precedes volitional motor control. For example, return of pain sensation is prognostic for motor return due to the proximate lateral locations in the spinal cord of the spinothalamic tract and the lateral CST. The American Spinal Injury Association (ASIA) examination includes segmental dermatomal examination of pinprick (pain), light touch sensation, and motor function of one muscle selected from each myotome. For myotomes such as the trunk, with multiple segmental innervation (i.e., T2–L1), the motor level is considered the same as the sensory level.

Once the bulbocavernosus reflex has returned, terminating the initial phase of spinal shock, the spinal injury can be classified as complete or incomplete, based on function of the sacral segments. ASIA has developed an internationally accepted classification that describes traumatic spinal cord injuries, using categories including complete, incomplete, and level of injury. A complete neurologic impairment is defined as total absence of all sacral sensation and voluntary motor function. An incomplete lesion includes sacral sparing of either sensory or motor function, and carries potential for recovery above the lesion, in contrast to a complete lesion. Lesions are further categorized by strength quality of remaining motor function distal to the level of spinal cord injury. It is also common to see isolated improvement of nerve root function about the level of the injury, called root escape, which represents recovery of a concurrent peripheral nerve injury. Root escape is often clinically significant, providing additional function to the recovering patient.

Spinal cord injury varies depending on the local anatomy, with lower cervical spine injury typically more severe than upper, due to cord diameter changes from cephalad to caudad. Over half of upper cervical spine injuries result in no cord damage because the cord is smaller in the upper segments, occupying a third of the spinal canal, expanding to occupy half the canal in the lower cervical spine. When spinal cord damage does occur, the upper cervical spine produces the most severe clinical picture, causing loss of all motor and sensory function in the descending and ascending tracts. Visceral function is also impaired in a high cervical complete lesion, requiring use of a mechanical ventilator to replace the paralyzed diaphragm and alternative management of bowel and bladder function.

Upper Motor Neuron versus Lower Motor Neuron Lesions

Cortical motor neurons and their descending corticospinal tract axons, which drive effector (motor) neurons, comprise what are generally known as upper motor neurons. The ventral horn α-motor neurons (effector neurons) are then referred to as the lower motor neurons. Injury to upper motor neurons compared to lower motor neurons produces significant and predictably different motor sequelae: upper and lower motor neuron syndromes. Upper motor syndrome characteristics include elevated deep tendon reflexes (hyperreflexia); hypertonicity that delays muscle atrophy; and spasticity indicated by the presence of clonus, involuntary rhythmic contractions elicited by a brief passive stretch by the examiner. In addition, lesions of the CST result in the reemergence of primitive reflexes. The most commonly tested is the cutaneous Babinski sign, which is normally present in infancy, before maturation of the CST. In contrast, the characteristics of a lower motor neuron syndrome are diminished or abolished reflexes (hyporeflexia or areflexia), hypotonicity or flaccidity with rapid muscle atrophy, and a negative Babinski sign.

Determining Laterality of Deficits after Spinal Cord and Supraspinal Injuries

The spinal cord level and the side on which injury occurs (laterality) can be determined by comparing the distribution of sensory loss. Spinal injury at any single level results in different patterns of sensory impairments for touch and pain sensations, producing dissociated sensory loss. Loss of touch sensation occurs on the side ipsilateral to the injury. The most rostral dermatome in which sensation is impaired corresponds to the level of injury in the spinal cord. For pain sensation, the most rostral dermatome in which sensation is impaired is about two segments lower than the injured spinal cord level and on the side contralateral to the injury. This is because the axons of the anterolateral system decussate over a distance of one or two spinal segments before ascending through the brain stem to the diencephalon. A caudal extension of spared pain sensitivity is significant for patients with spinal cord injuries, serving a protective role, notifying the person of a wound or other injury.

Spinal Cord Injury Syndromes

There are several common clinical presentations after specific lesions to the spinal cord. These are central cord, anterior cord, Brown-Séquard, posterior cord, cauda equina, and conus medullaris syndrome. The syndromes relate to the area of spinal cord damage (Figure 5.22). Central cord syndrome occurs most frequently in people over age 65 with degenerative narrowing in the spinal canal, although it can happen in any population. The cause is severe neck hyperextension, producing swelling and damage to the central spinal cord. Due to the lateral orientation of the lower extremity and sacral tracts within the spinothalamic tract and the CSTs, this syndrome produces greater upper extremity deficits than lower extremities. The clinical presentation of the syndrome can vary from mild weakness or sensory changes, to severe paralysis.

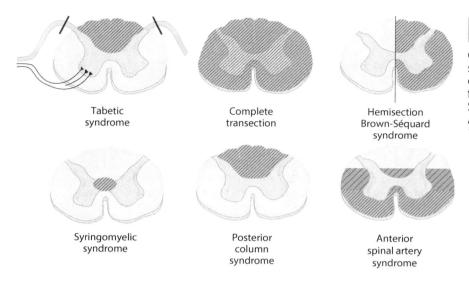

FIGURE 5.22

Characteristic spinal cord sensory syndromes (shaded areas indicate regions of damage). (Reproduced with permission from Ropper AH, et al. Chapter 9. Other Somatic Sensation. In: Ropper AH, et al, eds. Adams & Victor's Principles of Neurology, 10e. New York, NY: McGraw-Hill; 2014).

Trauma to the anterior spinal cord is typically produced by a flexion injury and occurs more often among younger people under age 35. In anterior cord syndrome the dorsal columns are preserved while the spinothalamic tract, the ventral horns, and often the CSTs are affected, abolishing pain and temperature sensation and volitional movement, with preserved proprioception, vibration, and deep pressure sensation.

A hemisection of the spinal cord produces Brown-Séquard syndrome, causing ipsilateral motor weakness associated with an upper motor neuron syndrome, and dissociated sensory deficits below the level of injury: ipsilateral loss of fine touch beginning at the level of injury, and contralateral loss of pain beginning one or two segments below the level of injury. Brown-Séquard syndrome is commonly due to a penetrating injury such as a stab wound, or a closed injury involving bony fracture and dislocation.

Posterior cord syndrome, rare among spinal cord injuries, is most commonly due to vascular disruption from trauma or disease. Patients present often with bilateral loss of discriminatory touch, vibration, and proprioception, sparing nociceptive and motor function. Once more common than today, tabes dorsalis, or tertiary syphilis, produces extensive demyelination in the dorsal column axons and impairment of those functions.

Injury to the caudal end of the spinal cord can produce either a conus medullaris or cauda equina syndrome. Injury to the fibers in the cauda equina produces radicular pain (radiating down the limb) and muscular weakness, both from involvement of lumbar level connections. Saddle anesthesia and bowel and bladder dysfunction arise from sacral segment damage. A lesion injuring the conus medullaris damages only sacral segments and produces back pain and bowel and bladder dysfunction without motor loss or anesthesia.

Frontiers of Research
Pharmacological and Nonpharmacologic Management of Spasticity

Spasticity is a complex and common clinical finding after spinal cord disruption. The loss of central inhibition produces an upper motor neuron syndrome with a classic presentation of increased reflexes, uncontrolled oscillatory motions (clonus), and increased resting muscle tone. This velocity-dependent resistance to motion provides challenges during motor control, as it can render the person unstable while reducing volitional control of the affected area. This commonly results in loss of function due to instability from weak muscles. Conversely, inherent muscle hypertonicity and resistance to movement limits joint motion and is associated with painful muscle contractions and permanent contractures. Clinically, many people living with upper motor neuron syndrome find a way to use the motion and elevated muscle tone produced by spasticity to produce motion or to create temporary stability during function. Therefore, controlling the amount of, rather than eliminating, spasticity is an area of ongoing medical research and interest.

All current treatment for spasticity management produces only temporary results. The most common management strategy is pharmacologic, with use of CNS inhibitors such as baclofen, diazepam, dantrolene, and tizanidine. These produce short-term reduction in muscle activation but carry side effects such as drowsiness, cognitive impairment, and muscle weakness. Treatment with the sedative baclofen at the local spinal level, called intrathecal baclofen, uses a programmable indwelling pump that is more specific and carries less general sedation; it is costly, however, and requires surgical implantation, which carries risk. Physical therapists are often involved in baclofen trials, which require several hours of observation. The physical therapist evaluates spasticity using a standardized measure several times over the trial, sharing findings with the patient and surgeon so that the ideal dosage can be determined. Use of Botulinum toxin A (BoNT) is also common, as this paralytic can be applied locally for management of focal spasticity. However, it also produces concurrent temporary paralysis, which limits function. Nonpharmacological management of spasticity is less effective; however, side effects are nearly absent. These physical interventions for treatment attempt to alter spasticity by affecting viscoelastic properties of connective tissue or altering the neural patterns of spasticity or spasms via gating, such as with pain. Examples of such physical interventions include use of sustained ice baths to the affected muscles and use of inhibitory compression or weight bearing on affected limbs, such as with prolonged standing.

CASE 5 DISCUSSION: Spinal Cord Injury

Bobby is now 30 years post spinal cord injury, and he reports his entire life has been changed in entirely unexpected ways by the injury. He credits his athletic background for his coping skills; as a child he excelled in individual sports and brought this desire to excel to the recovery process. His parents and friends were supportive and provided both emotional and social support. Bobby was fortunate to be at an inpatient rehabilitation facility that specialized in spinal cord injury recovery, with peer support groups and a multidisciplinary team. His physiatrist was warm and engaging, working to develop rapport and personalize his young patient's experience. His physical therapist knew just how hard to push him, keeping it fun and light. His intuitive occupational therapist provided emotional support and candid feedback during sessions that included learning bowel and bladder management. Bobby's level of injury at C5 made independent function particularly challenging due to absence of triceps function. His therapists taught him to externally rotate his shoulders with innervated scapular musculature and then use passive motion to lock his elbows into extension, either via gravity assistance or by placing his hands against a surface and pulling his torso away to extend his elbows.

Finally, his recreational therapist helped Bobby organize a wheelchair rugby team, which provided an athletic outlet and an entirely new social life. The first 15 years his spasticity was mild and very controllable, with occasional increase in response to irritations such as a mild skin burn or urinary tract infection. In recent years, the spasticity increased, waking him at night. He continues to refuse any medications for spasticity due to concerns regarding possible side effects including nerve pain. When interviewed for this textbook, Bobby offered the following advice to future health care providers.

Remember your patients are human. Get to know them by looking at personal items around the room and how they interact with their own friends and family. You can push your patient hard, but remember not everyone has good days in rehab and it's okay to acknowledge that as well.

REFERENCES

Al-Chaer ED, Feng Y, Willis WD. Comparative study of viscerosomatic input onto postsynaptic dorsal column and spinothalamic tract neurons in the primate. *J Neurophysiol.* 1999;82:1876–1882.

Altschuler SM, Bao XM, Bieger D, Hopkins DA, Miselis RR. Viscerotopic representation of the upper alimentary tract in the rat: sensory ganglia and nuclei of the solitary and spinal trigeminal tracts. *J Comp Neurol.* 1989;283(2): 248–268.

Amatya B, Khan F, La Mantia L, Demetrios M, Wade DT. Non pharmacological interventions for spasticity in multiple sclerosis. *Cochrane Database of Systematic Reviews.* 2013, Issue 2.

Andrew D, Craig AD. Spinothalamic lamina I neurons selectively sensitive to histamine: a central neural pathway for itch. *Nat Neurosci.* 2001;4:72–77.

Apkarian AV, Bushnell MC, Treede RD, Zubieta JK. Human brain mechanisms of pain perception and regulation in health and disease. *Eur J Pain.* 2005;9(4): 463–484.

Appelberg AE, Leonard RB, Kenshalo DR Jr., et al. Nuclei in which functionally identified spinothalamic tract neurons terminate. *J Comp Neurol.* 1979;188:575–586.

Arendt-Nielsen L, Svensson P. Referred muscle pain: basic and clinical findings. *Clin J Pain.* 2001 Mar;17(1): 11–19.

Belmonte C, Viana F. Molecular and cellular limits to somatosensory specificity. *Mol Pain.* 2008;4:14.

Benz EN, Hornby TG, Bode RK, Scheidt RA, Schmit BD. A physiologically based clinical measure for spastic reflexes in spinal cord injury. *Arch Phys Med Rehabil.* 2005;86:52–59.

Berkley KJ, Hubscher CH. Are there separate central nervous system pathways for touch and pain? *Nat Med.* 1995;1(8): 766–773.

Blomqvist A, Zhang ET, Craig AD. Cytoarchitectonic and immunohistochemical characterization of a specific pain and temperature relay, the posterior portion of the ventral medial nucleus, in the human thalamus. *Brain.* 2000;123(part 3): 601–619.

Boulenguez P, Liabeuf S, Bos R, et al. Down-regulation of the potassium-chloride cotransporter KCC2 contributes to spasticity after spinal cord injury. *Nat Med.* 2010;16(3): 302–307.

Brown AG. *Organization in the Spinal Cord: The Anatomy and Physiology of Identified Neurons.* New York: Springer, 1981.

Bushnell MC, Duncan GH, Hofbauer RK, Ha B, Chen JI, Carrier B. Pain perception: is there a role for primary somatosensory cortex? *Proc Natl Acad Sci USA.* 1999;96:7705–7709.

Chakrabarty S, Shulman B, Martin JH. Activity-dependent codevelopment of the corticospinal system and target interneurons in the cervical spinal cord. *J Neurosci.* 2009;29(27): 8816–8827.

Collins RD. *Illustrated Manual of Neurologic Diagnosis.* Philadelphia: Lippincott, 1962.

Cortright DN, Krause JE, Broom DC. TRP channels and pain. *Biochim Biophys Acta.* 2007;1772(8): 978–988.

Côté M-P, Gandhi S, Zambrotta M, Houle JD. Exercise modulates chloride homeostasis after spinal cord injury. *J Neurosci.* 2014;34(27): 8976–8987.

Cowie RA, Hitchcock ER. The late results of antero-lateral cordotomy for pain relief. *Acta Neurochir.* (Wien). 1982;64(1–2): 39–50.

Craig AD, Bushnell MC. The thermal grill illusion: unmasking the burn of cold pain. *Science.* 1994;265:252–255.

Crosby EC, Humphrey T, Lauer EW. *Correlative Anatomy of the Nervous System.* New York: Macmillan, 1962.

Danek A, Bauer M, Fries W. Tracing of neuronal connections in the human brain by magnetic resonance imaging in vivo. *Eur J Neurosci.* 1990;2: 112–115.

Dib-Hajj SD, Yang Y, Black JA, Waxman SG. The Na(V)1.7 sodium channel: from molecule to man. *Nat Rev Neurosci.* 2013 Jan;14(1): 49–62.

Dietz V. Spinal cord pattern generators for locomotion. *Clinical Neurophysiology.* 2003; (114): 1379–1389.

Ditunno JF, Little JW, Tessler A, Burns AS. Spinal shock revisited: a four-phase model. *Spinal Cord.* 2004;42, 383–395.

Dum RP, Strick PL. Medial wall motor areas and skeletomotor control. *Curr Opin Neurobiol*. 1992;2:836–839.

Dum RP, Strick PL. The origin of corticospinal projections from the premotor areas in the frontal lobe. *J Neurosci*. 1991;11:667–689.

Dum RP, Levinthal DJ, Strick PL. The spinothalamic system targets motor and sensory areas in the cerebral cortex of monkeys. *J Neurosci*. 2009, Nov 11;29(45):14223–14225.

Ellaway PH, Taylor A, Durbaba R. Muscle spindle and fusimotor activity in locomotion. *J Anat*. 2015 Aug;227(2): 157–166.

Fowler C, Griffiths D, de Groat WC. The neural control of micturition. *Nat Rev Neurosci*. 2008 Jun;9(6): 453–466.

Fitzgerald M. The development of nociceptive circuits. *Nat Rev Neurosci*. 2005;6(7): 507–520.

Friedman DP, Murray EA, O'Neil JB, Mishkin M. Cortical connections of the somatosensory fields of the lateral sulcus of macaques: evidence for a corticolimbic pathway for touch. *J Comp Neurol*. 1986;252:323–347.

Gandevia SC, Burke DA. Peripheral motor system. In: Paxinos G, Mai JK, eds. *The Human Nervous System*. London: Elsevier, 2004.

Gebhart GF. Descending modulation of pain. *Neurosci Biobehav Rev*. 2004;27(8):729–737.

Giboin LS, Lackmy-Vallée A, Burke D, Marchand-Pauvert V. Enhanced propriospinal excitation from hand muscles to wrist flexors during reach-to-grasp in humans. *J Neurophysiol*. 2012;107:532–543.

Giesler GJ Jr., Nahin RL, Madsen AM. Postsynaptic dorsal column pathway of the rat. I. Anatomical studies. *J Neurophysiol*. 1984;51:260–275.

Haeberle H, Lumpkin EA. Merkel cells in somatosensation. *Chemosens Percept*. 2008, Jun 1;1(2): 110–118.

Haggard P. Sensory neuroscience: from skin to object in the somatosensory cortex. *Curr Biol*. 2006, Oct 24;16(20): R884–R886.

Hakan Seçkin H, Ates O, Bauer A, Baskaya M. Microsurgical anatomy of the posterior spinal artery via a far-lateral transcondylar approach. *J Neurosurgery: Spine*. 2009;10 (3): 228–233.

Hall AC, Guyton JE. 2005. *Textbook of Medical Physiology*, 11th ed. Philadelphia: W.B. Saunders. pp. 687–690.

Han BS, Hong JH, Hong C, et al. Location of the corticospinal tract at the corona radiata in the human brain. *Brain Res*. 2010;1326:75–80.

Hayward V. A brief taxonomy of tactile illusions and demonstrations that can be done in a hardware store. *Brain Res Bull*. 2008, Apr 15;75(6): 742–752.

He SQ, Dum RP, Strick PL. Topographic organization of corticospinal projections from the frontal lobe: motor areas on the medial surface of the hemisphere. *J Neurosci*. 1995;15(5 Pt 1): 3284–3306.

Hendrik HD. Sucking pads and primitive sucking reflex. *J Neonatal Perinatal Med*. 2013, Jan 1;6(4): 281–283.

Holodny AI, Watts R, Korneinko VN, et al. Diffusion tensor tractography of the motor white matter tracts in man:current controversies and future directions. *Ann NY Acad Sci*. 2005;1064:88–97.

Hong JH, Son SM, Jang SH. Somatotopic location of corticospinal tract at pons in human brain: a diffusion tensor tractography study. *Neuroimage*. 2010;51(3): 952–955.

Hucho T, Levine JD. Signaling pathways in sensitization: toward a nociceptor cell biology. *Neuron*. 2007;55(3): 365–376.

Ikoma A, Steinhoff M, Stander S, Yosipovitch G, Schmelz M. The neurobiology of itch. *Nat Rev Neurosci*. Jul 2006;7(7): 535–547.

Jang SH. A review of corticospinal tract location at corona radiata and posterior limb of the internal capsule in human brain. *NeuroRehabilitation*. 2009;24(3):279–283.

Jankowska E, Lundberg A. Interneurons in the spinal cord. *Trends Neurosci*. 1981;4:230–233.

Jones EG. Organization of the thalamocortical complex and its relation to sensory processes. In: Darian-Smith I, ed. *Handbook of Physiology, Section 1: The Nervous System, Vol. 3: Sensory Processes*. Bethesda, MD: American Physiological Society, 1984:149–212.

Kass JH. Somatosensory system. In: Paxinos G, Mai JK, eds. *The Human Nervous System*. London: Elsevier, 2004.

Kim DG, Kim SH, Kim OL, Cho YW, Son SM, Jang SH. Long-term recovery of motor function in a quadriplegic patient with diffuse axonal injury and traumatic hemorrhage: a case report. *NeuroRehabilitation*. 2009;25(2):117–122.

Kumar A, Juhasz C, Asano E, et al. Diffusion tensor imaging study of the cortical origin and course of the corticospinal tract in healthy children. *AJNR Am J Neuroradiol*. 2009;30(10):1963–1970.

Kung C. A possible unifying principle for mechanosensation. *Nature*. 2005, Aug 4;436(7051):647–654.

Kuypers HGJM. Anatomy of the descending pathways. In: Brooks VB, ed. *Handbook of Physiology, Section 1: The Nervous System, Vol. 2, Motor Control*. Bethesda, MD: American Physiological Society, 1981:597–666.

Kuypers HGJM, Brinkman J. Precentral projections to different parts of the spinal intermediate zone in the rhesus monkey. *Brain Res*. 1970;24:151–188.

Kwon HG, Lee DG, Son SM, et al. Identification of the anterior corticospinal tract in the human brain using diffusion tensor imaging. *Neurosci Lett*. 2011;505:238–241.

Lackner JR, DiZio P.Vestibular, proprioceptive, and haptic contributions to spatial orientation. *Annu Rev Psychol*. 2005;56:115–147.

Langley JN. On axon-reflexes in the pre-ganglionic fibres of the sympathetic system. *J Physiol*. 1900, Aug 29;25(5): 364–398.

Latash M. Two archetypes of motor control research. *Motor Control*. 2010 July;14(3): e41–e53.

Liu M, Wood JN. The roles of sodium channels in nociception: implications for mechanisms of neuropathic pain. *Pain Medicine*. 2011;12:S93–S99.

MacKay-Lyons M. Central pattern generation of locomotion: a review of the evidence. *Phys Ther*. 2002;82:69–83.

Maricich SM, Wellnitz SA, Nelson AM, et al. Merkel cells are essential for light-touch responses. *Science*. 2009, Jun 19;324(5934): 1580–1582.

Mesulam MM, Mufson EJ. Insula of the old world monkey. Ill: Efferent cortical output and comments on function. *J Comp Neurol*. 1982;212:38–52.

Michael-Titus A. *Nervous System: Systems of the Body Series*. London: Churchill Livingstone, 2007.

Mirbagheri M, Alibiglou L, Thajchayapong M, Rymer WZ. Muscle and reflex changes with varying joint angle in hemiparetic stroke. *J NeuroEngineering and Rehabilitation*. 2008;5:6.

Morecraft RJ, Herrick JL, Stilwell-Morecraft KS, et al. Localization of arm representation in the corona radiata and internal capsule in the non-human primate. *Brain*. 2002;125:176–198.

Muratori LM, Lamberg EM, Quinn L, Duff SV. Applying principles of motor learning and control to upper extremity rehabilitation. *J Hand Ther*. 2013;26(2): 94–103.

Nicolson T. Fishing for key players in mechanotransduction. *TINS*. 2005 Mar;28(3):140–144.

Noble R, Riddell JS. Cutaneous excitatory and inhibitory input to neurones of the postsynaptic dorsal column system in the cat. *J Physiol*. 1988;396:497–513.

Olausson H, Lamarre Y, Backlund H, et al. Unmyelinated tactile afferents signal touch and project to insular cortex. *Nat Neurosci*. 2002;5(9):900–904.

Palecek J. The role of dorsal columns pathway in visceral pain. *Physiol Res*. 2004;53(Suppl 1):S125–S130.

Penfield W, Rasmussen T. *The Cerebral Cortex of Man: A Clinical Study of Localization of Function*. New York: Macmillan, 1950.

Percheron G. Thalamus. In: Paxinos G, Mai JK, eds. *The Human Nervous System*. London: Elsevier, 2004, pp. 592–676.

Picard N, Strick PL. Imaging the premotor areas. *Curr Opin Neurobiol*. 2001;11:663–672.

Pierrot-Deseilligny E, Burke D. *The Circuitry of the Human Spinal Cord*. Cambridge, UK: Cambridge University Press, 2005.

Purves D, Augustine GJ, Fitzpatrick D, Hall WC, LaMantia A, McNamara JO, White LE. *Neuroscience*, 4th ed. Sunderland, MA: Sinauer. 2008.

Review of Clinical and Functional Neuroscience. n.d. Site editor: Rand Swenson, Dartmouth Medical School. https://www.dartmouth.edu/~rswenson/NeuroSci/.

Roland PE, Zilles K. Functions and structures of the motor cortices in humans. *Curr Opin Neurobiol.* 1996;6:773–781.

Ross ED. Localization of the pyramidal tract in the internal capsule by whole brain dissection. *Neurology.* 1980;30:59–64.

Schell GR, Strick PL. The origin of thalamic inputs to the arcuate premotor and supplementary motor areas. *J Neurosci.* 1984;4:539–560.

Solinski HJ, Gudermann T, Breit A. Pharmacology and signaling of MAS-related G protein-coupled receptors. *Pharmacol Rev.* 2014 Jul;66(3):570–597.

Szolcsányi J. Capsaicin and sensory neurones: a historical perspective. *Prog Drug Res.* 2014;68:1–37.

Taricco M, Adone R, Pagliacci C, Telaro E. Pharmacological interventions for spasticity following spinal cord injury. *Cochrane Database of Systematic Reviews.* 2000;2:CD001131.

Tremolizzo L, Susani E, Lunetta C, Corbo M, Ferrarese C. Appollonio I. Primitive reflexes in amyotrophic lateral sclerosis: prevalence and correlates. *J Neurol.* 2014;261:1196–1202.

Wang CC, Willis WD, Westlund KN. Ascending projections from the area around the spinal cord central canal: a Phaseolus vulgaris leucoagglutinin study in rats. *J Comp Neurol.* 1999;415(3):341-367.

Willis WD, Al-Chaer ED, Quast MJ, Westlund KN. A visceral pain pathway in the dorsal column of the spinal cord. *Proc Natl Acad Sci USA.* 1999;96(14):7675–7679.

Willis WD, Kenshalo DR Jr., Leonard RB. The cells of origin of the primate spinothalamic tract. *J Comp Neurol.* 1979;188:543–574.

Willis WD Jr., Westlund KN. The role of the dorsal column pathway in visceral nociception. *Curr Pain Headache Rep.* 2001;5(1): 20–26.

Woolf CJ, Ma Q. Nociceptors—noxious stimulus detectors. *Neuron.* 2007;55(3):353–364.

Woolf CJ, Salter MW. Neuronal plasticity: increasing the gain in pain. *Science.* 2000;288:1765.

Yousif N, Cole J, Rothwell J, Diedrichsen J. Proprioception in motor learning: lessons from a deafferented subject. *Exp Brain Res.* 2015 Aug;233(8): 2449–2459.

 REVIEW QUESTIONS

1. Which of the following receptors mediates vibration sense?
   A. Thermal receptor
   B. Pacinian corpuscle
   C. Ruffini corpuscle
   D. Meissner's corpuscle

2. A 30-year-old male was driving a motorcycle when he swerved off the road and suffered a severe spinal cord injury. On neurological examination he was noted to have lost the sense of touch on his right leg and lower abdomen to the level of the umbilicus. He also lost pain sensation. Select from the following to describe the side of cord injury and lowest dermatomal level of remaining pain sensation: side of spinal cord at the ___ spinal segment.
   A. Left, T10
   B. Left, L1
   C. Right, L1
   D. Right, T10

3. Pain signals from caudal visceral structures ascend within which spinal pathway?
   A. Cuneate fascicle
   B. Gracile fascicle
   C. Anterolateral column
   D. Ventral column

4. Small-diameter afferent fibers terminate within which region of the spinal cord gray matter?
   A. Ventral horn
   B. Superficial laminae of the dorsal horn
   C. Deep layers of the dorsal horn
   D. Intermediate zone

5. Which of the following statements best describes a key feature of the reticulospinal tracts?
   A. They are components of the lateral descending pathways.
   B. They descend to the cervical spinal cord only.
   C. They originate from the medulla.
   D. They regulate autonomic behaviors.

6. The enlargement segments correspond to which of the following?
   A. Thoracic segments
   B. Segments containing the dorsal nucleus of Clarke
   C. Segments innervating the trunk
   D. Segments innervating the limbs

7. Occlusion of cortical branches of the anterior cerebral artery would disrupt motor control of which of the following regions?
   A. Foot
   B. Arm
   C. Neck
   D. Face

8. Your patient with low back pain reports use of adult diapers due to intermittent loss of bladder control. You suspect:
   A. injury to the thoracic spine.
   B. central cord syndrome.
   C. compression of the cauda equina.
   D. conus medullaris syndrome.

9. A proper reflex requires all of the following *except*:
   A. α-motor neuron.
   B. γ-motor neuron.
   C. Golgi tendon organ.
   D. annulospiral ending.

10. Hours after cutting his finger on a small piece of glass, a boy notices that the area around the cut burns and aches. What aspect of pain perception is active?
    A. Activation of C-fiber nociceptors associated with secondary hyperalgesia
    B. Activation of Aδ nociceptors associated with primary hyperalgesia
    C. Sharp, well localized pain sensation
    D. Activation of thickly myelinated axons with fast conduction

CHAPTER 6

The Brainstem, Cranial Nerves, and Visual Pathways

Maryke Neiberg*, Victoria Graham, and Tony Mosconi

> **CASE 6** **Cavernous Malformation in the Pons**

Sean thought it was odd when the tip of his right thumb went numb. He was playing soccer at San Jose State University, looking forward to getting one of the two coveted goalkeeper scholarships in the upcoming year. Over the next few weeks, he was increasingly tired and less athletic, and couldn't focus or jump. The numbness spread down the entire right side of his body, becoming painful, like someone digging into him. He rapidly lost the ability to walk, and his right hand "shriveled up." His family flew out to be with him, as he was initially diagnosed with a possibly fatal brainstem tumor. A subsequent MRI found a cavernous malformation in his pons. A cavernous malformation is a mass of abnormal blood vessels that appear as distended or dilated chambers. They tend to bleed slowly due to inadequate connective tissue support and poor quality smooth muscle and elastin that normally maintain vascular integrity. This low-flow lesion is differentiated from a high-flow cerebral arteriovenous malformation (AVM), which occurs when the normal capillary bed separating arteries and veins is absent, causing high-pressure distention of veins, which can burst, causing headaches, seizures, or stroke. Heavily sedated after the surgery, Sean barely recalls the four days in the hospital. However, the two weeks in the neurorehabilitation unit were miserable, with a bleak room, poor sleep quality, terrible food, and impossible therapy. Sean liked the therapists, but he couldn't do anything they asked, and it was frustrating to constantly fail. In retrospect, he is incredibly grateful for the rehabilitation and credits his early recovery to services received, which allowed him to return home and continue his progress. The rehabilitation team worked on his recovery from damage to structures located within the pons and surrounding tissues. Speech therapy focused on compensatory strategies to manage his slurred speech (dysarthria), as he lost motor and sensory function on the left side of his face and around the mouth. Occupational therapy focused on food management due to loss of distal tongue sensation. To this day, Sean feels no difference between a fork and a finger, and must be careful with hot beverages that simply feel warm and cold beverages that register as painful. Fortunately, taste sensation was preserved. On the right side of his body, he had altered perception of pain and temperature, arm weakness, and spasticity. Postoperatively he reported poor balance and experienced a change of vision in his left eye, describing it as perceiving only color, but not image, when looking through that eye.

*Maryke Neiberg, OD, FAAO, Massachusetts College of Pharmacy and Health Sciences, School of Optometry, Boston, MA

I OVERVIEW OF KEY CONCEPTS

This chapter continues the ascension toward the brain. The brainstem extends from the rostral midbrain through the caudal medulla and contains, in addition to the long pathways described previously, nuclei associated with the lower 10 cranial nerves, embedded within the reticular formation. The reticular formation communicates extensively with ascending and descending long pathways as well as with the cranial nerve nuclei that are embedded within it.

Each cranial nerve (CN) has been given a numeric designation, I–XII in a rostral to caudal progression, starting with CN I (olfactory), which is an oft-neglected nerve with significant diagnostic value, and ending with CN XII (hypoglossal), which controls the tongue (Figure 6.1). Notably, half of the cranial nerves work together to control vision and eye movement. Eyelid opening and closing are carried on cranial nerves III (oculomotor) and VII (facial), respectively; tear production is also on CN VII. CN V, the trigeminal nerve, forms the sensory limb of the corneal (blink) reflex; and CN VII, the motor limb. Cranial nerves controlling eye movement include CN III (oculomotor), CN IV (trochlear), and CN VI (abducens), which incorporate positional sensory information regarding head motion, supplied by the vestibular division of CN VIII (vestibulocochlear), to place the image precisely on the retina. Finally, visual information is carried proximally along CN II, (optic) for processing and interpretation in the brainstem, diencephalon, and cortex. Development of such an intricate and accurate visual sensorimotor system, complete with protective reflexes, attests to the importance of sight in the success of our species. Understanding sensory and motor aspects of vision is essential for all healthcare providers; recently it as been reported that alterations in vision and eye movements can identify mild traumatic brain injury and concussion, even in the absence of other clinical findings. Thus, visual functions are discussed in detail in this chapter.

Assessment of cranial nerve function is important for tracking therapeutic progress after nervous system damage in addition to making clinical diagnosis. Pathology produces classic presentations based upon the laterality of the lesion and the anatomic distribution of long pathways and CN nuclei at the injury site, allowing for relatively precise localization of the damage based on clinical findings. Clinical assessment of cranial nerve function requires practice and a solid understanding of what is normal; refer to Appendix for cranial nerve testing procedures, along with video demonstrations.

II DESCENDING CONTROL OF MOTOR CRANIAL NERVES: THE CORTICOBULBAR TRACT

As discussed in Chapter 5, the corticospinal tract drives motor functions in the body. Most of the cranial nerves have significant motor components directed by the cerebral cortex through a descending pathway known as the corticobulbar tract (CBT),

arising from the portion of the primary motor cortex containing the face representation (Figure 6.2). The CBT descends through the genu of the internal capsule, continues through the medial portion of the middle two-fourths of the crus cerebri into the medial part of the pons, and ends part way down the medulla in the medial part of the pyramids.

Among the motor nuclei receiving CBT innervation are the oculomotor (CN III), trochlear (CN IV), and the abducens (CN VI), all of which control extraocular eye movements; the motor component of the trigeminal nerve (CN V), which directs primarily the muscles of mastication; the facial nerve (CN VII), which controls muscles of facial expression; the glossopharyngeal (CN IX) and vagus (CN X) nerves supplying muscles of deglutition and phonation; and the hypoglossal nerve (CN XII), which has its complete distribution to tongue muscles CN nuclei. Cranial nerve XI, the spinal accessory nerve, is an atypical cranial nerve that has most of its motor neurons in the upper cervical spinal cord; it is supplied by the corticospinal tract.

The facial motor nucleus has two divisions, one containing motor neurons to the upper half of the face, innervating the orbicularis oculi as well as the muscles moving the eyebrows and forehead. The lower division contains neurons that control the muscles of the lower half of the face, including muscles that produce the nasolabial fold and those that move the mouth (Figure 6.3). The CBT provides bilateral innervation to CNs III and IV, the motor division of CN V, CN VI, and to the upper division of CN VII. Because of this redundant bilateral innervation of the nuclei associated with control of extraocular eye muscles, CBT lesions typically do not produce clinically observable deficits in eye movements. This bilateral CBT innervation also preserves eye-protective reflexes such as the corneal (blink) reflex. Thus observation of eye movement provides significant information about the localization of the lesion. Peripheral lesions produce classic motor deficits; eye turned "down-and-out," lateral gaze palsy for example. Motor problems associated with central lesions are often subtler and may be related to aberrant sensorimotor processing, such as impaired convergence seen after concussion. From the lower division of CN VII down through the CN XII, CBT projections are predominantly contralateral.

Knowledge of this connectivity provides profound diagnostic value, as a lesion of the CBT above the upper face division in CN VII motor nucleus will paralyze only the contralateral lower half of the face, whereas facial nerve injury can produce a complete ipsilateral facial paralysis (Figure 6.4).

This diagnostic presentation differentiates a central facial palsy due to injury to the CBT from a peripheral facial palsy produced by injury to the facial nerve. Presentation of a lower face paralysis will, therefore, provide laterality to the lesion (contralateral) as well as exclude the medulla from potential localization of the lesion.

A CBT lesion also generates paralysis of contralateral pharyngeal and laryngeal muscles from denervation of nucleus ambiguus and loss of CN X somatic motor function. Normally, upon phonation,

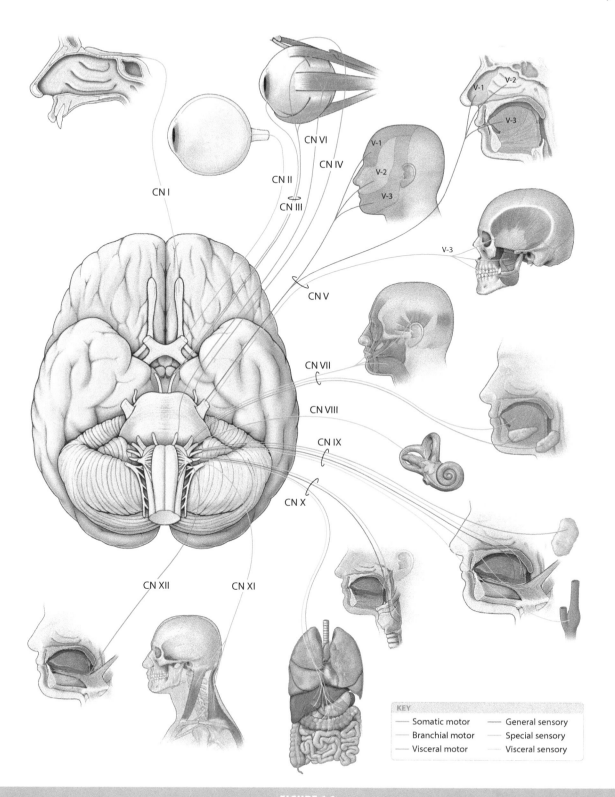

KEY
— Somatic motor — General sensory
— Branchial motor — Special sensory
— Visceral motor — Visceral sensory

FIGURE 6.1

Overview of the Cranial Nerves. Twelve cranial nerves with schematic of their basic functions. (Reproduced with permission from Chapter 17. Cranial Nerves. In: Morton DA, Foreman K, Albertine KH. eds. *The Big Picture: Gross Anatomy* New York, NY: McGraw-Hill; 2011).

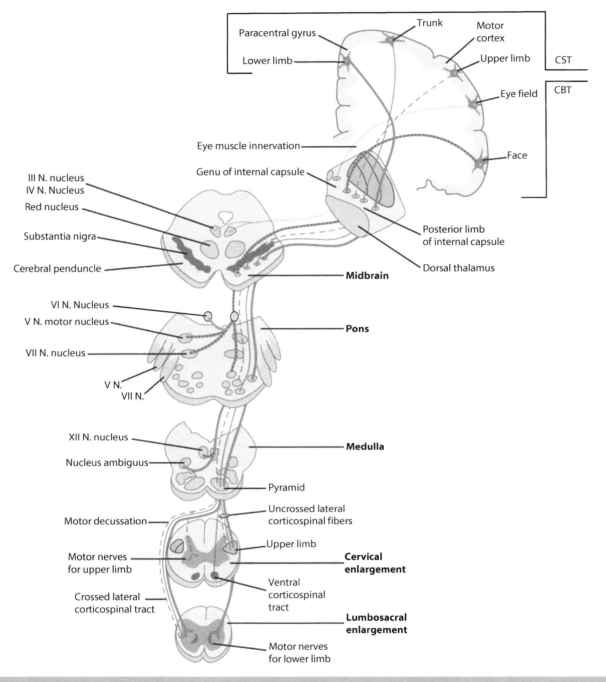

FIGURE 6.2

Schematic illustration of upper motor neuron pathways. CST = corticospinal tract; CBT = corticobulbar tract. (Reproduced with permission from Chapter 3. Motor Paralysis. In: Ropper AH, Samuels MA, Klein JP. eds. *Adams & Victor's Principles of Neurology*, 10e New York, NY: McGraw-Hill; 2014).

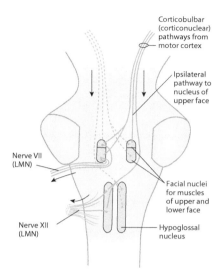

FIGURE 6.3

Corticobulbar pathways to the nuclei of cranial nerves VII and XII. Notice that portion of the facial nucleus representing muscles of the upper face receives bilateral descending input, whereas the portion representing lower facial muscles receives input from only the contralateral cortex. (Reproduced with permission from Chapter 7. The Brain Stem and Cerebellum. In: Waxman SG. eds. *Clinical Neuroanatomy*, 27e New York, NY: McGraw-Hill; 2013).

both palatoglossal arches rise, with the uvula maintained in the midline. With a CBT lesion, the contralateral vagus innervation of the palate is lost, producing paralysis of the palatoglossal arch. Upward movement of only one side of the palate draws the uvula toward the healthy side of the palate, and deviation of the uvula toward the side of the central lesion. In contrast, a peripheral lesion of CN X generates ipsilateral paralysis and deviation of the uvula contralateral to the vagus nerve injury. Weakness of palatal and pharyngeal muscles produces difficulty swallowing and a tendency to choke on food or water, called dysphagia. In addition, reduced function of laryngeal muscles produces a hoarse voice with diminished volume, which is called dysphonia.

Movements of the tongue can be somewhat more confusing, particularly when discussing deficits. The main muscle for protrusion of the tongue is the genioglossus, innervated, as are nearly all of the glossal muscles, by the hypoglossal nerve, CN XII. The genioglossus muscle pulls the tongue forward (protrudes it). When one side of the tongue is paralyzed, only the healthy genioglossus can pull the tongue forward, and the weak side of the tongue remains behind. Neuroanatomists often describe "deviation of the tongue" toward the impaired side upon protrusion, a behavior not typically

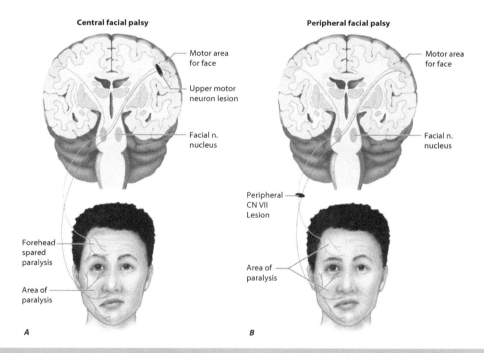

FIGURE 6.4

Cranial nerve VII central and peripheral facial palsies. *A.* Central CBT Lesion. Loss of crossed fiber innervation only to the lower face representation in the facial nucleus produces contralateral lower face paresis, sparing forehead function in an upper motor neuron lesion while, identifying this presentation as a central facial palsy. *B.* Peripheral CN VII lesion causes ipsilateral paresis of both upper and lower facial muscles. (Reproduced with permission from Jauch EC, White DR, Knoop KJ. EAR, NOSE, AND THROAT CONDITIONS. In: Knoop KJ, Stack LB, Storrow AB, Thurman R. eds. *The Atlas of Emergency Medicine*, 4e New York, NY: McGraw-Hill, 2016).

performed in polite company. Clinically, the patient loses the ability to clear food from the cheek on the same side as the weak tongue; this is due to loss of function of the more lateral tongue muscles, the styloglossus and hyoglossus. CBT lesions produce weakness in the *contralateral* half of the tongue, while peripheral injury of CN XII produces difficulties of movement on the *ipsilateral* side. In both central and peripheral lesion locations, tongue paralysis causes dysarthria, and prolonged paralysis of tongue muscles leads to substantial atrophy visible upon examination.

BRAINSTEM

The brainstem acts as an information superhighway, relaying ascending sensory and descending motor information related to virtually all somatic functions. Named for its stalklike (bulbar) shape, the brainstem extends from the midbrain rostrally down through the medulla caudally. Cranial nerve nuclei are distributed in functionally related, discontinuous columns through the brainstem in a pattern developed embryonically, as discussed in Chapter 4 (Figure 6.5).

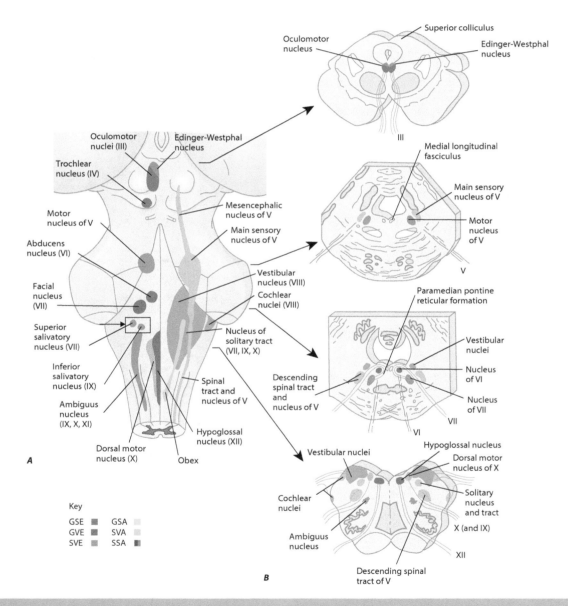

FIGURE 6.5

Cranial nerve nuclei. A. Dorsal view of the human brain stem with the positions of the cranial nerve nuclei projected onto the surface. Motor nuclei are on the left; sensory nuclei are on the right. **B.** Transverse sections at the levels indicated by the arrows. The Key details the colors of the different functional nuclear columns. (Reproduced with permission from Chapter 7. The Brain Stem and Cerebellum. In: Waxman SG. eds. *Clinical Neuroanatomy*, 27e New York, NY: McGraw-Hill; 2013).

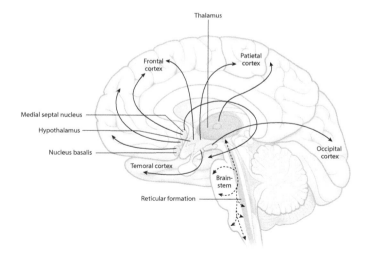

Reticular activating system. Sagittal section through the human brain showing the ascending reticular activating system in the brainstem, with projections to the intralaminar nuclei of the thalamus, and the output from the intralaminar nuclei to many parts of the cerebral cortex. (Reproduced with permission from Electrical Activity of the Brain, Sleep–Wake States, & Circadian Rhythms. In: Barrett KE, et al., eds. *Ganong's Review of Medical Physiology*, 25e New York, NY: McGraw-Hill, 2016).

Reticular Formation

The brainstem neuropil, the relatively homogeneous core of the brainstem, contains a collection of cell clusters (subtle nuclei) and an extensive cellular and axonal network that comprises the reticular formation (RF). Virtually all ascending sensory, descending motor, and local circuit pathways interact with the broadly distributed RF nuclei. The cranial nerve nuclei, which is discussed in greater detail below, are also embedded within this scaffold. The RF can be divided into functionally distinct portions: rostrally related to consciousness, awareness, and arousal (the reticular activating system) (Figure 6.6); and caudally to regulation of vital functions and patterned behaviors. It can be further organized into medial, intermediate, and lateral nuclear columns employing different neurotransmitters to accomplish those different functions. More than 60 neurotransmitters have been identified, with the major neurotransmitters discussed in Table 6.1.

TABLE 6.1 Major Neurotransmitters

Chemical Group	Neurotransmitter	Mechanism of Action	Function	Pathology
Acetylcholine	Acetylcholine	Excitatory	Muscle contraction Cortical neuroplasticity Hormone excretion Short term memory Emotion, learning, sleep, and wakefulness	Alzheimer's disease
Catchecolamines	Epinephrine	Excitatory	Flight-or-fight response	Anxiety disorders, social withdrawal, and depression
	Norepinephrine	Excitatory	Blood vessel constriction Increase in heart rate Attentiveness, emotions, circadian rhythm, sleeping, dreaming, and learning	Mood disorders, PTSD, and Parkinson's disease
	Dopamine	Excitatory and Inhibitory	Movement and posture control Mood modulator Cognitive control and working memory Reward/reinforcement and dependency	Parkinson's disease ADHD Schizophrenia
Monoamine	Serotonin	Excitatory/Inhibitory	Body temperature regulation Sleep, mood, appetite, and pain Decision making behaviors	Depression, suicide, impulsivity, and aggression

(continued)

TABLE 6.1 Major Neurotransmitters (*continued*)

Chemical Group	Neurotransmitter	Mechanism of Action	Function	Pathology
Amino Acids	Glycine	Mainly inhibitory, some excitatory	Processing of motor and sensory information for movement, vision, and hearing	Inborn errors of metabolism
	Gamma-Aminobutyric acid (GABA)	Inhibitory	Motor control Vision	Epilepsy, sleep disorders
	Glutamate and Aspartate	Excitatory	Learning and memory	Alzheimer's disease Autism OCD Schizophrenia Neurotoxicity
Neuropeptides	Substance P, somatostatin, neuropeptide-Y, calcitonin-related gene product (CGRP), etc.	Neuromodulators	Enhance or inhibit the effects of neurotransmitters	
	Histamine	Neuromodulator	Controls arousal, gastric secretion, cardiac stimulation, learning, memory, and peripheral allergic response	
Soluble gasses	Nitrous Oxide			

IV REGIONAL OVERVIEW

The brainstem is composed of three regions, from rostral to caudal, the midbrain, the pons, and the medulla. The cerebral aqueduct is the ventricular structure associated with the midbrain. The pons lies inferior to the midbrain, and the medulla below that, with the fourth ventricle extending posteriorly from rostral pons through caudal medulla (Figures 6.7 and 6.8).

Midbrain

The external features that define the midbrain include the crus cerebri anteriorly and the corpora quadrigemina (paired superior and inferior colliculi) posteriorly. The midbrain can be divided into three regions: the tectum, tegmentum, and basis pedunculi. The tectum (roof) can be found at the dorsal surface of the midbrain, where the superior and inferior colliculi reside. The superior colliculus is a layered structure that acts as a visual reflex center. The superficial layers primarily receive information from the retina and visual cortex, and the deeper layers receive projections from auditory and somatosensory systems, resulting in a complex interaction of motor and sensory information to orient the head and eyes in response to stimuli. Its function is primarily a reflexive response to turn the head in the same direction as a perceived flash of light, via a crossed spinotectal pathway, to facilitate foveation (aligning the most sensitive part of the eye, the macula or fovea, with the object of interest).

The inferior colliculi are involved in processing sounds and localization of sounds in space. The pineal gland is located between the two superior colliculi, just above the tectum. The function of the pineal gland is primarily to secrete melatonin, a hormone associated with sleep regulation and our circadian rhythm. It has also been associated with reproductive and immune function. Cranial nerves III and IV emerge from their nuclei in the midbrain.

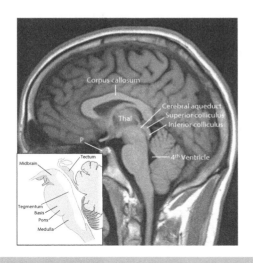

FIGURE 6.7

Midsagittal MRI of a normal brain. Midline sagittal T1-weighted MRI of the brain. Note that white matter appears brighter than gray matter and the corpus callosum is well defined. The pons, medulla, and cervicomedullary junction are well delineated, and the pituitary gland is demonstrated with a normal posterior pituitary bright spot (P). The cerebral aqueduct is seen between the ventral midbrain and the tectum with the superior and inferior colliculi. *Inset.* Drawing of the divisions of the brain stem in a midsagittal plane. The major internal longitudinal divisions are the tectum, tegmentum, and basis. The major external divisions are the midbrain, pons, and medulla. (Image: Reproduced with permission from Chapter 2. Imaging, Electrophysiologic, and Laboratory Techniques for Neurologic Diagnosis. In: Ropper AH, Samuels MA, Klein JP. eds. *Adams & Victor's Principles of Neurology*, 10e New York, NY: McGraw-Hill; 2014.; Inset: Reproduced with permission from Chapter 7. The Brain Stem and Cerebellum. In: Waxman SG. eds. *Clinical Neuroanatomy*, 27e New York, NY: McGraw-Hill; 2013).

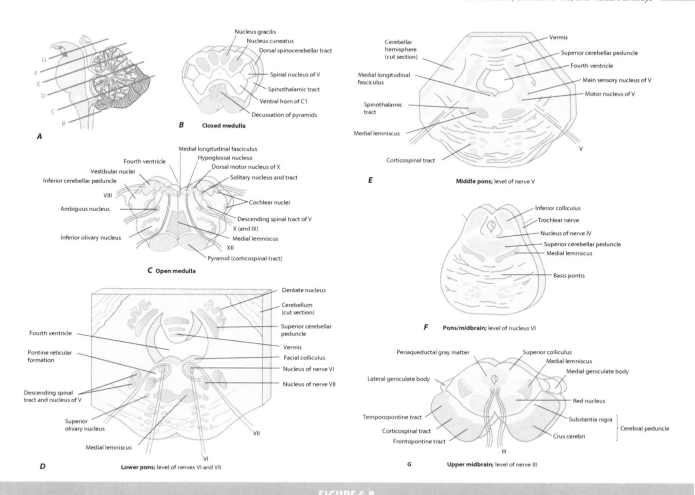

FIGURE 6.8

Brain stem. A. Key to levels of sections. **B–G.** Schematic transverse sections through the brain stem. The corticospinal tracts (blue) and the dorsal column nuclei/medial lemnisci (pink) are shown in color so that they can be followed as they course through the brain stem. (Reproduced with permission from Chapter 7. The Brain Stem and Cerebellum. In: Waxman SG. eds. *Clinical Neuroanatomy,* 27e New York, NY: McGraw-Hill; 2013).

Pons

The midbrain is connected caudally to the pons at the pontomesencephalic junction. The dorsal border of the pons is the fourth ventricle, which separates the pons from the cerebellum. It has a large ventral protrusion, the basilar pons, which contains the pontine nuclei and the fasciculated fibers of the CST and CBT. The superior, middle, and inferior cerebellar peduncles attach the pons to the cerebellum. From the pons originates four cranial nerves, CNs V–VIII. CN V (trigeminal) is a mixed sensory and motor nerve located in the mid- to rostral pons. CN VI (abducens), VII (facial), and VIII (vestibulocochlear) are located at the pontomedullary junction. The dorsolateral part of the tegmental region contains the three major ascending somatosensory pathways—the medial lemniscus, the spinothalamic tract, and the ventral trigeminothalamic tract—as well as the auditory pathway, the lateral lemniscus.

Medulla

The medulla extends from pontomedullary junction caudally to merge with the spinal cord. On its dorsal medullary surface,

the obex (the inferior apex of the fourth ventricle) marks the end of the medulla and the beginning of the spinal cord (see Figure 6.5). The CST descends from the pontomedullary junction and coalesces ventrally in the medulla to form the pyramids. Corticospinal (pyramidal) axons cross at the pyramidal decussation at the caudal end of the medulla to enter the lateral spinal cord; from there the pathway is referred to as the lateral corticospinal tract. A lesion rostral to the decussation causes a hemiplegia or hemiparesis on the contralateral side of the body, while a lesion caudal to the decussation (i.e., in the spinal cord) causes a deficit on the ipsilateral side of the body. Externally, just lateral to the pyramids, the rostral medulla has a pair of bulges, called the olives, which contain the inferior olivary nuclei. Each side of the dorsal surface of the medulla, slightly rostral to the pyramidal decussation, is decorated with a pair of bulges in the floor of the fourth ventricle, the gracile and cuneate tubercles, which mark the locations of the gracile and cuneate, or dorsal column, nuclei. The nuclei and peripheral nerves associated with CNs IX–XII are located in the medulla.

V ■ BRAINSTEM CRANIAL NERVES

Cranial nerves can be grouped according to their specificity of function as general or special, somatic or visceral, and afferent or efferent. General refers to components that carry motor or sensory information to or from the body or face. Special refers to components whose function pertains specifically to the head and neck. Somatic refers to the muscles and sensory innervation of the body, and visceral refers to interoceptors or autonomic motor neurons. Special somatic afferents are those related to the special senses: smell, taste, vision, hearing, and equilibrium. Special visceral efferents supply muscles derived from the embryonic branchial arches. General visceral efferents are the cranial parasympathetics (Table 6.2).

Cranial Nerve Functional Overview

A general feature of the anatomic layout of cranial nerve nuclei, introduced in Chapter 4, is that the cranial nerve nuclei are organized into functionally related discontinuous columns extending along the brainstem axis. Motor columns, basal plate derivatives, are found ventromedial to the remaining sulcus limitans, and sensory columns are dorsolateral. The brainstem houses three columns of cranial nerve motor nuclei. Most medially located are the nuclei of the somatic skeletal motor column (general somatic efferent). This column contains motor neurons that innervate consciously controlled striated muscle and include the extraocular muscles and the tongue.

Table 6.2 Cranial Nerves

	Nerve	Name	Cranial Foramina	Functional component	Nucleus	Target	Function
FOREBRAIN	I	Olfactory	Cribriform Plate	SVA	Connects directly with forebrain	Nose: Olfactory mucosa	Smell
	II	Optic	Optic	SSA	Thalamus, lateral geniculate nucleus	Eye: Retina	Vision
MIDBRAIN	III	Oculomotor	Superior Orbital Fissure	GSE	Oculomotor nucleus	Eyelid: Levator palpebrae superioris	Lid movements
						Eye muscles: superior rectus, inferior rectus, medial rectus, inferior oblique	Eye movements
				GVE (Parasympathetic)	Edinger-Westphal Nucleus	Pupil: Sphincter pupillae Intraocular lens: Ciliary muscles	Pupillary constriction Accommodation (focus of the eye)
	IV	Trochlear	Superior Orbital Fissure	GSE	Trochlear Nucleus	Superior oblique muscle	Eye movement
	V	Trigeminal	V3, Foramen Ovale	GSA	Mesencephalic Nucleus	Muscles of mastication	Proprioception
PONS	V	Trigeminal		GSA	Principal Sensory Nucleus	Face	Discriminative touch and vibration sense
				SVE	Motor Nucleus	Muscles of mastication	Movement of mandible
	VI	Abducens	Superior Orbital Fissure	GSE	Abducens Nucleus	Eye: Lateral Rectus	Abduction of the eye
	VII	Facial	Internal Auditory Meatus	SVE	Facial Nucleus	Face	Movement of muscles of facial expression; stylohyoid and posterior belly of digastric; stapedius
				GSA	Spinal Nucleus of CN V	Ear	Sensation from external acoustic meatus and skin posterior to ear
				GVE (Parasympathetic)	Superior salivatory Nucleus	Lacrimal, sublingual, and submandibular glands	Lacrimation and salivation
				SVA	Nucleus Solitarius	Anterior 2/3 of tongue	Taste
MEDULLA	VIII	Vestibulocochlear	Internal Auditory Meatus	SSA	Vestibular nuclear complex	Vestibulospinal tracts, vestibular nuclei, and cerebellum	Balance and reflex eye movements
				SSA	Cochlear nuclei	Inner ear: organ of Corti	Hearing
	IX	Glossopharyngeal	Jugular	GSA	Spinal Nucleus of V	Posterior 1/3 of tongue, tonsil, external ear, internal tympanic membrane, pharynx	Somatic sensation
				GVA	Nucleus Solitarius	Tongue and pharynx Carotid body	Gag reflex Chemoreceptors and baroreceptors
				SVA	Nucleus Solitarius	Posterior 1/3 tongue	Taste
				SVE	Nucleus Ambiguus	Stylopharyngeus	Motor
				GVE (Parasympathetic)	Inferior Salivatory nucleus	Parotid Gland	Salivation

(continued)

Table 6.2 Cranial Nerves *(continued)*

	Nerve	Name	Cranial Foramina	Functional component	Nucleus	Target	Function
MEDULLA	V (cont.)	Trigeminal		GSA	Spinal Nucleus of V	Face	Pain and temperature
	X	Vagus	Jugular	GSA	Spinal Nucleus of CN V	Posterior meninges, external acoustic meatus, skin posterior to ear	Somatic sensation
				GVA	Nucleus Solitarius	Larynx, trachea, esophagus, thoracic viscera, abdominal viscera	Somatic sensation
						Aortic arch	Stretch and chemoreceptors for cardiopulmonary system reflexes
				SVA	Nucleus Solitarius	Taste buds in epiglottis	Taste
				SVE	Nucleus Ambiguus	Pharyngeal muscles and intrinsic muscles of the larynx	Muscles of phonation and deglutition
				GVE (Parasympathetic)	Dorsal motor nucleus of vagus	Cervical, thoracic, and abdominal viscera; ganglion neurons located in/near target organ	Smooth muscle and glands of pharynx, larynx, thoracic viscera, abdominal viscera
				GVE	Nucleus Ambiguus	Cardiac muscle	Decrease heart rate and blood pressure
	XI	Accessory	Jugular	SVE	Spinal Accessory Nucleus; Nucleus Ambiguus	Sternocleidomastoid and trapezius	Shoulder and neck movement
	XII	Hypoglossal	Hypoglossal canal	GSE	Hypoglossal Nucleus	Hyoglossus, genioglossus, styloglossus, intrinsic muscles of tongue	Movement of the tongue

Autonomic Nuclei—General Visceral Efferents

The nuclei of the autonomic motor column (general visceral efferent) lie lateral to the general somatic efferent column. The autonomic motor column contains the preganglionic parasympathetic neurons that regulate cranial exocrine glands and smooth muscles in the head and neck, or that descend to supply thoracic and abdominal viscera. Axons from the preganglionic nuclei project along the cranial nerves to synapse on neurons in parasympathetic ganglia in or near their targets. The autonomic motor column contains four nuclei located from the midbrain to the medulla. The first is the parasympathetic Edinger-Westphal nucleus located in the pretectal area surrounding the nucleus of CN III. Its fibers travel on CN III, the oculomotor nerve, to synapse in the ciliary ganglion within the orbit, whose postganglionic axons drive pupil constriction.

The next two parasympathetic nuclei are the superior and inferior salivatory nuclei in the pons and medulla. These supply the nasal mucosa, lacrimal glands, and salivary glands. The superior salivatory nucleus fibers exit on the facial nerve and approach one of two peripheral parasympathetic ganglia. Some fibers pass from CN VII in its greater petrosal nerve branch to innervate cells in the pterygopalatine ganglion. Postganglionic fibers innervate the lacrimal glands and the nasal mucosa. Other parasympathetic fibers from the superior salivatory nucleus innervate the submandibular ganglion, from which postganglionic axons pass to the submandibular

and sublingual glands. The preganglionic fibers course along the chorda tympani, a facial nerve branch that also carries fibers mediating taste from the anterior two-thirds of the tongue. Fibers from the inferior salivatory nucleus project peripherally on the glossopharyngeal nerve (CN IV), branching off it into the lesser petrosal nerve to innervate the otic ganglion situated within the foramen ovale. Postganglionic fibers pass along the auriculotemporal nerve to supply the parotid gland.

Lastly, the dorsal motor nucleus of the vagus (CN X) is located below the fourth ventricle in the medulla. The vagus nerve descends through the neck into the thorax, where it contributes to cardiac and pulmonary plexuses supplying the lungs and heart. It regulates heart rate, blood pressure, and overall cardiovascular function. CN X continues to descend through the aortic hiatus in the diaphragm to enter the abdomen. There, its fibers enter the prevertebral plexuses to distribute along blood vessels with postganglionic sympathetic fibers to innervate the abdominal organs, including the liver and gall bladder, the pancreas and spleen, the kidneys, and most of the digestive system, in order to increase gut motility.

Branchiomeric Motor Column—Special Visceral Efferents

The branchiomeric motor column (special visceral efferent) originates from the branchial arches, and this nuclear column is constituted by the trigeminal motor nucleus, the facial motor nucleus, and the nucleus ambiguus. The trigeminal motor nucleus, located in mid-to-rostral pons, innervates the muscles of mastication along with a few small muscles in the palate and the middle ear. Axons from the facial motor nucleus contribute to the complex facial nerve and innervate the muscles of facial expression, a couple of small muscles in the neck, and the stapedius muscle in the middle ear. Nucleus ambiguus is a large nucleus extending over most of the rostrocaudal extent of the medulla. Its cells contribute to three cranial nerves, the glossopharyngeal, vagus, and spinal accessory nerves. Nucleus ambiguus supplies muscles of phonation (larynx) and deglutition (soft palate and pharynx) that are under volitional control. The glossopharyngeal nerve special visceral efferent supply is to the small, nearly insignificant stylopharyngeus muscle; function of this muscle cannot even be tested by typical cranial nerve assessment. Vagus supply innervates the muscles of the soft palate and the pharynx. It also emits two pairs of nerves that innervate the larynx, the superior laryngeal, and recurrent laryngeal nerves. The superior laryngeal nerve innervates the only external laryngeal muscle, the cricothyroid muscle. The right recurrent laryngeal nerve loops around the subclavian artery and ascends to enter the larynx as the inferior laryngeal nerve and to supply the remaining internal laryngeal muscles. Because of the development of the heart in the left thoracic cavity, the left recurrent laryngeal nerve loops under the aortic arch before ascending and terminating as the left inferior laryngeal nerve.

Taste and Visceral Sensation—Special Visceral Afferent

The solitary nucleus and its tract are located in the medulla. Its rostral end is expanded and receives inputs from taste receptors via the facial, glossopharyngeal, and vagus nerves. CN VII receives taste inputs from the anterior two-thirds of the tongue, which are carried on the chorda tympani along with preganglionic parasympathetic innervation from the superior salivatory nucleus. CN IX carries taste from the posterior third of the tongue, and CN X from taste receptors around the epiglottis. The caudal portion of the solitary nucleus receives visceral afferent inputs from chemoreceptors and baroreceptors associated with CNs IX and X and mediate reflex responses to CO_2 and O_2 in blood, pressure in vascular walls, mediate cough and gag reflexes, and contribute to efferent regulation of gut motility.

Facial Sensation—General Somatic Afferent

The trigeminal nerve (CN V) comprises the primary system of sensory input from the face. Its sensory components include, from rostral to caudal, the mesencephalic nucleus ascending to the midbrain, the principal sensory nucleus in the mid-rostral pons, which serves discriminative touch from the face, and the spinal trigeminal nerve extending from midpons downward into the upper cervical spinal cord. It receives nociceptive input from the ipsilateral face.

Audition and Equilibrium—Special Somatic Afferent

The most dorsolateral CN nuclei column contains nuclei related to CN VIII, the vestibulocochlear nerve, serving the special senses of audition and equilibrium. The vestibular nuclei comprise four separate centers that have extensive communication with the cerebellum, the brainstem, and the spinal cord. The dorsal and ventral cochlear nuclei mediate the sense of hearing. Much of its output ascends as part of the lateral lemniscus to the inferior colliculus.

VI CRANIAL NERVES

There are 12 pairs of cranial nerves that emerge from under the brain and brainstem. The cranial nerves are numbered in order; they have sensory, motor, or mixed functions and serve mainly the head.

Cranial Nerve I, The Olfactory Nerve

Cranial nerves are numbered from CN I, olfactory, most rostrally, to CN XII, hypoglossal, most caudally. CNs I and II are purely sensory cranial nerves; their functions are smell (olfaction) and vision, respectively. They are the only cranial nerves that have no connections to the brain stem. Instead, they connect directly to the forebrain. CN I (olfactory) is responsible for the sense of smell, and each nostril can detect odors independently. The olfactory epithelium is comprised of specialized nasal epithelium, a modified nasal mucosa that lines the roof and walls of the nasal cavity and sequesters the primary olfactory neurons (see Figure 6.9).

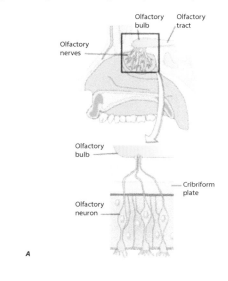

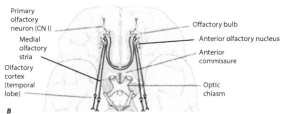

FIGURE 6.9

Cranial nerve I, the olfactory system. **A.** Medial view of the olfactory bulb, tract, nerves, and mucous membranes. **B.** Diagram illustrating the relationships between the olfactory receptors in the nasal mucosa and neurons in the olfactory bulb and tract. Cells of the anterior olfactory nucleus are found in scattered groups caudal to the olfactory bulb and make immediate connections within the olfactory tract. They project centrally via the medial olfactory stria and to contralateral olfactory structures via the anterior commissure. (Reproduced with permission from Neurophysiology. In: Kibble JD, Halsey CR. eds. *Medical Physiology: The Big Picture*. New York, NY: McGraw-Hill; 2009).

Bipolar olfactory neurons contain cilia projecting from their apical surfaces into the mucus in the nasal cavity, where they conduct the chemical interactions required for odorant signal transduction. Each bipolar neuron expresses only one olfactory receptor type that transduces the chemical interaction of only one odorant. Myelinated bundles of axons from the olfactory neurons, comprising the olfactory nerve, ascend through the perforations in the cribriform plate, converging onto a small population of glomeruli within the olfactory bulb. Axons synapse with second-order relay neurons and interneurons within a glomerulus; each set of glomeruli respond to only one specific odorant. Projection neurons send axons via the olfactory tracts that travel within the olfactory sulci along the ventral surface of the frontal lobes to directly enter the telencephalon.

There is no thalamic relay nucleus for olfaction as there is for most other sensory systems. The sense of smell and its counterpart, taste, are phylogenetically older than the other senses, and they have direct ipsilateral projections to the brain. Whereas taste provides the basic appreciation of sweet, sour, salty, bitter, and umami (savory), smell serves to add depth to the basic perceptions of taste. Loss of smell due to the common cold or head trauma seems to dull the taste of food, despite the preservation of the basic percepts.

Olfactory as well as gustatory information is processed broadly in the cortex within the limbic system or adjoining paralimbic cortices, including in the anterior olfactory nucleus, the olfactory tubercle, the amygdala, the piriform and periamygdaloid cortical areas, and the rostral entorhinal cortex. The piriform cortex projects via the medial dorsal nucleus to the orbitofrontal cortex. Thus, olfactory and gustatory information is processed directly in areas associated with emotions, emotion-driven behaviors, and memory, and it is well known that some smells are emotionally charged and deeply seated in long-term memory. Recently, the clinical relevance of understanding olfactory function has become clearer. In progressive neurodegenerative diseases, in particular, Alzheimer disease and Parkinson's disease, the anterior olfactory nucleus undergoes characteristic structural changes that might underlie the decreased sense of smell in patients with these diseases.

If the sense of smell is lost on one side (unilateral anosmia), the other side typically compensates, and the patient may be unaware of the sensory loss. Tumors of the frontal lobe, such as meningioma, or sarcoid granuloma, can also lead to unilateral anosmia with very few other signs or symptoms. Frontal lobe tumors are generally quiet tumors with limited symptomology; therefore, patients presenting with optic nerve atrophy in one eye and a swollen optic nerve in the other eye (Foster Kennedy syndrome) should also be screened for unilateral loss of smell.

Bilateral anosmia often manifests as decreased taste and is most commonly caused by damage to the delicate cribriform plate by head trauma, viral infections, or neurodegenerative disease, including Parkinson's and Alzheimer's diseases. Other neurological diseases known to cause olfactory dysfunction are schizophrenia, epilepsy, Huntington's chorea, and multiple sclerosis.

Migraine is associated with odor sensitivity or osmophobia that is more prominent during the acute phase of the migraine. During migraine, the piriform cortex and the amygdala are significantly activated, perhaps explaining the significant osmophobia associated with some migraine sufferers. Osmophobia is possibly one of the single most important differentiators of a migraine from other types of headache.

Cranial Nerve II, The Optic Nerve

CN II, the optic nerve, is not a true cranial nerve; it is an outgrowth of the developing forebrain serving the sensory component of vision. It transmits the chemoelectric signal (action potential) transduced from light waves impinging on retinal neurons. Motor cranial nerves (GSE) CNs III, oculomotor; IV, trochlear; and VI, abducens control eye movements that precisely align both eyes to focus an image onto the part of the retinas designed for maximal visual acuity and depth perception. Much of the brain, including cortical and subcortical locations, is dedicated to processing the visual input, with mechanisms that enable perception of shape, color, movement, and depth, as well as higher level processing to identify objects and integrate the new objects into cognitive experience.

Retinal anatomy

The lenses project light reflected off an object onto the retina, where photoreceptors transduce the energy of light waves into the chemoelectric energy of an action potential. The retina is a complex, layered structure (Figures 6.10 and 6.11) containing a large number

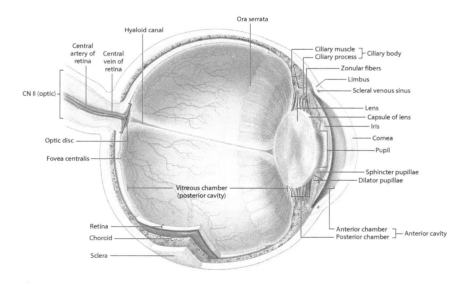

FIGURE 6.10

Anatomy of the eye. Image showing the anatomical structures of the eye, including CN II, posterior and anterior cavities, and intraocular muscles. (Reproduced with permission from The Eye & Ear: Special Sense Organs. In: Mescher AL. eds. *Junqueira's Basic Histology*, 14e New York, NY: McGraw-Hill, 2016).

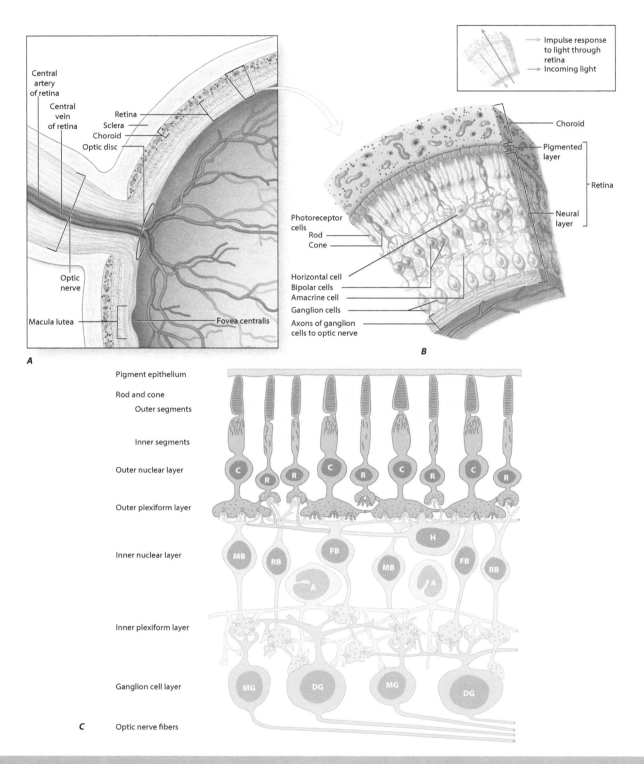

FIGURE 6.11

Retinal cell layers. A. Retinal blood supply and posterior eye structures. **B.** Enlarged view of the six retinal cell layers. The inset shows that the light travels through all six layers and is reflected forward off of the pigmented epithelium through the layers. Retinal ganglion cells lie most anterior in the retina. **C.** Illustration of the cell types within each layer. (A,B, Reproduced with permission from The Eye & Ear: Special Sense Organs. In: Mescher AL. eds. *Junqueira's Basic Histology*, 14e New York, NY: McGraw-Hill, 2016; C, Reproduced, with permission, from Dowling JE, Boycott BB: Organization of the primate retina: Electron microscopy. Proc Roy Soc Lond Ser B [Biol] 1966;166:80.)

of cell types and subtypes with extensive arrays of neurites and synapses. Counterintuitively, light travels through cells and axons in all of the layers before initiating the cascade of reactions producing sight. The retina has six layers from anterior to posterior: the optic nerve axon layer, ganglion cell layer, inner plexiform, inner nuclear, outer plexiform, and outer nuclear layers. The inner retina (the deepest layers) contains the ganglion cell layer with the fibers that constitute the optic nerve emitted superficially and the inner synaptic (plexiform) layer deeply; the inner nuclear layer contains the cell bodies of amacrine, interplexiform, bipolar, and horizontal cells; the outer synaptic (plexiform) layer; and the outer nuclear layer, which contains the rod and cone segments. Photoreceptors activate primary afferent bipolar neurons that then activate second-order retinal ganglion cells whose axons pass proximally toward the brain as the optic nerve. Horizontal cells and amacrine cells in the retina modify the signal from the light input and influence bipolar and retinal ganglion cell activity.

Photoreceptors

Retinal photoreceptors contain columns of flattened discs of light-sensitive pigment. Changes in light affect the release of the neurotransmitter, glutamate, in an inversely proportional relationship. In response to increased darkness (e.g., shadows moving across the receptive field), the membrane depolarizes, releasing glutamate. Conversely, increasing light intensity hyperpolarizes the membrane and reduces glutamate release. This relationship relates to center-surround physiological responses in bipolar cells that are discussed below.

Retinal photoreceptor cells are either rod or cone shaped, and each functions best under specific lighting conditions (Table 6.3). Photoreceptor distribution in the retina reflects their response characteristics. Located peripherally in the retina, rods are exquisitely sensitive to dim light and function best in low-light (scotopic) conditions; a single photon of light is sufficient to create an electrophysiological response in rod membrane potentials. Many rods converge their input onto a single rod bipolar cell. Such extensive convergence amplifies the dim light but sacrifices visual acuity and color perception.

Cones are less sensitive to light, that is, they are activated best by bright (photopic) light. Three types of cones have been identified by their responses to different wavelengths of light, thus cones

also confer color vision. They are concentrated in the central part of the eye, known as the macula. At the macula, the retinal neurons, axons, and blood vessels are oriented away from the photoreceptor layer, clearing the pathway for light to reach the photoreceptors. This orientation leaves a depression in the surface of the retina, called the foveal pit, or fovea. At the fovea, the neural pathway is essentially direct; one cone feeds information directly to a single cone bipolar neuron, optimizing visual acuity and spatial resolution. Macular nerve fibers form the papillomacular bundle; it enters the optic disc on the temporal side of the optic nerve. The presence of the emerging optic nerve creates a blind spot located temporally and slightly inferiorly to the visual axis. Processing in the visual cortex fills in the vacant portions of the visual field, and the blind spot is never perceived.

Retinal neurons and interneurons. Cones and rods synapse onto bipolar neurons, the first-order sensory afferents of the visual pathway. A bipolar cell's receptive field includes inputs from of all its converging photoreceptors, generating large receptive fields for rod bipolar cells, and small receptive fields for cone bipolar cells. Peripherally in the retina, many rods converge onto single rod bipolar cells. Convergence of the signals of a large number of photoreceptors, each activated by low-intensity light, increases the total excitation of the bipolar neuron, that is, it amplifies the light. The same convergence, however, dilutes the precision (acuity) of the inputs; it is no longer possible to distinguish the precise location of the object of interest within the receptive field because activating any of the photoreceptors informs only one bipolar cell. In the fovea, one, or very few, cones synapse onto a single cone bipolar neuron, sacrificing light sensitivity (no amplification) for increased spatial resolution and color vision (nearly 1-to-1 spatial relationship between photoreceptors and bipolar cells). Each photoreceptor occupies its own unique point on the retina by activating one bipolar cell.

Bipolar neurons synapse in the inner synaptic (plexiform) layer onto retinal ganglion cells. More than 22 ganglion cell types have been identified in the primate retina, yet only 3 of them are involved with visual perception: midget, parasol, and bistratified cells. In the macular region of the retina, midget cells, politically incorrectly named for their diminutive size, receive inputs from one or very few cone bipolar cells. Similarly to the manner with which one or a few cones synapse onto one cone bipolar cell, single cone bipolar cells synapse onto individual midget cells; thus spatial resolution of midget cell activation is extremely high.

Parasol-type retinal ganglion cells have extensive and elaborate dendritic arbors that receive inputs from many rod bipolar neurons. Once again, the high degree of convergence reduces the retinal capacity for precise localization of the object of interest.

Bistratified retinal ganglion cells and their dendritic arbors are distributed in the inner synaptic (plexiform) layer. Its output to the lateral geniculate nucleus projects to the koniocellular regions situated between the six layers. The function of the bistratified neurons seems to include contribution to color vision.

Retinal refinement of vision is nothing short of magnificent; processing condenses the information gathered by photoreceptors onto optic nerve fibers by a ratio of 125:1. Destruction of a single retinal ganglion cell therefore carries a significant consequence in the quality of information sent to the visual cortex and explains the devastating effect on vision caused by ganglion cell loss in various disease processes.

Table 6.3 Comparing Photoreceptors

Cones	Rods
Day vision	Night vision
Low light sensitivity	High light sensitivity
High visual acuity	Low visual acuity
Recognizes changes in visual field	Dim light amplifiers
Little/no convergence onto bipolar cells	Convergence onto bipolar cells amplifies light
Foveal concentration in retina	More prevalent peripherally within the retina
3 types with 3 different pigments responding maximally to 3 wavelengths of light; trichromatic	1 type; achromatic

Not all of the retinal ganglion cell axons in the optic nerve are involved in processing visual information. Some are destined for the diencephalon or the brain stem instead of the lateral geniculate nucleus and contribute little or nothing to vision. These are the photosensitive retinal ganglion neurons, and their central projections pass to the superior colliculus to regulate reflexive head movement in response to visual cues in three-dimensional space. Another contingent of fibers from photosensitive retinal ganglion neurons innervates the supraoptic nucleus of the hypothalamus and the pineal gland, regulating cyclic body processes. Other non–vision central projections innervate the superior colliculus. These retino-tectal fibers contribute to subconscious spatial awareness.

Horizontal cells and amacrine cells are retinal interneurons. They interject themselves in the synaptic (plexiform) layers and affect the responses of bipolar and retinal ganglion cells. Horizontal cells are distributed in the outer plexiform layer and interact with photoreceptors and bipolar cells. Interactions among the photoreceptors, bipolar, and horizontal cells confer center-surround physiological properties that are discussed below. Amacrine cells come in dozens of varieties disposed in the inner plexiform layer, where bipolar and retinal ganglion cells synapse. They appear to have a wide array of functions that are continually being updated in the literature, including integrating information vertically through the retina, modulating retinal ganglion cell sensitivity in light and dim conditions, and secreting dopamine, which augments cell synaptic activity in the dark.

The metabolic and structural functions of the retina are performed by the Müller cells that stretch from the outer to inner nuclear layer. Their cell bodies are located in the inner nuclear layer. The blood supply to the inner retina is provided by branches of the ophthalmic artery. The ophthalmic artery branches off from the internal carotid artery.

Some ganglion cells are lost through normal aging; others deteriorate from diseases that affect the optic nerve, such as optic neuritis from multiple sclerosis, or glaucoma. When axonal injury occurs, the axons distal to the injury, isolated from the neuronal cell body, undergo Wallerian degeneration. Ganglion cells are susceptible to small inciting events that induce programmed cell death (apoptosis). Cell death in posterior brain centers, such as with Alzheimer disease or cortical injuries, can deprive ganglion cells of their tropic target interactions, which promote retrograde cell death in healthy retinal ganglion cells. This is unfortunate because these highly specialized neurons do not regenerate, and vision is permanently lost.

Formation of the optic nerve. The ganglion cell axons exit the eye in a highly organized fashion. During development, the macular nerve fibers almost immediately migrate into the center of the optic nerve, where they are more protected. Once the ganglion cell axons leave the globe (eyeball) at the lamina cribrosa, they become myelinated, insulating the nerve and improving conduction. As CNS axons, the myelin on optic nerve axons is formed by oligodendrocytes. The optic nerve exits the orbit via the optic canal and continues posteriorly to the midbrain and thalamus, crossing below the frontal lobes of the brain and above the maxillary sinus, exiting into the cranium through the optic foramina. From the globe to the optic foramen, the optic nerve is approximately 20 mm long, with redundancy to allow motion for normal eye excursions without being pulled taut.

The meningeal sheath of the optic nerve is continuous with the globe and cerebrospinal fluid percolates through the subarachnoid space. An increase in intracranial pressure manifests in both optic nerves by creating bilateral optic disc edema or papilledema (Figure 6.12).

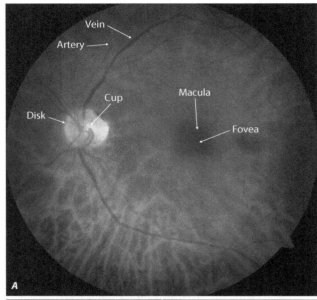

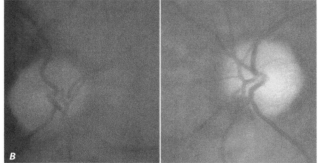

FIGURE 6.12

Fundoscope of the optic disc. *A.* Normal fundus. The disk has sharp margins and is normal in color, with a small central cup. Arterioles and venules have normal color, sheen, and course. Background is in normal color. The macula is enclosed by arching temporal vessels. The fovea is located by a central pit. (Photo contributor: Jeffrey Goshe, MD.). ***B.*** Papilledema (both eyes represented). The images below show swelling of both optic nerves of the eye associated with increased intracranial pressure (papilledema). The swelling in the images below is as a result of the mass effect of a large frontal tumor. The paler, atrophic nerves indicate that the papilledema is longstanding. The bright light reflex lines that can be seen next to the optic nerve in the right eye is as a result of the advanced swelling of the optic nerve, and are known as Patton's lines. The background color of the retina is determined by the coloring of the patient. In the case below, the photos are of a young Caucasian patient. (Photo contributor: Maryke Neiberg, OD)

Visual processing in the retina: center-surround physiology

Processing of visual information starts at the retina, more specifically, with the retinal ganglion cells. Retinal ganglion cells are each surrounded by an area, known as the receptive field of the cell, from which light stimuli influence cell activity. Each receptive field is divided into two concentric circles, known as "center" and "surround" receptive fields. Center-surround characteristics are produced in great part by the activity of the horizontal cells (Figure 6.13).

Two types of ganglion cell receptive fields have been identified: "on-center" and "off center." Whatever the designation of the center field, the properties of the surround field are opposite: "on-center, off-surround" and "off-center, on-surround" bipolar cells. An on-center, off-surround bipolar cell is depolarized when light is shone on the photoreceptors in its center receptive field; light shone in the surrounding outer circle hyperpolarizes the on-center cell. The off-center cells have a center circular receptive field that is off and a surrounding receptive field that is on when light is shone on the photoreceptors.

Dim light maintains the photoreceptors in a tonic state of partial depolarization, releasing glutamate at their synapses onto bipolar cells; this is referred to as the dark current. Glutamate is inhibitory to the on-center bipolar cell; in dim light and darkness, activity in the on-center bipolar cells is suppressed by glutamate, reducing activity in its target retinal ganglion cell. Increasing light intensity on photoreceptors in the center receptive field hyperpolarizes the photoreceptor, reducing release of glutamate and depolarizing of the on-center bipolar cell and therefore exciting its retinal ganglion cell.

In the surround receptive field of the on-center bipolar cell, tonic partial depolarization in dim light releases glutamate from the photoreceptors at a synapse with horizontal cells. Glutamate excites inhibitory GABAergic horizontal cells that presynaptically inhibit the center photoreceptor, further controlling photoreceptor glutamate release to the on-center bipolar cells. Light shone on the surround field photoreceptors hyperpolarizes them and curtails glutamate release. Loss of glutamate reduces release of GABA from horizontal cells, disinhibiting the center photoreceptor. Increased

glutamate release from the center photoreceptor of the on-center bipolar cell hyperpolarizes the cell and reduces activity in its target retinal ganglion cell. Ganglion cells with these types of on-center and off-center receptive fields are interspersed across the retina, forming a mosaic of overlapping receptive fields essential for appreciating relative illumination changes in our visual target and its background, also known as contrast.

Visual processing in the retina: color vision

Color vision is a highly complex function whereby visible light is encoded by cones and transmitted centrally for interpretation as color images. Two major theories have been proposed to explain color vision in humans: the trichromatic theory of Young and Helmholtz presented in the 19th century; and the opponent-process theory of Hering in 1878. The trichromatic theory is based on the premise (since demonstrated physiologically in human retinas) that there are three types of cone cells, each of which has a peak sensitivity to a specific wavelength of light: short wavelength sensitive (red/orange-red); middle wavelength sensitive (green/yellow-green); and short wavelength sensitive (blue). Because there is substantial overlap in the overall sensitivities of the three-photoreceptor categories, it is the balance of activity in the cones in response to the complete spectrum of reflected light wavelengths that permits us to perceive all colors. Color information is thus encoded, especially by foveal retinal ganglion cells, and the information propagated centrally.

Trichromatic coding of incoming light wavelengths is not yet color perception; rather, it is simply differentiation among light wavelengths. Hering noted that there were color combinations that are never perceived, such as greenish-red or yellowish-blue. He postulated that cone photoreceptors link to form opposing color pairs, specifically forming red/green, blue/yellow and black/white. Activation of one of the cones in the pair serves to inhibit the other and leads to the perception of color. Although Helmholtz and

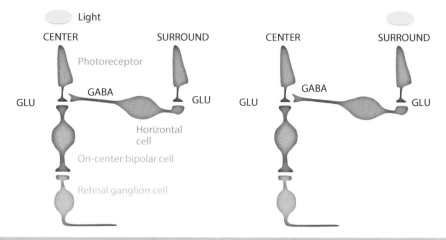

FIGURE 6.13

On-center off-surround retinal circuitry. On–center bipolar cells are hyperpolarized by glutamate (GLU). With light shone on the center of the on–center bipolar cell receptive field (left), the center photoreceptor is hyperpolarized, reducing GLU release and leading to depolarization of the bipolar cell and thereby its retinal ganglion cell. Horizontal cells confer the opposing suppression of on–center bipolar cell activity when light is shone in the surround receptive field (right). Reduced GLU release by the hyperpolarized surround photoreceptor reduces GABA release by the horizontal cell, disinhibiting the release of GLU by the center photoreceptor. Elevated GLU hyperpolarizes the on–center bipolar cell thereby reducing retinal ganglion cell activity. (Image provided by Tony Mosconi, 2017.)

Hering spent much of their lives as professional, philosophical, and personal mortal enemies, more equable researchers have recognized that the theories are complementary: trichromatic photoreceptors process light inputs within the retina to encode color; and opponent-processing acts centrally to perceive color at a conscious level.

Visual receptors and central pathways

As implied from the description of different photoreceptors, bipolar, and retinal ganglion cell types, the information carried from the retinas back to the brain is extraordinarily complex. Inputs are

influenced by the position on the retina from which the signal originated, the types of photoreceptors activated, and the anatomical and functional characteristics of the retinal ganglion cells. Central projections and the information they carry remain segregated all the way through the visual cortex.

Three distinct visual pathways can be identified, between the retina and the lateral geniculate nucleus (LGN): the parvocellular, magnocellular, and koniocellular pathways (Figure 6.14).

Access to each pathway depends on activation of specific sets of retinal ganglion cell types. The parvocellular pathway originates from midget cells in the retinal fovea and carries information about color, in particular red-green opponency. Midget cells have high spatial resolution and small receptive fields; however, they do not detect motion. They project to parvocellular layers (layers 3–6) of the LGN. Because they synapse on parvocellular layers in the LGN, midget cells are also called P-cells.

The magnocellular pathway originates from the parasol ganglion cell in the retina, which have large receptive fields and low spatial resolution and detect motion. These ganglion cells project to magnocellular layers (1–2) of the LGN and are also called M-cells. The koniocellular pathway originates from the bistratified ganglion cells of the retina. Like the magnocellular pathway, they have large receptive field and low spatial resolution. This pathway conveys information concerning blue-yellow spectral opponency.

The LGN emits third-order axons that travel posteriorly to the primary visual cortex in the occipital lobe. This large geniculocalcarine tract is more commonly referred to as the optic radiations (Figure 6.15), which comprise part of the extensive cortical white matter. Optic radiations are composed of two adjacent fascicles that

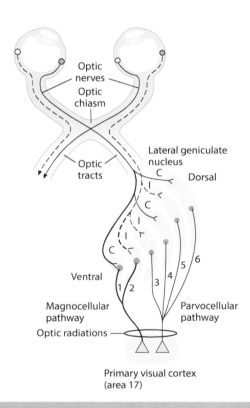

FIGURE 6.14

Projections to the lateral geniculate nucleus. Ganglion cell projections from the right temporal hemiretina of the ipsilateral eye and the nasal hemiretinal of the left eye to the right lateral geniculate body; this arrangement conveys images from the left visual hemisphere. From this nucleus, the optic radiations carry inputs to to the right primary visual cortex. Note the six layers of the geniculate body. P-ganglion cells project to layers 3–6, and M-ganglion cells project to layers 1 and 2. The ipsilateral (I) and contralateral (C) eyes project to alternate layers. Not shown are the interlaminar area cells, which project via a separate component of the P-pathway to blobs in the visual cortex. The magnocellular pathway conveys visual inputs with low acuity but high light sensitivity and engage the dorsal stream or "where" pathway described in Chapter 10. The parvocellular pathway conveys visual inputs with high acuity but low light sensitivity and engage the ventral stream or "what" pathway described in Chapter 10. (Reproduced from Vision. In: Barrett KE, Barman SM, Boitano S, Brooks HL. eds. Ganong's Review of Medical Physiology, 25e New York, NY: McGraw-Hill, 2016).

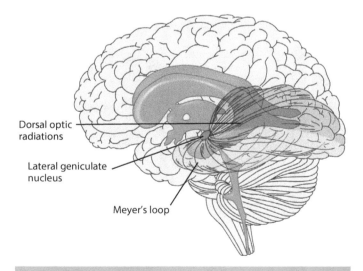

FIGURE 6.15

Optic radiations. Output fibers from the LGN pass posteriorly toward the primary visual cortex. Meyer's loop descends ventrally a short distance before turning posteriorly to innervate the lingual gyrus. Dorsally the dorsal optic radiations pass straight backwards to the cuneate gyrus. The optic radiations lie close to the lateral ventricles and are therefore endangered by lesions affecting the ventricle. (Image provided by Jamie Graham, 2017).

proceed to the cuneate (superior to the calcarine sulcus) and lingual (inferior to the calcarine sulcus) gyri. Axons emerging from the dorsal part of the LGN pass posteriorly as the dorsal optic radiations and terminate in the cuneate gyrus; dorsal optic radiations carry visual input arising from the contralateral lower visual field. Ventral axons exit the LGN and curve ventrally before turning posteriorly. This portion of the optic radiations is referred to as Meyer's loop (or the loop of Archambault), and the fibers carry information related to the contralateral upper visual field.

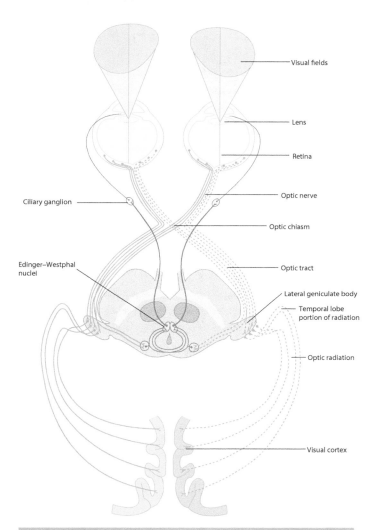

FIGURE 6.16

Sensory and motor visual pathways. The solid blue lines represent optic nerve fibers that extend from the retina to the occipital cortex and carry afferent visual information from the right half of the visual field (blue portion). The broken blue lines show the pathway from the left half of the visual fields (pink portion). Note that nasal hemiretinal fibers contribute to the contralateral optic tract by decussating in the optic chiasm, while temporal fibers pass directly into the ipsilateral optic tract. The green lines represent the efferent pathway for the pupillary light reflex. (Reproduced with permission from The Visual System. In: Waxman SG. eds. *Clinical Neuroanatomy*, 28e New York, NY: McGraw-Hill; 2017).

The visual field

The visual field is the subjective appreciation of the external world. It can be described and quantified by bisecting fixation, creating nasal and temporal hemifields that have superior and inferior quadrants for each eye. The visual field can also be divided into superior and inferior visual fields with nasal and temporal quadrants. The information from each quadrant and the information from the macula are carried to the cortex in a highly organized fashion (Figure 6.16).

The normal monocular visual field extends nasally by 60 degrees, superiorly by 60 degrees, inferiorly 70–75 degrees and temporally 100–110 degrees. It includes a small blind spot in the temporal field of each eye, corresponding to the optic nerve located in the nasal retina. When both eyes are open, the fields overlap and create a central binocular field that extends approximately 180 degrees. The overlap ensures that the blind spots are no longer visible and allow stereoscopic (three-dimensional) vision. Two small temporal crescents are present on each side of the visual field, where the fields do not overlap; these are called monocular crescents since images in this portion of the visual field are only received by the ipsilateral eye (Figure 6.17).

The visual field is projected onto the retina after passing through several structures. In order, these are the tear layer, cornea, anterior chamber, intraocular lens, and vitreous humor. Light rays are focused as they pass through the tear layer, cornea, and lens, directing light onto the retina. Each of these structures is essential

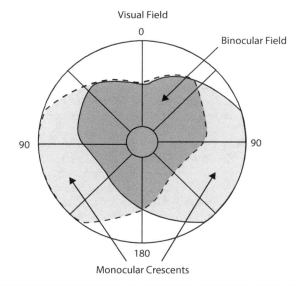

FIGURE 6.17

Monocular and binocular portions of the visual field. The dotted line encloses the visual field of the left eye; the solid line encloses that of the right eye. The common area (heart-shaped darker blue zone in the center) is viewed with binocular vision (binocular field). The lighter blue shaded areas are viewed with ipsilateral monocular vision (monocular crescents). (Reproduced from The Visual System. In: Waxman SG. eds. Clinical Neuroanatomy, 28e New York, NY: McGraw-Hill; 2017).

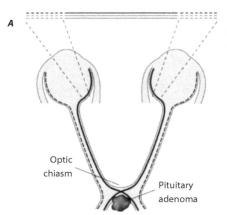
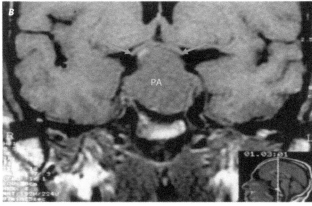

FIGURE 6.18

Pituitary adenoma. A. Diagram of a pituitary adenoma (PA) and its relationship to the optic chiasm. Reproduced with permission from Toy, EC, et al. *Case Files: Pathology* 2E. New York, NY: McGraw-Hill, 2008. **B.** Coronal MRI showing large pituitary adenoma elevating and distorting the optic chiasm (between the arrows). (Reproduced with permission from Riordan-Eva P, Hoyt WF. Chapter 14. Neuro-Ophthalmology. In: Riordan-Eva P, Cunningham ET, Jr. eds. *Vaughan & Asbury's General Ophthalmology*, 18e New York, NY: McGraw-Hill; 2011).

for normal vision. For example, dry eye may reduce corneal surface moisture, causing loss of acuity. Normally, an even layer of tears maintains a smooth corneal surface. With dry eye, the tear layer over the corneal surface has irregular patches that can distort the image, like looking through a frosted shower door.

Each retinal field is independent of the other and receives distinct inputs that overlap centrally. The lens refracts and focuses light onto the retina as an upside-down and backward image. The image is represented in the retinal field with the nasal region of the visual image projected to the temporal part of the retina and the temporal part of the image onto the nasal retinal field. The upper part of the image is projected onto the lower part of the retinal field, and vice versa for the lower part of the image. Subsequent cortical processing ensures that the image is perceived in its proper orientation.

The optic chiasm

Axons from the retina emerge from the posterior aspect of the eye and form the optic nerve. Each optic nerve carries the image received by the ipsilateral eye, with an image largely representing the contralateral visual hemisphere. Decussating optic nerve fibers form the X-shaped optic chiasm, located in the forebrain, directly inferior to the hypothalamus. The internal carotid arteries flank each side of the optic chiasm; the anterior cerebral arteries and the anterior communicating artery in front of the chiasm. Posteriorly, the pituitary stalk borders the chiasm and is almost completely surrounded by CSF. The pituitary gland lies directly beneath the hypothalamus in a depression of the bony skull that resembles a saddle and is known as the sella turcica.

In the optic chiasm, axons carrying the image only from the nasal retinal field decussate and contribute to the contralateral optic tract. Temporal fibers pass directly posteriorly to the ipsilateral optic tract. Nasal hemiretinal fibers carry inputs from the ipsilateral temporal (monocular) crescent as well as part of the binocular visual field. The decussation thus brings the image from the ipsilateral monocular crescent to the contralateral optic tract. Temporal hemiretinal fibers carry inputs from the nasal part of the ipsilateral eye's visual field

into the ipsilateral optic tract. Thus the optic tracts contain the complete image received from the contralateral visual hemisphere. This organization persists all the way back to the visual cortex. For this reason, a lesion of any part of the visual pathway behind the optic chiasm will impair vision only in the contralateral visual hemisphere.

The visual pathway at the optic chiasm is at the mercy of the pituitary gland. Enlargement of the pituitary gland from a tumor, most often a benign adenoma, not only creates abnormal hormone secretion, but it also compresses the decussating nasal fibers at the optic chiasm (Figure 6.18).

The visual field present in the chiasm includes both monocular crescents (temporal parts of the visual field), and a lesion damaging these fibers eliminates temporal visual fields of each eye. This is known as a bitemporal hemianopia (or "hemianopsia"). The patient may notice that side vision is reduced, but the nasal visual fields of each eye, which overlap in the presence of single binocular vision, persist. Because the loss occurs on opposite sides of the individual fields, the visual field loss is described as heteronymous. Slow-growing tumors can produce a gradual loss of peripheral vision, and patients fail to notice the loss. It is much like the old story of the frog in the pot of water. If a frog is placed in a pot of hot water, he immediately jumps out. If he is put in a pot of cool water that is being slowly heated, he never notices the heat and soon boils without even knowing why. Gradual behavioral or sensory changes are often missed or denied until visual field loss is severe, with less than 10 degrees of peripheral vision remaining. Patients may unfortunately discover their bitemporal hemianopia after a collision with an object from the side. When examined for head injury by computed tomography (CT) or magnetic resonance imaging (MRI), the tumor and compression of the optic chiasm is discovered.

An interesting anatomical misdirection is seen in patients with albinism. Ganglion cell growth in the retina is regulated by melanin, which is absent in this population. The ganglion cell growth therefore arrives late to the optic chiasm and is misdirected, primarily contralaterally, so that the right and left visual fields are cortically projected as mirror reversed.

Clinical differential diagnosis

By understanding the very precise way by which the axons of the ganglion cells traverse the optic nerve, optic chiasm, and optic tract, and by understanding the pathway from the LGN to the occipital cortex, the clinician can use the defects in the patient's visual field caused by the lesions to locate the lesion along the visual pathway. Differential diagnoses of neurological disease can be made on the bases of the presentation of the optic nerve, the deficit in the visual field, and the associated neurological signs and symptoms (Figure 6.19).

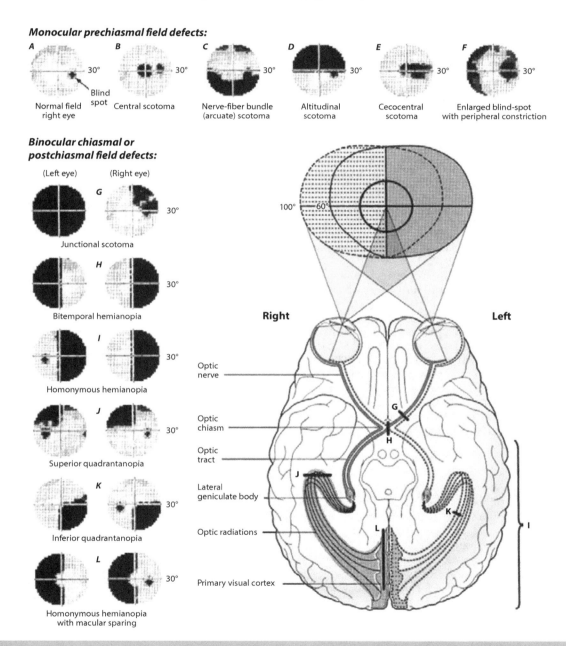

FIGURE 6.19

Visual field loss. Ventral view of the brain, correlating patterns of visual field loss with the sites of lesions in the visual pathway. The visual fields overlap partially, creating 120° of central binocular field flanked by a 40° monocular crescent on either side. The visual field maps in this figure were done with a computer-driven perimeter (Humphrey Instruments, Carl Zeiss, Inc.). It plots the retinal sensitivity to light in the central 30° by using a gray scale format. Areas of visual field loss are shown in black. The examples of common monocular, prechiasmal field defects are all shown for the right eye (*A-F*), and binocular postchiasmal deficits (*G-L*). By convention, the visual fields are always recorded with the left eye's field on the left and the right eye's field on the right, just as the patient sees the world. (Reproduced with permission from Horton JC. Disorders of the Eye. In: Kasper D, et al., eds. *Harrison's Principles of Internal Medicine*, 19e New York, NY: McGraw-Hill; 2014).

Visual deficits can present in a single visual field (monocularly) or in both visual fields (binocularly). Because the visual fields overlap, the patient may not be aware a deficit is present, or the deficit may be mitigated or changed. If the patient closes one eye, the deficit may become more apparent. Visual fields are always measured one eye at a time, but the results are evaluated as a pair. Neurological visual field defects occur along the vertical fixation line, creating hemifield deficits (hemianopia, hemianopsia), or an inferior or superior section of a hemianopia (quadrantanopia, quadrantopsia) in response to a lesion along specific and predictable sites along the visual pathway. For example, a lesion in the optic tract or LGN produces a loss of vision from the contralateral visual hemisphere, called a contralateral homonymous hemianopia. If a lesion occurs in either the dorsal optic radiations or the cuneate gyrus of the visual cortex, the deficit will appear as a contralateral homonymous inferior quadrantopsia.

Vascular visual field deficits typically occur along the horizontal fixation line. The laminar and prelaminar optic nerve blood supply is provided by the circle of Zinn-Haller, which arises from the short posterior ciliary arteries. Acute obstruction of these branches in older patients, known as anterior ischemic optic neuropathy, creates a distinctive type of visual field loss that may involve the top half or the bottom half of the visual field of the involved eye. This is known as an "altitudinal visual field defect."

Visual field loss can be described as relative or absolute. Absolute loss means no vision in the field, or total visual blindness. Relative loss may present as reduction in the visual sensitivity, or low vision. Most loss of vision is on a spectrum; training and low vision aids may serve to enhance the remaining functional vision.

A lesion along the visual pathway anywhere from the cornea to the prechiasmal area will produce a visual field defect only in the ipsilateral eye. At the chiasm, a lesion produces a bitemporal visual field defect. Depending on the extent and duration of the chiasmal compression of the visual pathway, the visual field loss may be relative or absolute. Lateral expansion of the tumor into the cavernous sinus may lead to other cranial nerve involvement, producing oculomotor misalignment resulting in double vision (diplopia) or loss of sensation on the face.

Three essential functions of the superior colliculus

Optic tracts contain primary afferent fibers from the retinal ganglion cells. The main central target of these fibers is the lateral geniculate nucleus. As described above, optic radiations carry the LGN neuron axons back to the primary visual cortex. About 5% of the axons from the optic tract bypass the LGN, form the brachium of the superior colliculus, and innervate the ipsilateral superior colliculus. Afferent nerve fibers headed for the superior colliculus have three essential functions. These functions are alignment of the head, control of pupillary diameter, and production of conditions for optimal near vision (accommodation).

The first of the functions of the fibers to the superior colliculus include alignment of the head based on coordinated information from both visual and auditory input (auditory inputs are also similarly processed in the inferior colliculus). Ascending sensory information from the eyes and ears is aggregated at the brachium of the superior colliculus and then transported upward to higher-order visual areas and the parietal-temporal-occipital association area via ascending axons to the lateral posterior and pulvinar nuclei of the thalamus.

The second essential function serves to reflexively control the pupils (Figure 6.20). Some of the visual input continues directly via the brachium of the superior colliculus to the pretectal nuclei. The tectum is the dorsal surface of the midbrain, and the pretectal nuclei receive binocular (from both eyes) inputs via the decussating fibers of the posterior commissure. This bilateral innervation ensures that illumination of only one eye will cause both eyes to constrict. Bilateral output from the pretectal nuclei innervate the preganglionic parasympathetic neurons in the Edinger-Westphal nucleus associated with CN III. Preganglionic fibers synapse on the parasympathetic neurons in the ciliary ganglion posterior to the eye within the orbit. Postganglionic fibers innervate two muscles that mediate pupil size, the sphincter, and the dilator (see Figure 6.10). The sphincter muscle is located within the iris, and when it contracts, it pulls the iris toward it, narrowing pupillary diameter in response to increasing light intensity; that is, the pupil constricts. Associated with pupillary constriction driven by increased light

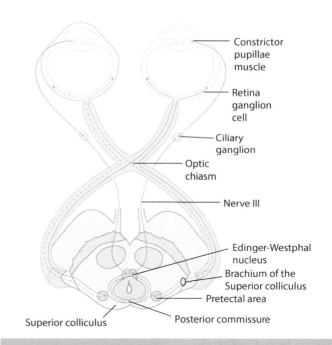

Constrictor pupillae muscle

Retina ganglion cell

Ciliary ganglion

Optic chiasm

Nerve III

Edinger-Westphal nucleus

Brachium of the Superior colliculus

Pretectal area

Superior colliculus

Posterior commissure

FIGURE 6.20

The path of the pupillary light reflex. Binocular inputs project via the brachium of the superior colliculus to the pretectal nucleus in the superior colliculus. Pretectal nuclei communicate across the posterior commissure and project bilaterally with the Edinger-Westphal nuclei, part of the oculomotor complex. Bilateral innervation of the constrictor pupillae muscles produces binocular pupillary constriction with increasing light intensity. (Reproduced with permission from Cranial Nerves and Pathways. In: Waxman SG. eds. Clinical Neuroanatomy, 28e New York, NY: McGraw-Hill, 2017).

intensity, the lens changes shape to become smaller in diameter and greater in thickness in a process called accommodation.

To reopen the pupil, the dilator muscle contracts. The dilator muscle is arranged radially around the pupil. Dilation of the eye occurs primarily by the action of the sympathetic branch of the central nervous system, or when the parasympathetic pupil pathway described above is inhibited (Figure 6.21). The hypothalamus, which also receives primary optic nerve inputs, regulates sympathetic activity in the mesencephalic pretectal nuclei. Output descends as the hypothalamospinal pathway. In its descent, it passes near the spinal trigeminal nucleus and the anterolateral system pathway in the lateral medulla; thus it is endangered with a lateral medullary syndrome and accompanies the loss of nociception from the ipsilateral face and contralateral body. The hypothalamospinal pathway descends through the lateral funiculus of the cervical spinal cord to synapse on preganglionic sympathetic neurons in the lateral horn of the first two or three thoracic segments. Preganglionic axons ascend in the sympathetic trunk to the superior cervical ganglion. Postganglionic outputs ascend on the external carotid arteries to

distribute to sweat glands, blood vessels, and the levator palpebrae superioris. Fibers destined for the pupillary dilators continue their ascent along the internal carotid artery and pass anteriorly through the superior orbital fissure. They continue forward riding on the long ciliary nerve, passing through without synapsing on the ciliary ganglion to innervate the pupillary dilators.

Various lesions may impair pupillary dilation. A lesion in the hypothalamospinal pathway in the lateral medulla, in the lateral funiculus of the cervical spinal cord, or in the superior cervical ganglion or its postganglionic output can leave the ipsilateral eye poorly responsive to decreasing light intensity and partially constricted, a state called miosis. Miosis, ptosis, and anhydrosis (dryness of the skin) form the triad of symptoms associated with a Horner's syndrome. Because blood vessels in the face are then left dilated, with loss of sympathetic innervation, flushed skin also is often associated with Horner's syndrome (Figure 6.22).

The sympathetic and parasympathetic systems continuously adjust the pupil in response to light stimuli; slight changes in the dominance of each system leads to natural fluctuations in pupil size. Unequal pupils are known as anisocoria. Twenty percent of the population has a natural size difference between pupils (anisocoria) of 0.5 mm or less; anisocoria of more than 0.5 mm is considered pathologic and requires additional examination to determine the cause.

As discussed previously, a reflex requires intact sensory and motor limbs to produce a motor response. In the visual system, pupillary constriction has a single sensory limb, the optic nerve, and two motor limbs, the bilateral Edinger-Westphal output carried on CN III. Light shone onto one eye will produce ipsilateral direct pupillary constriction and accommodation. Because of the bilateral input to the Edinger-Westphal nuclei, the contralateral pupil will show a consensual (indirect) response.

In certain disease conditions, the optic nerve of one eye does not relay the afferent stimulus bilaterally to the Edinger-Westphal nuclei and therefore does not cause pupil constriction in either eye. If the other (healthy) eye is then illuminated, it still relays the light to the Edinger-Westphal nuclei, and the pupils both constrict normally. Although the pupil itself is healthy, the response depends on the afferent signal received from the Edinger-Westphal nucleus.

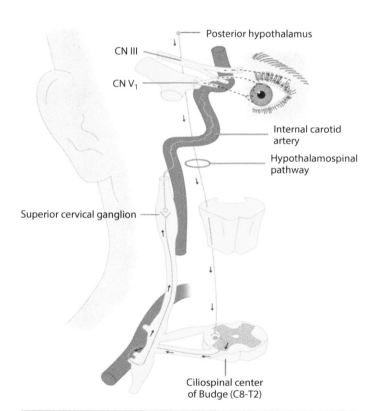

Posterior hypothalamus

CN III

CN V₁

Internal carotid artery

Hypothalamospinal pathway

Superior cervical ganglion

Ciliospinal center of Budge (C8-T2)

FIGURE 6.21

Sympathetic nerve pathway of the eye. An interruption anywhere along this pathway can cause Horner's syndrome. (Reproduced with permission from Walker RA, Adhikari S. Eye Emergencies. In: Tintinalli JE, et al., eds. *Tintinalli's Emergency Medicine: A Comprehensive Study Guide*, 8e New York, NY: McGraw-Hill; 2016).

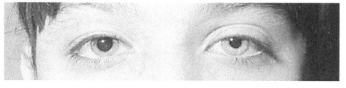

FIGURE 6.22

Congenital Horner syndrome. Ptosis, miosis, and heterochromia (lighter colored iris) are seen on the patient's affected left side. (Reproduced with permission from Braverman R. Eye. In: Hay WW, Jr., Levin MJ, Deterding RR, Abzug MJ. eds.CURRENT Diagnosis & Treatment Pediatrics, 23e New York, NY: McGraw-Hill, 2016).

This phenomenon is known as an afferent pupillary defect (APD), or Marcus-Gunn pupil (Figure 6.23).

Visual acuity alone is not a reliable measure of CN II function. A more sensitive measure of nerve function requires evaluating for an afferent pupillary defect. The presence of this defect often indicates subtle disease long before diminished visual acuity reflects the ganglion cell loss. Lesions posterior to the lateral geniculate nucleus do not present this APD phenomenon (see Appendix).

The third function of the superior colliculus is to produce the near triad, three conditions for optimal near vision related to changes in the focal distance. When objects come closer to the eye, both eyes converge, the pupils constrict, and the lens becomes smaller in diameter and thicker (accommodates). The visual cortex, motor neurons of CN III, and Edinger-Westphal parasympathetics must coordinate to achieve this near triad. When the pupillary changes of the triad are lost in response to increasing light intensity, but the accommodative response to near vision is present, it is known as light-near dissociation. This presentation accompanies a dorsal midbrain syndrome or Parinaud's syndrome, which is often caused by a pineal tumor

Cranial Nerve III, The Oculomotor Nerve

Cranial nerves III, IV, and VI together are responsible for the control of eye movements (Figure 6.24). These cranial nerves are

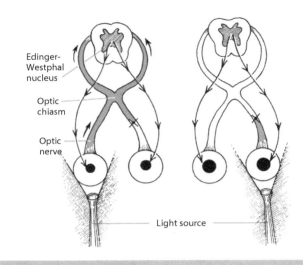

FIGURE 6.23

Afferent pupillary defect. Schematic representation of an afferent pupillary defect (APD) due to neurologic lesion (X) in the anterior visual pathway. (Reproduced with permission from Birinyi F, Mauger TF, Hendershot AJ. Ophthalmic Conditions. In: Knoop KJ, Stack LB, Storrow AB, Thurman R. eds. *The Atlas of Emergency Medicine*, 4e New York, NY: McGraw-Hill, 2016).

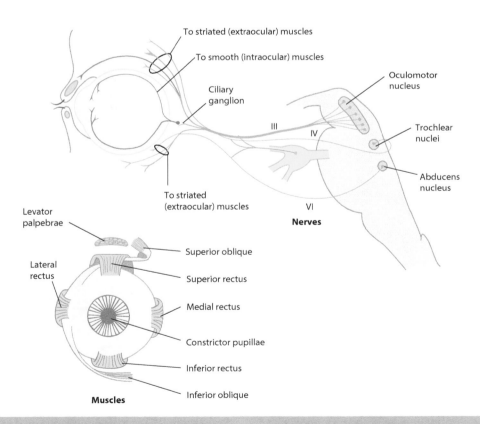

FIGURE 6.24

Cranial nerves innervating extraocular eye muscles. The oculomotor (III), trochlear (IV), and abducens (VI) nerves; anterior view of ocular muscles. (Reproduced with permission from Cranial Nerves and Pathways. In: Waxman SG. eds. *Clinical Neuroanatomy*, 28e New York, NY: McGraw-Hill, 2017).

responsible for ensuring that the eyes are optimally directed to receive input to the most sensitive part of the eye, the macula. They arise from general somatic efferent nuclei and serve only motor functions. Cranial nerve III, the oculomotor nerve, innervates most of the extraocular muscles, including the superior rectus, medial rectus, inferior rectus, and the inferior oblique muscle, as well as the levator palpebrae superioris, the muscle of the upper eyelid elevation. The superior oblique muscle is innervated by CN IV, the trochlear nerve; and the lateral rectus is supplied by CN VI, the abducens nerve (Figure 6.25).

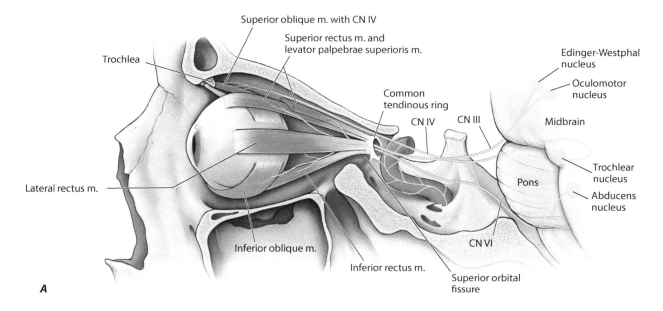

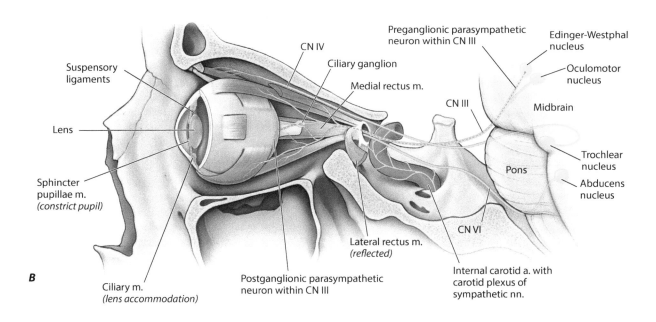

FIGURE 6.25

Extraocular eye muscles and their cranial nerve innervation in situ; lateral view. A. Somatic motor innervation from the oculomotor, trochlear, and abducens nerves (CNs III, IV, and VI, respectively). **B.** Visceral motor parasympathetic component of CN III. (Reproduced with permission from Chapter 17. Cranial Nerves. In: Morton DA, Foreman K, Albertine KH. eds. *The Big Picture: Gross Anatomy* New York, NY: McGraw-Hill; 2011).

The oculomotor nucleus or nuclear complex is wedge shaped and located in the midbrain. It sits at the level of the superior colliculus, ventral to the periaqueductal gray. The superior colliculus is a layered structure that acts as a visual reflex center. Its superficial layers primarily receive information from the retina and visual cortex, but the deeper layers receive auditory and somatosensory input, resulting in a complex interaction of motor and sensory information creating an egocentric three-dimensional representation of the self and surround to orient the head and eyes in response to external stimuli. The inferior colliculi are involved in processing sounds.

Subnuclei of CN III are each responsible for innervating a particular extraocular muscle (Table 6.4). The cell group of the levator palpebrae superioris is situated medially and sends fibers to both eyes, facilitating bilateral lid closure. The cell nucleus for the superior rectus sends information to the contralateral side, whereas those to the medial rectus, inferior rectus, and inferior oblique project only to the ipsilateral side.

This is of clinical significance because a rare lesion of the nucleus of CN III may be diagnosed when the presenting signs include contralateral superior rectus paresis and bilateral ptosis.

Voluntary movement of one eye is known as duction; the movement of two eyes in a similar direction is known as version. Adduction describes the movement of a single eye toward the nose, and the movement of a single eye away from the nose is known as abduction. Both eyes adducting produces a movement known as convergence. When an object comes toward the eyes, both eyes converge. Divergence describes the motion of the eyes in the opposite direction, away from the nose. When eye movement occurs in concert, it is known as conjugate eye movement. The muscles controlling conjugate gaze are known as yoked muscles that contract together to keep the object focused on the maculae of each eye. Dysconjugate (not moving in the same direction) movement occurs normally during near point convergence testing. After asking the patient to focus on an object moving toward the nose (convergence), the object is next moved farther away, and the eyes abduct (diverge) back to primary gaze. This concurrent abduction, a movement of the eyes in opposite directions back to their central resting place, is a normal divergent motion. Any other dysconjugate motion indicates the presence of a palsy.

Along with convergence and divergence, there are changes in pupil diameter and shape called accommodation. As the object moves closer, the pupil becomes smaller and thicker. As it moves away, it becomes wider and thinner. Convergence and accommodation are directed by the accommodation center in the visual association cortex through connections with the pretectal area in the superior colliculus.

The oculomotor CN III carries with it preganglionic parasympathetic innervation from the rostral midbrain to the ciliary ganglion in the orbit, and then to the iris sphincter via a postganglionic pathway within the ciliary nerves. The cell bodies of these neurons are located in the Edinger-Westphal nucleus, a subnucleus of the oculomotor nuclear complex (Figure 6.21). From the brainstem to the mid-cavernous sinus, the pupillary fibers are located around the superior surface of the oculomotor nerve. At the anterior cavernous sinus and the orbit, the pupillary fibers are carried with the inferior division of the oculomotor nerve.

Cranial nerve III palsy

When CN III is injured, ocular alignment and motility is affected. With unopposed action of CN VI and CN IV, the eye is positioned in partial abduction and depression with intorsion, which causes the eye to be turned "down and out." Because the levator palpebrae superioris is also innervated by CN III, ptosis may be present. Injury to the parasympathetic innervation to pupillary constrictors also produces a fixed dilated pupil or one that poorly responds to light (Figure 6.26).

The fascicles of CN III within the brainstem pass through the red nucleus and the medial cerebral peduncles, and exit the brainstem ventrally in the interpeduncular fossa. Vascular disorders, compressive lesions, or demyelination may affect the nerve fascicles in this location.

As the nerve continues its journey to the extraocular muscles, it enters the subarachnoid space and runs between the posterior cerebral and superior cerebellar arteries. It travels alongside the posterior communicating artery and exits the cranium by passing through the superior orbital fissure, in the lateral wall of the cavernous sinus. An aneurysm of the posterior communicating artery, which often occurs at the junction of the posterior communicating artery and the internal carotid, is the most common cause of a nontraumatic isolated CN III palsy. Another common cause of CN III palsy is microvascular disease, such as in diabetes or hypertension. A CN III palsy may be described as congenital or acquired, complete or partial, pupil sparing or pupil involving, isolated or accompanied by neurological involvement.

A dilated pupil associated with a CN III palsy is always assumed to be due to an aneurysm until proven otherwise, and is a medical emergency. A fixed dilated pupil or one that is unresponsive or poorly responsive to light indicates that the parasympathetic

Table 6.4 Oculomotor Subnuclei

Subnucleus	Muscles Supplied
Dorsal	Inferior Rectus
Intermediate	Inferior Oblique
Ventral	Medial Rectus
Edinger-Westphal	Pupil sphincter and lens ciliary muscle
Central Caudal	Levator palpebrae superioris
Medial	Superior Rectus

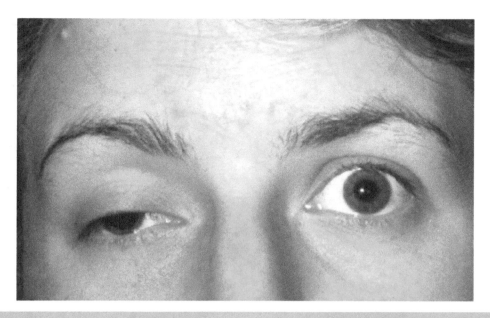

FIGURE 6.26

Ptosis and ophthalmoparesis seen with third nerve palsy. Note dilation of the right pupil; this is not pharmacologic. (Reproduced with permission from Moshiri A, Subramanian, PS. Disorders of the Eye. In: McKean SC, Ross JJ, Dressler DD, Scheurer DB. eds. *Principles and Practice of Hospital Medicine,* 2e New York, NY: McGraw-Hill, 2017).

fibers that travel on CN III are injured. Because clinicians know that pupillary involvement often may lag the motor signs of CN III palsy and only appear several days later, patients are carefully monitored during this period. A patient may also notice that near vision is blurry in the affected eye due to involvement of the ciliary nerves.

Abnormal eye deviation, such as that seen with CN III palsy, is known as strabismus (or tropia) of an eye. If the eye is turned inward toward the nose, it is known as an esotropia, or internal strabismus. If the eye is turned outward toward the ear, it is known as an exotropia, or external strabismus. An eye turn upward is known as a hypertropia, and by the same token, a downward eye turn is known as a hypotropia.

Acquired strabismus, such as in CN III palsy, causes misalignment of the visual axes that lead to double vision (diplopia). Congenital tropias are not usually associated with diplopia, as the brain adapts to eye deviation. In either case, the ability to appreciate perception of depth, or stereovision, is reduced, more so in the patient with frank diplopia.

When the eyelid is involved in CN III lesions, the patient may not complain of diplopia, because the lid covers the affected eye and acts as a patch. It is only when the lid is elevated by raising it with a finger that the patient experiences diplopia, and reports that it is worse when looking at near objects.

Cranial Nerve IV, The Trochlear Nerve

The nucleus of CN IV contains the cell bodies for the trochlear nerve. It is located in the tegmentum of the caudal midbrain. CN IV is predominantly motor but carries afferent proprioceptive fibers from the muscle it innervates (superior oblique). From its origin, CN IV is destined to innervate the superior oblique muscle on the contralateral side of the head. The right cranial nerve travels in the midbrain and then crosses in the anterior medullary velum, the roof of the Sylvian aqueduct, below the inferior colliculus. The anterior medullary velum is a thin white matter sheet that, together with the white matter of the vermis of the cerebellum, forms the anterior wall of the roof of the fourth ventricle.

Once the nerve exits the brainstem, it descends slightly, then travels in the periaqueductal gray, coursing anteriorly between the superior cerebellar and posterior cerebral arteries and laterally separated from CN III. The nerves emerge at the level of the inferior colliculus, pierce the dura, and pass through the wall of the cavernous sinus with several other cranial nerves, including CN VI (abducens) and the ophthalmic and maxillary divisions of the trigeminal nerve (CN V). It passes into the orbit via the superior orbital fissure, above the common tendinous ring. A CN IV lesion in the cavernous sinus typically affects the other cranial nerve functions.

CN IV travels with CNs III and VI, the abducens nerve, into the medial aspect of the orbit, and innervates the superior oblique muscle. The superior oblique muscle tendon passes through a pulley, or trochlea, at the superior nasal quadrant of the orbit. Movement of the muscle is afforded by the pulley system, but also by tendon elongation. The superior oblique muscle has the longest scleral contact arc of all the extraocular muscles. It functions as an intorter and depressor of the eye.

CN IV has connections with the vestibular system that are critical for, among other things, the orientation of the eyes associated with head tilt. When the head is tilted to the right shoulder, the right eye intorts slightly while the left eye extorts slightly. This is controlled by input from the vestibular system, with a precise disynaptic pairing of each of the three semicircular canals with the extraocular muscles (refer to CN VIII below for further discussion).

Excitatory connections run in the contralateral medial longitudinal fasciculus (MLF), and inhibitory connections run in the ipsilateral MLF. The action of the pairing is approximately in the plane of the semicircular canal stimulated. If the posterior canal is stimulated, it excites the depressors and inhibits the elevators, and the resulting eye movement is oblique and downward. With bilateral stimulation, both posterior canals create downward movement, but the oblique or torsional movements are effectively cancelled by the equal and opposite excitation created in each eye. By the same mechanism, if the anterior canal is stimulated, the resulting eye movement is upward and oblique.

CN IV is the thinnest of the cranial nerves and has the longest intracranial course. It travels 75 mm intracranially before it exits from the dorsal aspect of the brain stem. It is unprotected for most of its journey and is the cranial nerve most susceptible to injury, trauma, and increased intracranial pressure. CN IV palsy affects the superior oblique muscle, resulting in a slight extorsion or outward rotation of the eye, and a slight hyper deviation or elevation of the eye. Each of these actions is due the unopposed actions of the other extraocular muscles, such as the inferior oblique and the superior rectus. Patients complain of double vision and flex their neck to bring the elevated eye down into a primary gaze position for function. Additionally, many patients present with a subtle head tilt away from the side of the muscle palsy to compensate for the slight extorsion (Figure 6.27).

Loss of unilateral vestibular function can mimic a CN IV palsy, creating a torsion and resulting in double vision. The lesion can be

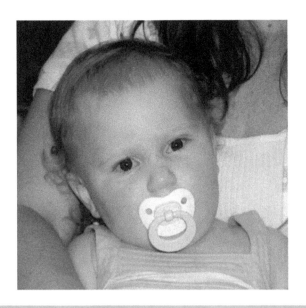

FIGURE 6.27

Head tilt due to congenital left superior oblique palsy. (Reproduced with permission from Motley W, Asbury T. Chapter 12. Strabismus. In: Riordan-Eva P, Cunningham ET, Jr. eds. *Vaughan & Asbury's General Ophthalmology*, 18e New York, NY: McGraw-Hill; 2011).

located centrally or peripherally in the vestibular pathway and is known as a "skew deviation." Abnormal torsional eye movement results from a lack of cancellation of the oblique movement by the affected side when the semicircular canal input from both sides is disrupted.

Trauma is the most common cause of CN IV damage. A lesion caused by hemorrhage, infarction, demyelination, or trauma affects the fascicles of CN IV. If the injury occurs before the decussation of the nerve, the effect is observed in the contralateral muscle; if en route to the orbit, it affects the ipsilateral eye. In addition, the sympathetic pupillary pathway that descends near the trochlear nucleus may also be injured and may present with features of a Horner's syndrome, miosis, ptosis, and anhydrosis on the ipsilateral side.

> ## > Neuroplasticity
> **Neuroplasticity: Aberrant Regeneration of CN III**
>
> The process of neuroplasticity allows adaptation or new learning to occur, holding promise for recovery after injury from disease or trauma. However this regeneration can also be functionally maladaptive. One fairly common example of peripheral neuroplasticity occurs after CN III injury. After a cavernous sinus lesion
>
> affecting CN III, the nerve may regenerate, or sprout axons, aberrantly, and connect incorrectly to another structure. If this aberrant regeneration follows a palsy, it is known as secondary aberrant regeneration. If it occurs without a preceding palsy, it is known as primary aberrant regeneration, and indicates an intracavernous lesion such as tumor or aneurysm. Common syndromes are described in Table 6.7.

Table 6.7 Aberrant Regeneration

Structure	Muscle	Action	Name
Lid	Inferior Rectus	Lid retracts when patient looks up	Pseudo-Von Graefe sign
	Medial Rectus	Lid retracts when patient looks to nose	Inverse Duane Syndrome
Pupil Sphincter	Inferior Rectus	Pupil constricts when looking down	
	Medial Rectus	Pupil constricts more briskly to convergence than to light	Pseudo-Argyll Robertson Pupil

Cranial Nerve V, The Trigeminal Nerve

The trigeminal nerve (CN V) is the largest of the cranial nerves (Figure 6.28). It emerges from the ventrolateral pons and contains general somatic afferent sensory and special visceral efferent motor components. CN V is the somatosensory nerve of the face, oral, and nasal cavities. Nearly all sensation, discriminative touch, proprioception, pain, and temperature from the face is carried on trigeminal fibers. In addition, it contains a smaller motor component that supplies primarily the muscles of mastication. The name arises from the three nerves that emerge from the trigeminal ganglion: the ophthalmic, maxillary, and mandibular nerves. These three nerves are often designated V_1, V_2, and V_3, respectively. Each of the three divisions contains afferent axons that carry sensory

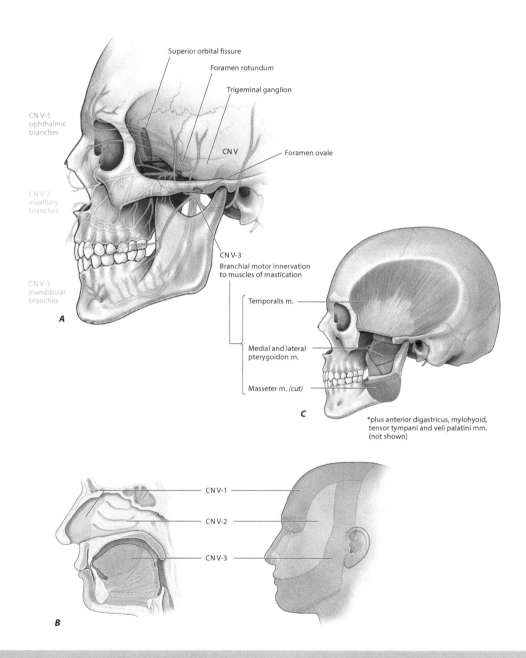

FIGURE 6.28

Trigeminal nerve (CN V) distribution. *A.* Boney relationships of the general sensory innervation from CN V. ***B.*** General sensory distribution of CN V divisions. ***C.*** Branchial motor distribution of the mandibular division of the trigeminal nerve (CN V_3) to muscles of mastication. (Reproduced with permission from Chapter 17. Cranial Nerves. In: Morton DA, Foreman K, Albertine KH. eds. *The Big Picture: Gross Anatomy* New York, NY: McGraw-Hill; 2011).

innervation from distinct regions of the face. Only the mandibular division contains motor fibers.

The three trigeminal divisions supply sensation to very specific areas on the head and face. Unlike the spinal dermatomes, the borders between areas supplied by each of the trigeminal divisions have little or no overlap in their somatosensory zones. V_1 and V_2 are purely sensory nerves. V_1, the ophthalmic division, receives sensations from the anterior scalp, the forehead, the upper eyelids, the conjunctiva and cornea of the eye, and parts of the nose, including the bridge (where glasses rest), dorsum nasi (length of the nose), and apex of the nose, excluding the ala (the wing of the nose lateral to the nostril). It also supplies the mucosa of the nasal cavities. Its innervation of the cornea contributes the sensory limb of the corneal reflex. V_2, the maxillary division, supplies the cheeks, the lower eyelids, the lateral aspect of the nose including the ala, the upper lip, upper teeth and gums, the palate, the nasal mucosa, and the mucosa of the maxillary sinuses.

V_3, the maxillary division, is a mixed sensory and motor nerve. It supplies sensory innervation to the skin of the mandible except at the angle and most of the skin of the external ear, which are supplied by branches of the cervical plexus. V_3 also innervates the lower lip, the lower teeth and gums, and much of the oral cavity, including sensory innervation from the anterior two-thirds of the tongue. Sensation from the posterior third and the epiglottis are supplied by the glossopharyngeal and vagus nerves, respectively. V_3 does not provide taste sensation from the anterior tongue; the chorda tympani of the facial nerve carries gustatory sensation. CN V is also the main supply of the meninges and the innervation of cerebral vasculature. A peripheral lesion of CN V is likely to cause a band of paresthesia or numbness within the distribution of V_1, V_2, or V_3 and can present as decreased sensation or frank pain.

The motor component of CN V, carried on the mandibular division, supplies branchiomeric muscles derived from embryonic pharyngeal arches. Thus the CN V motor nucleus is part of the special visceral efferent nuclear column in the brainstem. The major motor supply is to the muscles of mastication, the masseter, temporalis, and the medial and lateral pterygoid muscles. Several smaller muscles also receive V_3 innervation: the mylohyoid and anterior belly of the digastric muscles in the floor of the mouth; the tensor veli palatini in the soft palate; and the tensor tympani in the middle ear.

Sensory trigeminal nuclei

The sensory nuclei of the CN V comprise a discontinuous column of second-order neurons as well as a small complement of primary cells rostrally in the mesencephalon, extending from the mesencephalon caudally to the first one or two segments of the upper cervical spinal cord (Figure 6.29). As with the other sensory cranial nerve nuclei derived from the embryonic alar plate, the trigeminal nuclear complex ascends dorsolateral to the sulcus limitans in the floor of the fourth ventricle. It is composed of the mesencephalic nucleus rostrally, the principal (main or chief) nucleus in the pons, and the spinal nucleus descending from the pons downward into the cervical spinal cord. Each of these nuclei serves a specific sensory function.

The mesencephalic nucleus contains a set of ectopic primary afferent neurons serving a proprioceptive function. Its receptive field includes proprioceptors from the muscles of mastication and pressure receptors from the teeth and jaws. Output from the mesencephalic nucleus project to the cortex and to the spinocerebellum

through ill-defined pathways. It also mediates the masseter, or jaw-jerk, reflex.

The principal nucleus processes primarily the finest discriminative sensory input from the ipsilateral face. It lies approximately at the entry of the trigeminal root into the pons. Its second-order neurons receive inputs from sensitive mechanoreceptors mainly carried on Aβ axons. Lesions affecting the principal nucleus produce deficiencies in fine tactile information processing from the ipsilateral face.

The spinal trigeminal nucleus (SpV) is extremely long, extending from the pons into the spinal cord. Its major function is processing nociceptive input from the ipsilateral face. Just lateral to the nucleus

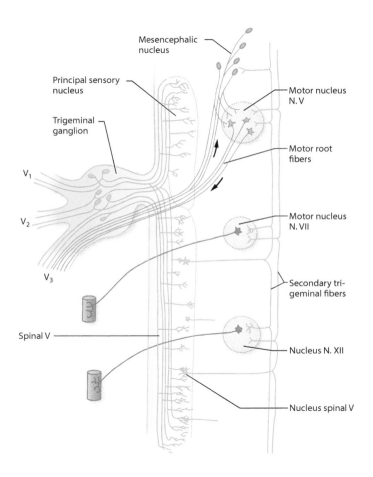

FIGURE 6.29

Scheme of the trigeminal nuclei and some of the trigeminal reflex arcs. V_1, ophthalmic division; V_2, maxillary division; V_3, mandibular division. Mesencephalic neurons innervate motor neurons in the motor nucleus of CN V to form the masseter reflex loop. Second-order neurons in the spinal trigeminal nucleus supplied by V_1 innervate CN VII motor nuclei bilaterally to form the corneal reflex loop. (Reproduced from Chapter 47. Diseases of the Cranial Nerves. In: Ropper AH, Samuels MA, Klein JP. eds. Adams & Victor's Principles of Neurology, 10e New York, NY: McGraw-Hill; 2014.)

throughout its entire length, primary afferent axons from neurons in the trigeminal ganglion create the SpV tract. Its axons dive deep from the tract to synapse on second-order neurons in the nucleus. SpV consists of three subnuclei: pars oralis, pars interpolaris, and pars caudalis. Pars oralis receives input from the oral cavity, especially from nociceptors. Pars interpolaris supplies extensive internuclear, brainstem, and cerebellar connections. Pars caudalis is most directly responsible for nociceptive transmission into the ascending trigeminal circuitry. Lesion of the SpV nucleus or its associated tract can produce reduction or loss of nociception from the ipsilateral face.

The motor trigeminal nucleus

The motor nucleus, a derivative of the embryonic basal plate, is situated slightly ventromedial to the principal sensory nucleus. Unilateral lesions of the descending CBT pathway, or cortical lesions, do not typically produce deficits because of the bilateral supply of motor nuclei above the upper representation of the face in the facial motor nuclei. Lesion of the motor root or the peripheral V3 paralyzes the ipsilateral muscles of mastication, producing weakness of bite and deviation toward the lesioned side, with mouth opening or protrusion. The masseter reflex, or jaw-jerk reflex, only seen under pathological conditions, presents as a sharp elevation of the mandible (bite) in response to a tap on the point of the chin. It indicates a lesion of the upper motor neurons supplying the motor trigeminal nucleus, and it tests the functional status of the mesencephalic nucleus and the mandibular division of CN V.

Cranial nerve V discriminative and nociceptive pathways

CN V's sensory pathway is a three-neuron sequence like that of the spinal level dorsal column-medial lemniscus and the anterolateral systems (Figure 6.30). The first-order neuronal cell bodies reside in the trigeminal ganglion and emit sensory axons that form the three divisions of the nerve. The second-order neurons in the principal and spinal nuclei receive synapses from the primary afferents. Lesions of the central primary afferent axons or the second-order neurons in the nuclei produce ipsilateral loss of sensation. A lateral medullary syndrome often damages both the SpV and the anterolateral system. With this injury, nociception is lost from the ipsilateral face and the contralateral body; this is an alternating hemianalgesia. Lesions in the SpV, most commonly attributable to ischemia or demyelination, result in loss of nociception in different patterns of distribution. Injury of the most caudal portion of the SpV eliminates nociception from the skin of the posterior face adjacent to the skin supplied by branches of the cervical plexus.

Deficits of nociception in the face demonstrate a somatotopy that is independent of the divisional distribution of V_1, V_2, and V_3. A lesion in SpV pars caudalis in the lower medulla and upper spinal cord produces a circle of analgesia that includes the scalp, ears, and chin. Injury to SpV pars interpolaris creates an analgesic area across the forehead, upper eyelids, cheeks, and the point of the chin. Lesions of SpV pars oralis eliminates nociception from the nose, lips, and oral cavity. Collectively, the concentric rings of analgesia produce an "onion-skin" pattern of loss of nociception that crosses divisional boundaries. Deficits appear on the half of the face ipsilateral to the SpV lesion.

Second-order trigeminal axons, like those in the spinal cord and dorsal column nuclei in the caudal medulla, decussate and ascend as the ventral trigeminothalamic tract, or trigeminal lemniscus, to

synapse on third-order cells in the ventroposteromedial (VPM) nucleus of the thalamus. A small dorsal trigeminothalamic tract ascends to the ipsilateral VPM, originating only from the principal nucleus, carrying discriminative touch and conscious proprioception from the oral cavity.

Output from the VPM thalamus ascends to the face representation in the lateral part of the contralateral SI cortex through the anterior portion of the posterior limb of the internal capsule. A lesion in the internal capsule can abolish all sensation from the contralateral face, but a lesion of the face area in SI eliminates only discriminative touch, vibration, and conscious proprioception from the contralateral face. Nociceptive inputs are widely distributed in the thalamus and cortex. The characteristics of pain sensation might be somewhat altered, but not completely lost.

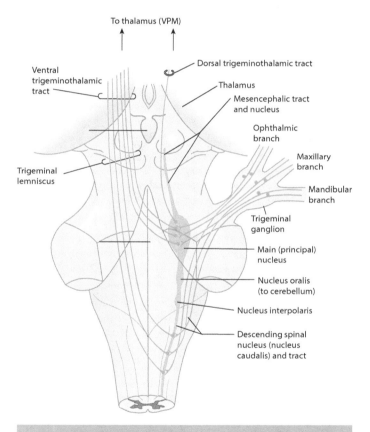

FIGURE 6.30

Schematic drawing of the trigeminal system and the ventral trigeminothalamic tract (trigeminal lemniscus). The trigeminal nuclei are projected onto the surface (green). The spinal trigeminal nucleus caudalis processes nociceptive input; the principal nucleus processes discriminative tactile inputs. A lesion of the ventral trigeminothalamic tract below the principal nucleus abolishes only nociception from the contralateral face. Above the principal nucleus, the ventral trigeminothalamic tract carries both nociceptive and s=discriminative inputs; lesions here eliminate all sensation from the contralateral face. (Reproduced with permission from The Brain Stem and Cerebellum. In: Waxman SG. eds. *Clinical Neuroanatomy*, 28e. New York, NY: McGraw-Hill, 2017).

Construction of the ventral trigeminothalamic tract has implications in the presentation of sensory deficits with central injury. In the medulla and caudal pons, lesions that damage the ventral trigeminothalamic tract produce contralateral sensory deficits. At this level, the only information carried on the ventral trigeminothalamic tract is nociceptive from the contralateral face. The pathway in the medulla lies adjacent to the lateral aspect of the medial lemniscus.

At the level of entry of the CN V root, the second-order axons from the principal nucleus decussate and join ventral trigeminothalamic tract on its ascent to the VPM thalamus. As it ascends, it assumes a position dorsal to the medial lemniscus, which, at the level of the rostral pons appears as a horizontal band. The dorsal relationship with the medial lemniscus persists until both pathways reach the thalamus. Lesions of the ventral trigeminothalamic tract from the level of the principal nucleus upward to the thalamus produce a total loss of touch and pain sensation from the contralateral face. Contralateral loss of nociception from the face is often associated with a medial medullary syndrome. Dorsolateral pontine or midbrain lesions abolish all sensation from the contralateral face, along with the loss of fine touch and pain from the contralateral body due to injury to the medial lemniscus and the anterolateral system pathway.

Synkinesis of cranial nerve V and cranial nerve III

During embryonic development, abnormal synkinetic connections ("miswiring") may form between CN III and CN V. The manifestation of this synkinesis is characterized by presence of a slightly drooping lid at rest that elevates in response to CN V activity of the medial and lateral pterygoids. The lid rises due to shared innervation with the pterygoid muscles that contract to protrude and depress the jaw. As the pterygoids relax, the eye returns to a slightly drooping position. This phenomenon is fairly common and known as Marcus-Gunn jaw winking.

Cranial Nerve VI, The Abducens Nerve

The abducens nerve supplies only one muscle, the lateral rectus, which is responsible for abduction (external deviation) of the eye. It emerges near the anterior midline at the pontomedullary junction. Its fascicle passes upward and forward through the cavernous sinus and through the superior orbital fissure into the orbit to access the lateral rectus muscle. The nucleus of the abducens nerve, in the general somatic efferent column, is located in the caudal portion of the pontine tegmentum beneath the floor of the fourth ventricle. The nucleus of cranial nerve VII is situated inferior to that of CN VI, but the motor fascicle of CN VII wraps over and around the CN VI nucleus and is referred to as the genu of the facial nerve (Figure 6.31).

Nuclear lesions of CN VI commonly also affect CN VII due to its anatomical proximity. Several syndromes have been identified based on the anatomical involvement of the brainstem and nuclei. The fascicle of CN VI crosses anteriorly through the caudal pontine tegmentum, passing lateral to the ventral trigeminothalamic tract, the medial lemniscus, and the CST. In this location, a lesion can damage both CN VI and the CST, producing a middle alternating hemiplegia, which presents as contralateral hemiparesis in the body with ipsilateral internal strabismus (medial deviation due to unopposed action primarily of the medial rectus). Of course this also produces diplopia. A lesion in this area may affect both CN VI and cause contralateral hemiparesis due to the proximity of the pyramidal tract in this area.

The nerve emerges from the pons in the pontomedullary sulcus, travels within the subarachnoid space, ascends the pons, where it is crossed by the anterior and inferior cerebellar artery and pierces the dura at the clivus, 2 cm below the posterior clinoid, to enter Dorello's canal. This route gives CN VI its S-shaped course, and in this area, the unprotected nerve is highly susceptible to increased intracranial pressure.

CN VI passes above the inferior petrosal sinus, runs under the petroclinoid ligament, and makes a sharp bend as it passes

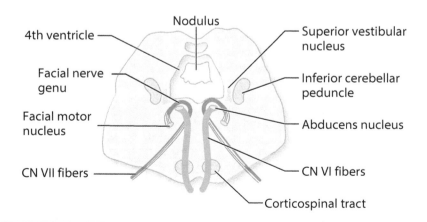

FIGURE 6.31

Brainstem at the level of the sixth-nerve nuclei. The genu of the facial nerve loops around the CN VI nucleus. CN VII exits the brainstem into the pontocerebellar angle; CN VI exits ventrally near the midline. (Reproduced with permission from Chapter 14. Disorders of Ocular Movement and Pupillary Function. In: Ropper AH, Samuels MA, Klein JP. eds. *Adams & Victor's Principles of Neurology*, 10e New York, NY: McGraw-Hill; 2014).

over the petrous tip of the temporal bone to enter the cavernous sinus. Disease of the petrous bone can affect the CN VI in this location. Localized inflammation or an extradural abscess of the petrous apex following complicated otitis media can also affect CN VI.

The nerve passes through the cavernous sinus lateral to the internal carotid and enters the superior orbital fissure to innervate the lateral rectus muscle. The lateral rectus is responsible for abduction of the eye. This muscle is responsible for turning the eye laterally (abducting), toward the ear.

Within the CN VI nucleus, there are two types of neurons, motor and internuclear (Figure 6.32). Motor neurons emit axons that create the abducens nerve, and internuclear neurons emit axons that decussate and ascend in the contralateral medial longitudinal fasciculus (MLF). Internuclear axons innervate cells in the trochlear nucleus before terminating in the CN III nucleus among the group of cells that innervate the medial rectus. In this way, activation of the abducens nucleus simultaneously directs ipsilateral abduction and contralateral adduction to deviate both eyes toward the abducting side. Thus the CN VI nucleus drives ipsilateral horizontal gaze.

Eye movements

As a visually oriented species, we rely heavily on our ability to focus on relevant objects in our visual field. Whether we are hunting prey, hiding from predators, searching for mates, or recognizing kin, we look, seek, watch, read, and view our world, directing the movements of our eyes by engaging specific cortical and subcortical circuits. We employ coordinated head and eye movements to direct our gaze so that we maintain the interesting image in focus on the region of highest acuity on retina, the fovea, situated in the middle of the macula. Directing view in this way is called foveation.

Complex eye movements ensure that an object remains foveated on our retinas, even while the object moves relative to us or we move relative to the object. Brainstem centers associated with CN III control disconjugate vergence movements and accommodation. Horizontal gaze is controlled by CN VI and its associated paramedian pontine reticular formation (PPRF); vertical gaze by the brainstem vertical gaze centers in the rostral midbrain reticular formation. The vestibular system drives reflex eye movements in response to changes in body and head position. Eye movement occurs along the horizontal or vertical axis, but oblique movement is generated by coordinated activation of the horizontal and vertical gaze centers. Saccades and smooth pursuit represent conjugate eye movements that allow us to examine and identify stationary objects and to follow moving objects through space.

One of the most important cortical areas directing volitional eye movements is the frontal eye field (FEF), Brodmann's area 8, in the frontal lobe. As described earlier in this chapter, it directs contralateral horizontal gaze through projections to the paramedian pontine reticular formation and its associated abducens nucleus. The FEF also directs vertical gaze through connections with centers in the rostral midbrain reticular formation. It prepares and triggers all saccades to visible objects, to the memory of those objects, and also to the predicted position of a moving object. Further examination has revealed that the FEF is a complex region with distinct but associated subcenters, including distinct horizontal and vertical saccades and smooth pursuit regions, as well as an anterior region that directs vergence movements.

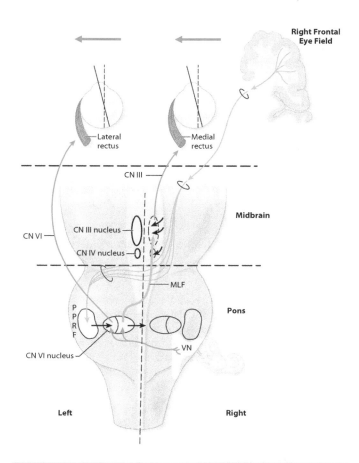

The internuclear pathways subserving saccadic horizontal gaze to the left. The pathway originates in the right frontal eye field, descends in the internal capsule, decussates at the level of the rostral pons, and descends to synapse in the left pontine paramedian reticular formation (PPRF). Connections with the ipsilateral CN VI nucleus and contralateral medial longitudinal fasciculus (MLF) are also indicated. Cranial nerve nuclei III and IV are labeled on left; nucleus of VI and vestibular nuclei (VN) are labeled on right. The right MLF (green line) contains axons from internuclear neurons in the left CN VI nucleus ascending to the right CN III nucleus. Contraction of the left lateral rectus (LR) and the right medial rectus (MR) deviate eyes to the left. The same eye movements occur reflexively (the vestibuloocular reflex) with head turn to the right and activation of the right VN. (Reproduced with permission from Chapter 14. Disorders of Ocular Movement and Pupillary Function. In: Ropper AH, Samuels MA, Klein JP. eds. *Adams & Victor's Principles of Neurology*, 10e New York, NY: McGraw-Hill; 2014).

Horizontal and vertical gaze

Eye movements can be grouped into two categories: volitional (voluntary) and reflexive. Because reflexive movements are primarily driven by activity in the vestibular system, those movements are discussed later. Volitional movements can be further categorized. Movements that focus an object onto the fovea (i.e., foveate the image) include horizontal and vertical gaze, convergence and divergence. Movements that stabilize the image on the retina include saccades and smooth pursuit.

In gazing, both eyes are directed either to the left or right in horizontal gaze, or upward or downward in vertical gaze. Voluntary horizontal gaze is known as saccades, and the pathway originates in the frontal eye fields of the frontal motor cortex. Projections from the frontal eye field travel directly or via the basal ganglia to the superior colliculus on the same side, cross over in the lower midbrain and upper pons, and terminate in the contralateral PPRF. The PPRF is situated anteromedial to the CN VI nucleus and anterolateral to the MLF. Its activation controls the ipsilateral abducens nucleus to abduct the ipsilateral eye, and, via axons from activated internuclear neurons ascending in the contralateral MLF, drives adduction of the contralateral medial rectus, acting as the yoke or bridge between the two eyes during conjugate horizontal gaze. Input from the frontal field drives gaze to the contralateral side via activation of the PPRF-abducens nucleus complex and the abducens nerve contralateral to the FEF, and the MLF and the CN III nucleus and nerve ipsilateral to the FEF.

The FEF, in collaboration with inputs from more diffuse cortical locations, also directs vertical gaze. Inputs that regulate downgaze descend to the midbrain rostral interstitial nucleus of the MLF and the interstitial nucleus of Cajal; and projections to the nucleus of Darkschewitz, in the posterior commissure mediate upgaze (Figure 6.33). Lesions of the dorsal midbrain can impair upgaze while sparing downgaze and horizontal eye movements.

Vergence

Vergence movements occur when the target moves toward (convergence) or away from the observer (divergence). These movements are slow, at about 20 degrees per second. Vergence occurs in parallel with accommodation due to connections between the Edinger-Westphal nucleus (the hub for accommodation) and the midbrain oculomotor nucleus (see CN III above).

Saccades

Saccades are rapid eye movements that combine a fixated phase with a ballistic movement phase. When we examine an object, we do not maintain unmoving focus on a single part of the object. For example, when we examine a face, we do not simply look at the eyes, but also at the nose, ear, chin, and other parts. Our eyes jump from one part to another. This movement accomplishes two things. First, it presents an overall impression of the object by foveating on a series of individual features; visual cortex integrates the separate images into a single object. Second, prolonged focus on a fixed object produces a form of adaptation that causes the image to fade from our perception. We must continually shift our point of focus to ensure that the image is not stationary on our retina for an extended period. This, in turn, ensures that the object remains, perceptually, in high resolution. Paradoxically, we do not perceive the movement during the saccade. There is speculation that visual input through the optic nerve is suppressed by the visual cortex during the movement phase of the saccade.

When reading a page, we do not simply track across a sentence; rather, we make small saccadic jumps covering an average of 7–9 characters taking about 20–40 ms with a fixation time of around 250 ms (a quarter of a second). Visually guided saccades, as when exploring the surrounding environment, also known as scanning, are of a much greater amplitude and of longer duration, on the order of 100 ms, although still with about 20–40 ms fixation.

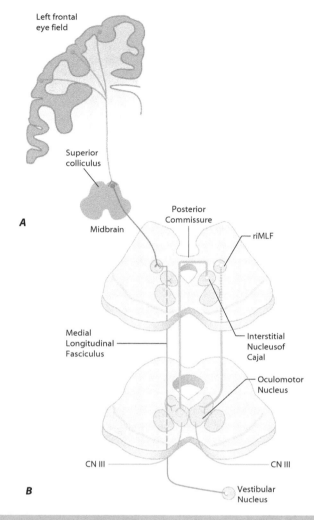

FIGURE 6.33

Pathways for the control of vertical eye movements. The main structures are the interstitial nucleus of Cajal (INC), the rostral interstitial nucleus of the medial longitudinal fasciculus (riMLF), and the subnuclei of the third nerve, all located in the dorsal midbrain. Voluntary vertical movements are initiated by the simultaneous activity of both cortical frontal eye fields. The riMLF serves as the generator of vertical saccades and the INC acts tonically to hold eccentric vertical gaze. The INC and riMLF connect with their contralateral nuclei via the posterior commissure, where fibers are subject to damage. Projections for upgaze cross through the commissure before descending to innervate the third nerve nucleus, while those for downgaze may travel directly to the third nerve, thus accounting for the frequency of selective upgaze palsies. The MLF carries signals from the vestibular nuclei, mainly ipsilaterally, to stabilize the eyes in the vertical plane (VOR) and maintain tonic vertical position. (*A*, Reproduced from Cranial Nerves and Pathways. In: Waxman SG. eds. *Clinical Neuroanatomy*. 28th ed. New York, NY: McGraw-Hill; 2017; *B*, Reproduced with permission from Chapter 14. Disorders of Ocular Movement and Pupillary Function. In: Ropper AH, Samuels MA, Klein JP. eds. *Adams & Victor's Principles of Neurology*. 10th ed. New York, NY: McGraw-Hill; 2014).

Control of saccades. Projections from the frontal eye field travel directly or via the basal ganglia to the superior colliculus on the same side, to determine accuracy, frequency, and velocity of the saccades. The superior colliculus in the midbrain regulates reflexive movements and is a center for reflexive head and neck movements, such as head and eye movements to a flash of light or loud sound. Visually guided reflexive saccades are known as prosaccades.

Inputs to the superior colliculus from the retina create an orderly three-dimensional map of the surround visual world perceived by the retina. This visual map coordinates with the motor map also present in the superior colliculus to create a reflex loop that produces the saccade. Similar auditory maps from the inferior colliculus and somatic information from the spinal cord, cerebral cortex, and substantia nigra also register with the superior colliculus motor map and coordinate eye and head in responses to a variety of stimuli. The superior colliculus projects to the PPRF and midbrain reticular formation and cervical spinal cord.

Activation of the visual map represented in the FEF and superior colliculus causes a saccade that is independent of the initial position of the eye. The direction of eye movement is determined by which muscles are stimulated; the amplitude of the eye movement is determined by the duration of the burst of neuronal activity in the muscle. A steady firing will hold the eye in its position. The FEF therefore stimulate the superior colliculus and control eye movements without input from the retinal fibers that terminate in the superior colliculus. Because the superior colliculus determines the accuracy, frequency, and velocity of the saccades, with loss of superior colliculus input, the saccade will still occur, but the eye will no longer be able to make very short latency reflex saccades (express saccades). Additionally, with loss of input from the FEF the eyes will not be able to move to the contralateral side, causing them to briefly deviate to the side of the lesion. This transient finding soon disappears as the superior colliculus compensates for loss of cortical input. We are able to voluntarily look away from a suddenly appearing peripheral stimulus; this movement is referred to as an antisaccade. Antisaccades have a longer latency, less perfect amplitude, and are a little slower than saccades. This ability is lost with injury to the FEF.

The natural aging process slows both antisaccades and prosaccades. This reflects a loss of grey matter in several frontal lobe areas in addition to the FEF (Figure 6.34). Loss of parietal cortices caused by degeneration or post-trauma, or with some psychiatric disorders, may also alter saccades.

Loss of inhibition is thought to be associated with higher antisaccade error rates and longer antisaccade latencies in schizophrenia and Korsakov syndrome. This patient population also shows higher fixation and prosaccade error rates. Patients with freezing gait in Parkinson's disease show a similar deficit in inhibitory control that leads to antisaccade errors. The antisaccade task and its relationship to inhibition has been used in rehabilitative training to reduce impulsivity, such as in patients with binge eating disorder and drug addiction.

Smooth pursuit

Besides the FEF, the supplementary eye field (SEF, Brodmann area 8) and dorsolateral prefrontal cortex (dlPFC, area 46) are two additional critical areas in the frontal cortex that regulate saccades and pursuits. The SEF is located in the superior part of the paracentral gyruson, the medial surface of the frontal lobe. These two areas have roles in the inhibition of reflexive saccades. They also contribute to sequencing eye movements based on spatial memory

of object position, and with predictive saccades toward where a moving object is likely to be. Brodmann area 9 in the frontal cortex, anterior to the supplementary eye field, acts along with the dlPFC in memory-guided saccades. The temporoparietal area is involved in spatial integration, directing attention toward the target. Attention is mediated by the anterior cingulate eye field (area 24). This cortical area also controls the dlPFC, influencing intentional eye movements. Visual attention is commonly viewed as a critical feature in pursuit, allowing us to concentrate on the image of one moving object among many that might be moving together.

Saccades must be suppressed when tracking (pursuing) an object, such as prey or predator, as it moves through visual space. For most people, it is not possible to suppress saccades to produce smooth tracking movements across visual space without having some moving object upon which to focus. Pursuits are relatively slow, involuntary conjugate eye movements covering several minutes per second to about 100 degrees per second, with a latency of 100–150 msec, which is about 50 msec shorter that the latency of a saccade. Pursuit movements, therefore, can be initiated before the initiation of the ballistic saccade.

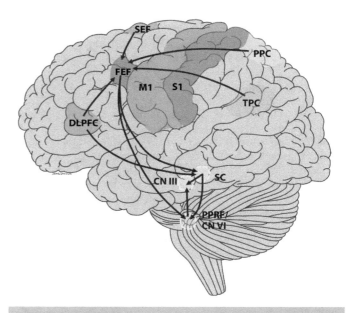

Cortical areas for eye movement. In addition to the frontal eye field (FEF), several other cortical centers contribute to the control of eye movement. Many emit inputs to the FEF for deeper integration of information required to predict or anticipate object position in space, or to direct various aspects of saccade production. The superior colliculus (SC) contains a three-dimensional egocentric map that guides the speed and accuracy of eye movements. Ultimate control over eye muscle contraction is exerted through the interaction of cells in the oculomotor nucleus (CN III), trochlear nucleus (not shown), and the paramedian pontine reticular formation/abducens nucleus complex (PPRF/CN VI). SEF, supplemental eye field; DLPFC, dorsolateral prefrontal cortex; PPC, posterior parietal cortex; TPC, temporo-parietal cortex; M1, primary motor cortex; S1, primary somatosensory cortex. (Image provided by Jamie Graham and Tony Mosconi, 2017).

Smooth pursuit movements compensate for small drifts in fixation and serve to keep a stationary target steady under static conditions. When the target is stationary, pursuits hold the eyes steady in fixation. As described above, the eyes typically drift slowly off a target, and the drifting is much faster and of larger range in the dark. The slow control of pursuits compensates for these drifts.

Pursuits also stabilize the image under dynamic conditions when the target is moving, suppressing the vestibulo-ocular reflex (VOR) and optokinetic reflex. The VOR controls eye movements that stabilize foveation of an image on the retinas during head or body movement. Head movement when tracking an object normally induces the VOR and causes a counter-roll of the eyes that disrupts fixation. When the eyes track a target, smooth pursuits suppress the VOR and optokinetic reflexes and permit an increase in the perception of optic flow, or the perception of relative movement in three-dimensional space.

Control of smooth pursuit. Pursuit movements are described in two phases, an open loop followed by a closed loop. The open loop describes the initial response to the acquisition of a target. The early component of the pursuit movement generates a rapid acceleration of the eyes independent of the stimulus velocity and retinal image position. Acquisition of the target initiates the fixation reflex, which is the ability to fixate and lock visually on a moving target. The end of the open loop phase correlates with the beginning of the closed loop phase, and this requires constant visual feedback and ongoing correction of pursuit movements.

The retinal images change as the eyes attempt to track a moving target. Without correction, the lag between slightly slower eye movement and movement of the target produces retinal slip, which degrades visual acuity and three-dimensional perception. Correction is made through feedback, which directs the eyes to move faster to compensate for the lag. During the closed loop component, pursuit is modified to match the velocity of the target and the retinal image position from the fovea. The velocity and direction of eye movements match movements of the target throughout the closed loop phase.

Once the target is locked in with fixation and there is no remaining retinal slip, the eye continues to track the target accurately. This is possible because the eye tracks the target relative to the head, using an egocentric three-dimensional map maintained in the extrastriate occipital cortex located near the junction of the occipital, posterior parietal, and temporal lobes in the middle temporal (MT) and middle superior temporal (MST) cortices. These cortices are connected to the pontine nuclei. Pontocerebellar fibers carry the signals to the flocculus of the cerebellum. Cerebellar outputs through the vestibular nuclear complex direct minute ongoing corrections in eye movements to generate smooth pursuit movements to the ipsilateral side.

Optokinetic nystagmus

Optokinetic nystagmus is a normal phenomenon that is substantially different from vestibular nystagmus, which is discussed later in this chapter. Optokinetic nystagmus produces reflexive eye movements that can be seen under certain conditions, such as when a patient is staring out of a window at a passing train. It is induced by visual stimuli. The eyes attempt to fixate on an object or feature, causing them to move with the target. As the train continues to move, the image drifts off the fovea, causing a quick

correction saccade back to the target to correct the fixation. This type of nystagmus is physiological. The optokinetic pathway shares the pathway for smooth pursuit, from area 18 and 19, the visual association areas, to the horizontal gaze center in the pons, which is essentially the PPRF-abducens nucleus complex.

The fast phase of the saccade is generated in the frontal cortex; therefore, if the corrective saccade is abnormal, the lesion is most likely located in the frontal cortex. The cerebellum is not involved in the initiation of saccades and eye movements. It controls and regulates, and is related to recovery of, saccades after disruption. The middle cerebellar zone, through the fastigial nucleus, controls the speed and accuracy of horizontal saccades. Vertical saccades are also regulated by the medial zone, however, through the interposed nuclei.

Lesions affecting gaze

Injuries of the visuomotor system produce distinctly different deficits depending on which part is injured. The ensuing section will discuss several common conditions.

Frontal eye field (FEF) injury. A lesion of the frontal eye field will cause paresis of contralateral gaze with drift of the eyes toward the side of the lesion. This is known as "right-way eyes." Cortical seizures, thalamic hemorrhage, and lesions of the base of the pons and tegmentum that damage the PPRF or CN VI nucleus can cause "wrong-way eyes," with the eyes deviated away from the side of the lesion.

Lateral rectus palsy. If the CN VI fascicle is injured in its passage through the brainstem (e.g., with the middle alternating hemiplegia) or anywhere along its course to the lateral rectus muscle, it produces an inability to abduct the ipsilateral eye, often with slight inward deviation, internal strabismus, or esotropia. This deficit is called a lateral rectus palsy, and it produces diplopia. With long-standing esotropia, cortical processing typically suppresses input from one eye, so the patient no longer experiences double vision.

Lateral gaze palsy. Injury to the nucleus of CN VI damages both the motor neurons and the internuclear neurons. This lesion prevents ipsilateral abduction and also eliminates contralateral adduction due to loss of ascending internuclear fibers. This injury produces a lateral gaze palsy preventing both eyes from deviating toward the side of the damaged CN VI nucleus. With a lateral gaze palsy, convergence and accommodation are spared, as there is no actual damage to the oculomotor neurons supplying the medial rectus muscle.

Internuclear ophthalmoplegia. Internuclear ophthalmoplegia results from a unilateral MLF lesion that interrupts sensorimotor integration in the pathway controlling horizontal eye movement. During evaluation, you ask your patient to gaze to his left. His left eye abducts, and his right eye adducts—both normal responses. Next you ask him to look to the right. His left eye remains at midline, staring straight ahead, while the right eye oscillates toward the right, indicating a left internuclear ophthalmoplegia. Internuclear ophthalmoplegia produces monocular nystagmus seen only in the abducting eye. This differentiates it from other types of nystagmus that typically involve binocular oscillation.

The vestibular nuclei integrate sensory information into control of horizontal gaze. When attempting to gaze contralateral to the injured MLF, internuclear fibers that drive ipsilateral adduction through CN III are lost, so the ipsilateral eye is unable to adduct. The contralateral abducens nucleus, the driver of the desired horizontal gaze, remains intact, and that eye abducts, but irregularly. Normal bilateral sensory impulses carried on the MLFs from the vestibular nuclei are now asynchronous, producing monocular nystagmus in the abducting eye. Gaze toward the side ipsilateral to the MLF lesion is unaffected, as are convergence and accommodation.

One-and-a-half syndrome. Occasionally, both the CN VI nucleus and the MLF are injured together on the same side (Figure 6.35). This lesion produces combined lateral gaze palsy and internuclear ophthalmoplegia. When trying to gaze ipsilateral to the lesion, the presentation is a lateral gaze palsy, and neither eye can deviate to the ipsilateral side. Gazing away from the lesion presents as an internuclear ophthalmoplegia. The ipsilateral eye is unable to adduct while the contralateral eye shows nystagmus on abduction. This disturbing condition is called a one-and-a-half syndrome. In some cases, the genu of the facial nerve is also injured with the injury to the nucleus of CN VI and the MLF. In this case, the deficit is the same as the one-and-a-half syndrome, plus paralysis of the entire face ipsilaterally; this is called an eight-and-a-half syndrome. Although rarer, the eight-and-a-half syndrome is sometimes seen in patients with multiple sclerosis.

Vertical gaze palsy. Vertical gaze is controlled by brainstem vertical gaze centers in the rostral midbrain reticular formation. Ventrally, the rostral interstitial nucleus of the MLF and the interstitial nucleus of Cajal regulate downgaze, and dorsally, the nucleus of Darkschewitz in the posterior commissure mediates upgaze. These anatomically discrete areas that mediate up- and downgaze create an important clinical tool localizing midbrain lesions. One of the more common lesions producing a vertical gaze palsy is the dorsal midbrain syndrome, or Parinaud's syndrome, most often caused by a pineal tumor, ischemic stroke, or multiple sclerosis. Among the symptoms presented with Parinaud's syndrome are paralysis of upgaze, sparing downgaze, pseudo–Argyll Robertson pupil (light-near dissociation in which the pupil constricts poorly in response to increased light intensity but properly with accommodation), and convergence-retraction nystagmus, in which attempted upgaze causes the eyes to deviate medially and the orbs to retract (Figure 6.36).

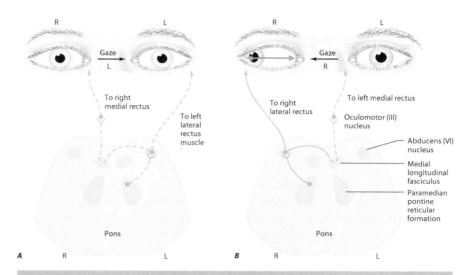

FIGURE 6.35

One-and-a-half syndrome. This results from a pontine lesion (blue shaded area) involving the paramedian pontine reticular formation (lateral gaze center) and medial longitudinal fasciculus, and sometimes also the abducens (VI) nucleus, affecting the neuronal pathways indicated by dotted lines. **A.** On attempted gaze toward the lesion, the left lateral gaze center cannot be activated, and the eyes do not move. **B.** Attempted gaze away from the lesion activates the uninvolved right lateral gaze center and abducens (VI) nucleus; the right lateral rectus muscle contracts, and the right eye abducts, although there is nystagmus indicted by the two-headed arrow. Involvement of the medial longitudinal fasciculus interrupts the pathway to the left oculomotor (III) nucleus, and the left eye fails to adduct. There is a complete (bilateral) gaze palsy in one direction (toward the lesion) and one-half (unilateral) gaze palsy (internuclear ophthalmoplegia) in the other direction (away from the lesion), accounting for the name of the syndrome. (Reproduced with permission from Neuro-Ophthalmic Disorders. In: Aminoff MJ, Greenberg DA, Simon RP. eds.*Clinical Neurology*, 9e New York, NY: McGraw-Hill; 2015.)

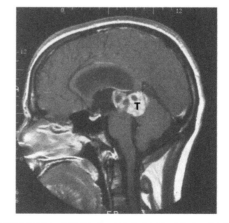

FIGURE 6.36

Pineal tumor. A midline sagittal T1-weighted contrast-enhanced MR image depicts a large tumor (T) in the region of the pineal gland. Lesions of this type can produce dorsal midbrain syndrome or Parinaud's syndrome. (Reproduced with permission from Chen MM, Whitlow CT. Chapter 1. Scope of Diagnostic Imaging. In: Chen MM, Pope TL, Ott DJ. eds. *Basic Radiology*, 2e New York, NY: McGraw-Hill; 2011).

Cranial Nerve VII, The Facial Nerve

The primary function of the facial nerve (CN VII) (Figure 6.37) is to provide motor innervation to the muscles of facial expression, which are derivatives of the primitive branchial arch. In addition to the large motor branch, CN VII includes a smaller component called the intermediate nerve that contains preganglionic parasympathetic, taste, and a small contingent of somatic sensory fibers. The facial nerve emerges from the brainstem at the pontomedullary junction into the cerebellopontine angle. It exits the cranium passing through the posterior cranial fossa in the company of the vestibulocochlear nerve, entering the internal auditory meatus in the petrous temporal bone. At different locations along its length, individual components emerge from the nerve.

As it passes through the facial canal through the petrous temporal bone, the facial nerve makes a sharp bend into the middle ear. At this point, along the nerve there is the geniculate ganglion containing primary somatic sensory neurons. Here, the intermediate

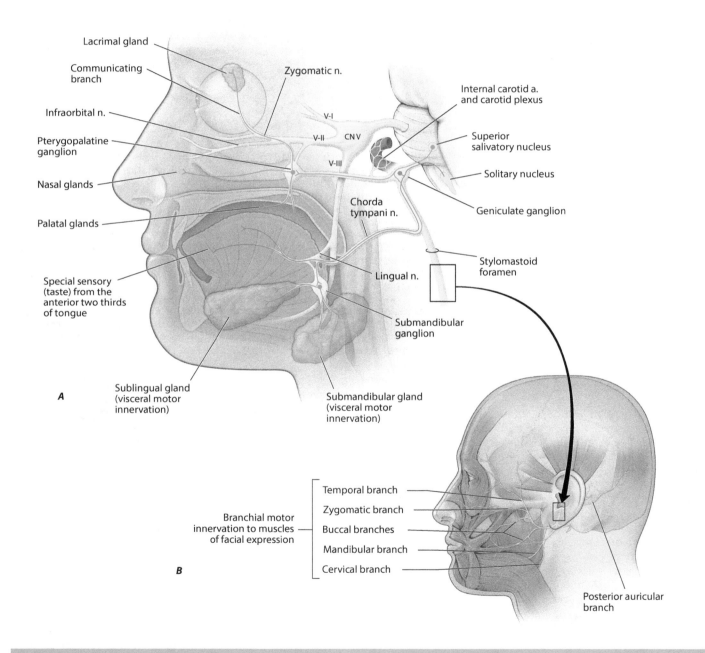

FIGURE 6.37

Facial nerve (CN VII) distribution. *A.* The facial nerve (CN VII). ***B.*** Branchial motor innervation to muscles of facial expression. (Reproduced with permission from Chapter 17. Cranial Nerves. In: Morton DA, Foreman K, Albertine KH. eds. *The Big Picture: Gross Anatomy* New York, NY: McGraw-Hill; 2011).

nerve branches from the motor portion of CN VII. The intermediate nerve contains the central axons of sensory neurons and preganglionic parasympathetic axons. GVE axons derive from neurons in the superior salivatory nucleus in the caudal pons just lateral to the abducens nucleus. Preganglionic parasympathetic axons do not synapse on cells in the geniculate ganglion. Instead, they pass through the ganglion and emerge as the greater petrosal nerve that courses rostrally to synapse on the pterygopalatine ganglion. Postganglionic parasympathetic axons innervate the lacrimal gland and the mucosal glands in the sinuses, nasal cavity, palate, and pharynx.

The facial nerve makes another sharp bend within the middle ear slightly medial to the incus bone. From this portion of the facial nerve, there emerges a small branch to the stapedius muscle. Damage to this innervation is thought to be one of the causes of hyperacousis, decreased tolerance to sounds. The stapedius muscle, along with the tensor tympani muscle innervated by CN V, dampen loud sounds by reducing movement of the incus and the tympanic membrane.

The motor portion of CN VII arises from a large nucleus located in the SVE cell column ventrolaterally in the caudal pons near the border with the medulla. Its fascicle passes dorsomedially and loops around the abducens nucleus as the genu of the facial nerve. At this location, a lesion of the abducens nucleus can also produce ipsilateral facial paralysis along with a lateral gaze palsy. An even larger lesion that damages the MLF produces a condition referred to as an eight-and-a-half syndrome, which combines a simultaneous lateral gaze palsy, an internuclear ophthalmoplegia, and a peripheral facial palsy.

The motor facial nerve emerges from the facial canal onto the face through the stylomastoid foramen. As it emerges, it emits the posterior auricular nerve to supply motor innervation to the posterior auricular and occipitalis muscles. Before CN VII enters the posterior margin of the parotid gland, it emits small branches to the posterior belly of the digastric and the stylohyoid muscles.

Within the substance of the parotid gland, the motor facial nerve divides into superior and inferior branches. The superior branch typically emits temporal, zygomatic, and buccal branches supplying muscles of facial expression in the areas for which they are named. The lower branch gives off marginal mandibular and cervical branches that supply muscles around the lower lip and the platysma muscle. A lesion of the motor facial nerve near its emergence from the stylomastoid can paralyze the entire ipsilateral face, impairing the corneal reflex and the ability to raise the eyebrow; it can also flatten the nasolabial fold, producing drooping of the corner of the mouth and an inability to smile or show the teeth on that side. Bell's palsy is the most common cause of facial paralysis. It is not caused by a stroke, but rather is thought to be caused by a virus, possibly the herpes virus (HSV-1), or other source of irritation of the facial nerve. If the irritation progresses proximally, patients might also experience loss of taste. Bell's palsy usually resolves itself within three weeks, but recovery can be hastened by early treatment with corticosteroids.

Of significantly more concern, a stroke or other lesion that damages the CBT above the facial motor nucleus causes a central facial palsy, which produces facial paralysis in a characteristic pattern. The facial motor nucleus is functionally divided into parts representing the upper face, including the forehead and periorbital muscles, and the lower face, including muscles of the cheek and mouth. Because the upper face representation is bilaterally supplied by the CBT, and the lower face primarily contralaterally supplied,

a CBT lesion above the facial motor nucleus produces paralysis of only the lower face contralaterally. Drooping of the corner of the mouth, flattening of the nasolabial fold, and inability to smile or show the teeth on the impaired side, while sparing forehead and periorbital movement, including sparing the corneal reflex, represents an emergent condition.

Geniculate ganglion

The geniculate ganglion contains sensory neuron cell bodies associated with CN VII. Somatic afferent (GSA) neurons in the geniculate ganglion emit peripheral fibers that course with the posterior auricular nerve to supply the skin of part of the external ear, a slip of skin behind the ear, and contributes, with CN V, to innervation of the external auditory meatus. Central somatic geniculate axons terminate in the spinal trigeminal nucleus.

The chorda tympani emerges from CN VII in the middle ear, exiting through the petrotympanic fissure and descending into the infratemporal fossa, where it joins the lingual nerve from the mandibular division of CN V and travels into the oral cavity. It carries special visceral afferent axons mediating taste from the anterior two-thirds of the tongue and the hard and soft palate. The axons from receptors in the taste buds travel on the chorda tympani and synapse on cells in the geniculate ganglion. Central projections are carried on the intermediate nerve and enter the tract of the solitary nucleus to terminate on the rostral bulb of the solitary nucleus, called the gustatory nucleus. The chorda tympani also carries preganglionic parasympathetic axons from the superior salivatory nucleus that innervate the submandibular ganglion attached to the lingual nerve. Postganglionic axons supply both the submandibular and sublingual salivary glands.

Cranial Nerve VIII, The Vestibulocochlear Nerve

CN VIII (the vestibulocochlear nerve) carries information from two different, highly specialized sensory systems originating in the inner ear (Figure 6.38). The vestibular division monitors head position in space, and the cochlear division responds to sound stimulation. Because they are separate sensory systems with completely different anatomic structures and pathways, each nerve division is discussed separately as either the cochlear nerve or the vestibular nerve. Located together in the membranous labyrinth of the inner ear are the sensory end organs for each system. Transducing cells in both systems are called hair cells, so called for the collection of stereocilia projecting from their apical surfaces. Hair cells differ subtly in anatomy and function, but in both systems they are innervated by primary afferent neuronal endings. The auditory hair cells are located within the organ of Corti in the snail-shaped cochlea. Hair cells for vestibular function are found in the utricle, saccule, and three semicircular canals. The cochlea and vestibular apparatus lie within the bony labyrinth of the inner ear cavity. The bony labyrinth encloses the membranous labyrinth that contains the cellular structures for generating auditory and vestibular signals. In the temporal bone, it is situated within the dense and protective petrous portion.

The two separate nerve divisions join at the lateral part of the internal auditory canal and briefly ascend together as the vestibulocochlear nerve, accompanied by CN VII. Of clinical note, fibers of both nerves may interweave with each other in this small space before separating again upon entering the brainstem at the pontomedullary junction. This may explain the unexpected vestibular

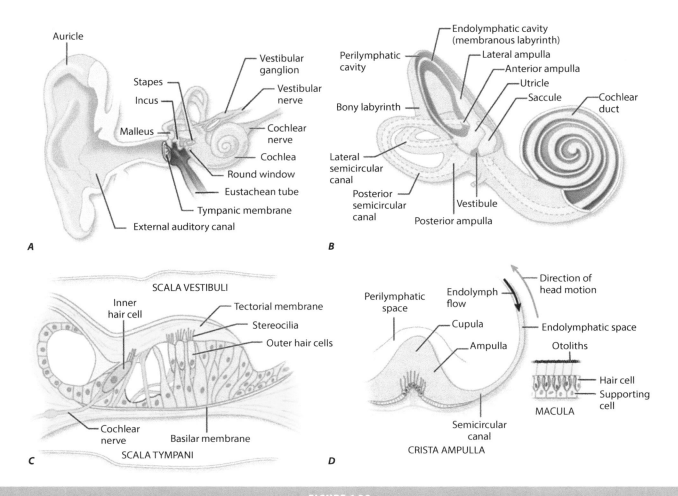

The auditory and vestibular systems. A. The right ear, viewed from the front, showing the external ear and auditory canal, the middle ear and its ossicles, and the inner ear. **B.** The main parts of the right inner ear, viewed from the front. The perilymph is located between the wall of the bony labyrinth and the membranous labyrinth. In the cochlea, the perilymphatic space takes the form of two coiled tubes—the scala vestibuli and scala tympani. The endolymph is located within the membranous labyrinth, which includes the three semicircular canals, utricle, and saccule. **C.** The organ of Corti. This is the end organ of hearing; it consists of a single row of inner hair cells and three rows of outer hair cells. The stereocilia of the hair cells are embedded in the tectorial membrane. **D.** Diagram of a crista ampulla, the specialized sensory epithelium of a semicircular canal. The crista senses the displacement of endolymph during head rotation. The direction of head rotation is indicated by the large arrow, and endolymph flow by the small arrow. The macula is the locus of the sensory epithelium in the utricle and saccule. Note that the tips of the hair cells are in contact with the otoliths (calcareous material), which are embedded in a gelatinous mass called the cupula. (Reproduced with permission from Chapter 15. Deafness, Dizziness, and Disorders of Equilibrium. In: Ropper AH, Samuels MA, Klein JP. eds. Adams & Victor's Principles of Neurology, 10e New York, NY: McGraw-Hill; 2014).

disturbance in facial paralysis and the persistence of tinnitus after cochlear neurectomy. The cochlear nerve ends at the cochlear nuclei on the rostral medulla, and the vestibular nerve terminates at four separate vestibular nuclei in the dorsolateral medulla and pons.

The cochlear nerve

Auditory function begins with activation of unique sensory end organs, located on the organ of Corti in the cochlea, a coiled structure about 30 mm long. The sensory end organs transform mechanical vibrations produced by sound waves into electrochemical signals transmitted centrally to the brainstem. These signals travel proximally on the cochlear nerve to the cochlear nuclei and ascend through the auditory pathway, decussating at multiple locations to innervate several nuclei and the auditory cortex for sound localization and contextual processing.

Peripheral receptors for hearing. A series of specific anatomic structures relay sound waves from the tympanic membrane (ear drum), through the middle ear, to the hair cells in the organ of Corti in the inner ear. Sound waves change the air pressure in the external auditory canal and vibrate the tympanic membrane. Ossicles in the middle ear, the malleus, incus, and stapes (the smallest bones in the body) conduct vibrations of the tympanic membrane across the space of the middle ear. The footplate at the distal end of the stapes inserts into to the oval window of the cochlea in the inner ear. The vibration of the stapes pushes the footplate in and out of the oval window like a piston, producing pressure changes that create waves in the fluid within the cochlea.

Within the bony labyrinth is a membrane containing the cochlea as well as five vestibular sensory organs that are discussed later. Much of the membranous labyrinth is filled with endolymph, an extracellular fluid resembling intracellular fluid in its ionic constituents. Three endolymph-filled compartments coil inside the cochlea: scala vestibuli, scala media, and scala tympani. The organ of Corti, the neural portion of the cochlear apparatus, resides in the scala media. Perilymph, a fluid resembling extracellular fluid and cerebrospinal fluid, fills the space between the membranous labyrinth and the temporal bone.

Pistoning of the stapes footplate in the oval window creates waves in the endolymph inside the cochlear compartments. The organ of Corti is composed of several parts that create a system in which fluid waves, generated by sound waves of varying wavelength and amplitude, activate tone-specific (tonotopic) auditory receptors (Figure 6.39). This traveling wave of fluid vibrates the basilar membrane, which rests on the floor of the scala medius; it contains the hair cells. Above the basilar membrane, fixed to the wall of the scala media, the tectorial membrane protrudes into the scala media endolymph.

The tectorial membrane is a gelatinous structure into which the stereocilia of the hair cells are embedded. The tectorial membrane is less compliant than the basilar membrane, so as the fluid wave vibrates the basilar membrane, the difference in movement between the membranes causes shearing of the hair cells, depolarizing them. The tonotopic organization of the hair cells on the organ of Corti is very specific, with receptors sensitive to high frequencies located near the cochlear base, and those sensitive to low frequencies located near the apex. The temporal lobe primary auditory cortex is also tonotopically organized.

High-frequency sounds generate vibrations on the basilar membrane, with a peak amplitude near the base of the cochlea; these sounds preferentially activate the basal hair cells. As the frequency of the sound decreases, the location of the peak amplitude of the wave on the basilar membrane shifts progressively toward the cochlear apex. This results in the preferential low-frequency activation of hair cells located at the cochlear apex. Although the mechanical properties of the basilar membrane are a key determinant of the auditory tuning of hair cells and

the tonotopic organization of the organ of Corti, other factors play important roles. For example, the length of the hair bundle varies with position within the cochlea. The bundles act as miniature tuning forks: The shorter bundles are tuned to high frequencies and are located on hair cells at the cochlear base, whereas the longer bundles are tuned to low frequencies and are located on hair cells at the apex.

Cochlear nuclei and pathways. The organ of Corti transduces sounds into neural signals through depolarization of hair cells. Each hair cell is innervated by fibers from primary afferent cells in the spiral ganglion within the cochlea. Central axons from these cells comprise the cochlear nerve. It exits the cochlea and travels through the internal auditory canal (IAC). The IAC is a 10–17 mm long bony

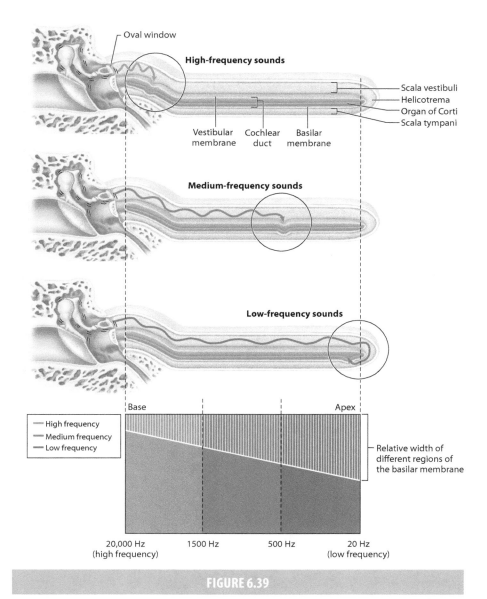

FIGURE 6.39

Interpretation of sound waves in the cochlea. In this figure, the cochlea is depicted as if uncoiled. (Reproduced with permission from The Eye & Ear: Special Sense Organs. In: Mescher AL. eds. *Junqueira's Basic Histology*, 14e New York, NY: McGraw-Hill, 2016).

canal in the temporal bone, containing the facial nerve, vestibular nerve, cochlear nerve, the vestibular ganglion, and the labyrinthine artery.

Upon exiting the IAC, the cochlear nerve enters the brainstem and synapses in the cochlear nucleus, which is composed of ventral and dorsal nuclei (Figure 6.40). The cochlear nuclei, located in the rostral medulla, are tonotopically organized, and ventral and dorsal nuclei have distinct functions. The ventral cochlear nucleus is important for horizontal sound localization and projects bilaterally to the superior olivary complex. The dorsal cochlear nucleus is thought to be important for vertical sound localization and for analyzing complex sounds. It projects directly to the contralateral inferior colliculus, bypassing the superior olivary complex.

The cochlear nucleus is the most central site in which a lesion can produce deafness in the ipsilateral ear. This is because it receives a projection from only the ipsilateral ear. Lesions of the other central auditory nuclei do not produce deafness; rather they produce partial hearing loss that is more prominent contralaterally, because more second-order axons decussate, and at each site along the central pathway there is convergence of auditory inputs from both ears (binaural). The anterior inferior cerebellar artery supplies the cochlear nuclei, and unilateral occlusion can produce deafness in one ear. Separate pathways of second-order axons from the cochlear nucleus ascend through the brainstem. Most fibers of the ventral acoustic stria, arising from the ventral cochlear nucleus, decussate

in the medulla as the trapezoid body; others ascend ipsilaterally, and both ascend to innervate the superior olivary complex. The dorsal acoustic stria from the dorsal cochlear nucleus, ascends mainly ipsilaterally, contributing to the lateral lemniscus, the main ascending fiber pathway of the auditory system. Every nucleus above the cochlear nucleus receives and processes binaural inputs.

An elegant mechanism exists in the superior olivary nucleus that integrates sound from both ears to precisely localize sound in three-dimensional space. When a sound is heard, especially when its source is from the side of the listener, there is a delay in activating auditory neurons such that the cochlear nucleus nearer the source is activated first. This is referred to as interaural time delay. The delay also means that sound waves in the near cochlear nucleus have higher intensity than those in the contralateral cochlear nucleus. Cochlear inputs from the near side arrive at the superior olivary nucleus and initiate activity in intensity-tuned cells in the superior olive. Later-arriving inputs activate cells in the superior olive as well. Activity is propagated through the nucleus, and when both inputs converge on the same cell, that cell's activity is maximal. That cell is integrated within the entire superior olivary nucleus in precise three-dimensional space. Loss of hearing impairs the ability to localize sound in space. Imagine that, in a large classroom, you ask a question of your professor, who, in her misspent youth, attended one too many loud rock concerts that damaged her ability to localize sound. The ability to process differences in sound intensity arriving at her superior olive is disturbed, and she looks around the classroom, trying to identify the student. You wave your hand and get her attention, much to her relief.

The lateral lemniscus carries auditory signals to the inferior colliculus, located on the dorsal surface of the midbrain tectum. The inferior colliculus is an auditory relay nucleus where most of the ascending fibers in the lateral lemniscal synapse. Inferior colliculus output projects to the medial geniculate nucleus located in the thalamus. The medial geniculate nucleus relays auditory information to the primary auditory cortex in the transverse temporal gyrus (Heschl's gyrus) on the superior surface of the superior temporal gyrus. As seen in subcortical auditory nuclei, the primary auditory cortex is tonotopically organized. Higher-order auditory areas encircle the primary area. Different sets of fibers emerge from the higher-order areas projecting to targets in the posterior parietal cortex and the dorsolateral prefrontal cortex processing sound localization. Another projection, important in processing complex sounds, including language, terminates in the ventral and medial prefrontal cortex. Wernicke's area (Brodmann's area 22), important in interpreting speech, is a part of the higher-order auditory cortex usually in the left hemisphere just posterior to Heschl's gyrus.

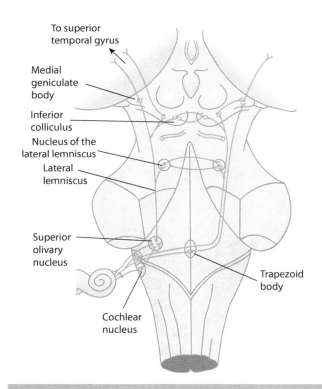

FIGURE 6.40

Diagram of main auditory pathways superimposed on a dorsal view of the brain stem. (Reproduced with permission from The Auditory System. In: Waxman SG. eds. *Clinical Neuroanatomy*, 28e New York, NY: McGraw-Hill, 2017).

The vestibular nerve

The vestibular system provides information regarding the location of the head in space, by continuously monitoring the exact position of each inner ear through activation of vestibular hair cells located in the five peripheral vestibular organs: the three semicircular canals, which signal angular acceleration; and the utricle and saccule, which signal linear acceleration (Figure 6.41). Head motion depolarizes the endings of bipolar neurons located in the vestibular ganglion.

The vestibular nerve relays messages to the brainstem, terminating in the four separate vestibular nuclei located beneath the floor of the fourth ventricle in the rostral medulla and caudal pons. Some vestibular axons project directly to the cerebellum and are the only primary sensory neurons that have this privileged access to the cerebellum because of the special relationship between the cerebellum and vestibular system in controlling eye, limb, and trunk movements.

Coordinating head and eye movements for stable vision during head motion ensures foveation to keep the desired image in the field where visual acuity is best. This requires significant interaction between the vestibular and visuomotor pathways, as well as ascending sensory feedback from cervical proprioceptors and descending motor pathways to the neck musculature, all coordinated in a complex network throughout the brainstem, diencephalon, basal nuclei, and cortex. The remaining vestibular system functions relate to the whole body, maintaining balance via the descending tracts to the neck, trunk, and extremities, and adjusting blood pressure during position changes.

Vestibular receptors for position sense. Neuroepithelial hair cells are vestibular transducers innervated by endings from bipolar primary vestibular neurons located in the vestibular (Scarpa's) ganglion situated within the internal auditory canal (IAC). As noted before, due to the close relationships among the facial nerve, auditory nerve, and vestibular nerve fibers in the IAC, damage to one nerve often affects the others. From Scarpa's ganglion the nerve enters the brainstem at the pons/medulla junction near the floor of the fourth ventricle. Most afferents project to the four vestibular nuclei (superior, inferior, medial, and lateral), with a few going directly to the cerebellum.

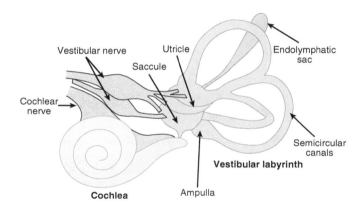

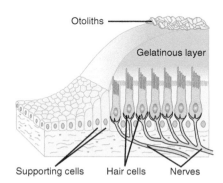

FIGURE 6.41

The membranous labyrinth of the inner ear has three components: semicircular canals, cochlea, and otolith organs. Hair cells in the semicircular canals are sensitive to angular accelerations that deflect the gelatinous cupula. Cochlea hair cells spiral along the basilar membrane within the organ of Corti. Airborne sounds set the eardrum in motion, which is conveyed to the cochlea by bones of the middle ear, and the membrane flexes up and down. Hair cells in the organ of Corti are stimulated by shearing motion. The otolithic organs (saccule and utricle) are sensitive to linear acceleration in vertical and horizontal planes. Hair cells are attached to the otolithic membrane. Information from the cochlear hair cells is carried by the cochlear division of the auditory (VIII cranial) nerve. Information from the hair cells in the semicircular canals and otolith organs is carried by the vestibular divisions of the auditory nerve. (Reproduced with permission from Hearing & Equilibrium. In: Barrett KE, et al., eds. *Ganong's Medical Physiology Examination & Board Review* New York, NY: McGraw-Hill, 2018).

Each hair cell has 50–100 stereocilia and a single long, thick kinocilium. The hair cells are distributed within the vestibular labyrinth in association with the vestibular organs. In the ampullae (dilatations) at the bases of the semicircular canals, the stereocilia and kinocilia of the hair cells protrude upward into a gelatinous mass called the cupula. Similarly, hair cells are distributed in a bed called the macula within the saccule and utricle, with the stereocilia and kinocilia extending into a gelatinous mass called the otolithic membrane. The surface of the gelatinous otolithic membrane is decorated with small calcium carbonate crystals, called otoliths or otoconia, that contribute extra mass and inertia to the otolithic membrane. This is why the utricle and saccule are often called the otolith organs.

Semicircular canals, utricles, and saccules are enclosed within a membranous labyrinth containing endolymphatic fluid. The three semicircular canals are arranged in orthogonal planes (at right angles to each other). Semicircular canals are paired with a complementary canal in the opposite labyrinth, and each pair responds to specific angular motion. The saccular and utricular maculae are also distributed at right angles; the saccular macula nearly vertical and the utricular macula horizontal. These are sensitive to linear acceleration and the force of gravity on the head.

In the semicircular canals, reactive flow of endolymph during head movement lags because of inertia. This inertia is augmented by resistance produced by the bulk of the gelatinous cupulae, and bends the cupula in the direction opposite head rotation. The stereocilia and kinocilium embedded in the cupula are deflected, and that transduces the motion to the vestibular afferent neurons.

Vestibular afferents innervating hair cells in all five peripheral vestibular organs have a resting firing rate of 70–100 spikes per second. Deflection of the hairs toward the kinocilium depolarizes (excites) the vestibular neurons, and deflection away hyperpolarizes (inhibits) afferent activity, thus the vestibular neurons instantaneously encode changes in head position (Figure 6.42).

This permits rapid processing of afferent input necessary for reflexive postural adjustments to maintain steady gaze or

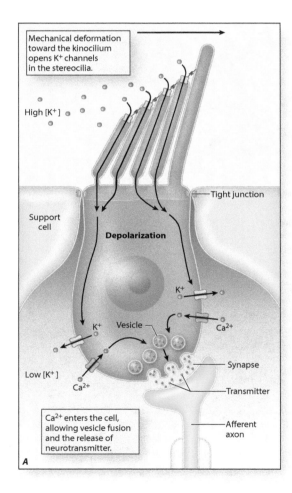
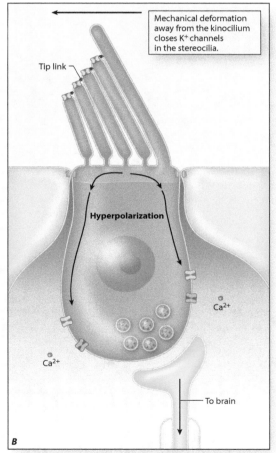

FIGURE 6.42

Vestibular afferents. Image demonstrating directional mechanical deformation of stereocilia and the kinocilium of a hair cell. **A.** Deflection toward the kinocilium activates K+ channels causing depolarization of the synapse. **B.** Deflection away from the kinocilium hyperpolarizes the synapse. (Reproduced with permission from The Eye & Ear: Special Sense Organs. In: Mescher AL. eds. *Junqueira's Basic Histology*, 14e New York, NY: McGraw-Hill, 2016).

trunk-righting reflexes. During angular head rotations, ipsilateral vestibular afferent excitation can increase firing rate up to 400 spikes per second, controlling responses over a range of head motion speeds. Inhibition of contralateral afferents increases the contrast between activating and inactivating directions of head movement. With cessation of head movement, the hairs return to their original positions and resume baseline firing rates.

Vestibular nuclei and pathways. The medial and inferior vestibular nuclei are located close to one another in the rostral medulla. The smaller lateral and superior nuclei lie within the pons. The four vestibular nuclei give rise to both ascending and descending tracts, sending projections to the cerebellum; brainstem nuclei, including the extraocular nuclei; and down to the spinal cord (Figure 6.43).

Lateral and medial vestibulospinal tracts carry vestibular output caudally to the spinal cord. Ascending tracts course primarily in the medial longitudinal fasciculus (MLF). Unlike the auditory and somatosensory systems, however, there is no single tract through which the ascending vestibular projection travels; some fibers travel in the MLF; some, in the lateral lemniscus; and others are scattered in the brainstem white matter.

The medial vestibular nucleus emits ascending and descending fibers that travel in the MLF. Axons descend bilaterally to the cervical and upper thoracic spinal cord via the medial vestibulospinal tracts to mediate head position by controlling the muscles of the neck and shoulder. Ascending fibers travel up the MLF, along with contributions from inferior and superior vestibular nuclei, and project bilaterally to all three extraocular eye muscle motor nuclei.

The lateral vestibular nucleus gives rise to the lateral vestibulospinal tract. Its fibers descend through the inferior vestibular nucleus and terminate on ipsilateral spinal interneurons near anterior horn cells at every spinal cord level to mediate trunk and limb muscle reflexes and postural control.

Cells in the superior vestibular nucleus are excited on the side to which the head is turned. Fibers from the superior vestibular nucleus cells decussate and ascend to the contralateral PPRF-abducens nucleus complex. This circuitry affects conjugate gaze opposite the activated superior vestibular nucleus. Therefore, turning the head to the left directs gaze to the right.

When we sit up quickly, blood must now flow against gravity. Maintenance of adequate blood flow to the brain is accomplished by a pressor reflex response.

Medial and inferior vestibular nuclei coordinate sensory input from viscera, muscle, skin, vestibular apparatus, and vision, regarding postural changes and resultant demands. This integrated information is used to influence the autonomic system to maintain stable blood pressure during postural changes by changing heart rate and vascular smooth muscle tone. When this response is inadequate, such as when a person is taking certain medications for reducing blood pressure, or diuretics, orthostatic hypotension ("postural" hypotension) can result and can cause fainting.

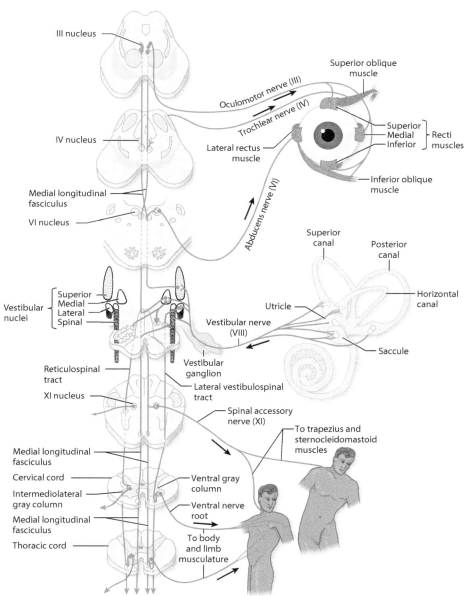

FIGURE 6.43

Vestibular nuclei and circuitry. Vestibular nuclei and vestibular reflex pathways for vestibulocular reflex, vestibulocollic and vestibulospinal reflex. (Reproduced from Chapter 15. Deafness, Dizziness, and Disorders of Equilibrium. In: Ropper AH, Samuels MA, Klein JP. eds. Adams & Victor's Principles of Neurology, 10e New York, NY: McGraw-Hill; 2014).

Reflex loops. A series of reflex loops involving vestibular system maintain head, trunk, and eye alignment during movements. There are three: the vestibulo-ocular and vestibulospinal reflexes, and the vestibulocollic reflex.

The vestibulo-ocular reflex (VOR). The VOR controls eye movements to stabilize foveation of the eyes on an image during head or body movement, and translates these velocity-generating movements into position sense. The mechanism of the VOR begins with head movement. The semicircular canals are paired, and movement in any direction depolarizes (excites) the vestibular neurons on the side to which the head turns, inhibiting contralateral neurons. Central projections from the depolarized ganglion cells excite the ipsilateral vestibular nuclei. Parallel outputs from the vestibular nuclei (particularly from the medial and lateral nuclei), combined with inhibition of the contralateral nuclei, produce a redundant connection that controls and coordinates binocular gaze opposite head movement. The vestibular nuclei emit axons into the MLF that ascend to the ipsilateral oculomotor nucleus cell cluster that innervates the medial rectus, adducting the ipsilateral eye. Simultaneously, output from the vestibular nuclei project to the contralateral PPRF/abducens nucleus, innervating both motor and internuclear neurons. The motor neurons drive contraction of the lateral rectus and abduction of the contralateral eye. Thus binocular gaze is directed opposite head movement. Axons from the internuclear neurons decussate and innervate oculomotor neurons that drive the ipsilateral medial rectus, reinforcing adduction. Inhibition of the contralateral vestibular nuclei acts to suppress antagonistic muscle contraction, preventing activity that would drive gaze ipsilateral to head rotation.

The orthogonal orientation (90 degree to one another) of the three semicircular canals in the vestibular labyrinth improves the three-dimensional resolution of head position. Each canal is paired with one from the contralateral labyrinth. Both horizontal canals are paired and are activated with horizontal head movements. Anterior canals are activated with forward head tilt, and inferior (posterior) canals with backward tilt. However, because the entire labyrinth is oriented about 45 degrees off the sagittal plane, the right anterior canal is paired with the left inferior, and vice versa, to detect angular head movements. Vestibular correlation of rotational and angular head movements is thus necessarily complex. Extraocular eye muscles are also attached in antagonistic pairs that move the eyes primarily in the same orthogonal planes. The pattern of activation in the vestibular system directs eye movements in predictable directions. For example, with bilateral stimulation of the posterior canals, the resulting eye movement is oblique and downward, as it excites the inferior recti and superior obliques and inhibits the superior recti and inferior obliques; medial and lateral recti contractions are effectively cancelled by the equal and opposite excitation created in each eye (Table 6.5).

This VOR is much faster than voluntary eye movements. Without the active stabilization provided by the VOR, patients experience oscillopsia in which the images from the retina appear to be blurred and seem to oscillate or jump. Unilateral loss can typically be compensated for by head movements. Bilateral loss leads to the sensation that the world is spinning or moving when the head moves, which leads to true vertigo.

Table 6.5 Physiological Activation of the Semicircular Canals

Semicircular Canal	Excitation	Inhibition
Horizontal	Ipsilateral MR Contralateral LR	Ipsilateral LR Contralateral MR
Anterior (Superior)	Ipsilateral SR Contralateral IO	Ipsilateral IR Contralateral SO
Posterior (Inferior)	Ipsilateral SO Contralateral IR	Ipsilateral IO Contralateral SR

The vestibulospinal reflex (VSR) and vestbulocollic reflex (VCR). The VSR and VCR are less well understood reflexes that use motion of the inner ear to produce motor responses. The VSR regulates full-body balance and postural responses, and the VCR coordinates vestibular activity, with input from proprioceptors in the neck to precisely coordinate and align head position during postural adjustments. Angular rotation of the head activates the medial vestibulospinal tract, which descends bilaterally through the cervical spinal cord, where it activates cervical axial muscles that coordinate head and neck movement to stabilize gaze. The lateral vestibulospinal tract descends to synapse on ipsilateral anterior horn interneurons at each level of the spinal cord. These interneurons innervate motor neurons in the anterior horn that excite antigravity muscles in the arms, trunk, and legs for specific stereotypical balance and posture responses. The reflexive motion produced is stereotypical due to monosynaptic activation of ipsilateral trunk and proximal limb extensors and polysynaptic inhibition of contralateral proximal extensors. Additionally, the cerebellum contributes to lateral vestibulospinal tract output to influence posture and equilibrium.

Caloric testing. Observing the VOR can reflect brainstem function in comatose patients, or definitively determine whether vestibular function is intact. Eye movements associated with the VOR can be produced by artificially stimulating movement of endolymph in the vestibular organ. To perform a caloric test, the patient is set supine, with her head tilted at an angle of 30 degrees to the bed, to orient the horizontal canals in the horizontal plane. Irrigating the right external auditory canal with cold water generates convection currents in the endolymph that mimic a head turn to the left. The VOR will then create a slow movement of the eyes to the right. Fast eye movement will be to the left, or left-beating nystagmus.

If the right external auditory canal is irrigated with warm water, the endolymph currents simulate a head movement to the right, causing a slow eye drift to the left and a quick right-beating corrective movement. The mnemonic, COWS, for this testing refers to the outcome of the direction of the nystagmus. Cold water causes fast-beating nystagmus in the opposite direction to the ear tested, and warm water calorics cause fast-beating nystagmus in the same direction as the ear tested.

Rotary chair test. To use the rotary chair test, a subject is placed in a chair that can spin in either direction. When rotation ceases, eyes oscillate, or show nystagmus. Like optokinetic nystagmus, vestibular nystagmus is also physiological and not under voluntary control. With slow (head) rotation to the left, the VOR drives slow eye movement to the right (i.e., in the direction *opposite* head movement). The rotary chair maintains the movement. As the rotation (head movement) continues, the eyes rapidly reset to the left. The alternating slow-rapid eye movements occur again and again while the rotation persists, demonstrating vestibular nystagmus named for the direction of the rapid phase. Thus the previous example represents a VOR; left-beating nystagmus. Rotation to the other side would, by the same token, produce right-beating nystagmus.

The oculocephalic reflex. The oculocephalic reflex is a form of the VOR typically used for testing comatose patients. Because it involves rotation of the head, the cervical spine must be uninjured before attempting the test. The patient's eyes are held open and the head turned rapidly left or right and briefly held in place. The oculocephalic reflex is positive when the eyes rotate opposite head rotation, indicating CNs III, VI, and VIII are intact (Figure 6.44).

The reflex is gradually suppressed in most normal infants by 11.5 weeks of age and masked by voluntary movements. Upward and downward movements are often accompanied by closing or opening of the eyelids, resembling a doll's eyes. Although an alert patient does not show the doll's head phenomenon, a comatose patient must have the doll's eye reflex; its abolition indicates the presence of a lesion in the afferent or efferent limb of the reflex arc, or within the connection of the two limbs. The afferent limb is composed of the labyrinth, vestibular nerve, and neck proprioceptors. The efferent limb is composed of CN III, CN VI, and CN VIII. Doll's eye testing is useful in patients with Parinaud's syndrome, where voluntary upgaze is diminished, but if the brainstem pathways are still intact, reflexive upgaze is possible. Absence of the doll's eye reflex is one of the criteria for determining brain death.

Cranial Nerve IX, The Glossopharyngeal Nerve

Although it is a relatively small nerve, the glossopharyngeal nerve, CN IX (Figure 6.45), contains neurons in five separate functional nuclear columns: SVE, GVE, GVA, SSA, and SVA. CN IX exits the brainstem as the most rostral of a series of nerve rootlets that protrude between the olive and the inferior cerebellar peduncle. It exits the cranium in the company of the vagus and spinal accessory nerves by passing through the jugular foramen into the cervical region. The superior and inferior ganglia of CN IX reside in the jugular foramen. The nerve descends between the internal jugular vein and the internal carotid artery, crossing superficial to the artery and passing deep to the styloid process. It descends across the stylopharyngeus muscle, innervating it and continuing rostrally deep to the hyoglossus muscle to distribute in the posterior oral cavity.

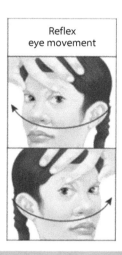

FIGURE 6.44

The oculocephalic reflex. Turning the head in either direction produces horizontal deviation of the eyes in the opposite direction. (From Durcan L. Coma and Disorders of Consciousness. In: McKean SC, Ross JJ, Dressler DD, Scheurer DB. eds. *Principles and Practice of Hospital Medicine*, 2e New York, NY: McGraw-Hill, 2017).

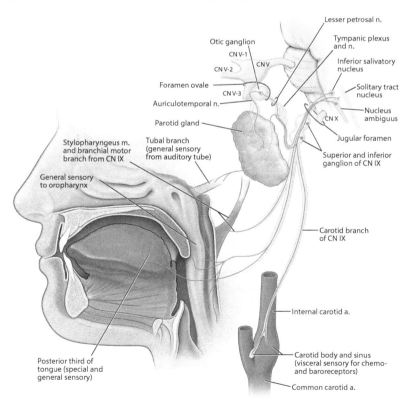

FIGURE 6.45

Distribution of the glossopharyngeal nerve (CN IX). (Reproduced with permission from Chapter 17. Cranial Nerves. In: Morton DA, Foreman K, Albertine KH. eds. The Big Picture: Gross Anatomy New York, NY: McGraw-Hill; 2011).

The SVE component of CN IX arises from the rostral end of nucleus ambiguus in the medulla. The few cells that contribute to the glossopharyngeal nerve provide the motor innervation of the stylopharyngeus muscle. The small muscle aids in elevating the pharynx for deglutition and phonation, but its effects are slight, and it is not possible to selectively test for stylopharyngeus function.

The inferior salivatory nucleus contains preganglionic parasympathetic neurons whose axons contribute to CN IX. GVE fibers pass through the superior and inferior ganglia without synapsing, emerging as the tympanic nerve. It enters the tympanic cavity, where it emits a few branches. One supplies general sensation to the middle ear. Another branch exits the cavity and passes into the middle cranial fossa, forming the lesser petrosal nerve. Axons in the lesser petrosal nerve synapse on cells in the otic ganglion situated within the foramen ovale. Postganglionic axons ride on the auriculotemporal branch of V_3 to terminate by supplying the parotid gland.

The inferior glossopharyngeal ganglion (petrous ganglion) contains the GSA, SVA, and GVA neurons of CN IX. The superior ganglion is sometimes considered an ectopic bit of the inferior ganglion. GSA and SVA axons are carried on the branch that enters the oral cavity. GSA fibers supply general sensation to the palatine arch, the pharynx, and the posterior third of the tongue behind the row of circumvallate papillae. This innervation contributes the sensory limb to the gag reflex. Branches also innervate the skin behind the ear and the internal surface of the tympanic membrane. As with the GSA fibers of CN VII, somatic sensation carried on CN IX enter the spinal trigeminal tract and synapse on second-order cells in the spinal trigeminal nucleus, from which axons of the ventral trigeminothalamic tract terminate in the VPM thalamic nucleus. Taste from the posterior third of the tongue is predominately bitter. Those axons also ascend into the solitary tract and synapse in the rostral gustatory nucleus.

GVA fibers exit the lesser petrosal nerve and descend into the neck. This fascicle arises from cells in the carotid body and carotid sinus, and they carry information concerning the oxygen and CO_2 tension and blood pressure changes. Central projections of this contingent also innervate the solitary nucleus. However, these end in the caudal portion of that nucleus responsible for sensorimotor integration of vital visceromotor functions regulating cardiovascular, respiratory, and gastrointestinal tract functions.

Cranial Nerve X, The Vagus Nerve

Cranial Nerve X, the vagus (Latin, "wandering") nerve, is the longest cranial nerve (Figure 6.46).

It descends through the neck, supplying cervical viscera; then through the thorax, supplying cardiorespiratory apparatus; and terminates by supplying most of the abdominal viscera. It exits ventrolaterally from the pontomedullary junction and

rostral medulla as several rootlets, into the pontomedullary junction alongside the CNs IX and XI between the inferior olive and inferior cerebral peduncle. It crosses the subarachnoid space and leaves the cranium via the jugular foramen accompanied by those nerves.

The vagus nerve descends through the jugular foramen, passing through the superior (jugular) and inferior (nodose) vagal ganglia and into the carotid sheath, lying posterior to and between the common carotid artery and internal jugular vein. During its descent, it emits thoracic branches and the superior laryngeal nerve that further divides into the internal and external laryngeal nerves. Caudal to these branches, the right and left vagal nerves take different courses. The right vagus descends between the subclavian artery and the sternoclavicular joint into the thorax. As it crosses anterior to the subclavian artery, it emits

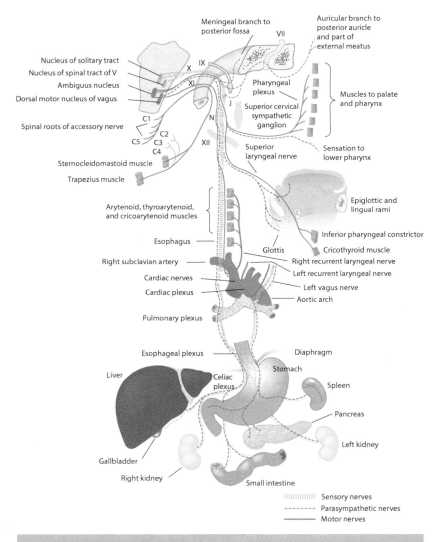

FIGURE 6.46

Distribution of the vagus nerve (CN X). Image shows vagus nerve and its many branches, as well as CN IX, XI and XII. (Reproduced with permission from Cranial Nerves and Pathways. In: Waxman SG. eds. *Clinical Neuroanatomy*, 28e New York, NY: McGraw-Hill, 2017).

the right recurrent laryngeal nerve that loops beneath the artery and ascends between the esophagus and the trachea to terminate inside the larynx as the inferior laryngeal nerve. The remainder of the vagus nerve enters the thorax and descends posterior to the root of the lung.

The left vagus descends between the common carotid and subclavian arteries, behind the sternoclavicular joint into the thorax. It first passes over the aortic arch, just anterior to the root of the lung. The left recurrent laryngeal nerve loops under the aortic arch, lateral to the ligamentum arteriosum, and ascends (recurs) back into the neck, where it distributes to the larynx like the right recurrent nerve.

The anterior vagal trunk, containing fibers mostly from the left vagus, and the posterior vagal trunk, mainly from the right vagus, pass into the abdominal cavity through the esophageal hiatus in the diaphragm. After this point, the trunks branch prolifically and distribute to the abdominal viscera.

Functional components of the vagus nerve

In its extensive descent through the neck, thorax, and abdomen, CN X emits numerous branches that supply sensory and motor functions to the head through the splenic flexure of the colon in the abdomen; many of these are named and described in Table 6.6. As was the case with CN IX, the vagus nerve employs several different functional nuclear columns, including GSA, SVA, GVA, SVE, and GVE. Several different brainstem nuclei account for these functions. GSA and SVA comprise relatively minor components of CN X function. SVE and GVE motor components utilize separate nuclei. Nucleus ambiguus, as described above, contains a few rostral neurons that contribute to CN IX. As will be discussed below, there might also be a few caudal neurons that contribute to the spinal accessory nerve (CN XI). By far, the greatest contribution from nucleus ambiguus is to the vagus nerve, supplying the muscles of phonation (speaking) and deglutition (swallowing). Parasympathetic (GVE) output associated with CN X derives from the dorsal motor nucleus of the vagus, and it supplies cervical, thoracic, and abdominal viscera.

Sensory innervation. Nearly 80–90% of the vagus nerve is sensory, the preponderance from thoracic and abdominal viscera. Sensory fibers in the pharyngeal and superior laryngeal nerves innervate pharyngeal and laryngeal mucosae. Lesions that damage the internal laryngeal nerve increase the possibility of choking because there is a loss of sensation in the uppermost part of the respiratory passage.

A small general somatic afferent portion of the vagus nerve supplies skin around the ear, the meninges of the posterior cranial fossa, and the mucosa of the epiglottis and at the root of the tongue. As with the minor GSA components of CNs VII and IX, central vagal GSA projections terminate in the spinal trigeminal nucleus. Central fibers of the auricular branch are carried on the vagus nerve while still within the posterior fossa of the cranium. Peripheral fibers of the auricular branch emerge in the neck from primary afferent neurons in the small superior vagal (jugular) ganglion in the jugular foramen. They pass posteriorly, ascend through a small canal in the mastoid bone, and soon merge with the posterior auricular nerve of CN VII, distributing to the external auditory canal and the auricle. A small contingent of vagal GSA fibers also innervates the meninges of the posterior cranial fossa, and additional somatic sensation innervates the epiglottis and root of the tongue.

Special visceral sensation, from taste buds in the root of the tongue and epiglottis, is also carried on vagal branches. The primary afferent neurons mediating vagal taste are located in the inferior (nodose) vagal ganglion in the neck, just below the smaller jugular ganglion. Three cranial nerves supply taste sensation from the

Table 6.6 Visceral Branches of CN X

Visceral Level	Nerve	Branches	Targets	Function
Cervical	Pharyngeal		Palate and Pharynx	Motor to Palate and Pharynx; Sensory to the Pharynx
	Superior Laryngeal	Internal Laryngeal	Inside the Larynx	Sensory and Parasympathetics to Internal Larynx
		External Laryngeal	Outside the Larynx	Motor to Cricothyroid Muscle
	Recurrent Laryngeal	Inferior Laryngeal	Larynx, Upper Esophagus, Trachea	Motor to all Intrinsic Laryngeal Muscle (not Cricothyroid); Sensory and Parasympathetics to Lower Larynx; Motor, Sensory, and Parasympathetics to upper Esophagus and Trachea
Thoracic	Thoracic Plexus Branches	Cardiac Plexus	Heart	Parasympathetics to Heart
		Pulmonary Plexus	Lungs	Parasympathetics to Bronchial Tree; Lungs
		Esophageal Plexus	Esophagus	Parasympathetics to Esophagus
Abdominal	Anterior and Posterior Vagal Trunks	Auerbach's Plexus	Between Circular and Longitudinal Muscle Layers in Gastrointestinal Tract	Motor, Parasympathetic, Sympathetic to most Abdominal Viscera; Peristalsis, Glandular Secretion
		Meissner's Plexus	Gastrointestinal Submucosal Tissue	Glandular Secretion

tongue (Figure 6.47); all of the central fibers innervate the rostral, gustatory, part of the solitary nucleus.

Vagal GVA innervation is most prominent in thoracic and abdominal regions. These sets of innervation are related to reflex activities that affect cardiovascular, respiratory, and gastrointestinal (GI) function. Generally, vagal parasympathetics have a depressive function, contributing to the "rest and digest" or "feed and breed" behavioral responses to extrinsic and intrinsic stimuli. CN X also carries sympathetic fibers to CNS locations mediating the balance between parasympathetic and sympathetic effects.

A small fascicle descends from the cervical vagus into the thorax and innervates the aortic arch. These afferents are baroreceptors, detecting changes in blood pressure, osmotic receptors monitoring changes in blood viscosity, and chemoreceptors sensing changes in O_2 and CO_2 partial pressure in the blood. Afferent innervation of the lower airways might be related to the rasping, burning sensations perceived with bronchial and lung irritation. Also within the thorax, CN X branches contribute extensively to the cardiac plexus; a substantial portion of the cardiac plexus is also sympathetic. It is from this plexus that the efferent regulation of heart rate and blood pressure is exerted.

Vagal afferents in the abdominal cavity are extensive, supplying the GI tract from the stomach to the splenic flexure of the colon, the liver, gall bladder, and pancreas, but not the spleen. The abdominal afferents include chemoreceptors monitoring the gut lumen contents for pH, glucose, fats, and peptides; interruption of vagal GI afferents can induce hyperphagia. Mechanoreceptors and nociceptors signal stretch of gut organs. Some recent work has suggested that nociception from the GI tract is not so much related to discriminating pain as to the affective-emotional responses to visceral pain through connections with brainstem and hypothalamic nuclei. Recent researchers have noted that abdominal vagal branches are in a position to detect peripheral (external) materials that can induce immune responses. With the massive rostral projection to brainstem and forebrain structures that mediate immune responses, the vagus could be a critical component of immune-mediated behavioral responses.

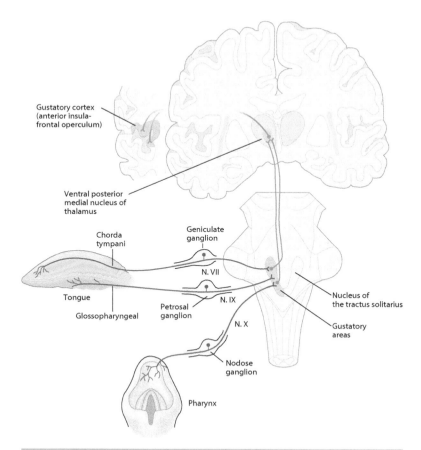

FIGURE 6.47

Special visceral sensation from the tongue. Diagram of taste pathways. Signals from the taste buds travel via different nerves to gustatory areas of the nucleus of the solitary tract, which relays information to the thalamus; the thalamus projects to the gustatory cortex. (Reproduced from Smell & Taste. In: Barrett KE, Barman SM, Boitano S, Brooks HL. eds. Ganong's Review of Medical Physiology, 25e New York, NY: McGraw-Hill; 2016).

SVE motor innervation. Vagal efferents innervate the muscles of deglutition and phonation as well as smooth muscles in the cervical, thoracic, and abdominal viscera. SVE output derives from cells occupying the bulk of nucleus ambiguus, and the GVE preganglionic parasympathetic neurons are located in the dorsal motor nucleus.

Axons from nucleus ambiguus innervate the muscles of the soft palate except the tensor veli palatini, innervated by CN V, and the palatoglossus, the only glossal (tongue) muscle not supplied by CN XII. A bulbar palsy (involving cranial lower motor neurons) of vagal innervation of the muscles of the palate produces paralysis of the ipsilateral palate, and that side will not rise upon phonation (such as when asking the patient to say "Ahhhh."). Only the rising of the contralateral palatoglossal arch deviates the uvula away from the side of the peripheral lesion. Compare this presentation with the description of the pseudobulbar (upper motor neuron) palsy

described above, in which the uvula deviates toward the side of the CBT lesion. Pharyngeal motor branches innervate the superior, middle, and inferior pharyngeal constrictors and the circular muscles guarding the opening of the esophagus. They also innervate the trachealis muscles in the trachea.

GVE motor innervation. Parasympathetic activity in CN X is not independent from sympathetic, somatosensory, and even cognitive activity. Proper function requires coordination of activity in brainstem autonomic centers, caudally in the spinal cord, and rostrally in the hypothalamus, thalamus, and cerebral cortex.

The nucleus of the solitary tract (solitary nucleus), in the medulla at the same level as the dorsal motor nucleus and nucleus ambiguus, is the primary target of visceral afferents. Its rostral end, the gustatory nucleus, receives SVA taste input from CNs VII, IX, and X.

Its caudal portion is the target for GVA inputs from CNs IX and X and from neurons in the dorsal root ganglia. This part of the solitary nucleus integrates sensorimotor input to regulate autonomic responses to visceral stimuli. Ascending output from the solitary nucleus projects to autonomic reticular formation centers, the thalamus, hypothalamus, amygdala, insular, and medial frontal cortices. These projections mediate complex autonomic functions such as the physiological changes associated with sexual arousal or fear.

Peripheral axons from DRG afferents travel on sympathetic nerves to innervate the abdominal viscera. They include stretch and pressure receptors to detect fullness in the gut and bladder, and nociceptors sensing potentially damaging stretch, ischemia, and irritation. There are relatively few sensory endings in the viscera, so sensation, particularly pain, is poorly localized. DRG visceral afferents terminate in the dorsal horn, and some end near the lateral horn close to parasympathetic and sympathetic neurons. These endings contribute to local visceral reflex circuitry. Second-order nociceptor fibers ascend in the anterolateral system, but others terminate on cells in the spinal cord gray matter near the central canal. Output from these cells ascend in the ventral dorsal columns and terminate in the dorsal column nuclei; outputs from there ascend to the contralateral VPL nucleus in the thalamus. Some hypothesize that a few of the DRG visceral afferents terminate in the dorsal horn onto neurons that also receive inputs from cutaneous receptors. These neurons are seldom activated by noxious input from the viscera. Noxious visceral stimulation is therefore perceived by the brain as deriving from a remote cutaneous target, providing a possible mechanism for referred pain.

The solitary nucleus receives cardiovascular inputs from CN IX derived from the carotid body, and from CN X from the aortic arch. These include baroreceptors monitoring vascular pressure, chemoreceptors detecting changes in the partial pressure (p) of O_2 and CO_2, and osmoreceptors that sense the osmolarity (the degree of hydration/dehydration) of blood. Changing pCO_2 and pO_2 signal the need to alter the rate of breathing. The solitary nucleus signals reticular centers that regulate inspiration and expiration; activation of inspiratory and expiratory centers is mutually exclusive. Outputs to spinal cord motor neurons stimulate diaphragmatic contraction and inspiration or intercostal and abdominal contraction for expiration. Lesions of the caudal solitary nucleus can lead to extremely dangerous breathing patterns such as ataxic (irregular), apneustic (deep inspiration with a prolonged stop—up to 90 seconds—followed by sudden expiration), or Cheyne-Stokes respiration ("crescendo-diminuendo" breathing pattern with progressively longer, deeper breathing, or hyperpnea, followed by shallower breaths, with intervening apnea). Each of these patterns is associated with significant brainstem damage and indicates life-threatening conditions.

Increasing blood pressure is monitored by glossopharyngeal baroreceptors in the carotid body that project to the solitary nucleus. For the baroreceptor reflex, solitary nucleus output projects to the dorsal motor nucleus cardioinhibitory neurons that innervate the sinoatrial (SA) node pacemaker cells to reduce heart rate. Simultaneously, the barosympthetic reflex reduces tonic constriction in peripheral blood vessels to reduce blood pressure. Decreasing blood pressure signals the solitary nucleus to excite inhibitory cells in the adjacent reticular formation that project to the lateral horn in the spinal cord, reducing sympathetic output to the arterioles and lowering peripheral arterial resistance.

Micturition (urination). Bladder control requires a complex interaction of somatic, autonomic, and cognitive functions. Somatic and sympathetic input from stretch receptors in the walls of the urinary bladder, carried on pelvic splanchnic nerves, innervate local spinal motor neurons, and the pudendal nerve, carrying somatic and sympathetic outputs, completing a reflex circuit that can stimulate bladder voiding. This reflex is usually under conscious control, and we can hold our water. Sympathetic output maintains relative high muscle tone in the external urethral sphincter, whereas parasympathetic innervation is suppressed, relaxing the detrusor muscle. In the rostral pons, there is a pontine storage center that maintains sympathetic output and allows the bladder to fill.

When the bladder wall receptors signal stretch (fullness) or pain (urgency), the ascending signal terminates in the pontine micturition center slightly dorsomedial to the storage center. The micturition center communicates with the frontal (orbitofrontal cortex: micturition decision center) and insular cortex, hypothalamus, and the midbrain periaqueductal gray. Descending projections from the micturition center inhibit sympathetics in T12–L2 pelvic and excite parasympathetics at S2-4. The result is descent of the bladder neck, relaxation of the sphincter, and contraction of the detrusor muscle for expulsion of urine.

The sensation of urine flow, carried on the pudendal nerve, reflexively maintains detrusor contraction and sphincter relaxation and a voiding phase. When the sensation ceases, the urethral reflex is activated, detrusor contraction is suppressed, and sphincter contraction is initiated, and micturition is halted. The pontine storage center is reactivated, and the bladder is prepared for storage until the next wave of stretch. If the pelvic floor is weak, as after childbirth or after prostate surgery, the sphincter muscles are insufficient to stem flow, especially against periodic increases in intra-abdominal pressure. This produces stress incontinence (loss of volitional control), which can interfere with activities of daily living.

Neurogenic bladder. Nervous system damage, through injury or disease, commonly produces impairment of bladder control. Loss of the complex neurological control of urinary storage/retention and volitional continence is not only embarrassing and uncomfortable, but can be life threatening due to infection, renal failure, and even sepsis. Neurogenic bladder is commonly classified by lesion location: in the brainstem, location in the spinal cord or peripheral nerve.

Lesions in the brainstem produce hyperactivity of the detrusor, as normal CNS inhibition is lost. Because sensory information from the bladder remains intact, patients report urinary urgency as well as increased frequency, and incontinence from detrusor overactivity. The bladder will not overfill because the sphincters remain functional and relax when the bladder contracts.

Lesions in the spinal cord above T12 produce an upper motor neuron lesion and spastic bladder. As seen with lesions in the brainstem, the detrusor becomes hyperactive. However the lesion also abolishes sensory input, so the reflexive emptying of the bladder is still possible, and unexpected and uncontrolled incontinence is a serious concern.

When the lesion is above T6, the patient is at risk for potentially life-threatening autonomic hyperreflexia, where a noxious stimulus (full bladder) triggers a dangerous hypertensive response. With this lesion, patients may have to self-catheterize, as spastic voiding is not always complete.

Lesions below T12, disconnecting lumbar and sacral spinal segments, produce a lower motor neuron flaccid bladder. During bladder filling, the denervated detrusor is dysfunctional, with variable muscle tone. Sensation may be intact or absent, depending on the type of lesion. Bladder leakage may be a concern, as is infection due to near constant presence of urine in the urethra, which is a perfect medium for bacterial growth. These lesions always require catheterization. With either spastic or flaccid bladder conditions, patients should be taught self-maintenance whenever they participate in social situations.

Sexual function. Like micturition, sexual function is a complex interaction of somatic, autonomic, cognitive, and emotional functions, with a decidedly different behavioral response. Behavioral responses vary among individuals, even within gender, due to the interaction of personal preferences and past experience. The neurological control of sexual reflexes is the same between genders, however, and the differences in responses are largely due to differences in sex organ anatomy. There are also well documented gender differences in response to different types stimuli; for example, visual stimulation generally appears to be less arousing for women. However, this aspect of behavior is outside the scope of this textbook. Overall, various somatic and special sensory inputs, in combination with memories of pleasurable experiences and erotic fantasies, initiate arousal and the sexual drive. The coordinated functions regulate such diverse physiological responses as vasodilation and constriction for erection, glandular secretion, and both autonomic and somatic muscular contraction, requiring visceral and somatic sensory input as well as higher-level responses affecting psychological and emotional responses.

Sexual reflexes consist of four stages: erection (due to vascular congestion of the tissues), emission, ejaculation, and orgasm. First, erection is initially stimulated by somatic input from genitalia carried on the pudendal nerve (S2-4 spinal segments), as well as from non-genital erogenous areas such as the neck and nipples. Special senses, sight, sound, and smell also contribute to the emotional/cognitive aspects of sexual arousal. Both sympathetic (from T12–L2) and parasympathetic (from S2-4) innervation combine in the pelvic plexus. Parasympathetic output is the main contributor to producing an erection by constricting the ischiocavernosus muscle to prevent outflow of blood from the penis or clitoris. A concomitant central suppression of sympathetic output helps produce and maintain the erection.

Second, parasympathetics further direct emission (fluid secretion) from vaginal glands in females, and primarily from the seminal vesicles and the prostate in males. Sympathetic activity produces the combined behaviors that occur during the third phase, ejaculation. The external sphincter of the bladder is constricted to prevent flow of ejaculate into the bladder, and a series of muscular contractions propels sperm along the vas deferens, collecting fluids from the seminal vesicles and the prostate, and expels seminal fluid out of the body through the urethra.

Finally, the orgasm, although inconsistently described in the literature, is accompanied by predictable physiological changes, including tachycardia, increased blood pressure, and flushing of the skin. Contractions of somatic muscles in the pelvic floor, as well as the bulbospongiosus muscle around the bulb of the penis or the female vestibular bulb, are driven by output from a collection of specialized neurons in the sacral spinal cord ventral horn called Onuf's nucleus, carried on the pudendal nerve. Shortly after orgasm, sympathetic innervation relaxes the ischiocavernosus muscle, allowing blood to flow out of the congested tissues, relaxing the erection in both sexes. In males, this is usually followed by a refractory period during which the penile sensory threshold is significantly elevated and production of another erection is more difficult.

The capacity for sexual function in patients after complete spinal cord injury is variable. Because much of sexual function is reflexive, and other contributions arise from mental eroticism, some patients retain some functional sexual capacity. This is more likely if the spinal cord injury occurs above the lumbar level, sparing the innervation of the pelvic plexus and the somatic afferent and efferent functions of the pudendal nerve. After injury above the lumbar cord, some women are still able to perceive sensation from clitoral stimulation, as well as discomfort during menstruation or uterine contractions. Functional MRI results demonstrate that brainstem areas associated with the vagus nerve remain active in these cases; injury to the vagus nerve can abolish these sensations. Priapism is an often painful, prolonged erection without sexual stimulation that is common after partial spinal cord injury and disruption of parasympathetic innervation.

Cranial Nerve XI, The Spinal Accessory Nerve

The spinal accessory nerve is a purely motor nerve to the sternocleidomastoid and trapezius muscles (Figure 6.48). It is peculiar in that the vast majority of its motor neurons lie within the spinal accessory nucleus in the cervical spinal cord. The rootlets of CN XI arise from cervical spinal segments: C1–2 supply the sternocleidomastoid, and C3–4 supply the trapezius. CN XI ascends through the foramen magnum to join CNs IX and X as they exit the skull through the jugular foramen. In many reports, there are a few CN XI neurons in the caudal-most part of nucleus ambiguus that ultimately distribute with CN X. Other reports deny that this population is part of CN XI, contending that the neurons simply contribute to the vagus nerve. One possible clue to the actual anatomy might lie in the branchiomeric origin of the sternocleidomastoid and trapezius muscles, suggesting that there could be a special visceral efferent component to CN XI.

The sternocleidomastoid muscle turns the head to the opposite side and is tested by turning the head against resistance. This is weak when turning to the side ipsilateral to a CN XI injury. The trapezius attaches extensively to the scapula, and it is tested by elevating (shrugging) the shoulders against resistance. With injury, there might be an ipsilateral shoulder drop. Corticobulbar tract innervation is said to be ipsilateral, contralateral, or bilateral. CBT lesions often produce slight or transient deficits.

Cranial Nerve XII, The Hypoglossal Nerve

The most caudal cranial nerve in the brainstem is the hypoglossal nerve (Figure 6.48). It emerges ventrally as a series of small rootlets extending over the lower two-thirds of the medulla from the preolivary sulcus between the pyramid anteriorly and the olive posteriorly. In its course anteriorly, it passes through the hypoglossal canal to emerge onto the lateral aspect of the neck, crossing the carotid triangle near its apex. It extends across the hyoglossus muscle and into the oral cavity to provide motor innervation to the tongue, supplying the muscles that assisting with chewing, drinking, and vocalization.

Axons of the motor neurons of CN XII innervate the four intrinsic (within the tongue) muscles and three of the four extrinsic (attaching the tongue to the mandible, the styloid process, and the hyoid bone) muscles, except for palatoglossus, which is innervated by the vagus nerve. The intrinsic muscles have no bony attachments and lie entirely within the tongue. Their action is determined by fiber alignment, with the superior longitudinal muscle contracting to shorten the tongue and also make the dorsal surface concave. Conversely, the inferior longitudinal muscle makes the dorsal surface convex. The tongue becomes narrow and elongated by the contraction of the transverse muscle, whereas the vertical muscle makes the tongue broad and flat.

The extrinsic muscles attach the tongue to bones of the jaw and cranium. The genioglossus is a large, fan-shaped muscle covering most of the volar surface of the tongue, with attachment to the mandible. The upper, middle, and lower fibers have different orientations that produce variable function. Upper fiber contraction retracts the tip of the tongue. Contraction of middle fibers depresses the central portion of the tongue (forming a cup), and the longitudinally oriented lower fibers pull the tongue toward the mandible,

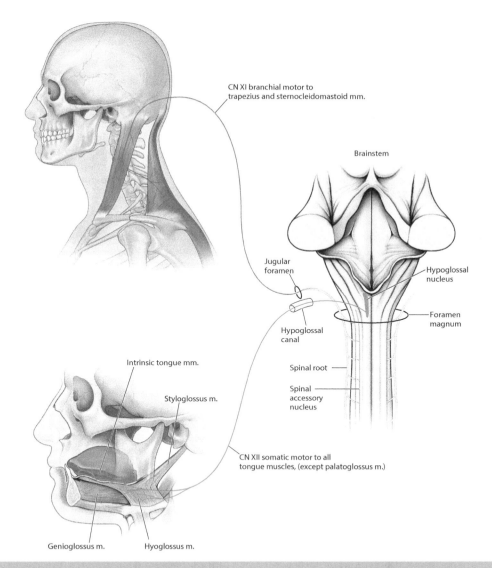

FIGURE 6.48

Distribution of the spinal accessory nerve (CN XI) and the hypoglossal nerve (CN XII). (Reproduced with permission from Chapter 17. Cranial Nerves. In: Morton DA, Foreman K, Albertine KH. eds. *The Big Picture: Gross Anatomy* New York, NY: McGraw-Hill; 2011).

protruding the tongue. The hyoglossus runs from the hyoid bone to the lateral surface of the inferior tongue. Contraction depresses the tongue, and once stretched into protrusion, the fibers become oriented anteriorly, producing retraction. The styloglossus attaches the lateral surface of the tongue (blending into the upper border of the hyoglossus) to the styloid process on the temporal bone. This muscle elevates and retracts the tongue during swallowing. The final extrinsic tongue muscle, the palatoglossus, has no bony attachment. It is innervated by CN X via the pharyngeal plexus and lies on the inferior surface of the palatine aponeurosis between the hard and soft palate, attaching to the lateral margin of the tongue. Contraction depresses the palate and elevates the back of the tongue.

The hypoglossal nucleus is the caudal-most part of the general somatic motor cell column. The nucleus lies near the midline in the hypoglossal trigone on the floor of the fourth ventricle, medial to the dorsal nucleus of CN X. Nerve fibers course through the medullary tegmentum, lateral to the ventral trigeminothalamic tract and the medial lemniscus, passing between the pyramids and the inferior olivary nucleus. This relationship jeopardizes CN XII with a middle medullary syndrome, typically caused by occlusion of branches of the anterior spinal artery. Sensory deficits associated with the middle medullary syndrome include loss of discriminative touch from the contralateral body and loss of pain from the contralateral face. Motor loss includes contralateral hemiparesis in the body, with ipsilateral paralysis of the tongue—an alternating hemiplegia.

The upper motor neurons for the tongue arise in the contralateral primary motor cortex and descend as part of the CBT, and a lesion in this innervation will cause contralateral tongue weakness. Typically, a lesion within the internal capsule causes a mild contralateral tongue weakness.

If there is a lesion within the hypoglossal nucleus or its nerve, the paralysis of the tongue is ipsilateral. The tongue rapidly atrophies, appearing fasciculated and wrinkled. When a patient is asked to protrude the tongue (or is simply rude!), it deviates toward the lesioned side. A more functionally relevant test is to ask the patient to try to clear food from the vestibule of the mouth (between the cheek and gums). The patient finds this movement difficult on the side ipsilateral to the lesion. Dysarthria (slurred speech) often results due to the inability to control the fine movements of the tongue necessary for articulated speech.

VII INTEGRATION OF SYSTEMS FOR MOTOR FUNCTION AND BALANCE

Complex, volitional human motor function depends upon successful integration of sensory systems to provide information about our environment. The visual, somatosensory, and vestibular systems provide information for central processing and evaluation based in large part on past experiences. These senses and their cognitive/perceptual interpretation serve as the foundation for normal movement; our four pillars of motor function (Figure 6.49).

The most dominant sense, vision, offers real-time information for advanced motor planning; scanning the environment for barriers, obstacles, or targets of our desire. Vision allows us to plan ahead, avoiding tripping over a rock on the ground. Somatosensory function provides rapid real-time feedback regarding changing external (environmental) and internal (joint position) during movements.

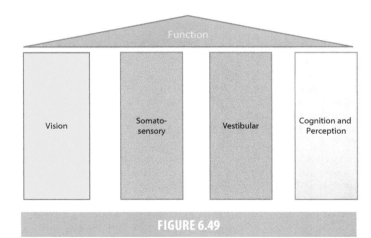

FIGURE 6.49

Four sensory pillars of motor function. (Image provided by Victoria Graham, 2016).

This allows us to adjust ankle muscle firing patterns while walking on an uneven surface. Vestibular system input to gaze centers ensures reflexive maintenance of image stability through eye and neck muscle adjustments. Information descending to postural muscles provides input for maintaining balance. Balance control involves the vestibular system, the visual system, and the somatosensory system acting upon cervical and extensor musculature. The cerebellum and cortex provide control over the sensorimotor processing that occurs predominantly in the brainstem. For example, normal balance processes act to keep the head upright. When falling asleep (for example, reading this textbook), the loss of cortical input reduces the tonic output of the vestibulocollic pathways, causing your head to fall forward. Additionally, long vestibulospinal pathways integrate sensory information to produce the proper sequence of trunk and leg musculature contraction to keep you upright, for example, while standing and walking on a swaying bridge.

Interpretation of these sensory inputs within the CNS is shaped by past experience and current cognition, which create perception of the experience and influence our response. During a hike, a small cylindrical object is seen on the path ahead; is the obstacle in the path a snake or a stick? Past experiences may sensitize us to incorrectly interpret a benign object as a cause of fear, altering our perception and prompting an exaggerated response. We discuss cognition and perception in future chapters, as they have a strong impact in fear avoidance behaviors commonly seen in chronic pain, as well as dysfunctional movements and misperceptions of body or visual perception common after stroke and traumatic brain injury.

VIII RESPONSE TO INJURY

The brainstem is often called the primitive brain, and loss of function can be life threatening. Brainstem damage may affect consciousness, muscle tone, respiration, and other basic life-sustaining functions coordinated through the cranial nerve pathways and nuclei, as well as reticular formation function.

Lesions of the ventral pons, usually associated with large basilar artery injury affecting bilateral corticospinal and corticobulbar tracts, can produce quadriplegia, loss of horizontal eye movements, and weakness of the lower face. This clinical presentation is known as locked-in syndrome. The reticular formation is spared, so the patient is fully aware; most somatic sensation is also preserved, but all ability to move or communicate is lost. Because the injury is below the nuclei of CNs III and IV, and the midbrain pretectum are spared, vertical eye movements and blinking may remain intact; therefore, communication might be accomplished with coded blinking and vertical eye movement.

Unilateral and bilateral brainstem injuries can produce pathological body posturing referred to as decerebrate and decorticate rigidity (Figure 6.50). Both can be caused by significant increases in intracranial pressure due to space-filling intracranial lesions, such as vascular injury or tumor, which compresses CST fibers in the midbrain or pons. Patients are usually comatose, and the posture is produced by applying noxious stimuli. Loss of CST regulation disinhibits extrapyramidal motor functions, producing rigid extension in the body and lower extremities due to elevated extensor activity from increased pontine reticulospinal and vestibulospinal output. Distinction between decerebrate and decorticate posturing is determined by the preservation of rubrospinal tract projection. If the lesion lies above the red nucleus, and rubrospinal output persists, the result is decorticate posture: rigid extension of body and lower extremities with flexion of the upper extremities. This occurs because there is combined facilitation of upper extremity flexion by combined rubrospinal and medullary reticulospinal output. Lesions below the red nucleus interrupt rubrospinal output; medullary reticulospinal output alone is insufficient to overcome extension generated by pontine reticulospinal and vestibulospinal output; upper extremities are also in extended posture. Transition from decerebrate to decorticate posturing suggests shrinking of the lesion and may be a positive sign.

The blood supply to the medulla is derived from the vertebral system (Figure 6.51). Damage to individual branches that supply distinct areas of the brainstem create signs and symptoms that are therefore clinically diagnostic. The ventral branches from each of the vertebral arteries combine to form the anterior spinal artery.

Medial medullary syndrome (inferior alternating hemiplegia) is also known as Dejerine syndrome. It is an extremely rare type of brainstem stroke that affects the small vessels of the vertebral or proximal basilar artery supplying the ventral medulla. It is characterized

by a triad of ipsilateral tongue weakness and atrophy (CN XII) and contralateral hemiplegia (pyramidal tract), representing an inferior alternating hemiplegia, and sensory loss (medial lemniscus).

The posterior inferior cerebellar arteries (PICA) are the most inferior brainstem vascular branches that emerge either from the vertebral arteries or from the basilar artery as it begins to snake up the ventral pons. These branches supply the posteroinferior cerebellum and the dorsolateral medulla. Cerebellar ischemia causes acute and severe vertigo, nausea, and vomiting, and due to its intimate relationship with the vestibular system, will cause three additional typical symptoms: ataxia, nystagmus, and tremor.

Occlusion of PICA presents with a complex set of findings, depending on the size and location of the infarct, producing a lateral medullary syndrome (Wallenberg syndrome). Classically, the syndrome includes six sensory and motor signs. Three are due to cranial nerve nuclei involvement: nucleus ambiguus (dysphagia and dysphonia), vestibular nucleus (vertigo and nystagmus), and the spinal trigeminal nucleus (decreased pain and temperature sensation from the ipsilateral face). Two additional signs are produced by damage to fiber tracts: decreased pain and temperature sensation from the contralateral limbs and body (spinothalamic tract), and Horner's syndrome (descending sympathetics in the hypothalamospinal tract). The final set of deficits arises from cerebellar involvement with a large lesion. Ipsilateral loss of facial pain with contralateral loss of pain from the body and limbs is called alternating hemianalgesia and is a strong indicator of the presence of a lateral medullary syndrome.

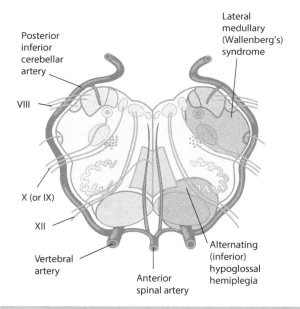

FIGURE 6.51

Clinical syndromes associated with vascular medullary lesions. Blood is supplied to the medulla from branches of the vertebral arteries. Injury to branches of the anterior spinal artery can produce an inferior alternating hemiplegia (middle medullary syndrome). A lesion of the posterior inferior cerebellar artery (PICA) can produce a lateral medullary (Wallenberg's) syndrome. (Adapted from The Brain Stem and Cerebellum. In: Waxman SG. eds. *Clinical Neuroanatomy*, 28e New York, NY: McGraw-Hill, 2017).

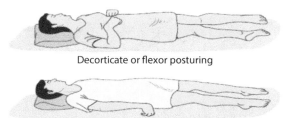

Decorticate or flexor posturing

Decerebrate or extensor posturing

FIGURE 6.50

Decerebrate and decorticate postures. (Reproduced with permission from Mariano GL, Fink ME, Hoffman C, Rosengart A. Intracranial Pressure: Monitoring and Management. In: Hall JB, Schmidt GA, Kress JP. eds. *Principles of Critical Care*, 4e New York, NY: McGraw-Hill; 2014).

The paramedian branches of the basilar artery supply the medial and basal pons, and interruption of these arteries will affect the corticospinal, corticobulbar, and corticopontine tracts and the descending root fibers of CN VI. This produces ipsilateral lateral rectus palsy (CN VI) and contralateral hemiparesis, known as middle alternating hemiplegia (Figure 6.52).

Interruption of the blood supply from the paramedian branches of the posterior cerebral or superior cerebellar arteries in the midbrain causes a contralateral hemiparesis (corticospinal tract) and an ipsilateral CN III (oculomotor) paresis. This is known as superior alternating hemiplegia. Because the optic tract passes posterior adjacent to the crus cerebri, where the motor fibers are located, a contralateral homonymous hemianopsia is also possible with Weber's syndrome (Figure 6.53).

Benedikt syndrome describes a lesion of the superior cerebellar peduncle, the red nucleus, and the oculomotor fibers. This leads to contralateral hyperkinesia, tremor, and ataxia in addition to oculomotor palsy.

The brainstem CN pathways are comprised of delicate nervous tissue at high risk for injury with neurological or vascular diseases or trauma. Their close proximity makes it likely that multiple cranial nerves will be injured with tumors or bleeding. Supratentorial herniation endangers rostral brainstem nuclei as well as the reticular activating system, which can cause coma. The high mobility of the upper cervical spine also places more caudal brainstem structures at risk for shearing during whiplash or head injuries. Routine screening and testing of the cranial nerves is an essential component of clinical care, easily integrated into patient examination. An overview of common cranial nerve conditions is described below.

CN I dysfunction may be an early sign of neurodegenerative disease. Anosmia is seen in patients with Alzheimer's and Parkinson's diseases, before any overt cognitive or motor signs appear.

CN II is exposed to tumors of the pituitary gland at the chiasm decussation; clinicians can use the resulting visual field defect (heteronymous bitemporal hemianopsia) to screen for tumor location. Like the white matter of the brain and spinal column, the optic nerve is susceptible to demyelinating disease. Optic neuritis is a common initial manifestation of multiple sclerosis. Anterior optic neuritis is characterized by visible swelling of the optic nerve and is associated with acute loss of visual acuity.

CN III is commonly affected by microvascular disease such as in diabetes or hypertension. Compression of CN III produces an oculomotor palsy. It can be caused by an aneurysm, usually at the junction of the posterior communicating artery and the internal carotid, but may occur at other junctions of the posterior communicating artery. It typically presents as an eye that deviates "down and out," accompanied by ptosis.

As the only dorsally exiting nerve, CN IV is very susceptible to trauma, with even mild injury potentially causing bilateral deficits. CN IV palsy leads to a hypertropia with a cervical torsional component; the eye is turned "up and in" with torticollis. A unilateral peripheral lesion of CN IV after it has decussated produces an ipsilateral CN IV palsy. If there is a lesion of the trochlear nucleus, it damages the fibers before decussation and produces a contralateral CN IV palsy.

CN V is often associated with infection by the herpes virus, causing eruption of a skin rash (shingles) along the dermatomal distribution of V1, V2, or V3 (Figure 6.54). The pain is known as postherpetic neuralgia and may precede the rash or linger long after the rash has

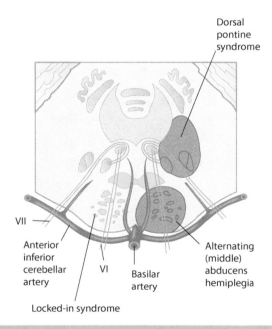

FIGURE 6.52

Clinical syndromes associated with vascular pontine lesions. Unilateral focal lesions of the penetrating branches of the basilar artery can damage the CST and the roots of CN VI, producing a middle alternating hemiplegia. A lesion farther dorsolaterally can produce a dorsal pontine syndrome that may affect some eye and face movements. A large basilar artery injury can deprive the ventral pons bilaterally, damaging the CSTs and CBTs on both sides. This produces a locked-in syndrome and bilateral quadriplegia. (Reproduced with permission from The Brain Stem and Cerebellum. In: Waxman SG. eds. *Clinical Neuroanatomy*, 28e New York, NY: McGraw-Hill, 2017).

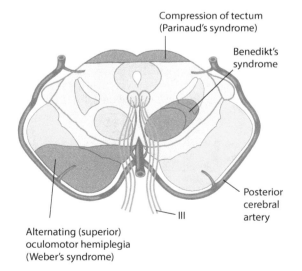

FIGURE 6.53

Clinical syndromes associated with vascular midbrain lesions. Lesions of the posterior cerebral artery include Weber's, Parinaud's, and Benedikt's syndromes. (Reproduced with permission from The Brain Stem and Cerebellum. In: Waxman SG. eds. *Clinical Neuroanatomy*, 28e New York, NY: McGraw-Hill, 2017).

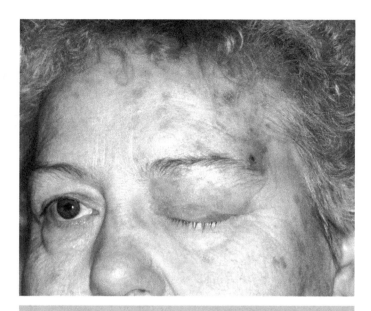

FIGURE 6.54

A 71-year-old woman developed typical pain and vesicles in the distribution of the first division of the left trigeminal nerve. An acute, profound left third cranial nerve palsy occurred 2 weeks after the onset of pain, when the vesicles were healing. A complete ptosis is evident in this clinical photograph, along with the healing vesicles. (Reproduced with permission from Pain and Sensation. In: Martin TJ, Corbett JJ. eds. *Practical Neuroophthalmology*, 1st New York, NY: McGraw-Hill; 2013).

cleared. CN V is also at risk for inflammation called trigeminal neuralgia, also known as tic douloureux, which may cause intense face and jaw pain along the nerve distribution. In the past, pain from trigeminal neuralgia caused many sufferers to commit suicide.

CN VI is longest cranial nerve, and with its length and sinuous trajectory, it is highly vulnerable to increased intracranial pressure. Many of the cranial nerves pass through the cavernous sinus. It is susceptible to many diseases and disorders that may affect the nerves to different extents.

CNs VII and VIII share the tiny internal auditory canal in the middle ear. This shared pathway places the structures at risk, and concurrent screening of hearing, vestibular function, and facial weakness or sensory changes is essential. Involvement of CNs V and VI, with otitis media, is known as Gradenigo syndrome and is characterized by esotropia (cross-eyes), facial pain, and an ear infection.

Integration of Systems
Benign Paroxysmal Positional Vertigo

Benign paroxysmal positional vertigo (BPPV), first described in 1980 by Epley, is the most commonly reported cause of vertigo. It is a peripheral condition in which calcium carbonate crystals, normally embedded in the gelatinous masses capping the hair cells in the ampullae, become dislodged and move freely within the semicircular canals. Changing head position causes the loose crystals to erroneously stimulate the hair cells, producing a sensation of rapid motion caused by kinocilia deflection. Diagnosis of BPPV is done by placing and maintaining the patient into a position that places each canal upside down, allowing the otoconia to become dislodged. A positive finding of BPPV is indicated by patient report of symptom reproduction after 10–30 seconds, and close monitoring of eye motion for VOR activation. Because each canal is linked to a specific eye muscle, stimulation of the VOR will produce stereotypical eye motion.

The most common location for these wandering otoconia to settle is in the inferior (posterior) semicircular canals, due to their inferior position during most upright postures. The examination is called the Dix-Hallpike maneuver (Figure 6.55) and involves placing the person's inferior canal into a specific angle to stimulate motion of the suspected misplaced otoconia.

The inferior semicircular canal SSC excites the ipsilateral superior oblique muscle and the contralateral inferior rectus, so a positive Dix-Hallpike maneuver indicating posterior canal BPPV will display rotary eye motion toward the canal of stimulus origin. A positive right posterior canal BPPV will produce rotation of eyes toward the right side (a right nystagmus).

Treatment for this benign condition via the Epley maneuver (Figure 6.56) involves moving the patient into several specific positions, resting in each to allow the otoconia to move along the canal, and finally ending with the otoconia returned back in the ampulla. Images in Figure 6.56A–D show treatment of a right inferior canal BPPV, beginning with the Dix-Hallpike maneuver, moving into the Epley canalith-repositioning maneuver. Image (A) begins with the patient seated, head turned 45 degrees into the plane of the canal. Next, move the patient's head (B) so that gravity will help dislodge the otoconia. Once the nystagmus and symptoms of vertigo resolve, the patient is moved into position (C), moving the otoconia further around the canal. Moving the patient into the next position (D) allows the otoconia to drift up and over the apex of the canal so that when the patient is returned to sitting, the otoconia may drop down into the ampulla.

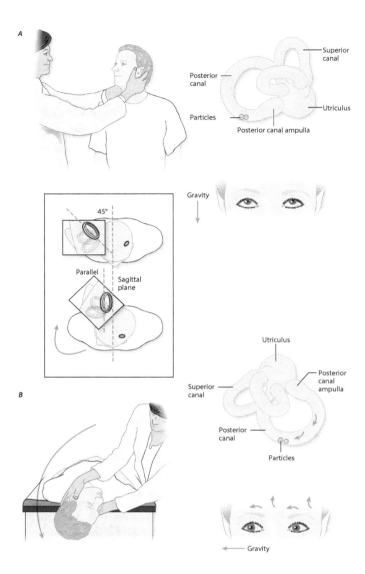

FIGURE 6.55

Dix-Hallpike maneuver to diagnose BPPV. Examination of benign paroxysmal positional vertigo (BPPV) using the Dix-Hallpike maneuver shown for vertigo originating in the right posterior semicircular canal. **A.** The maneuver begins with the patient seated and the head turned to one side at 45 degrees, which aligns the right posterior semicircular canal with the sagittal plane of the head. **B.** The patient is then helped to recline rapidly so that the head hangs over the edge of the table, still turned 45 degrees from the midline. Within several seconds, this elicits vertigo and nystagmus that is right beating with a rotary (counterclockwise) component. An important feature of this type of "peripheral" vertigo is a change in the direction of nystagmus when the patient sits up again with his head still rotated. If no nystagmus is elicited, the maneuver is repeated after a pause of 30 seconds, with the head turned to the left. (Reproduced with permisson from Chapter 15. Deafness, Dizziness, and Disorders of Equilibrium. In: Ropper AH, Samuels MA, Klein JP. eds. *Adams & Victor's Principles of Neurology*, 10e New York, NY: McGraw-Hill; 2014).

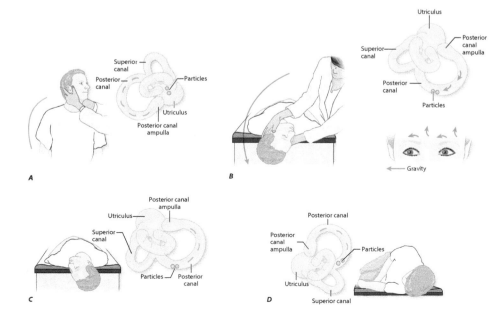

FIGURE 6.56

Canalith repositioning (Epley) maneuver to treat BPPV. Treatment with the canalith repositioning maneuver shown for a right posterior canal BPPV. (Reproduced with permisson from Chapter 15. Deafness, Dizziness, and Disorders of Equilibrium. In: Ropper AH, Samuels MA, Klein JP. eds. *Adams & Victor's Principles of Neurology*, 10e New York, NY: McGraw-Hill; 2014).

Frontiers in Research
Finding Cancer In Situ

Olfaction is important for survival; it is linked to emotions and the emetic pathway to assist in keeping us safe from eating harmful food, and attracts us to friends and potential mates via the complexities of pheromone (body scents) detection. Additionally, loss of smell can be used to detect onset of Alzheimer's and Parkinson's diseases.

An interesting new application of olfaction to health care is medical detection dogs. In 1989, a case involving a border collie mix was reported in the United Kingdom. The family dog was unusually attentive to a mole on her owner's leg, constantly sniffing and biting at it. This prompted the owner to seek medical attention, and a subsequent biopsy revealed malignant melanoma at an early stage; her dog may have saved her life. This observation encouraged researchers to investigate the mechanism of cancer detection through smell, and they discovered that tumors produce organic compounds excreted via urine, breath, and sweat. This led to exploration of new technologies, including nanotechnological "super noses," based on the superior smell capabilities of our canine friends. Additional studies reveal that all dogs may have this innate ability, and many can be trained to detect and notify humans when tumors are detected in body fluid samples. Early detection of cancer in situ (in place in the body) promotes earlier treatment and improves outcomes.

A dog's sense of smell is tremendously more sensitive than human olfaction, with vastly more peripheral receptors and greater central representation (Figure 6.57). A dog's olfactory nerves are twice as wide as humans', with olfactory epithelium containing over 500 million receptors (compared to 5 million in humans). As in humans, these receptors contain cilia that produce the chemical reaction to appreciate different odors. However, dogs also have a unique, specialized olfactory chamber called the vomeronasal organ. This remarkable sense of smell is now being used to detect early stages of cancer. This large, fluid-filled chamber is located above and behind the incisors bilaterally and has microvilli rather than cilia. Another interesting anatomic structure, a shelf above the ethnoturbinate bones, creates a large collecting area for odor molecules. This creates a gathering space for molecules, and more time to perform detailed identification of various smells. Dogs divide up their nasal function to share respiration and smell, which further optimizes sensory input, a behavior easily observed by watching a dog's nostrils gyrate as a scent is detected. Additionally, the areas for central processing of olfaction, which includes temporal lobe structures, limbic and paralimbic areas, the amygdala, and the hypothalamus, have a greater area of activation in dogs than humans.

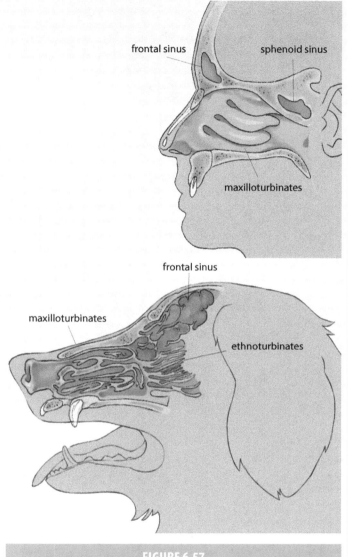

FIGURE 6.57

Human and canine olfaction. Note the difference in complexity of maxilloturnbinates, as well as the special collecting chamber, the vomeronasal organ, found only in the dog. (Image provided by Jamie Graham, 2017).

> **CASE 6 DISCUSSION: Cavernous Malformation in the Pons**

Sean's cavernous malformation created specific clinical findings that were direct results of the damage to his pons. Loss of distal tongue sensation, weakness, and sensory changes on the left side of his face and around the mouth were due to trigeminal nerve damage. These impairments contributed to his dysarthria. Fortunately, taste sensation, carried on the facial nerve, was preserved due to the more caudal location of the gustatory portion of the solitary nucleus in the medulla. Perception of pain and temperature, carried along the spinothalamic tract as it ascends through the pons, were lost on the right side of his body. Damage to the corticospinal tract produced right arm weakness and spasticity (a contralateral upper motor neuron hemiparesis).

Diagnosing a cavernous malformation is more difficult than diagnosing an AVM, as symptoms may be mild, with normal angiogram findings. Slow leaking may be episodic and cause mild, variable clinical findings, further confounding diagnosis. However, bleeding may also cause serious symptoms, including seizure or hemorrhagic stroke. Medical management varies from clinical observation for worsening symptoms, medication to treat seizures or pain, and surgical resection of the malformed vessels. Location and depth of the malformed vessels increases surgical risk. His additional post-operative symptoms from extended involvement of local tissues were unfortunate, but not surprising, due to delicate nervous system structures located close to the pons. Because light input carried on the second cranial nerve was preserved, Sean's altered left eye perception of only color and not image was due to damage in higher cortical centers involved with visual perception. Finally, his new symptom of poor balance was likely caused by damage extending locally into the cerebellum.

One year later, Sean has a positive outlook and perspective on the experience. His strong family support and close friendships sustained him during recovery, and he returned to the training room as soon as possible, once discharged from the hospital. His trainers and teammates welcomed him back and were supportive and encouraging during the early days as he worked to gain strength and coordination. Fortunately, a friend, active in adapted sports, told him about competitive adaptive paralympic soccer, open to male athletes with cerebral palsy or acquired brain injury. The game follows the standard FIFA (Federation International of Football Association) rules for seven-a-side soccer, with minor changes to accommodate physical impairments. Sean tried out, earning a place on Team USA, and represented his country in the 2016 Rio de Janeiro Summer Paralympic Games.

REFERENCES

Ayling J. Managing head injuries. *Emerg Med Serv*. 2002 Aug;31(8):42.

Azarmina M, Azarmina H. The six syndromes of the sixth cranial nerve. *J Ophthalmic Vis Res*. 2013 Apr;8(2):160–171.

Baloh RW, Honrubia V. Clinical neurophysiology of the vestibular system. *Contemp Neurol Ser*. 1979;18:1–21.

Baraniuk JN, Merck SJ. Nasal reflexes: Implications for exercise, breathing, and sex. *Curr Allergy Asthma Rep*. 2008 Apr;8(2):147–153.

Behbehani R. Clinical approach to optic neuropathies. *Clin Ophthalmol*. 2007 Sep; 1(3): 233–246.

Berns GS, Brooks AM, Spivak M. Scent of the familiar: an fMRI study of canine brain responses to familiar and unfamiliar human and dog odors. *Behav Processes*. 2015 Jan;110:37–46.

Boyle R. Vestibulospinal control of reflex and voluntary head movement. *Ann N Y Acad Sci*. 2001 Oct;942:364–380.

Brandt T, Dieterich M. Skew deviation with ocular torsion: a vestibular brainstem sign of topographic diagnostic value. *Ann Neurol*. 1993 May;33(5):528–534.

Caria MA, Tavera C, Melis F, Mameli O. The vestibulospinal reflex in humans: effects on paraspinal muscle activity. *Acta Otolaryngol*. 2003 Sep;123(7):817–825.

Cevette MJ, Puetz B, Marion MS, Wertz ML, Muenter MD. A physiologic performance on dynamic posturography. *Otolaryngol Head Neck Surg*. 1995;112:676–688.

Chugh JP, Jain P, Chouhan RS, Rathi A. Third nerve palsy: an overview. *Indian J Clin Practice*. 2012 May; 22(12).

Cohen-Gadol AA, Bohnstedt BN. Recognition and evaluation of nontraumatic subarachnoid hemorrhage and ruptured cerebral aneurysm. *Am Fam Physician*. 2013 Oct 1;88(7): 451–456.

Craven BA, Paterson EG, Settles GS. The fluid dynamics of canine olfaction: unique nasal airflow patterns as an explanation of macrosmia. *J R Soc Interface*. 2010 Jun 6;7(47):933–943.

Doty RL, Bayona EA, Leon-Ariza DS, et al. The lateralized smell test for detecting Alzheimer's disease: failure to replicate. *J Neurol Sci*. 2014 May 15;340(1–2):170–173.

Eggers SD, Zee DS. Evaluating the dizzy patient: bedside examination and laboratory assessment of the vestibular system. *Semin Neurol*. 2003 Mar;23(1):47–58.

Gates P. The rule of 4 of the brainstem: a simplified method for understanding brainstem anatomy and brainstem vascular syndromes for the non-neurologist. *Intern Med J*. 2005 Apr;35(4):263–266.

Graham V, Napier-Dovorany K. Multifactoral measures of fall risk in the visually impaired population: A pilot study. *J Bodyw Mov Ther*. 2016;20(1):104–109.

Greer DM, Yang J, Scripko PD, et al. Clinical examination for prognostication in comatose cardiac arrest patients. *Resuscitation*. 2013 Nov;84(11):1546–1551.

Hamid MA, Hughes GB, Kinney SE. Specificity and sensitivity of dynamic posturography: a retrospective analysis. *Acta Otolaryngol Suppl (Stockh)*. 1991;481:596–600.

Horton JC. Wilbrand's knee of the primate optic chiasm is an artefact of monocular enucleation. *Trans Am Ophthalmol Soc*. 1997;95:579–609.

Jacobs DA, Galetta SL. Neuro-ophthalmology for neuroradiologists. *AJNR Am J Neuroradiol*. 2007 Jan;28(1):3–8.

Jacobson GP, Newman CW, Hunter L, Balzer GK. Balance function test correlates of the Dizziness Handicap Inventory. *J Am Acad Audiol.* 1991;2:253–260.

Kavoi BM, Jameela H. Comparative morphometry of the olfactory bulb, tract and stria in the human, dog and goat. *Int. J. Morphol.* 2011;29(3):939–946.

Khan S, Chang R. Anatomy of the vestibular system: a review. *NeuroRehabilitation.* 2013;32(3):437–443.

Kim C, Sohn JH, Jang MU, et al. Ischemia as a potential etiologic factor in idiopathic unilateral sudden sensorineural hearing loss: analysis of posterior circulation arteries. *Hear Res.* 2016 Jan;331:144–151.

Kim JS, Kim HG, Chung CS. Medial medullary syndrome. Report of 18 new patients and a review of the literature. *Stroke.* 1995 Sep;26(9):1548–1552.

Krusemark EA, Novak LR, Gitelman DR, Li W. When the sense of smell meets emotion: anxiety-state-dependent olfactory processing and neural circuitry adaptation. *J Neurosci.* 2013 Sep 25;33(39):15324–15332.

Lee JH, Lee HK, Lee DH, Choi CG, Kim SJ, Suh DC. Neuroimaging strategies for three types of Horner syndrome with emphasis on anatomic location. *AJR Am J Roentgenol.* 2007 Jan;188(1):W74–W81.

Macchi MM, Bruce JN. Human pineal physiology and functional significance of melatonin. *Front Neuroendocrinol.* 2004 Sep–Dec;25(3–4):177–195.

Mandal AK, Anandanadesan R, Missouris DG. The hazards of being a gentleman farmer: a case of transient Horner's syndrome. *JRSM Short Rep.* 2012 Aug;3(8):53.

Muncie HL, Sirmans SM, James E. Dizziness: Approach to evaluation and management. *Am Fam Physician.* 2017;95(3):154–162.

Nishino T. The swallowing reflex and its significance as an airway defensive reflex. *Front Physiol.* 2013 Jan 7;3:489.

Noback CR, Strominger NL, Demarest RJ, Ruggiero DA. Robotic control based on the human nervous system. *International Journal of Artificial Intelligence & Applications.* 2011 Oct;3(4):107–123.

Optic Neuritis Study Group. Multiple sclerosis risk after optic neuritis: final optic neuritis treatment trial follow-up. *Arch Neurol.* 2008 Jun;65(6):727–732.

Ozdoğmuş O, Sezen O, Kubilay U, et al. Connections between the facial, vestibular and cochlear nerve bundles within the internal auditory canal. *J Anat.* 2004 Jul; 205(1): 65–75.

Passi N, Degnan AJ, Levy LM. MR imaging of papilledema and visual pathways: effects of increased intracranial pressure and pathophysiologic mechanisms. *AJNR Am J Neuroradiol.* 2013 May;34(5):919–924.

Perlmutter JS, Mink JW. Deep brain stimulation. *Annu Rev Neurosci.* 2006; 29: 229–257.

Rascol O. Sabatini U, Fabre N., et al. Abnormal vestibuocolar reflex cancellation in multiple system atrophy and progressive supranuclear palsy but not in Parkinson's disease. *Mov Disord.* 1995 Mar;10(2);163–170.

Sah P, Faber ES, Lopez De Armentia M, Power J. The amygdaloid complex: anatomy and physiology. *Physiol Rev.* 2003 Jul;83(3):803–834.

Sanders RD. The trigeminal (V) and facial (VII) cranial nerves: head and face sensation and movement. *Psychiatry (Edgmont).* 2010 Jan;7(1):13–16.

Schmitz B, Krick C, Käsmann-Kellner B. [Morphology of the optic chiasm in albinism]. *Ophthalmologe.* 2007 Aug;104(8):662–665.

Schubert MC, Minor LB. Vestibulo-ocular physiology underlying vestibular hypofunction. *Phys Ther.* 2004 Apr;84(4):373–385.

Shams PN, Bremner FD, Smith SE, Plant GT, Matthews TD. Unilateral light-near dissociation in lesions of the rostral midbrain. *Arch Ophthalmol.* 2010 Nov;128(11):1486–1489.

Siéssere S, Vitti M, Sousa LG, Semprini M, Iyomasa MM, Regalo SC. Anatomic variation of cranial parasympathetic ganglia. *Braz Oral Res.* 2008 Apr–Jun;22(2):101–105.

Sires BS, Stanley RB Jr, Levine LM. Oculocardiac reflex caused by orbital floor trapdoor fracture: an indication for urgent repair. *Arch Ophthalmol.* 1998 Jul;116(7): 955–956.

Snir M, Hasanreisoglu M, Goldenberg-Cohen N, et al. Suppression of the oculocephalic reflex (doll's eyes phenomenon) in normal full-term babies. *Curr Eye Res.* 2010 May;35(5):370–374.

Stamps JJ, Bartoshuk LM, Heilman KM. A brief olfactory test for Alzheimer's disease. *J Neurol Sci.* 2013 Oct 15;333(1–2):19–24.

Thompson TL, Amedee R. Vertigo: A review of common peripheral and central vestibular disorders. *Ochsner J.* 2009 Spring;9(1):20–26.

Walker HK, Hall WD, Hurst JW. *Clinical Methods: The History, Physical, and Laboratory Examinations.* 3rd ed. Boston: Butterworths; 1990.

Wesson DW, Wilson DA. Sniffing out the contributions of the olfactory tubercle to the sense of smell: hedonics, sensory integration, and more? *Neurosci Biobehav Rev.* 2011 Jan;35(3):655–668.

Whiting AC, Marmura MJ, Hegarty SE, Keith SW. Olfactory acuity in chronic migraine: A cross-sectional study. *Headache.* 2015 Jan;55(1):71–75.

Willis CM, Church SM, Guest CM, et al. Olfactory detection of human bladder cancer by dogs: proof of principle study. *BMJ.* 2004 Sep 25;329(7468):712.

Wilson VJ, Boyle R, Fukushima K, et al. The vestibulocollic reflex. *J Vestib Res.* 1995 May–Jun;5(3):147–170.

Wu S, Li N, Xia F, et al. Neurotrophic keratopathy due to dorsolateral medullary infarction (Wallenberg syndrome): case report and literature review. *BMC Neurol.* 2014 Dec 4;14:231.

Yates BJ, Bronstein AM. The effects of vestibular system lesions on autonomic regulation: observations, mechanisms, and clinical implications. *J Vestib Res.* 2005;15(3):119–129.

Zhang X, Kedar S, Lynn MJ, Newman NJ, Biousse V. Homonymous hemianopias: clinical-anatomic correlations in 904 cases. *Neurology.* 2006 Mar 8;66(6):906–910.

> REVIEW QUESTIONS

1. A patient with an upper motor neuron lesion in the corticobulbar tract will have:
   A. ipsilateral weakness.
   B. bilateral weakness.
   C. contralateral weakness.
   D. no weakness.

2. The superior colliculus is a _____ center, and the inferior colliculi are involved in _____ processing.
   A. taste and sound; vision
   B. sound; vision
   C. visual reflex; sound
   D. motor processing; auditory

3. A lesion rostral to the pyramidal decussation causes _____ hemiplegia.
   A. alternating
   B. bilateral
   C. ipsilateral
   D. contralateral

4. Your patient has bitemporal visual field loss. You suspect a lesion
   A. of the left optic nerve.
   B. at the optic chiasm.
   C. at the left optic tract.
   D. at the optic radiation (Meyer loop).

5. Presence of consensual pupil response when shining a light in the right eye indicates
   A. intact CNs II and III bilaterally.
   B. intact CN III bilaterally.
   C. intact right CN II and left CN III.
   D. intact left CN II and left CN III.

6. With locked-in-syndrome, the paralyzed patient is awake, with intact cognition and vertical eye movements due to the following:
   A. Corticospinal and corticobulbar tract damage, with sparing of reticular formation and supranuclear ocular motor pathway
   B. Vestibulospinal and spinothalamic tract damage, with sparing of corticobulbar tract and upper cortical function
   C. Spinothalamic and corticospinal tract damage, with sparing of vestibulo-ocular pathways
   D. Brainstem stroke with sparing of spinothalamic and corticobulbar vision pathways

7. Differential diagnosis of your patient's head tilt to the right at rest, includes ruling out
   A. compensation for left CN IV muscle palsy due to slight extorsion and elevation of the eye.
   B. a contracture of the right sternocleidomastoid muscle producing ipsilateral head tilt.
   C. compensation for unilateral loss of CN VIII producing altered subjective visual vertical.
   D. all of the above.

8. A stroke affecting the corticobulbar tract will produce which of the following trigeminal motor impairments?
   A. Weakness or paralysis of ipsilateral muscles of mastication
   B. Weakness or paralysis of contralateral muscles of mastication
   C. Weakness or paralysis of muscles of mastication, bilaterally
   D. Minimal weakness because the trigeminal motor nucleus receives a bilateral corticobulbar tract innervation

9. Which of the following best indicates the location of lost facial muscle control after a corticobulbar tract stroke?
   A. Upper facial muscles contralaterally
   B. Upper and lower facial muscles ipsilaterally
   C. Lower facial muscles contralaterally
   D. Lower facial muscles bilaterally

10. A stroke that damages the caudal part of the nucleus ambiguus produces the most significant impairment of the following:
    A. Pharyngeal muscle control
    B. Taste from posterior third of the tongue
    C. Tongue muscle control
    D. Blood pressure regulation

CHAPTER 7

Cerebellum

> ## CASE 7 Cerebellar Stroke

VIDEO

Mali wriggled in her mother's arms, smiling and playing with her rattle as they sat on the couch in the small, furnished apartment the family was staying in during the remodel. Tabitha spoke of the harrowing events of the past year, her voice occasionally soft with emotion. Originally from the same small town, Tabitha and her husband reconnected after college and married soon after. Five months into marriage, they found she was pregnant with a baby girl. Tabitha was 33 weeks along at the baby shower. With another seven weeks left until full term, her husband was increasingly concerned about the health of his vivacious wife.

The first trimester had passed without complications. The onset of extreme fatigue early in her second trimester was unusual, but not a specific concern. As Tabitha entered the third trimester, she developed horrible headaches, so bad they disturbed her sleep. She was diagnosed with sinus headaches and initially responded to ephedrine with some reduction in pain, although a later episode brought her to the emergency room, and she was referred to an ear, nose, and throat specialist. The visit was on a rainy day, and she got confused and lost driving to the appointment. Her symptoms were too subtle for definitive diagnosis, and everyone attributed her confusion to "pregnancy brain." She tried using a neti pot (nasal irrigation with a saline mixture), with minimal benefit, again visiting the doctor when the headaches became worse, experienced as loud booming in the back of her head. She lay in a dark room in the physician's office, diagnosed with a migraine and given drops

for a sinus infection, which helped for a bit. Another emergency room visit was occasioned when Tabitha became concerned that she had developed preeclampsia. Eclampsia is a dangerous condition that can cause seizures and lead to coma during a pregnancy; increased blood pressure, swelling of the extremities, and albuminuria characterize preeclampsia. Tabitha drove herself to the drug store to take her blood pressure, and on the way home collapsed before the front door of her neighbor, who called Tabitha's husband.

Unfortunately for Tabitha, normal pregnancy brings many new and vague symptoms precipitated by dramatic hormonal changes, and her many symptoms were dismissed as the experiences of a young, dramatic first-time mother. So instead of continuing to reach out to the medical professionals in her life, who had been unable to explain her ongoing symptoms, Tabitha dismissed her loss of taste and sensation on one side of her tongue, increasing clumsy behavior, right leg weakness, and loss of balance to pregnancy side effects.

Tabitha could barely walk at the baby shower due to increasing right leg weakness. The next morning, Tabitha was so sleepy, her concerned husband asked her mother to come over before he left for work. Her mom helped her into the shower and got her to eat a little something. She threw up and had a seizure. That was the last thing Tabitha recalled before waking up with half her head shaved. She wrote about it in her blog:

My hair was gorgeous! I was rocking the natural look and my

hair had grown SO much from the pregnancy hormones, and they CUT IT! (I still have to let this go … lol) A CT/MRI scan was finally ordered and I was diagnosed with a benign brain tumor. WOAH—unbelievable, I was pregnant with a brain tumor! My family and I were devastated to say the least, no one in our family had experienced this before. My fight or flight response triggered and I had no choice but to survive, not just for myself but for my family, my husband, and our unborn child—you have to do what you have to do as a mommy! My OBGYN was amazing and transferred me to one of the best hospitals in the world to figure out a plan of action and to move quickly. I felt like Beyonce when I arrived, I had an entire team of doctors and nurses anticipating my arrival. Apparently being pregnant with a brain tumor is very rare, there are only 80 cases a year worldwide, so they were anxious to say the least. At the time I was 33 weeks pregnant with Mali, so in order to deliver a healthy baby and successfully remove my tumor, I had to WAIT—endure a little over a week in ICU and allow Mali to develop before having my surgery. Just to let you know even a day in ICU will drive anyone insane! There are all kinds of tubes plugged to you, nurses everywhere and no sleep from the constant beeping of the machines and medicine administration. Mali was born February 8, 2016 via C-section.

I was under complete anesthesia; I have no recollection of the birth of my daughter, and this makes me very sad. My brain surgery was February 10, 2015, 2 days after Mali's birth, and would last 7 hours. I woke up in immense pain, but the surgery was a success! I was in the hospital for a month, undergoing 4 surgeries and a week of rehab. My phenomenal husband, overflowing with faith, love and devotion, stayed in the hospital with me every night for a month—I didn't think I could love him anymore than when I said I do. I stand corrected.

I OVERVIEW OF KEY CONCEPTS

The cerebellum is the brain's comparator, monitoring sensory input throughout goal-oriented behavior and directing minute changes throughout the process. Dorsal and ventral spinocerebellar tracts carry proprioceptive information; dorsal columns carry stretch and pressure information; the spinothalamic tract carries noxious and thermal information; visual and vestibular systems carry information about spatial position; and all of these inputs are monitored in the cerebellum to make the small motor changes that produce fluid, efficient, even elegant movements. Much of the information is processed at an unconscious level since making such tiny instantaneous changes during movement could not be accomplished in a timely manner if they were driven by conscious cerebral control. Coordination of sensory input with motor output is an ongoing process that results in smooth movements of appropriate distance, power, and velocity. The cerebellum, along with the basal ganglia, controls how we learn and perfect skilled movement, known as motor learning and motor control. Loss of sensorimotor integration by damage to the cerebellum—to its input or output structures—can lead to characteristic motor malfunctions such as ataxia, dysmetria, or tremor on intention (volitional movement).

A useful mnemonic for understanding cerebellar organization is the "rule of threes" (Table 7.1). Primary among these are (1) three lobes or sagittal zones that organize cerebellar inputs and outputs; (2) three layers in the cerebellar cortex whose circuitry modulates overall cerebellar output; and (3) three cerebellar syndromes: ataxia, tremor, and hypotonia. The cerebellum influences virtually all movements, including eye movements and vocalization. Injury to the cerebellum, however, does not produce typical upper or lower motor neuron syndromes. Instead, it is the precision and accuracy of movements and the ability to learn novel complex multijoint movements that suffer from cerebellar injuries. Also, because cerebellar circuits involving other brain regions cross twice, the effects of cerebellar injury are observed ipsilateral to the damaged side.

Although still somewhat controversial, recent studies have assigned some cognitive function for the cerebellum, based on widespread anatomical projections including some to the cerebral cortex, as well as evidence from patients with cerebellar injury or degeneration. Patients with cerebellar injury can develop cerebellar cognitive affective syndrome, which produces neurobehavioral abnormalities such as impaired motor planning, verbal disturbances, and impaired abstract reasoning.

II CEREBELLAR ANATOMY

The cerebellum is the portion of the brain that lies posterior to the pons and medulla, separated from them by the fourth ventricle (Figure 7.1). Developmentally derived from the rhombencephalon and metencephalon (Chapter 4), it occupies the posterior cranial fossa within the skull. It lies inferior to the dural tentorium cerebelli, and a small vertical falx cerebelli incompletely separates its hemispheres.

Gross Anatomy

The cerebellar cortex is extensively convoluted, a mechanism for greatly increasing its surface area similar to the gyri/sulci seen in the cerebral cortex. The ridges in the cerebellar cortex are much smaller and more regular, and are called folia. If it were possible to flatten out the cerebellar cortex, it would cover about 500 cm^2, with a total cellular volume of 300 cm^3. The total number of neurons in the cerebellar cortex ranges from about 70 billion (out of 85 billion neurons in the whole brain) to 101 billion (out of approximately 120 billion total neurons). Whichever estimate one accepts, the cerebellum contains a disproportionately large number of the brain's total neurons.

The cerebellum's outer cortex contains a rich variety of neuronal types (Figure 7.2), and its deeper white matter region contains

Table 7.1 Cerebellar Regions

Cerebellar Lobe	Sagittal Zone	Phylogenetic Designation	Functional Designation	Function
Flocculonodular	Vermal; includes some anterior lobe	Archicerebellum	Vestibulocerebelum	Control of eye movements; axial musculature related to balance and posture
Anterior	Intermediate; includes some vermis and posterior lobe	Paleocerebellum	Spinocerebellum	Control of neck, trunk, and limb musculature
Posterior	Lateral; includes some anterior lobe	Neocerebellum	Cerebrocerebellum	Modulation of fine movements; motor learning

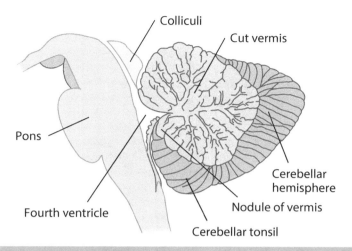

FIGURE 7.1

Midsagittal section through the cerebellum. (Reproduced with permission from Chapter 7. The Brain Stem and Cerebellum. In: Waxman SG. eds. Clinical Neuroanatomy, 27e New York, NY: McGraw-Hill; 2013).

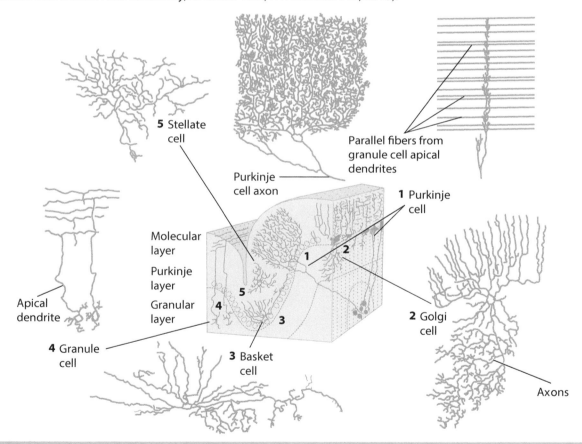

FIGURE 7.2

Location and structure of five neuronal types in the cerebellar cortex. Drawings are based on Golgi-stained preparations. Purkinje cells (1) have processes aligned in one plane; their axons are the only output from the cerebellum. Axons of granule cells (4) traverse and make connections with Purkinje cell processes in molecular layer. Golgi (2), basket (3), and stellate (5) cells have characteristic positions, shapes, branching patterns, and synaptic connections. (**1, 2**, Reproduced from Reflex & Voluntary Control of Posture & Movement. In: Barrett KE, et al, eds. Ganong's Review of Medical Physiology, 25e New York, NY: McGraw-Hill, 2016; **3-5** Reproduced with permission of Palay SL, Chan-Palay V: Cerebellar Cortex. Berlin: Springer-Verlag, 1975.)

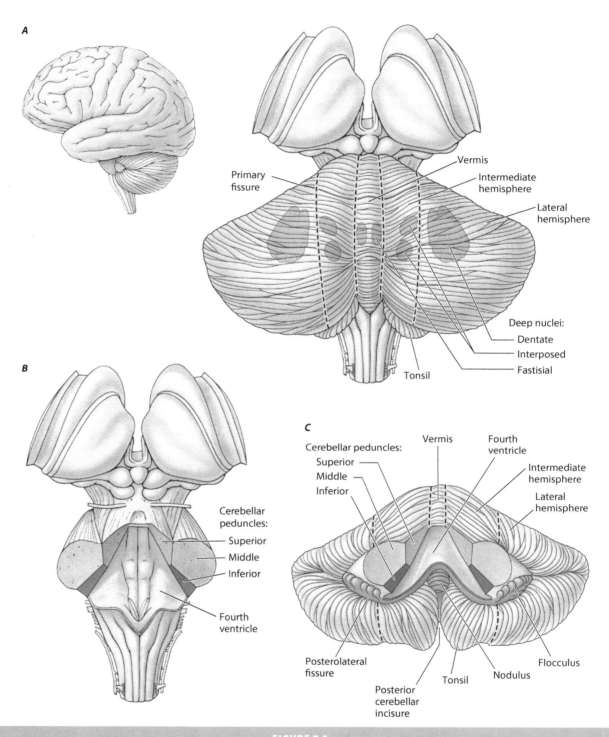

FIGURE 7.3

Brainstem and Cerebellum Relationships. **A.** Dorsal view of the brain stem and cerebellum. The borders between the vermis and intermediate and lateral parts of the cerebellar hemisphere are shown. These three parts of the cerebellar cortex also correspond to functional subdivisions. **B.** The three cerebellar peduncles are revealed when the cerebellum is removed. **C.** The cerebellum, viewed from the ventral surface. Inset (**A**) shows lateral view of brain. (Reproduced with permission from The Cerebellum. In: Martin JH. eds. Neuroanatomy Text and Atlas, 4e New York, NY: McGraw-Hill, 2012).

primarily myelinated axons. The cerebellar cortex is organized into groups of folia, or lobules, separated from one another by fissures (Figure 7.3).

Anatomists generally recognize 10 lobules, whose nomenclature is used largely by specialists studying the cerebellum and unnecessary detail for this text. Two particularly deep fissures divide the lobules into three distinct lobes: anterior, posterior, and flocculonodular. The primary fissure separates the anterior lobe from the posterior, and the posterolateral fissure separates the posterior from the flocculonodular lobe. The flocculonodular lobe consists of the nodulus (the anterior inferior part of the vermis) with two flocculi on either side. The anterior lobe coordinates limb and trunk movements; the posterior lobe integrates multisensory inputs with the cortical motor plan for movement precision; and the flocculonodular lobe regulates eye movements and affects balance and posture.

The three cerebellar lobes are also named for their phylogeny, which also correlates with their increasingly complex function (Table 7.1). The oldest part is the archicerebellum, which corresponds to the flocculonodular lobe. This portion, also referred to as the vestibulocerebellum, is intimately related to the vestibular nuclei and their primary afferent neurons. Of intermediate phylogenetic age, the paleocerebellum, corresponding mainly to the anterior lobe, is also referred to as the spinocerebellum. Spinal proprioceptors provide a major input to this lobe. The cerebrocerebellum (neocerebellum) is the newest cerebellar lobe. It corresponds mainly to the posterior lobe and receives a dense projection from contralateral motor cortices via synapses with the pontine nuclei.

Pontocerebellar efferents decussate and enter the cerebellum through the middle cerebellar peduncle.

Internal Anatomy

The complex circuitry of the cerebellum is better understood along functional bases by division into sagittal zones that contain functionally related parts of more than one lobe (Figure 7.4). The vermal zone lies on the midline and is composed primarily of the flocculonodular lobe. It functions in control of eye movements as well as axial musculature related to balance and posture. The intermediate zone consists of the anterior lobe, the vermis, and a portion of the posterior lobe. Through connections with the motor cortex and spinal proprioceptive pathways, the intermediate zone regulates control of neck, trunk, and limb musculature. It compares the changing relationship between the person and the environment throughout the planned movement and makes minor adjustments as needed. The lateral zone, made up mainly of the posterior lobe, with a small contribution from the anterior lobe, is involved with modulation of fine control of movements such as control of force and direction, speed and amplitude; it is involved in motor learning and may influence some aspects of cognition. Its only inputs are from the cerebral cortex, and its output influences premotor and primary motor cortex activity.

Beneath the cerebellar cortex is the white matter, which contains axons coursing to and from the cerebellar cortex. The branching pattern of the white matter in the cerebellum inspired early anatomists to refer to it as the arbor vitae (Latin for "tree of life");

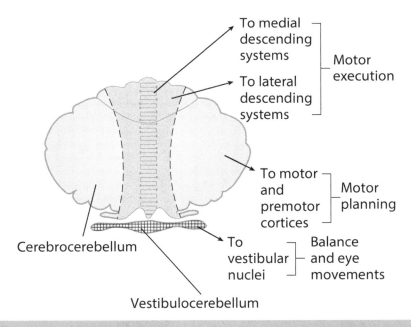

FIGURE 7.4

Three functional divisions of the cerebellum. The nodulus in the vermis and the flanking flocculus in the hemisphere on each side form the vestibulocerebellum which has vestibular connections and is concerned with equilibrium and eye movements. The rest of the vermis and the adjacent medial portions of the hemispheres form the spinocerebellum, the region that receives proprioceptive input from the body as well as a copy of the "motor plan" from the motor cortex. The lateral portions of the cerebellar hemispheres are called the cerebrocerebellum which interacts with the motor cortex in planning and programming movements. (Reproduced from *Reflex & Voluntary Control of Posture & Movement.* In: Barrett KE, et al, eds. *Ganong's Review of Medical Physiology,* 25e New York, NY: McGraw-Hill, 2016).

hence, the name folia (Latin for "leaves"), rather than gyri, is used to describe cerebellar cortex convolutions.

Four bilaterally paired nuclei, the deep cerebellar nuclei, are embedded within the cerebellar white matter (Figure 7.5). They are, from medial to lateral, the fastigial, the globose nucleus, the emboliform nucleus (together referred to as the interposed nuclei), and the dentate nucleus. These nuclei provide the only outputs from the cerebellum, and damage to these produce the most profound and predictable cerebellar deficits.

Axons projecting to and from the cerebellum course through three peduncles. The superior cerebellar peduncle contains mostly efferent axons; the middle cerebellar peduncle contains only afferent axons; and the inferior cerebellar peduncle contains both afferent and efferent axons.

Three arteries supply the cerebellum and adjacent brainstem (Figure 7.6). Circulation to the brain is described in more detail in Chapter 2, with only cerebellar circulation reviewed below. Arising from the vertebral artery, the posterior inferior cerebellar artery (commonly called PICA) provides support to the inferior posterior portion of the cerebellum as well as the adjacent lateral medulla and inferior cerebellar peduncle. Occlusion of PICA produces a lateral medullary, or Wallenberg, syndrome. The anterior inferior cerebellar artery, from the basilar artery, supplies the anterior inferior part of the cerebellum, anastomosing with the PICA. The superior cerebellar artery supplies the upper half of the cerebellum. It emerges from the basilar artery near its termination. The oculomotor nerve emerges from the midbrain between the superior cerebellar artery and the posterior cerebral artery.

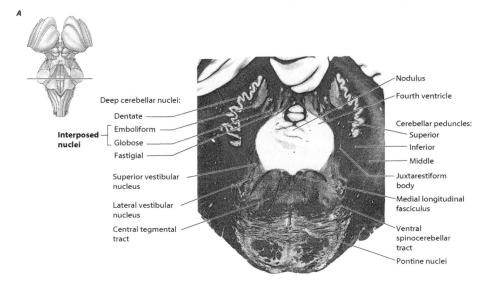

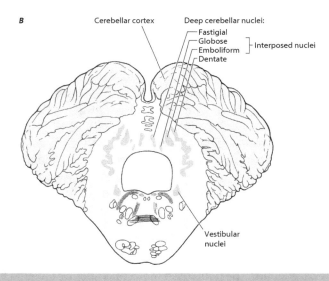

FIGURE 7.5

**Transverse sections through the cerebellar deep nuclei. Weigert stained (left) and cartoon (right) sections are from approximately the same brainstem level. *A.* Myelin-stained transverse section through the caudal pons and deep cerebellar nuclei. The inset shows the plane of section. *B.* Location of the deep cerebellar nuclei. The vestibular nuclei are also shown because they are anatomically equivalent to the deep cerebellar nuclei for the flocculonodular lobe. They receive inputs from Purkinje cells and the inferior olivary nucleus. (*A*, Reproduced with permission from The Cerebellum. In: Martin JH. eds. Neuroanatomy Text and Atlas, 4e New York, NY: McGraw-Hill, 2012; Photo used with permission from Howard J. Radzyner; *B*, Reproduced with permission from The Cerebellum. In: Martin JH. eds. Neuroanatomy Text and Atlas, 4e New York, NY: McGraw-Hill).

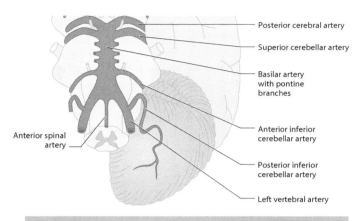

FIGURE 7.6

Principal arteries of the posterior fossa. (Reproduced with permission from Chapter 12. Vascular Supply of the Brain. In: Waxman SG. eds. Clinical Neuroanatomy, 27e New York, NY: McGraw-Hill; 2013.)

III CEREBELLAR CIRCUITRY

Cerebellar circuitry comprises three sets of connections: intrinsic cortical circuits and extrinsic afferent inputs, and efferent projections. In all there are feedback circuits that sculpt cerebellar output, eliminating extraneous or incorrect movements to produce controlled coordinated movement.

Cerebellar Cortex

The cerebellar cortex consists of three layers (Figure 7.7), in contrast to the six-layered cerebral cortex. The layers, from deep to superficial, are the granule cell layer, adjacent to the cerebellar white matter (medullary) region; the Purkinje cell layer; and the molecular layer. Each contains distinct cell types and participates in specific parts of cerebellar circuitry. Not every cell type is restricted completely to one layer; some have processes that extend across multiple layers

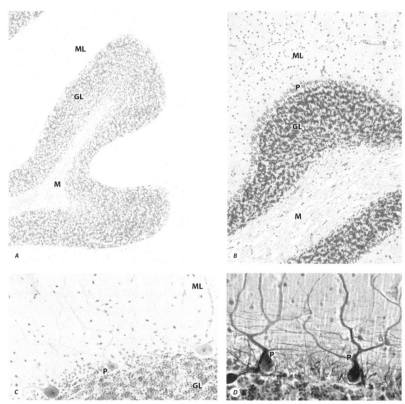

FIGURE 7.7

Photomicrographs of the cerebellar cortex. A. The cerebellar cortex is convoluted with many distinctive small folds, each supported at its center by tracts of white matter in the cerebellar medulla (M). Each fold has distinct molecular layers (ML) and granular layers (GL) (X6; Cresyl violet). **B.** Higher magnification shows that the granular layer (GL) immediately surrounding the medulla (M) is densely packed with several different types of very small rounded neuronal cell bodies. The outer molecular layer (ML) consists of neuropil with fewer, much more scattered small neurons. At the interface of these two regions a layer of large Purkinje neuron (P) perikarya can be seen (X20; H&E). **C.** A single intervening layer contains the very large cell bodies of unique Purkinje neurons (P), whose axons pass through the granular layer (GL) to join tracts in the medulla and whose multiple branching dendrites ramify throughout the molecular layer (ML). Dendrites are not seen well with H&E staining (X40; H&E). **D.** With appropriate silver staining dendrites from each large Purkinje cell (P) are shown to have hundreds of small branches, each covered with hundreds of dendritic spines. Axons from the small neurons of the granular layer are unmyelinated and run together into the molecular layer where they form synapses with the dendritic spines of Purkinje cells (X40; Silver). (Reproduced with permission from Nerve Tissue & the Nervous System. In: Mescher AL. eds. Junqueira's Basic Histology, 14e New York, NY: McGraw-Hill.)

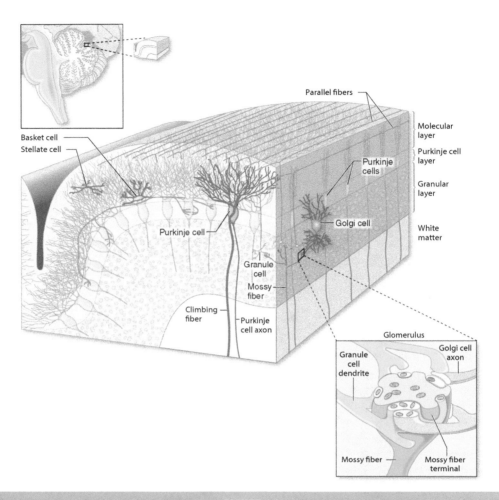

Anatomic organization of the cerebellar cortex in a longitudinal and transverse section of a folium. Shown are the relationships between climbing fibers and Purkinje cells, mossy fibers and both granule cells and Golgi cells, and the parallel fibers that course longitudinally and connect these three main cell types. (Reproduced with permission from The Cerebellum. In: Kandel ER, et al., eds. Principles of Neural Science, Fifth Editon New York, NY: McGraw-Hill; 2012.)

(Figure 7.8). This arrangement permits dispersion of inputs across multiple layers and cell types.

The granule cell layer contains a vast population of granule cells, the only excitatory type in the cerebellar cortex, as well as Golgi cells that participate in an inhibitory feedback circuit with the granule cells. The middle layer in the cerebellar cortex contains only the large cell bodies of Purkinje cells. These cells form the sole output from the cerebellar cortex, and they are inhibitory, using GABA (gamma-aminobutyric acid) as their neurotransmitter. The molecular layer is cell sparse, containing mainly the parallel fibers from the granule cells. There are also stellate and basket cells and Bergmann glia that primarily regulate Purkinje cell function.

Cerebellar Cortical Circuitry

All inputs to the cerebellum are excitatory. They arrive on one of two different fiber systems: climbing fibers and mossy fibers (Figure 7.9), each derived from different anatomic sources and using mainly glutamate as the neurotransmitter. As they enter the cerebellum, both fiber systems emit excitatory collaterals to the deep cerebellar nuclei before continuing to the cerebellar cortex, where they synapse on Purkinje cells (climbing fibers) or granule cells (mossy fibers).

Climbing fibers arise only from the inferior olivary nucleus, decussating and entering the cerebellum through the inferior cerebellar peduncle. The olivocerebellar climbing fibers are part of a feedback circuit involving the red nucleus. They are called climbing fibers because they ascend along the Purkinje cell axon and ramify (branch) profusely to synapse extensively on the cell body and dendritic arbor of the Purkinje cell, bringing massive excitatory input to a very small number of Purkinje cells. All other inputs to the cerebellum comprise the mossy fibers system. Mossy fibers are also excitatory and also emit collaterals to the deep nuclei before ascending in the cerebellar white matter to the deep granule cell layer of the cerebellar cortex.

The deep cerebellar nuclei comprise the only output centers from the cerebellum. The distribution of cerebellar efferents is broad, including ascending, descending, ipsilateral, and contralateral projections. All of the incoming excitatory axons entering the

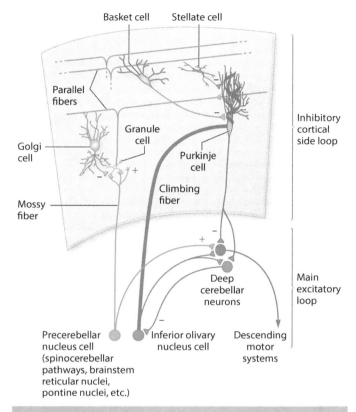

Basket cell   Stellate cell

Parallel fibers

Golgi cell

Granule cell

Purkinje cell

Climbing fiber

Mossy fiber

Inhibitory cortical side loop

Deep cerebellar neurons

Main excitatory loop

Precerebellar nucleus cell (spinocerebellar pathways, brainstem reticular nuclei, pontine nuclei, etc.)

Inferior olivary nucleus cell

Descending motor systems

FIGURE 7.9

The physiologic organization of cerebellar circuitry. The main output of the deep cerebellar nuclei is excitatory and is transmitted through mossy and climbing fibers. This "main loop" is modulated by an inhibitory cortical loop, which is effected by Purkinje cell output but indirectly includes the other main cell types through their connections with Purkinje cells. Recurrent pathways between the deep nuclei and cortical cells via mossy and climbing fibers complete the cerebellar servomechanism for motor control. (From Raymond JL, Lisberger SG, Mauk DM: The cerebellum: a neuronal learning machine? Science 1996; 272:1126-1131. Reprinted with permission from AAAS.)

cerebellum emit collaterals that excite the deep nuclei. The only output neurons in the cerebellar cortex are the inhibitory Purkinje cells, and their axons pass to the deep nuclei. Thus, the complex circuitry within the cerebellar cortex is designed to modulate deep cerebellar nuclei output by controlling Purkinje cell inhibition over deep nuclear neuronal activity.

The apical dendritic arbor of Purkinje cells is nearly two-dimensional, forming a flat plane oriented perpendicularly to the longitudinal axes of the folia. Climbing and mossy fiber inputs exert their excitatory influence on these cells in two different ways. As described, climbing fibers directly and robustly excite single Purkinje cells. Mossy fiber input is somewhat more complex. Within the molecular layer, there is a dense array of fibers derived from the apical dendrites of granule cells. These fibers, called parallel fibers,

course through the molecular layer parallel to the cortical surface. Each of the fibers passes through the plane of the Purkinje cell arbor, synapsing a few times on many Purkinje cells as it extends through the molecular layer. Thus the parallel fibers provide a large, broadly distributed excitatory input to the cerebellar cortex.

Granule cells are excited by mossy fibers. Each granule cell emits an apical dendrite that ascends into the molecular layer and bifurcates to form a "T." The arms of the T comprise the fibers running parallel to the long axis of the folium, which exert small bursts of excitation to a large number of Purkinje cells. Mossy fibers therefore bring massive excitatory input to the cerebellar cortex through small activation of a huge number of parallel fibers from the granule cells. Granule cell activity is governed by the circuitry in multisynaptic apparatus, called the glomerulus, consisting of a highly branched excitatory mossy fiber terminal synapsing on several granule cells. Glomerular excitation is regulated by a feedback circuit mediated by inhibitory Golgi cells. These cells are located superficially within the granule cell layer with dendritic arbors distributed in both the granule and molecular layers. Their molecular layer dendrites are excited by the parallel fibers arising from the granule cells. The deeper dendrites distribute in the granule cell layer, where they participate in the glomerulus. Golgi cells are excited by the parallel fibers and emit axons that modulate glomerular output.

Purkinje cell bodies comprise the entire middle layer of the cerebellar cortex. These cells are inhibitory, using GABA as their neurotransmitter. The Purkinje somata are aligned in a single plane, with their arbor extending through the molecular layer. Their axons descend through cerebellar white matter en route to the deep nuclei. Their inhibitory influence controls deep nuclear output and therefore modulates overall cerebellar function.

The molecular layer is mainly composed of the parallel fiber system, which synapses on both Purkinje and Golgi cell arbors. Activation of Golgi cells contributes to a cortical feedback loop regulating granule cell excitatory output. Small populations of stellate cells and basket cells in the molecular layer (Figures 7.8 and 7.9) are also excited by parallel fibers and create another feedback loop regulating excitation of Purkinje cells by parallel fibers. When excited by parallel fibers, both stellate and basket cells inhibit Purkinje cell activation through GABAergic synapses on the Purkinje cell dendritic arbor or its soma, respectively.

Feedback Circuitry within the Cerebellar Cortex

There are several feedback circuits in the cerebellar cortex that compare excitatory and inhibitory signals during execution of the motor plan. All cerebellar inputs excite the deep nuclei on entering the cerebellar white matter. Input fibers excite the Purkinje cells: climbing fibers directly, and mossy fibers indirectly through the parallel fibers. Purkinje axons, in turn, inhibit (regulate) deep nuclear output.

Mossy fiber input to granule cells activates the excitatory parallel fiber system. The entire parallel fiber system excites Purkinje cells broadly, but they also excite inhibitory Golgi, stellate, and basket cells. When the Golgi cells are excited, their inhibitory input to the glomerulus controls the excitation of the granule cells and regulates parallel fiber activation of Purkinje cells. Further, similar activation of stellate and basket cells control activation of Purkinje cells.

In addition, the cerebello-rubro-olivary circuit is active in making continuous fine adjustments to the motor plan. Motor cortical efferents transmit the initial motor plan, including directions relating the specific sequence of muscle contractions, to the pontine nuclei. Pontocerebellar fibers decussate and enter the lateral (posterior lobe) cerebellar cortex through the middle peduncle. Output through the dentate nucleus ascends through the superior cerebellar peduncle back to the parvocellular region of the red nucleus. Rubral efferents descend to the inferior olivary nucleus, which then transmits information back to the lateral cerebellar cortex through the inferior peduncle, completing the loop. This circuit seems to affect the timing of muscle contraction throughout complex, multijoint movements without conscious integration of sensory inputs. The inferior olive neurons are less active when adapting self-directed intended movements, such as while playing a piano or hitting a baseball. Interruption in this pathway interferes with the ability to make subtle corrections to movements for perfecting new behaviors.

Afferent and Efferent Connectivity through the Cerebellar Peduncles

Three cerebellar peduncles, thick axon fascicles, carry information into (afferent) or out of (efferent) the cerebellum (Figure 7.10).

These are: the inferior cerebellar peduncle (also known as the restiform body and juxtarestiform body); the middle cerebellar peduncle (brachium pontis); and the superior cerebellar peduncle (brachium conjunctivum). Inputs that pass through the peduncles comprise the mossy and climbing fiber systems; climbing fibers are derived solely from the contralateral inferior olivary nucleus; mossy fibers come from all other sources of cerebellar input. Each peduncle contains a predictable complement of afferent fibers from and efferents to select targets (Figure 7.11).

Vestibulocerebellar (Medial Zone) Circuitry through the Inferior Cerebellar Peduncle

The main cerebellar cortex targets of the inferior cerebellar peduncle include neurons in the flocculonodular lobe (vestibulocerebellum) and the intermediate zone (spinocerebellum). The inferior peduncle carries substantial inputs from the vestibular system and the spinal cord. The inferior cerebellar peduncle carries projections from cells in the vestibular nuclei, as well as direct afferent inputs from primary vestibular neurons in the vestibular ganglion (Scarpa's ganglion) located in the internal auditory meatus (Figure 7.12). All of these vestibular inputs are ipsilateral. Of note, in addition to connections to the fastigial nucleus, many flocculonodular lobe Purkinje cells emit efferent axons directly to the vestibular nuclei and so comprise

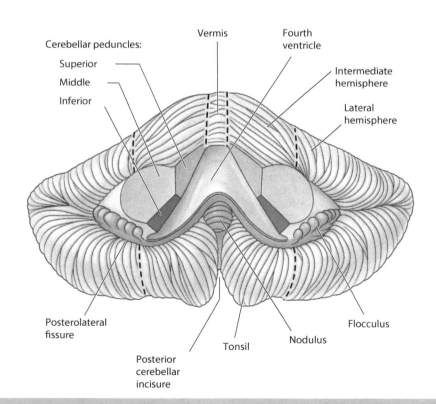

Cerebellar peduncles:
Superior
Middle
Inferior

Vermis
Fourth ventricle
Intermediate hemisphere
Lateral hemisphere

Posterolateral fissure
Posterior cerebellar incisure
Tonsil
Nodulus
Flocculus

FIGURE 7.10

The cerebellum, viewed from the ventral surface. The superior cerebellar peduncles, the main output fiber bundle related to fine movements, extend upward to the midbrain. The inferior cerebellar peduncle, main axon bundle regulating postural, axial, and activity in many motor cranial nerve s extends downward into the medulla. The middle cerebellar peduncle provides access for a large mass of pontocerebellar axons into the lateral zone. (Reproduced with permission from The Cerebellum. In: Martin JH. eds. Neuroanatomy Text and Atlas, 4e New York, NY: McGraw-Hill, 2012).

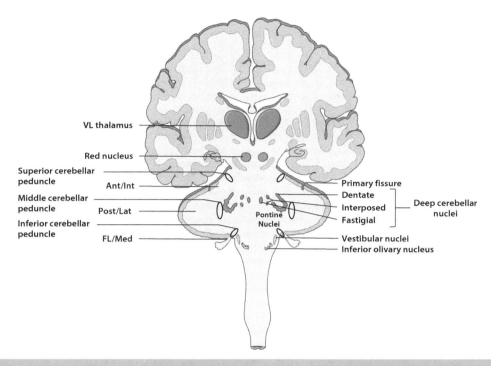

VL thalamus

Red nucleus

Superior cerebellar peduncle

Ant/Int

Middle cerebellar peduncle

Post/Lat

Inferior cerebellar peduncle

FL/Med

Primary fissure

Dentate

Interposed

Fastigial

Deep cerebellar nuclei

Pontine Nuclei

Vestibular nuclei

Inferior olivary nucleus

FIGURE 7.11

Diagram of CNS structures associated with cerebellar circuitry. VL thalamus – ventral lateral thalamic nucleus; Ant/Int – anterior lobe/intermediate zone; Post/Lat – posterior lobe/lateral zone; FL/Med – flocculonodular lobe/medial zone. Peduncles are represented as black ovals in their approximate anatomical positions. (Image provided by Jamie Graham, 2017.)

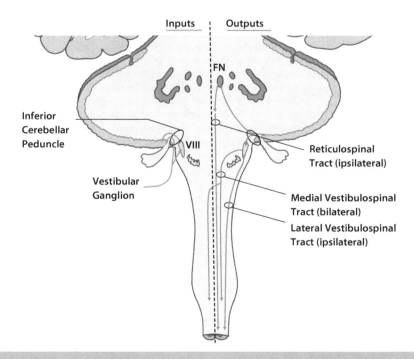

Inputs

Outputs

FN

Inferior Cerebellar Peduncle

VIII

Vestibular Ganglion

Reticulospinal Tract (ipsilateral)

Medial Vestibulospinal Tract (bilateral)

Lateral Vestibulospinal Tract (ipsilateral)

FIGURE 7.12

Flocculonodular lobe/middle zone inputs and outputs. Inputs are drawn in red on the left side of the figure; outputs in blue on the right side. FN – fastigial nucleus; VIII – vestibular nuclei. (Image provided by Jamie Graham, 2017.)

the only cerebellar outputs that bypass the deep cerebellar nuclei. This suggests why the functions of the vestibulocerebellum and the vestibular system are nearly inseparable. Cerebellar efferents to the lateral vestibular nucleus influence the medial and lateral vestibulospinal pathways. Medial vestibular nucleus outputs descend bilaterally with the medial longitudinal fasciculus through the cervical spinal levels. They influence neck muscle contraction (particularly of the sternocleidomastoid muscles) to position the head in response to changing posture. Fibers of the lateral vestibulospinal tract descend ipsilaterally through sacral spinal levels. Along with the pontine reticulospinal tract (Chapter 6), lateral vestibulospinal tract axons enhance excitation of antigravity postural muscles, helping to maintain muscle length and tone. Medullary reticulospinal tract spinal projections modulate extensor contraction and liberate antigravity muscle reflex contraction. Think of standing erect: extensor muscles maintain constant contraction to support the body in this posture. When it becomes necessary to flex the trunk, the medullary reticulospinal tract relaxes some of the extensors to permit flexion. Some extensor contraction persists, however, controlling flexion and preventing falling forward.

Spinal cord inputs also ascend through the inferior peduncle and project in great part to the intermediate zone that comprises the spinocerebellum. Spinocerebellar pathways were introduced in Chapter 5 and are reviewed in detail below in Figure 7.13. Primary proprioceptive neurons in the dorsal root ganglia encode changes in body position and carry that information centrally. Some collaterals ascend in the ipsilateral dorsal columns to synapse onto second-order neurons in the dorsal column nuclei. Afterward the information ascends to the contralateral somatosensory cortex and is processed for conscious appreciation of positional changes. Inputs to the cerebellum are processed at a subconscious level that is required to affect minute motor responses that must occur faster than conscious calculation would allow.

Spine-to-cerebellum connectivity for postural control involves a two-neuron circuit. Proprioceptors from ~C8–L2/3 emit collaterals that innervate cells in Clarke's nucleus dorsalis, distributed in the thoracic and upper lumbar spinal cord, relaying somatosensory input from muscles and joints as well as proprioceptive spatial information regarding the body's position in three-dimensional space. Output from neurons in Clarke's nucleus ascend uncrossed in the ipsilateral

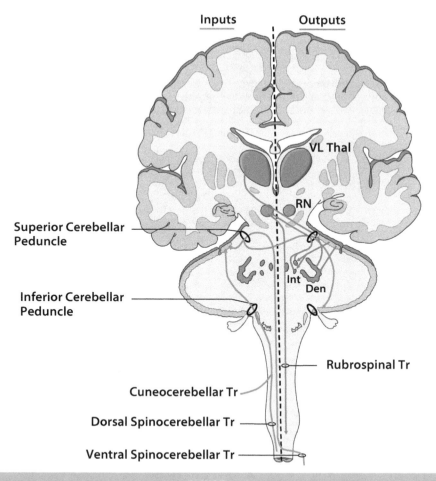

FIGURE 7.13

Anterior lobe/intermediate zone inputs and outputs. Inputs are drawn in red on the left side of the figure; outputs in blue on the right side. VL Thal – ventral lateral thalamic nucleus; RN – red nucleus; Int – interposed nuclei; Den – dentate nucleus; Tr – tract. (Image provided by Jamie Graham, 2017.)

dorsal (posterior) spinocerebellar tract and enter the cerebellar white matter through the inferior peduncle to the granule cell layer in the spinocerebellar cortex. Clarke's nucleus cells and the dorsal spinocerebellar tract are activated during active or passive movement. Rostrally, upper limb somatosensory and positional information ascends in the accessory cuneate nucleus in the caudal medulla, then into the ipsilateral cerebellum, also through the inferior peduncle.

Lower extremity position sense is relayed through the ventral (anterior) spinocerebellar tract. Primary afferent inputs from levels below ~L2/3 innervate spinal border cells, found laterally within the ventral horn, through inhibitory interneurons. Axons from the spinal border cells decussate in the anterior white commissure and ascend in the ventral part of the contralateral lateral funiculus to the upper pons, where they enter the cerebellar white matter through the superior cerebellar peduncle. Most ventral spinocerebellar tract fibers again decussate and reenter the contralateral cerebellum. They emit collateral fibers to the interposed nuclei before innervating the vermal and intermediate zones of the cerebellar cortex. This forms a "double crossed" system and may coordinate bilateral lower extremity function during gait. The spinal border cells emitting the ventral spinocerebellar pathway are activated primarily through inhibitory interneurons during volitional movement. They receive descending input indirectly from the motor cortex via reticulospinal projections, and from primary proprioceptive afferents whose cell bodies reside in the dorsal root ganglia. Processing at the spinal cord level integrates a premotor "copy" of the original motor plan with sensory feedback from changing limb position. This is important especially when controlling rhythmic antagonistic muscle contraction during the gait cycle.

Spinocerebellar outputs employ both the interposed and dentate nuclei. Interposed nuclei axons mainly innervate the contralateral red nucleus, comprising part of the decussation of the superior cerebellar peduncle. The decussation of the superior cerebellar peduncle is a thick fiber band composed of bilateral cerebellar projections to the thalamus crossing the midline in the midbrain, virtually enveloping the red nuclei. Red nucleus neurons innervated by the output of the interposed nuclei emit the rubrospinal tract that decussates and descends through cervical levels. It facilitates upper extremity flexion but is rudimentary in humans since the development of the corticospinal tract (CST). Its function is notable when there is a lesion affecting the CST above the level of the red nuclei, sparing the rubrospinal tract and producing decorticate posturing with extreme extension in the neck, torso, and lower extremities, and flexion of the upper extremities. Spinocerebellar outputs that use the dentate nucleus and dentatothalamic fibers, which also contribute to the decussation of the superior cerebellar peduncle, project to the contralateral ventral lateral motor thalamic nucleus. From there thalamocortical fibers project to the motor cortex and influence the CST, controlling limb musculature.

Cortical Input to the Cerebrocerebellum (Lateral Zone) through the Middle Cerebellar Peduncle

The middle cerebellar peduncle is composed almost entirely of axons arising from the contralateral pontine nuclei (Figure 7.14). Pontine nuclei are small clusters of neurons occupying the ventral basilar pons. They fasciculate the CST as it descends, dividing it into bundles that fuse caudally to form the medullary pyramids. Pontine nuclei receive descending inputs from frontal motor cortices. Decussating pontocerebellar fibers enter the contralateral cerebellum through the middle peduncle and distribute primarily

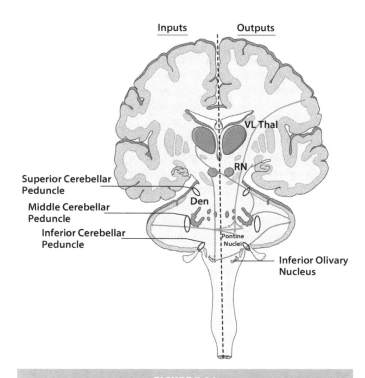

Posterior lobe/lateral zone inputs and outputs. Inputs are drawn in red on the left side of the figure; outputs in blue on the right side. VL Thal – ventral lateral thalamic nucleus; RN – red nucleus; Den – dentate nucleus. (Image provided by Jamie Graham, 2017.)

to lateral zone cerebellar cortex (primarily posterior lobes). Lateral zone output through the dentate nuclei project to contralateral ventral lateral thalamic nucleus and then to premotor and primary motor cortex. Injury to the middle cerebellar peduncle produces ataxic movements of limbs and trunk, speech, and eye movements, apparently related to mistiming of corrective movements.

Intermediate and Lateral Zone Output through the Superior Cerebellar Peduncle

The superior cerebellar peduncle is the principle cerebellar output related to regulation and refinement of dexterous multijoint movements, as well as development of novel motor skills (motor learning). The most significant afferent component of the superior peduncle is the ascending ventral spinocerebellar tract, but additional sensory afferent projections, such as trigeminocerebellar and tectocerebellar pathways, also enter the cerebellum through the superior peduncle. The remainder of its fiber complement is efferent and made of cerebellothalamic (also known as the dentatothalamic) tract and cerebellorubral pathways that form the decussation of the superior cerebellar peduncle. Similar to the output from the intermediate zone through the dentate nucleus, lateral zone dentatothalamic axons innervate the contralateral ventral lateral thalamus and, through the thalamocortical projections to frontal motor cortices, affect CST output; these influence complex distal multijoint movements on the same side as the cerebellum. Superior cerebellar peduncle injury produces a similar constellation of deficits to those seen with middle peduncle damage, such as ataxic movements of limbs, including intention tremor,

> Neuroplasticity
Cerebellar Plasticity with Cerebellar Transcranial Direct Current Stimulation

Pharmacological treatments for cerebellar dysfunction have been elusive. A novel noninvasive treatment has been examined that is aimed at promoting cerebellar plasticity and ameliorating the motor, cognitive, and emotional signs presented by patients with cerebellar injury. Therapeutic use of transcranial direct current stimulation (tDCS) of the cerebral cortex, to either inhibit or promote brain activity via electrodes using a machine very similar to an iontophoresis unit, directs beneficial plasticity in patients with brain injuries, without significant detrimental side effects. Studies are underway to determine whether it can produce positive changes in cerebellar function and reduce signs of cerebellar damage.

Recovery of motor function after cerebellar injury is a process called adaptation, which is a progressive reduction in error making. Adaptation is difficult after cerebellar damage, so a safe, effective treatment is needed to facilitate this process. In patients with visuomotor impairments, cerebellar tDCS (ctDCS) stimulation showed a faster reduction in erroneous movements during the adaptation process. Similar results have been found with gait adaptation, with a reduction in errors in spatial component of gait, that is, foot placement. Upper limb coordination was less improved with ctDCS, but combined ctDCS and tDCS of motor cortex reduced upper limb postural tremor, action tremor, and dysmetria.

Functional MRI studies demonstrated that the lateral zone of the cerebellum is involved in higher level non-motor functioning. With the observation that the lateral zone is most responsive to ctDCS, the technique was tested in normal subjects to determine if it could improve their cognitive function, learning, and ability to recognize emotional responses in others. Subjects' performance in all of the relevant tests supported the effectiveness of ctDCS to influence those higher-level functions that are impaired in patients with cerebellar injuries. A noninvasive treatment with no negative side effects that could help patients with cognitive, emotional, and learning disabilities after cerebellar injury, even in children with developmental cerebellar dysfunction, might be within reach.

dysdiadochokinesia, and discoordinated heel-to-shin motion with testing, scanning speech (words are broken into distinct syllables, often with pauses between syllables, and spoken at irregular volumes; also called explosive speech), and ataxic eye movements.

As mentioned above, there is a feedback circuit related to motor learning, which arises from lateral zone outputs through the dentate nucleus. Projections pass to the contralateral red nucleus. Red nucleus axons descend to innervate the inferior olivary nucleus. Olivocerebellar axons decussate and enter the contralateral cerebellum (where the original dentato-rubral fibers arose) through the inferior cerebellar peduncle to innervate lateral zone Purkinje cells as climbing fibers. This circuit appears to regulate mossy fiber excitation of Purkinje cell activation when refining a behavior.

IV   CEREBELLAR FUNCTION

The cerebellum is key for motor control and motor learning. Motor control incorporates sensory and motor information, with the use of feed forward and feedback information to regulate motion. The cerebellum does not appear to play a large role in movement initiation, but rather acts as an error sensor (difference engine), coordinating information in real time to modify motion. The neural substrates of motor learning include, most significantly, the motor cortex and dorsolateral prefrontal cortex. These areas are discussed in detail in Chapter 9. To allow readers to appreciate the neurologic underpinnings of motor learning, we begin with an overview of key concepts related to the subject.

Role in Motor Control and Motor Learning

Motor learning describes the process of how we gain control over the production of both simple and complex motions. This involves assessing the environment, generating a specific motor plan, then modifying the plan to create smooth, effective motions. There are

> Integration of Systems
> **Cerebellar Connectivity Includes Reciprocal Spinal, Brainstem, and Cortical Projections**

A new cerebellar atlas based on mapping of 20 healthy brains is available as an open source toolbox, thanks to the work of Diedrichsen and colleagues. The program is called SUIT, which loosely stands for spatially unbiased atlas template of the cerebellum and brainstem. This flat representation of the cerebellum will be used for research and diagnosis, expanding knowledge of specific normal cerebellar function and providing a common reference for describing and localizing cerebellar lesions.

different approaches to the study of motor learning, based on theories regarding central neurologic processes, use of feedback, skill acquisition, and progression with practice. There are two distinct types of motor learning, acquisition, and adaptation. Motor acquisition involves developing new patterns of muscle activation, contrasted with adaptation of a known motor skill to new conditions.

Stages of Motor Learning

Fitts and Posner (1967) described three advancing stages of acquiring the ability to move: cognitive, associative, and autonomous. The cognitive stage of motor learning involves the initial cortical instructions and produces slower movements as the motor plan is developed and tested. After practice, motor skills demonstrate greater efficiency, with less error of movement. This associative phase timeline is defined by greater fluidity of motion, and it varies dramatically among individuals and by motor complexity. Motor control at the associative phase is still difficult, requiring sustained attention, focus, and sufficient practice to progress. Motor learning is considered complete at the autonomous phase, when the movement is efficient, unconscious, and automatic. Additional motor or cognitive tasks may be layered onto the refined movements without interfering with performance. Achieving high-level motor performance requires thoughtful practice, which includes making, recognizing, and correcting errors in movement.

Types of Feedback

Error recognition provides information required for improved skill refinement. This recognition is considered feedback and falls into two main categories: knowledge of performance (KP) and knowledge of results (KR). Performance-based feedback provides moment-to-moment information regarding fluctuations away from the average motion trajectory. KP can be self-perceived or provided externally, such as during coaching, and allows the individual to make adjustments during the motion. Results-based feedback provides only information about task accomplishment. With KR feedback, an individual may choose from a variety of movement options to meet the goal. External feedback types are further defined as visual, proprioceptive, tactile, vestibular, and verbal, occurring during the task as KP or afterward as KR. Although feedback is helpful and may speed learning, it can also be limiting, as excess external feedback restrains random chance and useful errors. The ideal type and timing of feedback to improve motor learning and performance remains an area of robust investigation.

The cerebellum is a key neurologic structure in this feedback mechanism, modifying the force, direction, speed, and amplitude of movements. This can be seen during the simple task of drinking. When reaching for a cup, we use vision to identify the object shape. This visual information travels along the visual pathway to the occipital lobe to inform the motor pattern. Along with activating motor cortices to initiate the movement, information is relayed to the cerebellum so that even before contacting the target cup, the hand is preformed to match the shape.

Control of the movement during execution is supported by several types of KP, including conscious feedback from the somatosensory system (through the dorsal column-medial lemniscus pathway) and unconscious inputs from the proprioceptive system (traveling up the dorsal and ventral spinocerebellar tracts). While reaching for the cup, the hand is positioned by motor output information generated in the frontal lobe to match the cylindrical surface. As the arm extends, variations from the average trajectory can be monitored by vision and proprioception. KP feedback is coordinated in the cerebellum to produce a smooth, efficient motion toward and around the surface. New information regarding the temperature, weight, and stability collected by the tactile systems is sent to the spinal cord, where minor adjustments are made, and relayed to somatosensory, motor, and association cortices for further refinement. The cerebellum coordinates this flow of information, producing immediate minor modifications in muscle contraction timing and intensity.

V   RESPONSE TO INJURY

Different locations of cerebellar injuries produce stereotypical deficits that enable relatively precise diagnoses.

Frontiers in Research
Using Proprioceptive Input to Decrease Falls

Multiple sclerosis (MS) is an autoimmune disease of the nervous system, causing axon damage and demyelination. People with MS have reduced postural control and significantly more falls, most likely due to slowed neural impulses. An innovative therapy using proprioceptive input to the trunk through a customized weighted vest is decreasing falls in this population. The idea came to the originator, Cindy Gibson-Horn, when she was working in the home with a patient with poor balance. Ms. Gibson-Horn had just finished teaching a community exercise class for osteoporosis prevention that used weighted vests to increase the spinal load for enhanced bone density. She noticed the patient was leaning heavily backward. She decided to bring the patient forward with 1.5 pounds located anteriorly. Immediately the patient stood more vertically and walked with improved motor control and balance. The patient stated, "I don't have to think to move."

Researchers later developed rigorous studies to quantify the assessment techniques, verify her findings of improved postural control and balance with use of strategically weighted vests, and attempt to determine the mechanism. Initial studies support the use of the torso-weighted vest in people with peripheral and central nervous systems problems affecting balance. The vest is customized for each patient using a process called balanced body torso weighting (BBTW). A trained clinician observes quiet standing via the Romberg test, then detailed reactive control of static standing during light, 4–6 pound perturbations (0.15–0.25 sec) in multiple directions. Based on this assessment, the clinician strategically places small weights on the torso until stability is achieved. The weights range from one-eighth to one-half pound each, with placement and size proportional to the location and extent of balance loss.

Although the mechanism remains undetermined, the current theory is the BBTW system strategically reweights the somatosensory receptors, providing more useful afferent input to the cerebellum and basal ganglia. This improved sensory information allows for better calibration of timely, smooth motor responses and an improved feedback loop that reduces ataxia and postural instability.

Some theories of the underlying mechanism are listed here:

1. Altered postural angles, which alter weight distribution to the lower extremities relating to improved proprioception
2. Altered input to trunk, muscle spindles, touch receptors, or pressure receptors in the skin
3. Increased muscle firing rate due to tactile input altered pressure and pressure relationships through all the joints
4. Improved sense of stability, thereby decreasing co-contraction of the trunk or limbs during perturbation
5. Increased conscious attention to body position, which is less likely as patients report diminished perception over time, with no corresponding reduction in efficacy over time
6. Adjustments due to biomechanical shift in center of mass, also less likely as research shows no corresponding adjustment in center of pressure related to the weight

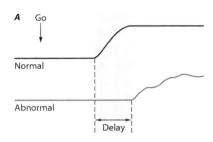

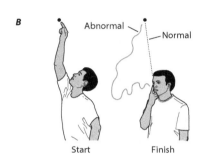

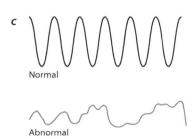

FIGURE 7.15

Typical defects associated with cerebellar disease.
A. Lesion of the right cerebellar hemisphere delays initiation of movement. The patient is told to clench both hands simultaneously; right hand clenches later than left (shown by recordings from a pressure bulb transducer squeezed by the patient). **B.** Dysmetria and decomposition of movement shown by patient moving his arm from a raised position to his nose. Tremor increases on approaching the nose. **C.** Dysdiadochokinesia occurs in the abnormal position trace of hand and forearm as a cerebellar subject tries alternately to pronate and supinate forearm while flexing and extending elbow as rapidly as possible. (Reproduced with permission from The Cerebellum. In: Kandel ER, Schwartz JH, Jessell TM, Siegelbaum SA, Hudspeth AJ, Mack S. eds. Principles of Neural Science, Fifth Editon New York, NY: McGraw-Hill; 2012.)

Classic Signs of Cerebellar Damage

There are three classic signs of cerebellar damage: ataxia, tremor, and nystagmus. Ataxia is inaccuracy in the speed, force, and distance of movement. In reaching for an object, a patient with cerebellar damage overshoots (hypermetria) or undershoots (hypometria) the target. Ataxia of gait produces staggering and lurching. Ataxia is due to impairments in interjoint coordination. Tremor is involuntary oscillation of the limbs or trunk. Cerebellar tremor is characteristically present when the patient is trying to perform a movement requiring skill, such as touching the examiner's finger or bringing a forkful of food to the mouth. Nystagmus is a rhythmic involuntary oscillation of the eyes. Ataxia and nystagmus typically occur after damage to cerebellar inputs, such as the spinocerebellar tracts or the inferior cerebellar peduncle. In contrast, tremor is more often a consequence of damage to the cerebellar output pathways, such as the superior cerebellar peduncle. However, combinations of signs typically occur with damage to the cerebellum, depending on the site and size of the lesion.

Deficits Appear Ipsilateral to the Lesion

Knowledge of the anatomy of the descending projection pathways is crucial for understanding why unilateral cerebellar damage typically produces ipsilateral limb motor signs. Ipsilateral signs occur because both the cerebellar efferent projections and the descending pathways (i.e., the targets of cerebellar action) are crossed. The combined decussations result in a system of connections that is "doubly crossed." Damage to cerebellar input from the spinal cord also produces ipsilateral signs because the principal spinocerebellar pathways, the dorsal spinocerebellar and cuneocerebellar tracts, ascend ipsilaterally. Thus, whether damage occurs to cerebellar inputs or outputs, or to the cerebellum itself, neurological signs are present on the ipsilateral side.

Typical motor defects associated with cerebellar disease include delayed motion, ataxia, dysmetria, intention tremor, and dysdiadochokinesia. These are shown during fine upper extremity motor tasks in (Figure 7.15).

Ataxia syndromes can be hereditary, genetic, or acquired, and are classified several ways by clinical incident as episodic, temporary, or progressive; or by clinical presentation as cerebellar, vestibular, or sensory ataxia. Localizing cerebellar lesions with careful examination of presenting deficits shows posterior cerebellum deficits produce eye movement disorders; midline lesions cause gait and trunk ataxia; and hemispheric lesions produce limb ataxias, reduced muscle tone (hypotonia), and difficulty with speech production (dysarthria).

> **CASE 7** **DISCUSSION: Cerebellar Stroke**

VIDEO

Tabitha had a grade I cerebellar pilocytic astrocytoma, with hydrocephalus. Unlike other cancers, which are staged by their location, size, lymph node involvement, and migration to other tissues, brain tumors (neoplasms) rarely spread outside the brain. Neoplasms

are instead graded I–IV based on biopsy analysis of tumor cell aggressiveness. Factors in grading include size, location, tissue type, potential for surgical removal, and likelihood of migration.

Fortunately for Tabitha, a grade I neoplasm has low mitotic activity, with low propensity to become malignant.

Named for the involved cell type, piloid astrocytes, and location, in the cerebellum, it is the most common brain tumor in children. Her tumor was most likely present for many years; cerebellar astrocytomas are typically slow growing and often develop in early childhood. Although brain tumors remain rare in young women, glial tumors are the most common. Pregnancy is believed to promote tumor growth due to hormonal growth factors and angiogenesis present for fetal development. Additional increase in maternal blood volume may also increase edema around the tumor, exacerbating symptoms through increased pressure on delicate nervous tissue.

Tabitha arrived at the hospital in her 33rd week of pregnancy, making her baby premature if delivered at that time. So the medical team put her on two weeks of bedrest, with an extraventricular drain to reduce pressure from the significant obstructive hydrocephalus, and steroids to manage edema. Her baby was successfully delivered via caesarian section at 35 weeks; then the neurosurgical team began in earnest to prepare for the surgery to remove her tumor, which was quite large (6.3 cm × 4.5 cm × 6.1 cm). A repeat CT scan showed ventriculomegaly in the third and lateral ventricles, but fortunately no other changes from the first scan two weeks prior. Preoperative testing was thorough to ensure her good health and identify possible complications caused by other health conditions such as cardiac problems.

Tabitha's tumor extended 17 mm down into her foramen magnum, with slight compression of the spinal cord at the medulla–cord junction and compression of the medulla and pons. Fortunately there was no spinal cord signal abnormality noted on the MRI, which meant that the cord remained intact and without damage. The team monitored neurologic status during the surgery with somatosensory-evoked potentials of ulnar and tibial nerve activity. During the delicate, microscopic dissection, the neurosurgeon found a large, predominantly solid mass with cystic components filling her right cerebellum, extending into the tentorial incisurae area and down to the medulla. He carefully cut the tumor, sending a sample to pathology for analysis, and removed the pieces of her right cerebellum until he exposed the floor of the fourth ventricle, leaving only the lateral wall.

During Tabitha's month of surgery, recovery, and rehabilitation, her mother came to care for the new baby. Over 90% of the benign cerebellar tumor was removed, but the lesion left her with specific impairments. She had physical therapy (PT), occupational therapy (OT), speech language pathology (SLP), and neuropsychiatric services during her week in the rehab unit, focusing on her self-care, mobility, and concentration, all of which were a challenge due to reduced cerebellar function. She was unsteady during gait, with ataxia and loss of strength in her right leg. Her right hand was weak and her movements ataxic during attempted fine motor function. Postoperatively, her vision became impaired, with diplopia at distance vision, and nystagmus likely due to cranial nerve VI compression. The surgery included extensive dissection of the tumor, and the long abducens nerve, which is particularly vulnerable, may have been stretched or compressed. Cognitive challenges included reduced tolerance to noises, possibly due to cochlear nuclei involvement, and difficulties in visually busy environments from dipolpia. She was unable to sustain attention for a film or even a short television program. Finally, her endurance was poor due to prolonged inactivity the prior months.

Once home, her mother continued as caregiver to baby Mali and to Tabitha during the next six months of her ongoing recovery. They decided as a family to wait until Tabitha could safely care for herself and the baby before she would take her role as primary caregiver—mommy—to her daughter. The transition was smooth and gradual, with Tabitha slowly taking on more of the duties. Now, several months later, everyone is thriving. Tabitha continues with weekly PT and is scheduled to start OT soon to work on her ability to write. She is planning to begin vision therapy with a neuro-optometrist, and will eventually start with a local driving reentry program when she is ready. Tabitha and her family are very close and share a strong faith. Their resilience is promising for a bright future with full recovery from this unexpected complication during what should have been a healthy pregnancy.

REFERENCES

Afifi A. *Functional Neuroanatomy*. New York: McGraw Hill; 1998

Alstermark B, Ekerot CF. The lateral reticular nucleus; integration of descending and ascending systems regulating voluntary forelimb movements. *Front Comput Neurosci*. 2015 Aug;9(102):1–12.

Andersen BB, Korbo L, Pakkenberg B. A quantitative study of the human cerebellum with unbiased stereological techniques. *J Comp Neurol*. 1992, Dec 22;326(4):549–560.

Babalian AL, Vidal PP. Floccular modulation of vestibuloocular pathways and cerebellum-related plasticity: an in vitro whole brain study. *J Neurophysiol*. 2000;84:2514–2528.

Bick SK, Eskandar EN. Neuromodulation for restoring memory. *Neurosurg Focus*. 2016 May;40(5):E5.

Chakravarthy DJ, Bapi RS. What do the basal ganglia do? A modeling perspective. *Biol Cybern*. 2010;103:237–253.

Crittendon A, O'Neill D, Widener G, Allen DD. Standing data disproves biomechanical mechanism for balance-based torso-weighting. *Arch Phys Med Rehabil*. 2014 January;95(1):43–49.

Diedrichsen J. A spatially unbiased atlas template of the human cerebellum. *Neuroimage*. 2006, Oct 15;33(1):127–138.

Diedrichsen J, Balsters JH, Flavell J, Cussans E, Ramnani N. A probabilistic MR atlas of the human cerebellum. *Neuroimage*. 2009, May 15;46(1):39–46.

Diedrichsen J, Maderwald S, Küper M, et al. Imaging the deep cerebellar nuclei: a probabilistic atlas and normalization procedure. *Neuroimage*. 2011, Feb 1;54(3):1786–1794.

Diedrichsen J, Zotow E. Surface-based display of volume-averaged cerebellar imaging data. *PLoS One*. 2015, Jul 31;10(7): e0133402.

Dietz V. Proprioception and locomotor disorders. *Nat Rev Neurosci*. 2002 Oct;3(10):781–790.

Dolciotti C, Nuti A, Cipriani G, et al. Cerebellar ataxia with complete clinical recovery and resolution of MRI lesions related to central pontine-myelinolysis: case report and literature review. *Case Rep Neurol*. 2010 Sep;2(3):157–162.

Fisher BE, Petzinger GM, Nixon K, et al. Exercise-induced behavioral recovery and neuroplasticity in the 1-methyl-4-phenyl-1,2,3, 6-tetrahydropyridine-lesioned mouse basal ganglia. *J Neurosci Res*. 2004, Aug 1;77(3):378–390.

Furuya S, Hanakawa T. The curse of motor expertise: Use-dependent focal dystonia as a manifestation of maladaptive changes in body representation. *Neurosci Res*. 2016 Mar;104:112–119.

Gorgas AM, Widener GL, Gibson-Horn C, Allen DD. Gait changes with balance-based torso-weighting in people with multiple sclerosis. *Physiother Res Int*. 2015 Mar;20(1):45–53.

Hawes SL, Evans RC, Unruh BA, et al. Multimodal plasticity in dorsal striatum while learning a lateralized navigation task. *J Neurosci*. 2015, Jul 22;35(29):10535–10549.

Haycock DE. *Being and Perceiving*. New York: Manupod Press; 2011:49.

Keeler JF, Pretsell DO, Robbins TW. Functional implications of dopamine D1 vs. D2 Receptors: A "prepare and select" model of the striatal direct vs. indirect pathways. *Neuroscience*. 2014;282:156–175.

Lange W. Cell number and cell density in the cerebellar cortex of man and some other mammals. *Cell Tissue Res*. 1975;157(1):115–124.

Llinas RR, Walton KD, Lang EJ. Ch. 7 Cerebellum. In: Shepherd GM, ed. *The Synaptic Organization of the Brain*. New York: Oxford University Press; 2004.

Manto M. Consensus paper: roles of the cerebellum in motor control-the diversity of ideas on cerebellar involvement in movement. *Cerebellum*. 2012 June;11(2):457–487.

Martin TA, Keating JG, Goodkin HP, Bastian AJ, Thach WT. Throwing while looking through prisms. I. Focal olivocerebellar lesions impair adaptation. *Brain*. 1996;119:1183–1198.

Middleton FA, Strick PL. Basal ganglia and cerebellar loops: motor and cognitive circuits. *Brain Res Rev*. 2000;31:236–250.

Nolte J. *The Human Brain—An Introduction to its Functional Anatomy, 6e*. London: Moby, 2008: 499–509.

Petzinger GM, Fisher BE, Van Leeuwen JE, et al. Enhancing neuroplasticity in the basal ganglia: the role of exercise in Parkinson's disease. *Mov Disord*. 2010;25(Suppl 1):S141–S145.

Pinzon-Morales RD, Hirata Y. A realistic bi-hemispheric model of the cerebellum uncovers the purpose of the abundant granule cells during motor control. *Front Neural Circuits*. 2015, May 1;9:18.

Preziosa P, Rocca MA, Mesaros S, et al. Relationship between damage to the cerebellar peduncles and clinical disability in multiple sclerosis. *Radiology*. 2014 Jun;271(3):822–830.

Purves D, Augustine GJ, Fitzpatrick D, et al., eds. *Neuroscience*. 5th ed. Sunderland, (MA): Sinauer Associates; 2001.

Siegel A, Sapru HN. *Essential Neuroscience*. 2nd ed. Philadelphia: Lippincott; 2011. 146–149.

Stoodley CJ, Schmahmann JD. Evidence for topographic organization in the cerebellum of motor control versus cognitive and affective processing. *Cortex*. 2010;46(7):831–844.

Swenson RS. *Review of Clinical and Functional Neuroscience*, Ch 8B, Cerebellar Systems. © Swenson 2006. Site editor: Rand Swenson, Dartmouth Medical School. https://www.dartmouth.edu/~rswenson/NeuroSci/index.html.

Temel Y, Blokland A, Steinbusch HWM, Visser-Vandewalle V. The functional role of the subthalamic nucleus in cognitive and limbic circuits. *Prog Neurobiol*. 2005;76:393–413.

Widener GL, Allen DD, Gibson-Horn C. Randomized clinical trial of balance-based torso weighting for improving upright mobility in people with multiple sclerosis. *Neurorehabil Neural Repair*. 2009 Oct;23(8):784–791.

Wieland S, Schindler S, Huber C, Köhr G, Oswald MJ, Kelsch W. Phasic dopamine modifies sensory-driven output of striatal neurons through synaptic plasticity. *J Neurosci*. 2015, Jul 8;35(27):9946–9956.

Xu D, Liu T, Ashe J, Bushara KO. Role of the olivo-cerebellar system in timing. *J Neurosci*. 2006;26:5990–5995.

> REVIEW QUESTIONS

1. The middle cerebellar peduncle carries _____ axons.
   A. cerebellar afferent
   B. cerebellar efferent
   C. an equal distribution of efferent and afferent
   D. neither efferent nor afferent

2. In which artery does occlusion produce lateral medullary syndrome?
   A. Posterior inferior cerebellar artery
   B. Superior cerebellar artery
   C. Anterior inferior cerebellar artery
   D. Middle cerebellar artery

3. The following statements regarding inputs to the cerebellum are true *except*:
   A. Glutamate is the main neurotransmitter.
   B. All inputs are excitatory.
   C. The two fiber systems are climbing and mossy.
   D. Mossy fibers are excitatory, and climbing fibers are inhibitory.

4. Feedback circuits in the cerebellar cortex serve to:
   A. provide inhibitory feedback to inhibitory Golgi cells.
   B. inhibit deep nuclei on entering the cerebellum.
   C. excite the deep cerebellar nuclei for motion control.
   D. compare excitatory and inhibitory signals during movement.

5. Classic signs of cerebellar damage include all of the following:
   A. Tremor, nystagmus, paresis
   B. Spasticity, ataxia, nystagmus
   C. Ataxia, tremor, nystagmus
   D. Nystagmus, paresis, tremor

6. The principle of disinhibition is best described by the following example:
   A. Excitation of an inhibitory neuron
   B. Inhibition of an inhibitory neuron
   C. Inhibition of an input neuron
   D. Excitation of an input neuron

7. The clinical consequence of combined cerebellar efferent and descending pathway decussations:
   A. Clinical signs will be ipsilateral to the lesion.
   B. Clinical signs will be contralateral to the lesion.
   C. Clinical signs will be bilateral even if the lesion is unilateral.
   D. Clinical signs only occur with bilateral damage.

8. The rule of threes in the cerebellum correlates to all *except* the following:
   A. Three sagittal zones
   B. Three spinocerebellar tracts
   C. Three cerebellar syndromes
   D. Three layers in the cerebellar cortex

9. These neurons provide the only efferent projections from the cerebellar cortex:
   A. Granule cells
   B. Golgi cells
   C. Purkinje cells
   D. Basket cells

10. The cerebellum performs the following functions *except*:
    A. eye movement coordination.
    B. coordination of sensory input with motor output.
    C. posture and gait control.
    D. motor control initiation.

Basal Nuclei

Harry's office is on the eighth floor, with a commanding view of campus, befitting a college provost. He was sitting on a couch in his office, a copy of Moby Dick open at his side, as he reflected on his 14-year journey with Parkinson's disease. Although medical care continues to improve, there remains no cure for PD. Receiving this diagnosis must be very difficult, and being a part of a patient's journey through this process is both an honor and a responsibility. Harry agreed to discuss his experience since his diagnosis, providing valuable insight for future healthcare providers.

Growing up in New York, Harry became interested in a vocation that allowed him to command his time, rather than following in the family business of politics and law. He studied modern thought and literature, and later became interested in Frederick Olmstead, the urban reformer. When Harry attended graduate school on the West Coast, he studied the enlightenment, writing his dissertation on Jefferson's educational model and his studies of architecture. After finishing his dissertation in the summer of 1980, Harry traveled back east for his first teaching job at Middlebury College in Vermont. He moved up the ranks in academia over the next few decades, relocating across the country for opportunities before finally settling in southern California. Studying literature grounded Harry in a pragmatism that, he says, helps him live with PD.

"Rigidity is my constant companion," Harry muses, as he now realizes some early symptoms of rigidity were signs of PD. He used to run an eight-mile course regularly with a running partner, who asked one day, "Why do you run with your right arm pinned to your chest?"

Harry was never flexible, and this observed stiffness was not especially odd or out of place, so he ignored the comment and explained it away as just normal for him. He also noticed that every now and then, before he'd deliver a speech, he'd tremble, and he felt new aches in his back, during long walks, that did not respond to a course of physical therapy or stretching. Because there was no recognizable history of neurologic disease in the family, the cause was assumed to be coming from the central nervous system. He underwent medical testing consisting of CT and MRI, which were both negative for tumor or other CNS diseases.

He finally went to see a neurologist, who suspected Parkinsonism, and carefully examined him to determine the definitive diagnosis. Harry was diagnosed with early onset PD and a central nervous system disorder after several years of increasing rigidity, which he describes as feeling like the "Tin Man after a rainstorm." He never had the resting tremor, or a family history of the disease, which may have delayed diagnosis somewhat.

Harry approached this diagnosis in his typical style—researching the disease enough to understand that determining the ideal treatment of his PD would take time—so he decided not to worry about it. This attitude was useful, particularly because diagnosis and management of PD is a complex process.

I OVERVIEW OF KEY CONCEPTS

The basal ganglia are a collection of subcortical nuclei that display a remarkable range of behavioral dysfunction associated with basal ganglia disease. The term *basal ganglia* is a misnomer, and the more accurate designation, *basal nuclei*, is becoming the more common form. In the past, much of basal nuclei function was deduced from the observation that these nuclei were notably damaged with conditions that produce significant motor disturbances ranging from the paucity and slowing of movement in Parkinson's disease, to the writhing movements of Huntington disease, to the bizarre tics of

Tourette syndrome, and distorted postures of dystonia. The discovery that basal nuclei project to nearly the entire cerebral cortex has revealed much more extensive function than previously appreciated. Indeed, basal nuclei disorders can produce sensory disturbances of smell and vision, as well as cognitive impairments, such as those seen in obsessive-compulsive disorder, which is often comorbid with Tourette syndrome, and in addiction. Further, dementia is an early disabling consequence of Huntington's disease and can be present in patients with advanced stages of Parkinson's disease.

Basal nuclear and cerebellar function, although related, are not the same. We have seen that firing in the cerebellum precedes

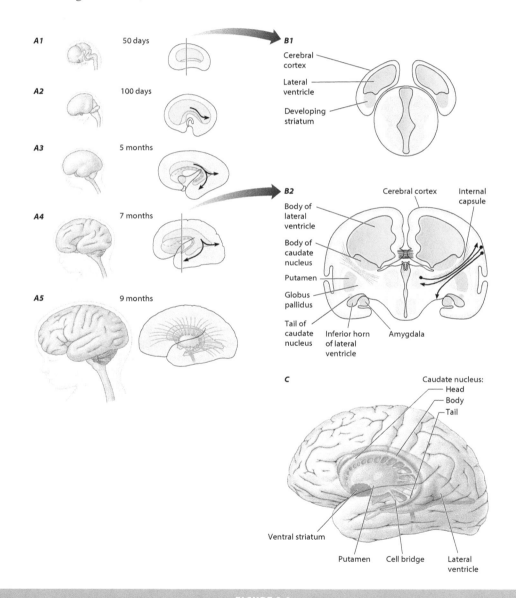

FIGURE 8.1

Development of the basal ganglia. *A.* Lateral views of the developing brain and head at different prenatal ages (**A1–A4**) and term. Schematic diagrams of the cerebral hemisphere, lateral ventricle, and striatum accompany each age. The fibers in **A5** (right) are of the internal capsule. ***B.*** Brain sections through 50-day embryo (**B1**) and 7-month embryo (**B2**). Schematic ascending and descending axons in the internal capsule are shown in **B2**. ***C.*** The striatum in relation to the ventricular system in the mature brain. The striatum consists of the caudate nucleus, putamen, and the ventral striatum. Only the caudate nucleus has a C shape, which is similar to that of the lateral ventricle. (Reproduced with permission from The Basal Ganglia. In: Martin JH. eds. *Neuroanatomy Text and Atlas*, 4e New York, NY: McGraw-Hill, 2012).

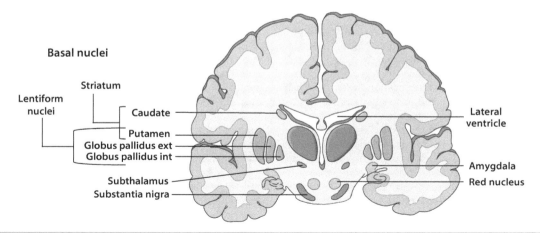

Basal nuclei

Striatum

Lentiform
nuclei

Caudate

Putamen

Globus pallidus ext

Globus pallidus int

Subthalamus

Substantia nigra

Lateral
ventricle

Amygdala

Red nucleus

FIGURE 8.2

Diagram of the basal nuclei and associated structures. (Image provided by Jamie Graham.)

that of primary motor cortex, suggesting that the cerebellum is related to the initiation of movement. Firing in the basal nuclei, on the other hand, is delayed until after firing in the cortex. Output from the cerebellum, in addition to the ventral lateral nucleus of the thalamus, also projects to other brainstem and spinal cord targets, whereas the basal nuclei have fewer brainstem projections and no direct projections to the spinal cord. Without spinal motor neuron connections, the basal nuclei are unable to directly affect muscle contraction. The extensive motor and sensory cortical connections allow the basal nuclei to influence executive motor functions, including action selection, the decision to activate particular behavior patterns appropriate to smoothly perform the intended movement.

II   BASAL NUCLEI ANATOMY

Nuclei comprising the basal nuclei have varied embryonic origins, and nuclei derived from a common source share histological and functional features (Figure 8.1).

The caudate nucleus and the putamen are forebrain (telencephalon) derivatives, and the thalamus and the subthalamic nucleus have diencephalic origins. The substantia nigra lies in the midbrain and is a mesencephalic structure.

There are five principal basal nuclei: the caudate nucleus, the putamen, the globus pallidus with internal and external segments, the substantia nigra, and the subthalamic nucleus. Additional nuclei typically considered with the basal nuclei include the ventral striatum, related to the input nuclei, the caudate and putamen, and the ventral pallidum, related to the output nucleus, the internal segment of the globus pallidus (Figure 8.2). Pathways involving these nuclei constitute a cerebro-basal nuclei-thalamo-cortical circuit that influences motor function as well as aspects of such diverse functions as personality, memory and learning, and emotion.

Reciprocal fiber connections between the thalamus and the cerebral cortex, as well as additional corticofugal (leaving the cortex) projections, contribute to the fiber complement in the internal capsule (Figure 8.3). The internal capsule is a cuplike structure with anterior

FIGURE 8.3

T1-weighted magnetic resonance image through the basal nuclei, showing the relationships with the internal capsule. (Reproduced with permission from Chapter 2. Imaging, Electrophysiologic, and Laboratory Techniques for Neurologic Diagnosis. In: Ropper AH, et al., eds. *Adams & Victor's Principles of Neurology*, 10e New York, NY: McGraw-Hill; 2014).

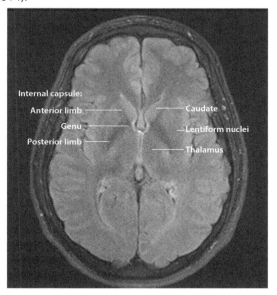

Internal capsule:

Anterior limb

Genu

Posterior limb

Caudate

Lentiform nuclei

Thalamus

and posterior limbs and a medial convexity. The lentiform nuclei fill the concavity. Major components in the anterior limb include connections between the caudate and putamen, as well as cortical inputs to the striatum. The posterior limb contains a large population of sensory thalamocortical fibers carrying both noxious and discriminative touch information from the contralateral body and face. The posterior limb also includes descending motor corticospinal axons destined for the contralateral lateral column that synapse on motor neurons in the ventral horn. At the genu, the deepest part of the cup at the inflection point transitioning from anterior to posterior limbs, corticobulbar fibers descend to innervate brainstem motor nuclei. The main arteries supplying the internal capsule are the lenticulostriate branches of the middle cerebral artery.

The caudate nucleus is found in the floor of the lateral ventricle and arches rostrocaudally through the same developmental processes that produced the C-shaped appearance of the lateral ventricles, corpus callosum, fornix, and the cerebral cortex. Together, the caudate nucleus and the putamen form the striatum that is the primary input center of the basal nuclei. These two nuclei are histologically related; thin cellular and fiber bridges connecting the nuclei across the anterior limb of the internal capsule give it its striated appearance and hence its name. Cells in the striatum predominately use GABA (γ-aminobutyric acid), an inhibitory neurotransmitter.

The thalamus (see Chapter 9 for details) is a large bilateral collection of nuclei that form the walls of the third ventricle and are joined by a small fiber bridge, the massa intermedia. Each thalamus is a major sensory relay center for somatic and special sensory pathways. There are, however, also thalamic motor nuclei that relay cerebellar and basal nuclei projections to frontal lobe motor cortices. As described above, most of the cerebellar output projects to the ventral lateral nucleus of the thalamus. Basal nuclei outputs also use the ventral lateral nucleus, as well as the ventral anterior and dorsal nuclei, to influence primary motor, premotor, supplementary motor, and limbic cortices.

The globus pallidus lies medial to the putamen. Collectively, the putamen and the globus pallidus comprise the lentiform ("lens-shaped") nuclei. The anterior limb of the internal capsule separates the head of the caudate nucleus from the lentiform nuclei. The posterior limb of the internal capsule separates the laterally positioned lentiform nuclei from the thalamus medially. The globus pallidus consists of an internal segment (GPi) that forms the principal output nucleus of the basal nuclei, and an external segment (GPe) that is part of the polysynaptic intrinsic basal nuclei circuitry.

Lying farther posteriorly and ventrally below the thalamus are two more intrinsic nuclei. The subthalamic nucleus receives inhibitory GABAergic projections from GPe and projects excitatory glutamatergic projections to GPi. Lying inferior to the subthalamic nucleus, the substantia nigra ("dark substance") is a large midbrain nucleus composed of two histologically, biochemically, and functionally distinct portions, the more superficial pars reticulata and the deeper pars compacta. Substantia nigra pars reticulata (SNpr) is histologically and functionally related to the GPi and separated from it by thin cellular bridges across the inferior part of the internal capsule, similar to the cellular bridges connecting the caudate and putamen. The GPi/SNpr nuclear complex emits GABAergic fibers to the motor thalamic nuclei. The substantia nigra pars compacta (SNpc) contains the brain's largest complement of dopaminergic neurons. These cells contain the dark pigment, neuromelanin, that gives the substantia nigra its name. SNpc output to the striatum is somewhat complex, both exciting and inhibiting different populations of striatal neurons. The dopaminergic neuron population in the SNpc is characteristically depleted in Parkinson's disease.

III DISINHIBITION

Before exploring basal nuclei circuitry in greater depth, the principle of disinhibition must be discussed (Figure 8.4). Inputs to a target neuron influence its rate of action potential firing, and those inputs can be either excitatory or inhibitory. When an input neuron acts independently, it maintains its target neuron action potential firing at a baseline rate (Figure 8.4A). The input neuron itself can be influenced, as it receives either excitatory or inhibitory synapses. Exciting an excitatory input neuron increases the

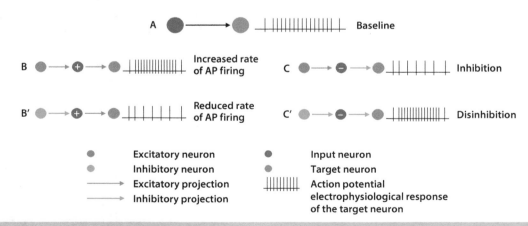

FIGURE 8.4

The principle of disinhibition. A. Input neurons (purple circles) regulate the activity of their target neurons (green circles) to produce a baseline rate of action potential firing. **B.** An excitatory synapse (blue circle; blue arrow) onto an excitatory input cell (white "+" inside the purple circle) increases the output of the excitatory input cell, which increases the rate of firing of the target cell. **B'.** An inhibitory synapse (red circle; red arrow) onto an excitatory input cell decreases the output of the excitatory input cell, which decreases the rate of firing of the target cell. **C.** An excitatory synapse onto an inhibitory input cell (white "-" inside the purple circle) increases the output of the inhibitory input cell, which decreases (inhibits) the rate of firing of the target cell. **C'.** An inhibitory synapse onto an inhibitory input cell decreases the output of the inhibitory input cell, which disinhibits the target cell and increases its rate of firing.

excitatory influence it exerts on its target neuron, increasing the target neuron's output (Figure 8.4B). Inhibiting the excitatory input neuron reduces its excitation of the target neuron, thus reducing its output (Figure 8.4B'). When an inhibitory input neuron is excited, it increases its inhibitory effects on the target neuron, suppressing (inhibiting) its action potential production (Figure 8.4C). If the same input neuron itself is inhibited, its level of inhibitory output to its target neuron is reduced (Figure 8.4C'). The rate of action potential firing in the target neuron is therefore disinhibited, allowing the target neuron to fire at an increased rate. This principle is significant in basal nuclei circuitry, and injury to different nuclei affect basal nuclei output, which can produce an array of deficits.

IV BASAL NUCLEI CIRCUITRY—DIRECT AND INDIRECT PATHWAYS

Excitatory glutamatergic fibers originate from various cortical motor, premotor, somatic sensory, and association areas and project to specific portions of the striatal input nuclei. Basal nuclei function engages anatomically and functionally distinct pathways that generally exert opposite effects on the control of face, limb, and trunk musculature. The direct pathway is an intrinsic monosynaptic circuit between the basal nuclei input nucleus, the striatum, and the output nucleus, the GPi/SNpr. Indirect basal nuclei circuitry is

an extrinsic polysynaptic circuit involving the GPe and subthalamic nucleus, initiated by cortico-nigral activation of SNpc neurons. The "go–no go" hypothesis states that the direct pathway facilitates movement, and the indirect pathway suppresses (i.e., modulates or regulates) movement. Direct or indirect pathways cannot function to the exclusion of the other and collaborate to produce coordinated volitional movement.

A recent hypothesis of basal nuclei function refers to "prepare and select" striatal circuitry. Increasing engagement of the direct, "prepare," circuit increases movement in response to stimuli. The indirect, "select," pathway is more active in the regulation of muscle contraction to produce meaningful motor activity relevant to the stimuli. Activity in the dopaminergic nigro-striatal output neurons in the SNpc to the striatum determines whether the direct or indirect pathway is dominant.

Striatal neurons are GABAergic, and they express D1- or D2-type dopamine receptors. The interaction between nigro-striatal inputs and D1 or D2 expressing striatal neurons is complex and incompletely understood. Briefly, and extremely simplified, SNpc dopaminergic synapses onto striatal neurons with D1 receptors, engages the direct pathway (Figure 8.5), and increases the inhibitory output from the striatum to GPi/SNpr. Reduced GPi/SNpr output reduces inhibition of thalamocortical output, which increases corticospinal tract activity and promotes movement. When movements must be reduced or refined through action of the indirect pathway, cortico-nigral output is reduced. The modulated nigro-striatal projection, acting through striatal neurons expressing D2 receptors, engages the indirect pathway (Figure 8.6). Striatal inhibitory output to GPe controls the degree of inhibition GPe cells exert on the subthalamic nucleus. Subthalamic output to GPi/SNpr controls the inhibition of the thalamus and refines thalamocortical and CST activity.

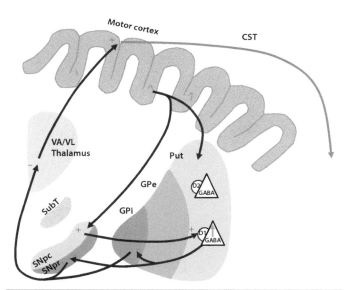

FIGURE 8.5

Direct basal nuclei circuitry. Depicted are the striatum, represented by the putamen (Put); globus pallidus external (GPe) and internal (GPi) segments; the substantia nigra pars compacta (SNpc) and pars reticulata (SNpr); the subthalamic nucleus (SubT), and the ventral anterior/ventral lateral thalamic nuclei (VA/VL Thalamus). Triangles represent GABAergic (GABA) striatal neurons with either D1 or D2 dopamine receptors. The small red upward arrow in the GABAergic striatal cell with the D1 dopamine receptor represents the increased activity produced by nigro-striatal inputs through D1 dopamine receptors. Note that the GPe and subthalamus are not engaged with activity in the direct basal nuclei pathway. +, excitatory synapses; −, inhibitory synapses (Image by Tony Mosconi, 2017).

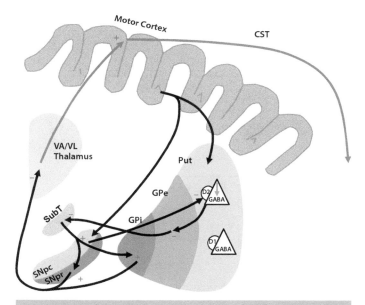

FIGURE 8.6

Indirect basal nuclei circuitry. The same conventions apply as those seen in Figure 8.5. The small red downward arrow in the GABAergic striatal cell with the D2 dopamine receptor indicates the reduced activity produced by nigro-striatal inputs through D2 dopamine receptors (Image by Tony Mosconi, 2017).

V PARALLEL CIRCUITS IN THE BASAL NUCLEI

Anatomical, physiological, and behavioral studies have described four primary parallel pathways, or loops, in basal nuclei-thalamus-cortex circuits: the skeletomotor, oculomotor, prefrontal cortical (or cognitive), and limbic loops (Figure 8.7). Integration among these four loops regulates and coordinates complex behaviors. Each loop includes reciprocal connections to different cortical areas and engages specific circuits within the basal nuclei. Cortical return pathways for each loop target separate portions of the frontal lobe.

The skeletomotor loop plays important roles in the control of facial, limb, and trunk musculature. Inputs originate from the primary somatosensory and frontal motor cortices including primary motor, supplemental motor, and premotor areas. Cortical inputs enter the skeletomotor loop through the putamen. Output from the putamen participates in the direct and indirect pathways, regulating GPi/SNpr inhibition of the ventral anterior and ventral lateral thalamic nuclei. Projections back to the frontal motor areas affect corticospinal tract output.

The oculomotor loop affects the control of saccadic eye movements. Key inputs derive from the frontal eye field, which is important in the production of rapid conjugate eye movements through

brain stem projections, and from the posterior parietal association cortex, which processes visual information for controlling the speed and direction of eye movements. Basal nuclei inputs of the oculomotor loop employ specifically the body of the caudate nucleus. GPi/SNpr output projects to the ventral anterior and medial dorsal thalamic nuclei. The oculomotor loop returns to the frontal eye movement control centers.

Recognizing cognitive difficulties in patients with basal nuclei injuries, including impaired executive motor control as well as emotional irregularities affecting behavior, has prompted examination of basal nuclei function beyond motor control. Studies have described an associative loop that plays a role in cognition and executive behavioral functions, such as strategic planning of behavior. Receiving inputs from diverse association areas including posterior parietal, middle, and inferior temporal association cortices, and prefrontal and premotor cortices, this loop projects primarily to the head of the caudate. Output is through the GPi/SNpr nucleus to the ventral anterior and medial dorsal thalamic nuclei. Thalamocortical projections pass to the dorsolateral prefrontal cortex and some premotor regions. Though principally involved in thought and reasoning and in the highest level of organizing goal-directed behaviors, the prefrontal cortex has relatively direct connections with premotor areas involved in movement planning.

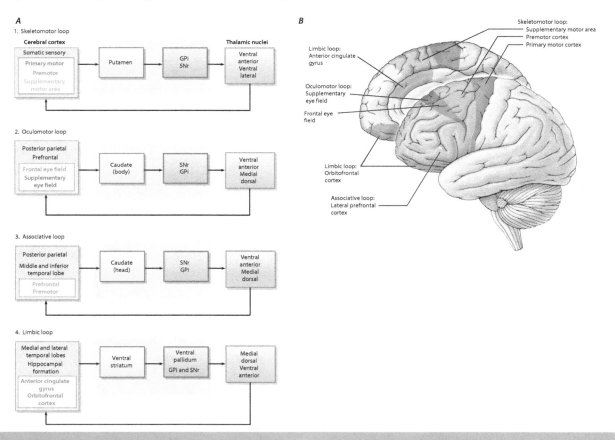

FIGURE 8.7

Four principal input-output loops through the basal ganglia. *A.* Block diagrams illustrating the general organization of the loops. (1) Skeletomotor loop, (2) oculomotor loop, (3) associative loop, and (4) limbic loop. GPi, internal segment of the globus pallidus; SNr, substantia nigra pars reticulata. ***B.*** Lateral and medial views of the cerebral cortex, illustrating the approximate location of the target regions in the frontal lobe. The medial orbitofrontal cortex is ventral to the lateral prefrontal cortex. (Reproduced with permission from The Basal Ganglia. In: Martin JH. eds. *Neuroanatomy Text and Atlas*, 4e New York, NY: McGraw-Hill, 2012).

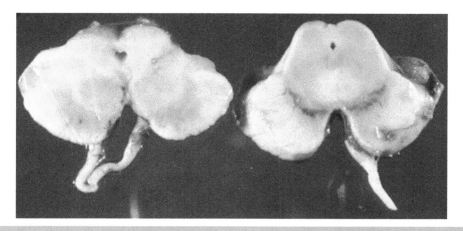

FIGURE 8.8

Substantia nigra in Parkinson's and normal midbrains. *(Left panel)* Pronounced loss of pigmentation of the substantia nigra in the midbrain in Parkinson disease. ***(Right panel)*** Normal substantia nigra. (Used with permission from Kinuko Suzuki, MD, Tokyo Metropolitan Institute of Gerontology; retired faculty, Department of Pathology and Laboratory Medicine, University of North Carolina, Chapel Hill, NC)

The limbic system comprises the principal circuitry for motivation, emotion, and learning, and it also participates in high-level regulation of behavior. The limbic association cortex, including the anterior cingulate gyrus and the orbitofrontal cortex, and the hippocampal formation provide the major inputs to the limbic loop, projecting to the ventral striatum. Output from the ventral striatum projects not only to the GPi/SNpr nucleus but also to the ventral pallidum. Output from those nuclei project to the ventral anterior and medial dorsal thalamic nuclei. The limbic loop is completed with thalamocortical return to the anterior cingulate gyrus in the frontal lobe.

VI   RESPONSE TO INJURY: LESIONS OF THE BASAL NUCLEI

Damage to different basal nuclei can produce striking and predictable movement disorders. Because interruption of the circuitry affects corticospinal tract output, deficits from some unilateral lesions appear contralaterally. Other well-known diseases and the associated pathological movements result from degeneration of neurons in particular nuclei. Interruption of the circuitry in the indirect pathway produces excessive (hyperkinetic) or reduced (hypokinetic) movement.

Parkinson's Disease

The most common neurodegenerative disease affecting the basal nuclei is Parkinson's disease (PD), characterized by bilateral degeneration of dopaminergic neurons in the substantia nigra pars compacta (Figure 8.8). It should be noted here that there are other dopaminergic systems that show functional degradation in PD, including the visual system. The loss of dopamine is gradual, with an estimated 20 years and loss of over 70% of dopamine neurons before producing the clearly observable behavioral changes. The classic movement signs of PD that develop over time are tremor, hypokinetic movements such as bradykinesia (slowness of movement) or akinesia (frozen movement), impaired postural control, and rigidity.

Studies focusing on early diagnosis are showing promise, including a simple skin test for abnormal protein biomarkers (as brain and skin share embryological tissue origins), or testing olfaction, as CN I function appears sensitive to mild neurodegenerative changes seen in early phases of both Alzheimer's and Parkinson's disease.

Over time, this gradual decline in dopaminergic neurons reduces SNpc modulation of D2-expressing inhibitory striatal cells of the indirect pathway. Striatal projections to GPe (Figure 8.9) are disinhibited, suppressing GPe output and releasing—disinhibiting—activity in the subthalamic nucleus. Increased excitatory subthalamic output to GPi/SNpr increase inhibition of the ventral anterior and ventral

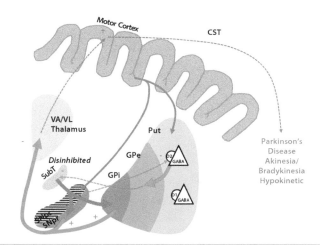

FIGURE 8.9

Impaired basal nuclei circuitry with Parkinson's disease. The same conventions apply as those seen in Figure 8.5. The hatched area represents damage to the dopaminergic SNpc. Red lines indicate inhibitory output; green lines represent excitatory output. Thin dashed lines indicate reduced output; thick lines indicate increased output. Loss of suppression of D2-GABAergic striatal cells due to loss of nigro-striatal inputs produces a relative increase in striato-GPe inhibitory output to the subtalamus. Suppressed GPe-subthalamus inhibition *Disinhibits* the subthalamic neurons to greatly excite the GPi/SNpr cells. The inhibition of VA/VL thalamus is increased; thalamocortical output is suppressed; and CST output is reduced, producing hypokinetic signs such as bradykinesia and akinesia (Image by Tony Mosconi, 2017).

lateral thalamic nuclei, reducing thalamocortical excitation of the primary motor cortex, producing the classic signs of Parkinson's disease.

Parkinson's disease is a progressive, degenerative disease, with no known cure at this time, that unfortunately progresses to death. The disease is divided into early, middle, and late phases, often using the Hoehn and Yahr Scale, with therapeutic interventions categorized by Dal Bello Haas as preventative, restorative, or adaptive (Table 8.1). Despite limitations, such as primarily using movement-based impairments to stage the disease, the Hoehn and Yahr Scale remains widely used to describe the progression of PD. Many decades ago, the administration of levodopa (L-dopa), a dopamine precursor able to cross the blood–brain barrier before converting to useable dopamine, produced remarkable results. Patients given L-dopa had a nearly complete reduction in clinical presentations. Unfortunately, after several years, patients adapted to the drug, limiting its effectiveness. More recent development of neuroprotective drugs, dopamine agonists, and other drug therapies are providing a longer window of treatment. Therapeutic interventions remain a central component of disease management.

Treatment during stages of Parkinson's disease

During early stages, treatment is focused on patient education toward prevention of secondary sequellae, such as loss of joint mobility and muscle strength due to paucity of motion.

Although most clinical findings in PD involve restrictions in motion, such as rigidity and hypokinesis, a common early finding in about 75% of people with PD is a resting, "pill-rolling" tremor that might begin unilaterally and progress to bilateral presentation. Some evidence suggests that damage to a cerebello-thalamo-cortical circuitry, in addition to the loss of dopaminergic cells, produces the tremors. Pharmacolgic treatment is somewhat effective,

Additional early symptoms include voice and speech difficulties in about 90% of people with PD, which do not respond to L-dopa. During early stages, people often develop hypophonia, a soft and breathy voice with reduced modulation of volume and pitch, as well as dysprosody (flat speech melody). Hypophonia persists even in loud environments, when people normally realize that their voices cannot be heard over the din and raise their voice. People with

Table 8.1 Parkinson's Disease Progression

Severity	Hoehn and Yahr Stage Description	Clinical Findings	Recommended Therapy Interventions
Early	1—Unilateral	Unilateral tremor Hypophonia Micrographia	**Preventative:** Neuroprotective drugs Stretching to prevent contractures—emphasis on ankle and spinal mobility **Restorative:** Dopamine agonists Progressive resistive exercises Cardiopulmonary and cardiovascular exercises Training in speaking loudly **Compensatory:** Education on disease progression, refer to support group Training in movement strategies useful in middle stages
Early	1.5—Unilateral and axial	Mild gait hypokinesia Axial rigidity	**Preventative:** As per Stage I **Restorative:** Continue with Stage I interventions Add training in larger amplitude motions (e.g., LSVT BIG) **Compensatory:** As per Stage I
Early	2—Bilateral involvement without balance impairment	Bilateral bradykinesia Postural instability Mild bilateral rigidity	**Preventative:** Improve balance reactions through training **Restorative:** Vestibular training LSVT BIG/LOUD **Compensatory:** L-dopa Strategies to increase parasympathetic function to decrease rigidity: relaxation, slow rocking, small rotations, inhibitory vibration Evaluate for assistive device as needed

(continued)

Table 8.1 (*continued*)

Severity	Hoehn and Yahr Stage Description	Clinical Findings	Recommended Therapy Interventions
Middle	3—Mild to moderate bilateral disease, postural instability, physically independent	Postural instability with gait and balance impairments Functional limitations Moderate bilateral and trunk rigidity Freezing Dysarthria Increasing assistance needed over time	**Preventative:** Patient and family/caregiver training in fall prevention and home safety **Restorative:** LSVT BIG/ LOUD Range of motion to reduce rigidity High-intensity muscle strengthening Task specific training: treadmill training, compensatory steps, gait training **Compensatory:** Strategies to bypass basal nuclei including auditory/ visual cues Evaluate for adaptive equipment such as assistive gait devices, grab bars, shower bench Deep brain stimulation
Late	4—Severe disability with some ability to walk or stand	Severe disability Pulmonary and swallowing impairments develop	**Preventative:** Caregiver training for safety with mobility Pulmonary hygiene Skin care and wound prevention **Restorative:** Balance training **Compensatory:** Deep brain stimulation Evaluate for adaptive equipment for self-care and mobility
Late	5—Wheelchair bound or bedridden	Requires assistance with all functions Severe pulmonary and swallowing impairments Bladder dysfunction, with incontinence	**Preventative:** As per Stage IV **Restorative:** N/A at this stage **Compensatory:** Evaluate for total care equipment needs Refer to hospice for end-of-life concerns

Staging of Parkinson's disease into early, middle, and late stages, as well as Hoehn and Yahr stages. The table presents commonly seen clinical findings and recommended therapeutic interventions.

this inability to hear their own voice while speaking have reduced striato-prefrontal cortex activity seen on fMRI.

Treatment during stage 3 focuses on compensatory strategies that bypass the basal nuclei pathways, accessing other systems such as sound, as well as interventions to promote neuroplasticity, now understood to be possible in early and middle stages of PD (see Neuroplasticity box for further discussion). Rigidity and postural instability worsen, due to progressive loss of dopaminergic pathways. During middle stages of PD, people often develop dysarthria (poor articulation of speech without loss of meaning) as well as restricted facial expression with a masklike appearance.

In the later stages of PD, progressive deterioration of dopaminergic neurons and interruption of the basal nuclei circuits produce impaired vision, psychosis, and cognitive decline, likely from damaged associative and limbic loops. Changes in vision are multifactorial and remain poorly understood. Vision changes can include reduced acuity and markedly reduced contrast sensitivity, loss of convergence impairing focus, loss of visual fields, impaired saccadic and smooth pursuit eye movements, disturbances in visuo-spatial perception, and hallucination. A classic clinical presentation in PD includes staring, due to impaired pupil reactivity, blink reflex, and frequency.

Vision changes are not well understood; however, there may be some better-known features of PD that might be related. Impaired basal nuclei associative and limbic loops that activate posterior parietal cortex provide a potential mechanism for disrupted visuo-spatial orientation. Interruption in the visual loop impacts the normal saccade and pursuit movements. Loss of dopamine in the retina causes optic nerve thinning seen in the parafoveal inner nuclear layer, without changes in other retinal layers or total macular thickness. This reduces overall vision, which has been proposed as part of the generation of hallucinations. Hallucinations can be caused by excessive dopaminergic activation of D2 striatal cells, which may underlie the observation that patients using L-dopa often experience hallucinations. Further, sleep disorders and interruption of REM sleep among patients with PD are well known, and many patients are somnolent (excessively sleepy) during the daytime. There is a possibility that hallucinations are related, therefore, to a sort of waking dream. Poor vision, impaired eye movements, and disturbances in visuo-spatial cortical centers might combine to produce visual anomalies.

Treatment in late stage IV and V requires interprofessional coordination to manage increasing caregiver burden due to severe disability with high fall risk; cognitive decline; loss of speech, respiratory function, and swallowing; onset of severe visual disturbances; and even psychosis. Each case is best addressed in a holistic manner that incorporates the needs and concerns of the entire family and care team to lessen the emotional, financial, and physical burden of this horrible disease.

Huntington's Chorea

Huntington's disease, or Huntington's chorea, is another basal nuclei

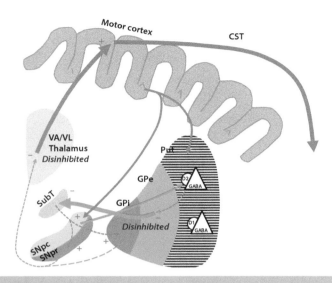

FIGURE 8.11

Impaired basal nuclei circuitry with Huntington's disease. The same conventions apply as those seen in Figure 8.9. The hatched area represents damage to the striatum. Loss of GABAergic striatal cell output decreases striato-GPe inhibition (*Disinhibition*). This increases inhibition of the subthalamus and reduced subthalamo-GPi/SNpr excitation. *Disinhibition* of VA/VL thalamus and increased thalamocortical output leads to elevated CST output, producing hyperkinetic signs such as such as choreoathetosis (Image by Tony Mosconi, 2017).

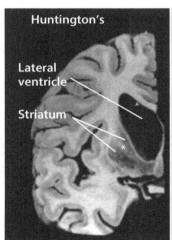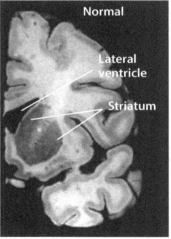

FIGURE 8.10

Striatum in Huntington's and normal coronal sections. *(Left panel)* Left hemispheric section shows severe atrophy of the caudate nucleus and putamen and expansion of the lateral ventricle in Huntington's disease. *(Right panel)* Right hemispheric section shows caudate nucleus and putamen and lateral ventricle in normal adult brain. (Used with permission from Kinuko Suzuki, MD, Tokyo Metropolitan Institute of Gerontology; retired faculty, Department of Pathology and Laboratory Medicine, University of North Carolina, Chapel Hill, NC)

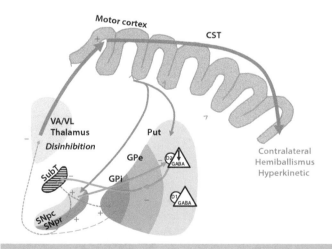

FIGURE 8.12

Impaired basal nuclei circuitry with hemiballismus. The same conventions apply as those seen in Figure 8.9. The hatched area represents damage to the subthalamic nucleus. Subthalamic excitatory activation of GPi/SNpc is reduced or lost, reducing suppression of (Disinhibition) VA/VL thalamus, increasing thalamocortical and CST output, producing hyperkinetic signs such as such as hemiballismus. Unlike Parkinson's and Huntington's diseases, which usually are bilateral degenerative diseases, subthalamic lesions are often caused by vascular injury and are unilateral. Deficits appear contralateral to the subthalamic nucleus injury (Image by Tony Mosconi, 2017).

degenerative disease. It is an autosomal dominant disease in which a genetic error results in producing an abnormal protein, huntingtin, that kills neurons especially in the striatum (Figure 8.10). It is characterized by a gradual loss of cognitive function and depression. With degeneration of striatal neurons, control over GPe cells is lost, disinhibiting the inhibitory cells of GPe which are then free to severely inhibit subthalamic neurons (Figure 8.11). Reduced subthalamic excitation of GPi/SNpr cells' inhibition of VA/VL thalamus disinhibits the thalamocortical projections, leading to elevated CST output and the hyperkinetic signs of Huntington's disease. Motor deficits associated with Huntington's disease begin as fidgeting and restlessness, progressing to unintentional, jerky, irregular movements that may affect limbs, speech, swallowing, and posture. Further deterioration may produce athetosis, slow writhing movements seen in distal limb muscles, possibly developing into choreoathetosis, uncontrollably flailing of the limbs, often accompanied by fast, forceful ballistic movement. Loss of striatal neurons produce hyperkinetic movements contrasting with those seen with Parkinson's disease.

Injury to the subthalamic nucleus produces another hyperkinetic movement disorder, hemiballismus (Figure 8.12). Hemiballismus presents as large-amplitude unilateral flinging of the contralateral limbs, which can be debilitating. Reduced subthalamic-GPi/SNpr excitation reduces regulation of VA/VL thalamic activity, increased thalamocortical excitation, and unwanted movement at rest. Symptoms may be reduced when the patient is asleep. Recently, effects of subthalamic lesions on cognition and motivation have been observed, primarily through the side effects of deep brain stimulation of the nucleus, a therapy that has been used successfully in treatment of Parkinson's disease. Effects range from mild personality changes and cognitive degradation to hypersexuality and severe depression. These results extend subthalamic nuclear influence beyond the well-known motor effects.

> Neuroplasticity

Experience-Dependent Principles and Basal Nuclei Function

Exercise and activity promote neuroplastic changes in the CNS, called experience-dependent plasticity. In 2008, Kleim and Jones described 10 principles of experience-dependent neuroplasticity, from basic science research with application to human clinical practice. They are (1) use it or lose it, (2) use it and improve it, (3) specificity, (4) repetition matters, (5) intensity matters, (6) time matters, (7) salience matters, (8) age matters, (9) transference, and (10) interference. These principles provide a useful foundation for clinical practice.

Neuroplasticity responds to behavioral demands, with ongoing long-term depression or potentiation based on demand, synaptic pruning, and cortical reorganization, supporting the principles of both "use it or lose it" and "use it and improve it." The caveat to this principle is the critical period, shown to create a limited window for change. Paucity of behavioral experience during the critical period in infancy can produce permanent functional loss due to synaptic pruning and dendritic atrophy in the quiescent circuitry. Principles related to activity dosing include specificity, repetition, and intensity, all shown to promote long-term potentiation of pathways specific to the task. Timing is a factor along with activity dosing because of critical periods in infancy and post injury; early intense behavioral challenges can be overwhelming to the developing and recovering nervous system. Selecting a task meaningful to the patient, salience, increases attention necessary to produce neurologic changes. This is supported by animal models, where loss of cholinergic neurons within the basal forebrain prevented central changes in association cortices with practice when compared to non-lesioned controls. The age of the patient is also critical, as young brains tend to be more plastic. However, older people benefit from a lifetime of experiences and more long-term learning and memories that often persist even with central nervous system disease or injury. Transference and interference relate to types of practice and their effect on the brain. With transference, training in one task may promote improvement in other, related tasks. An example is training in use of verbal self-talk to manage episodes of freezing in middle and late stage PD, which can also improve gait parameters when using self-cues or metronomes. Finally, the principle of interference relates to the competing nature of neuroplasticity. New or even existing plasticity may be impeded within local circuitry when too many stimuli are offered simultaneously during skill acquisition. This important principle offers considerations for the clinician when selecting training programs.

New basic science studies of the role of the basal nuclei in skill learning offer valuable insight to the clinician. Better understanding of the role of the dorsal striatum during stages of motor learning demonstrates that synaptic plasticity during learning is specific to striatal subregion, training stage, and involved hemisphere. Separate striatal subregions of the basal ganglia support specific stages of motor learning. The focused attention and decision-making required early in the process occur in the dorsomedial region; practice increases dorsolateral striatum activity, supporting automaticity and skill perfection. This synaptic plasticity during learning is quite specific. Dendritic pruning during training produces a more consistent, automatic movement.

Clinical application of this research is the next step. When training patients, it is important to understand the specificity of skill acquisition to task, the stage of learning, and the neurological pathways that must be reactivated. Research into neuroplasticity of basal nuclei function shows promise for rehabilitation, even in patients with PD. One recent study in a mouse model of PD looked at the role of exercise in changing basal ganglia function. It found that properly timed (4 days post-onset PD) and dosed exercise (high-intensity treadmill training gradually increased in intensity over a 4-week period) was neuroprotective, and animals with PD in the exercise group performed better than the sedentary control group. The researchers hypothesized that this was due to exercise-induced expression of proteins and genes involved in basal nuclei function, including upregulation of brain-derived neurotrophic factor, downregulation of the glutamate receptor, and increased expression of dopamine transport expression.

Integration of Systems
Complementary Approaches to Treatment for Parkinson's Disease Motor and Speech Impairments

Levodopa alone is not an effective treatment for speech deficits common in Parkinson's disease, which often worsen after deep brain stimulation of the subthalamic nucleus. Therefore speech therapy interventions combined with L-dopa are widely used to treat hypophonia, dysprosody, and dysarthria. One effective intervention uses specific feedback to increase the amplitude of respiratory and laryngeal function: LSVT (Lee Silverman Voice Therapy) LOUD. Early success using this approach inspired a complementary intervention, LSVT BIG, to improve motor function in PD. PD produces well-known motor signs, including tremor, hypokinesia, postural control, and rigidity, which lead to high fall risk; and even though L-dopa more effectively reduces motor function deficits, it has limitations over time.

These complementary approaches apply concepts of experience-dependent neuroplasticity, including specificity, repetition, intensity, transference, and interference. The training sessions emphasize task specificity, with singular focus on amplitude, using the patient's maximum effort each time. A month of weekly sessions and daily home exercises ensure adequate repetition. Interference is minimized through use of simple, easily repeated tasks with minimal instructions, which transfer to other associated motor skills such as speech and gait. The LSVT LOUD interventions focus on high-amplitude vocalization and speech, with quality in various pitches. Training uses modeling or tactile/visual cues: "watch me and do what I do." The singular focus on amplitude keeps the practice simple, limiting cognitive load. Increasing vocal volume improves the person's ability to self-monitor, and recalibrates perception of improved vocal volume, so he or she can avoid the problem of downscaling motion due to bradykinesia. Improving vocal amplitude also improves articulation, intonation, and vocal quality. LSVT BIG focuses on high-amplitude movements of all four limbs, with quality and ease of motion. Motions are demonstrated during the practice, and taught using mirroring: "watch me and do what I do." The focus on amplitude rather than velocity is more effective in managing bradykinesia, as faster motions can tend to become smaller and less accurate. The training seeks to improve movement perception by recalibrating perception of movement execution so the person can avoid the problem of downscaling motion due to bradykinesia. The exercises transfer to improved motor control, including ambulation.

Frontiers in Research
Medical Marijuana

Use of medical marijuana is expanding due to several factors. The discovery of cannabinoid receptors in the central nervous system, combined with the ability to isolate cannabidiol (the nonpsychoactive compound), as well as changing societal views with increasing legalization, has stimulated research into the therapeutic use of marijuana.

Marijuana use as treatment for central nervous system disorders has been studied for decades, providing valuable information regarding risk versus benefit for specific diseases. Endogenous ligands are found in the hippocampus, association cortices, basal nuclei, and cerebellum. At the spinal level, the receptors are highly concentrated in the neurons in the dorsal root ganglia (DRG). Notably, the thalamus and brainstem do not appear to express cannabinoid receptors. Marijuana causes direct inhibition of adenosine triphosphate (ATP) production and release of certain neurotransmitters, with indirect effects on other receptors, producing physiologic responses including reduction in nociception, emesis, spasticity, locomotion, and cognitive processing.

Considering the concentration of receptors in the DRG cells, it is not surprising that marijuana is commonly taken for pain management. Its use is also recommended for treating central pain in multiple sclerosis, a CNS autoimmune demyelinating disease. Use of medical marijuana in treating spasticity, an upper motor neuron condition related to loss of central inhibition of the local reflex loop, is also supported in patients with multiple sclerosis and may be effective in patients with spinal cord injuries.

Marijuana use in treating motor disorders is more complicated. The presence of endogenous cannabinoid receptors in association cortices, basal nuclei, and cerebellum holds promise for targeted treatment; however, the drug inhibits release of key neurotransmitters, such as acetylcholine and dopamine, essential to movement. Unfortunately, there appears to be little value in using medical marijuana to treat the writhing movements of Huntington's chorea, levodopa-induced dyskinesia in late stages of Parkinson's disease, or tremor seen in multiple sclerosis.

> **CASE 8** **DISCUSSION: Parkinson's Disease**

Our patient case, Harry, has an atypical presentation of PD, and even after 15 years he lacks the commonly seen resting tremor and has never experienced freezing. Rather than spend all his time researching the disease, Harry stays broadly familiar with the evidence, keeps abreast of drug developments, and works to maintain his physical health. He is pleased with his care plan, keeping the same neurologist for the past 10 years, visiting several times annually to monitor disease progression and discuss any needed adjustments to his regimen.

Harry and his physician changed treatment regimens four or five times over the years, the most recent adjustment in response to a new onset of midday fatigue. Between the hours of 12 and 2 p.m., Harry became lethargic, and his shuffling became worse. His physician adjusted his medication schedule to accommodate for the fatigue. This treatment plan is working well, allowing him to meet the demands of part-time work and live a relatively normal life.

He found that massage helps slightly with the stiffness, although not permanently. The most powerful thing he does to manage his PD symptoms is his daily three- to four-mile walk. Although not as strenuous as his regular run of years ago, he remains committed to the routine of regular exercise, which includes not only the run but also a series of push-ups, sit-ups, and stretching. When walking, he focuses on swinging his arms so that it will become routine through regular practice. This begins well but becomes challenging at four miles. He also stretches before walking, which helps.

Harry's rehab consisted of physical and speech therapy, where he received some good strategies. He continues to monitor his speech closely, speaking slowly, breathing well, standing to speak, and trying not to go on too long (5–10 minutes maximum). Before he teaches or does any public speaking, he lies on the floor to loosen up his back in all directions.

Coping with a progressive degenerative disease like Parkinson's disease is never easy and carries a long, slow burden of daily reality. Harry's lifelong study of philosophy and literature provided him with a solid and unique perspective on the struggles in life. He reflects, "Ultimately, we have no control. Nature wants everything to go south tomorrow, that's what it is." He finds value in maintaining personal and public dignity, and practicing compassion for others. By revealing his symptoms, those around him have permission to express their emotions. Additionally, he strives to be gracious in accepting help when others want to help, feeling it insults them if he rejects their kindness. Six years ago, Harry chose to give up driving because he "didn't want to kill someone." He also decided to take advantage of the university early retirement program, which allows people to transition to part time and begin drawing early retirement for up to five years prior to retiring.

When he married, Harry became stepfather to three teenagers who are now grown, giving him eight grandchildren. His wife was there when he received the initial news, which was hard to hear and even harder to reveal to their children. Harry said it was the first time in his life he was up against something he couldn't conquer. His pragmatic approach was not to despair, but rather to consider what he could do and adjust his horizons. He and Donna, his wife of 29 years, figured it out eventually. She now handles the driving and takes charge of the medication as well. The neurologist gave them a variety of options for the course of care, which included diet, medications, and emotional support groups. Donna tried the support group, but it was not appealing to Harry, who found the general information regarding coping to be sufficient. The diagnosis has changed their future plans, prompting them to put their financial plans in order so that there are no surprises. Neither of them are big travelers, so their plan to retire to Pismo Beach, where they have a second home, remains on track.

Harry's advice for others living with PD is "to keep doing things you like to do, and don't leave any blank spaces in your life." That's why he's taking early retirement. He tries to devote the same amount of time to exercise as before, just less intensely. "Emotionally, try not to get upset," he says. "This situation is like the weather—you just have to deal with it." He has been open, telling people what's going on with him. He is fortunate, he says, to be in a position of power, with no fears of job loss.

Finally, Harry's advice to future clinicians is to go beyond dispensing technical advice. "Attitude is key, so try to remain positive with your patients. Look as far down the road as practical; rather than trying to look at the end, focus on now, the reasonable near future." He learned much from reading the Stoics, the Greek philosophers. They taught acceptance of mortality; that change and decay are part of life. "The key is to find equilibrium, neither too much joy nor despair."

REFERENCES

Afifi A. *Functional Neuroanatomy*. New York: McGraw Hill; 1998.

Ahlskog JE. Does vigorous exercise have a neuroprotective effect in Parkinson disease? *Neurology*. 2011 Jul 19;77(3):288–294.

Alstermark B, Ekerot CF. The lateral reticular nucleus; integration of descending and ascending systems regulating voluntary forelimb movements. *Front Comput Neurosci*. 2015 Aug;9(102):1–12.

Armstrong RA. Visual symptoms in Parkinson's disease. *Parkinson's Dis*. 2011;1–9.

Arnold C, Gehrig J, Gispert S, Seifried C, Kell CA. Pathomechanisms and compensatory efforts related to Parkinsonian speech. *Neuroimage Clin*. 2013 Oct 31;4:82–97.

Chakravarthy DJ, Bapi RS. What do the basal ganglia do? A modeling perspective. *Biol Cybern*. 2010;103:237–253.

Clarke CE. Medical management of Parkinson's disease. *J Neurol Neurosurg Psychiatry*. 2002;72:i22–i27.

Davidsdottir S, Cronin-Golomb A, Lee A. Visual and spatial symptoms in Parkinson's disease. *Vision Res*. 2005 May;45(10):1285–1296.

Dibble LE, Cavanaugh JT, Earhart GM, Ellis TD, Ford MP, Foreman KB. Charting the progression of disability in Parkinson disease: study protocol for a prospective longitudinal cohort study. *BMC Neurol.* 2010 Nov 3;10:110.

Dietz V. Proprioception and locomotor disorders. *Nat Rev Neurosci.* 2002 Oct;3(10):781–790.

Fisher BE, Petzinger GM, Nixon K, et al. Exercise-induced behavioral recovery and neuroplasticity in the 1-methyl-4-phenyl-1,2,3, 6-tetrahydropyridine-lesioned mouse basal ganglia. *J Neurosci Res.* 2004 Aug 1;77(3):378–390.

Fox C, Ebersbach G, Ramig L, Sapir S. LSVT LOUD and LSVT BIG: behavioral treatment programs for speech and body movement in Parkinson disease. *Parkinson's Dis.* 2012;2012:1–9.

Furuya S, Hanakawa T. The curse of motor expertise: use-dependent focal dystonia as a manifestation of maladaptive changes in body representation. *Neurosci Res.* 2016 Mar;104:112–119.

Goetz CG, Poewe W, Rascol O, et al. Movement Disorder Society Task Force report on the Hoehn and Yahr staging scale: status and recommendations. *Mov Disord.* 2004 Sep;19(9):1020–1028.

Hawes SL, Evans RC, Unruh BA, et al. Multimodal plasticity in dorsal striatum while learning a lateralized navigation task. *J Neurosci.* 2015 Jul 22;35(29):10535–10549.

Haycock DE. *Being and Perceiving.* New York: Manupod Press; 2011: p. 49.

Herd CP, Tomlinson CL, Deane KHO, et al. Comparison of speech and language therapy techniques for speech problems in Parkinson's disease. *Cochrane Database Syst Rev.* 2012; 8. Art. No.: CD002814.

Keeler JF, Pretsell DO, Robbins TW. Functional implications of dopamine D1 vs. D2 receptors: A "prepare and select" model of the striatal direct vs. indirect pathways. *Neuroscience.* 2014;282:156–175.

Kelm-Nelson CA, Brauer AF, Ciucci MR. Vocal training, levodopa, and environment effects on ultrasonic vocalizations in a rat neurotoxin model of Parkinson disease. *Behav Brain Res.* 2016 Jul 1;307:54–64.

Kleim JA, Jones TA. Principles of experience-dependent neural plasticity: implications for rehabilitation after brain damage. *J Speech Lang Hear Res.* 2008 Feb;51(1): S225–S239.

Lee JM, Derkinderen P, Kordower JH, et al. The search for a peripheral biopsy indicator of α-synuclein pathology for Parkinson disease. *J Neuropathol Exp Neurol.* 2017 Jan 9;76 (1):2–15.

Lee JY, Kim JM, Ahn J, Kim HJ, Jeon BS, Kim TW. Retinal nerve fiber layer thickness and visual hallucinations in Parkinson's disease. *Mov Disord.* 2014 Jan;29(1):61–67.

Middleton FA, Strick PL. Basal ganglia and cerebellar loops: motor and cognitive circuits. *Brain Res Rev.* 2000;31:236–250.

Miyasaki JM. Treatment of advanced Parkinson disease and related disorders. *Continuum (Minneap Minn).* 2016 Aug;22 (4 Movement Disorders):1104–1116.

Nolte J. *The Human Brain—An Introduction to Its Functional Anatomy,* 6e 2008:499–509.

Petzinger GM, Fisher BE, Van Leeuwen JE, et al. Enhancing neuroplasticity in the basal ganglia: the role of exercise in Parkinson's disease. *Mov Disord.* 2010;25 (Suppl 1): S141–S145.

Purves D, Augustine GJ, Fitzpatrick D, et al. eds. *Neuroscience.* 5th ed. Sunderland, MA: Sinauer Associates; 2001.

Quinn L, Busse M, Dal Bello-Haas V. Management of upper extremity dysfunction in people with Parkinson disease and Huntington disease: facilitating outcomes across the disease lifespan. *J Hand Ther.* 2013 Apr–Jun;26(2):148–154.

Saltychev M, Bärlund E, Paltamaa J, Katajapuu N, Laimi K. Progressive resistance training in Parkinson's disease: a systematic review and meta-analysis. *BMJ Open.* 2016 Jan 7;6(1):1–9.

Satue M, Rodrigo MJ, Obis J, et al. Evaluation of progressive visual dysfunction and retinal degeneration in patients with Parkinson's disease. *Invest Ophthalmol Vis Sci.* 2017 Feb 1;58(2):1151–1157.

Siegel A, Sapru HN. *Essential Neuroscience.* 2nd ed. Philadelphia: Lippincott; 2011:146–149.

Swenson RS. *Review of Clinical and Functional Neuroscience,* Chapter 8B—Cerebellar systems. © Swenson 2006. Site editor: Rand Swenson, Dartmouth Medical School. https://www.dartmouth.edu/~rswenson/NeuroSci/index.html.

Varanese S, Birnbaum Z, Rossi R, Di Rocco A. Treatment of advanced Parkinson's disease. *Parkinson's Dis.* 2011 Feb 7;2010:1–9.

Wieland S, Schindler S, Huber C, Köhr G, Oswald MJ, Kelsch W. Phasic dopamine modifies sensory-driven output of striatal neurons through synaptic plasticity. *J Neurosci.* 2015 Jul 8;35(27):9946–9956.

> REVIEW QUESTIONS

1. Injury to which of the basal nuclei is associated with Huntington's disease?
   A. The striatum
   B. The subthalamic nucleus
   C. The substantia nigra pars compacta
   D. The globus pallidus internus

2. The most well-known and best-studied basal nuclei circuit is the:
   A. associative loop.
   B. motor loop.
   C. visual loop.
   D. limbic loop.

3. Developmentally, which nuclei are most closely related?
   A. The substantia nigra pars compacta and the globus pallidus externa
   B. The putamen and the subthalamic nucleus
   C. The substantia nigra pars reticularis and the globus pallidus interna
   D. The caudate and the subthalamic nucleus

4. Output from the subthalamic nucleus:
   A. is inhibitory to the globus pallidus externa.
   B. is excitatory to the striatum.
   C. is inhibitory to the thalamus.
   D. is excitatory to the globus pallidus interna.

5. Loss of which neurotransmitter is associated with Parkinson's disease?
   A. Serotonin
   B. Glutamate
   C. Dopamine
   D. GABA

6. Lesions in the basal nuclei:
   A. produce tremors on intention.
   B. produce contralateral deficits.
   C. produce only motor deficits.
   D. produce ataxia, tremor, and nystagmus.

7. Which of the following statements concerning the direct and indirect basal nuclei pathways is correct?
   A. The indirect pathway reduces movement and "selects" meaningful motor activity.
   B. The direct pathway involves activation of the globus pallidus externa and subthalamic nucleus.
   C. The indirect pathway activates striatal neurons that express the D1 dopamine receptor.
   D. Direct and indirect pathways are mutually exclusive and cannot act simultaneously.

8. Cognitive impairment after basal nuclei injuries is from damage to the following basal nuclei pathway:
   A. Limbic loop
   B. Prefrontal cortical loop
   C. Skeletomotor loop
   D. Globus pallidus internus loop

9. The skeletomotor loop pathway consists of the following *except*:
   A. primary somatosensory and frontal motor cortices.
   B. putamen.
   C. globus pallidus internus.
   D. ventral striatum.

10. Which of the following statements regarding Parkinson's disease and Huntington's chorea is false?
    A. Both are basal nuclei degenerative diseases.
    B. Both produce cognitive decline.
    C. Both involve disinhibition (suppression) of subthalamic nuclei.
    D. Both produce significant motor impairments.

CHAPTER 9

Diencephalon

Norma B. was shocked when the doctor gave her the diagnosis of mild, late onset Alzheimer's disease (AD) at age 91. Her husband Georg was not; it explained her increasingly strange behavior over the past few years. She had been ever more dependent on him for names and details of events, repeating the same information several times in a short period, misplacing kitchen and other items, and losing hundreds of dollars.

They phoned each of their grown children to share the sad news. They were determined that this would not change their lives. In fact, Georg became more patient now that he understood Norma's behavior. Georg and Norma had only just found each other again, college sweethearts reunited in their 70s after a lifetime apart. Norma admitted to her daughter the early difficulties: "It's really hard because I'm losing my friendships." She told her, "I feel lonely; I can't talk to them because I forget the words. They are so kind and make an effort to include me, but I'm ashamed. It's embarrassing."

Late-onset Alzheimer's disease, the most common form, begins with age-related free radicals, generated in the mitochondria, cause oxidative stress which further damages the mitochondria, disrupting ATP production. With loss of ATP to fuel maintenance of the membrane resting potential, the disrupted mitochondrial cell membrane becomes permeable to an influx of damaging levels of calcium while leaking large proteins into the surrounding cell. Leaked proteins are neurotoxic and produce senile plaques and neurofibrillary tangles, two pathological findings in AD. Senile plaques are extracellular deposition of beta amyloid-Aβ, causing neuron death, synapse damage, and loss of long-term potentiation. New diffusion tensor imaging to view white matter axon tracts reveals selective early degeneration within the limbic–diencephalic network. This causes early disruption in memory, behavior, and emotion due, in part, to loss of acetylcholinergic cells. MRI imaging shows selective early damage from plaques to the entorhinal cortex and hippocampus, disrupting path-finding directionality (such as whether to turn left or right) and memory loss. Secondary damage from intracellular accumulation of tau protein disrupts axon transport and is found extracellularly in neurofibrillary tangles. Abnormal tau first appears in the entorhinal cortex, then in the hippocampus, and at later stages in the association cortex.

Norma's clinical findings were consistent with the early damage to the limbic system pathways involving memory, behavior, and emotions. Her symptoms progressed very slowly over the next few years. She was the choir director at their church, and when this became too difficult to manage, she cut back to just playing the piano during service, which remained easy due to years of practice. However, she noticed that she would forget the song order and constantly have to check the printed schedule, something that had never happened before. She became focused on earlier events in her own life as recent memory faded; she replaced the photos of her grandchildren with a photo of her own grandfather. She no longer recognized or even thought of her own grandchildren in her daily life. Over time, Norma became more confused, putting dishes away in the wrong place, insisting on a cup of salt in a recipe rather than a cup of sugar because she wanted to be useful. Simple tasks such as dressing became overwhelming, as she could not manage the little decisions regarding jewelry, shoes, and so on. She asked her oldest daughter to come for a visit to help her get organized, and described the challenge, "I've been trying to clean out my desk, and get lost with little cards people send." She would get distracted by the emotional connection to an item, become overwhelmed, and lose focus on the task for several hours, while she sat at the desk or puttered around the room. It was during that visit that her daughter found the stash of misplaced money and coin purses. The tangled mess perfectly mirrored the disease; under the sink Norma had stashed neatly rolled bills and coin purses, surrounded by crumpled towels, washcloths, and tissues.

I OVERVIEW OF KEY CONCEPTS

The diencephalon is a bilaterally symmetrical collection of structures found at the core of the brain. The term *diencephalon* means "between brain," an apt description, as it anatomically and functionally bridges the gap between the phylogenetically older brainstem, with its vital function control and maintenance, and the newer forebrain, in which are situated the "higher" functions such as cognition, language, creativity, and those thought processes that, in many ways, distinguish humans from the rest of the animal kingdom.

Developmentally, as discussed in Chapter 3, the diencephalon derives originally from the rostral primary vesicle, the prosencephalon. Later in embryonic life, the diencephalon divides from the telencephalon, the progenitor of the cerebrum. The diencephalon is a forebrain structure, retaining extensive connection with the cerebral cortex. Optic cups emerge from its surface to differentiate into the eyes, and the optic nerves and tracts remain attached to the diencephalon.

All but the ventral surface of the diencephalon is enclosed by cerebral cortex. Ventrally, it is continuous with the rostral midbrain. Its parts, particularly the thalamus and the hypothalamus, communicate rostrally with the cortex, as well as caudally with the rest of the brainstem, receiving afferent inputs and emitting efferent outputs in both directions. The thalamus was once considered a simple relay center for sensory and motor circuits, but its function has been greatly expanded by recent study. The hypothalamus is well known for its regulation of autonomic function and for its influence on hormonal function through its control over the pituitary gland. It too has an expanded role in modern neuroscience, with implications in cognitive functions such as memory and emotions.

The diencephalon also includes smaller regions, the subthalamus and the epithalamus. The motor functions of the subthalamus and its inclusion in the basal nuclei have been discussed in Chapter 7. Epithalamus function remains poorly elucidated; however, one of its major components, the pineal gland, is key in sleep/wake cycle maintenance and might be involved with development of sexual characteristics.

II MAJOR COMPONENTS OF THE DIENCEPHALON

The diencephalon is a roughly ovoid structure at the core of the forebrain, extending anteriorly to the region of the optic chiasm and posteriorly just past the superior colliculus (Figure 9.1). Medially, it forms the walls of the third ventricle. The superior margin of the thalamus forms part of the floor of the lateral ventricles, and it sits on the midbrain. Within the medial wall of the diencephalon is a shallow furrow, the hypothalamic sulcus, running from the foramen of Monro to the cerebral aqueduct. It forms a faint divide between the superior thalamus and the inferior–anterior hypothalamus. The epithalamus lies above and behind the thalamus. The pineal gland is suspended off its posterior aspect in the space between the superior colliculi. The small subthalamus lies between the thalamus and the midbrain substantia nigra; its nucleus is described with the basal nuclei (Chapter 8).

Anatomy of the Thalamus

The thalamus comprises the bulk of the diencephalon. In 70% of the population, the medial surface lining the wall of the third ventricle contains a decussating fiber bundle—the massa intermedia,

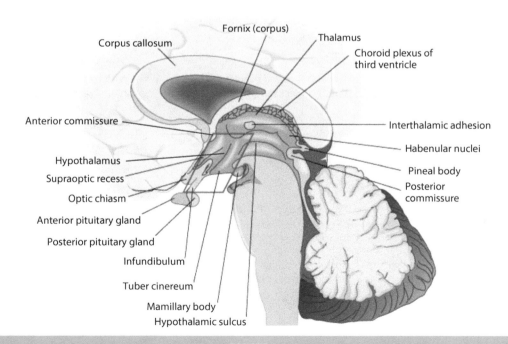

Corpus callosum
Fornix (corpus)
Thalamus
Choroid plexus of third ventricle
Anterior commissure
Interthalamic adhesion
Habenular nuclei
Hypothalamus
Pineal body
Supraoptic recess
Posterior commissure
Optic chiasm
Anterior pituitary gland
Posterior pituitary gland
Infundibulum
Tuber cinereum
Mamillary body
Hypothalamic sulcus

FIGURE 9.1

Diagram of midsagittal section through the diencephalon. (Redrawn from Chusid JG. Correlative Neuroanatomy and Functional Neurology, 19th ed. Originally published by Lange Medical Publications. Copyright © 1985 by The McGraw-Hill Companies, Inc).

or interthalamic adhesion—that joins the two thalami. The anterior tubercle is an anterior protrusion of the thalamus and contains the anterior nuclear group (Figure 9.2). Its most posterior part is the pulvinar. Lying laterally to the midbrain under the pulvinar is the medial geniculate body, containing the thalamic nucleus, relaying auditory information to the primary auditory cortex in the transverse temporal gyrus. Lateral to the medial geniculate body, separated from it by the brachium of the superior colliculus, is the lateral geniculate body, containing a nucleus that receives the majority of the primary visual system axons from the optic tract.

The lateral border of the thalamus is formed by the posterior limb of the internal capsule. Reciprocal axon connections with the cerebral cortex, called thalamic radiations, pass within the posterior limb of the internal capsule. The reticular nucleus is distributed as a sheet of cells situated between the thalamus and the internal capsule; the external medullary lamina lies between the reticular nucleus and the lateral thalamic nuclei. The myelinated fibers of the internal medullary lamina divide the thalamus into anterior, medial, and lateral nuclear groups. The lateral group is further subdivided into dorsal and ventral tiers. The pulvinar is the largest and most posterior representative of the dorsal tier, accompanied by the lateral dorsal and lateral posterior nuclei. The ventral tier contains the relay nuclei: the ventroposterolateral and ventroposteromedial nuclei (comprising the ventrobasal complex receiving somatic sensory inputs) and the ventral anterior and ventral lateral nuclei (motor thalamic nuclei receiving cerebellar and basal nuclei inputs). The anterior end of the internal medullary lamina bifurcates to enclose the anterior nucleus.

Within the substance of the internal medullary lamina are intramedullary nuclei and the centromedian nucleus.

Anatomy of the Hypothalamus

The hypothalamus lies anterior and ventral to the thalamus (Figure 9.1). It is bordered rostrally by the anterior commissure and caudally by the cerebral aqueduct. The medial hypothalamic area contains numerous nuclei; the lateral hypothalamic area contains more diffuse clusters of cells embedded within fiber bundles comprising the medial forebrain bundle. Medial hypothalamic nuclei can be divided into anterior, middle, and posterior groups. The anterior group is also known as the suprachiasmatic region, and it lies above the optic chiasm. Emerging ventrally from the middle region is the tuber cinereum, a funnel-shaped area that extends into the infundibular (pituitary) stalk connecting the hypothalamus with the neurohypophysis, or the posterior pituitary gland. The posterior region contains the mammillary bodies which which are functionally more related to the limbic system than to the rest of the hypothalamus.

Anatomy of the Epithalamus and Subthalamus

Both the epithalamus and subthalamus are small regions. The epithalamus contains the habenula and its decussating connecting fiber bundle, the habenular commissure. The stria medullaris connects the habenula with the thalamus and hypothalamus as well as

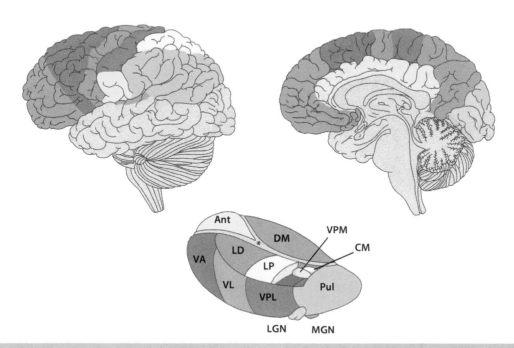

FIGURE 9.2

Diagram of thalamus with cortical connectivity. Internally, the thalamic nuclei are segregated into anterior, medial, and lateral groups by band of myelinated axon, the internal medullary lamina (*). Thalamic nuclei are color-coded to the cortical location to which they project. ANT = anterior nucleus; DM = dorsomedian; LD = lateral dorsal; LP = lateral posterior; VA = ventral anterior; VL = ventral lateral; VPL = ventroposterolateral; VPM = ventroposteromedial; CM = centromedian embedded within the internal medullary lamina; Pul = pulvinar; LGN = lateral geniculate nucleus; MGN = medial geniculate nucleus. (Image provided by Jamie Graham, 2017.)

the septal area pleasure region. The pineal gland suspends from the posterior portion of the epithalamus, dangling between the two superior colliculi. The subthalamus lies between the lower fibers of the internal capsule and the substantia nigra, ventral to the thalamus; the role of the subthalamic nucleus in basal nuclei circuitry has been discussed previously (Chapter 6). Several significant pathways cross the subthalamus. The ansa lenticularis and the lenticular fasciculus combine to form the thalamic fasciculus. Each connects different parts of the GPi/SNpr with the VA and VL nuclei in the thalamus. Cerebellothalamic fibers ascend from the cerebellum to the VA nucleus. The reticular formation extends rostrally into the subthalamus as the zona incerta and intervenes between the subthalamic nucleus and the thalamus, partially enclosed by the fibers of the ansa lenticularis.

III FUNCTIONAL DIENCEPHALON

The simplistic description of the thalamus as a collection of relay nuclei, and of the hypothalamus as the autonomic control center, is inadequate to an understanding of the circuitry of the diencephalon. Below, we elaborate on the much more extensive activities influenced by the thalamus, hypothalamus, and epithalamus.

Functional Thalamus

All of the thalamic nuclei communicate with the cerebral cortex, except the reticular nuclei, which provide intrathalamic connections.

These connections between the thalamic nuclei and the cerebral cortex are reciprocal; thus the thalamus does not merely relay information, but it receives corticothalamic feedback that likely regulates thalamocortical throughput. The thalamic radiations include the thalamocortical and corticothalamic fibers coursing through the internal capsule, utilizing both the anterior and posterior limbs.

The information processed in the thalamus is complex, incorporating ascending basal forebrain and subcortical information as well as descending cortical inputs that influence behavior (Figure 9.3). This includes inputs from primary afferent neurons from the visual system; second-order somatosensory inputs from the dorsal column nuclei; brainstem sensory nuclei; spinal cord nociceptors; ascending motor projections from both the cerebellum and basal nuclei; and descending inputs from widespread cortical sites. Therefore, the thalamus engages an information-processing loop wherein it processes information from subcortical sensory and motor centers, forwards the information to the cerebral cortex, receives feedback from those same cortical sites, and reintegrates the information with new inputs for entry back into the loop. Imagine being in a car wash, blissfully unaware of the details of your situation. You look up from your phone and see the brushes moving past your window. For an instant you feel as though you are moving forward and hit the brakes. Your visual inputs activated your lateral geniculate nucleus, and from there, via optic radiations, to your visual cortex. Additional inputs to the hypothalamus and the limbic loop produced autonomic responses and images of hitting the car in front of you. However cortical processing through parietal-temporal-occipital association

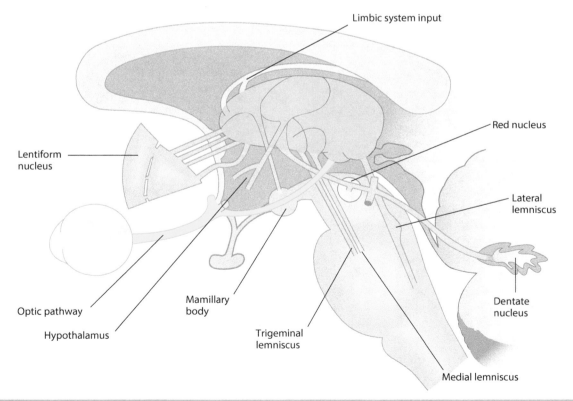

Limbic system input

Red nucleus

Lentiform nucleus

Lateral lemniscus

Optic pathway

Hypothalamus

Mamillary body

Trigeminal lemniscus

Dentate nucleus

Medial lemniscus

FIGURE 9.3

Schematic lateral view of the thalamus with afferent fiber systems. (Reproduced with permission from Chapter 9. Diencephalon. In: Waxman SG. eds. *Clinical Neuroanatomy*, 27e New York, NY: McGraw-Hill; 2013).

areas manage the details, informing the thalamus that the situation is only an illusion. The thalamus now processes the new information, along with new visual and somatic inputs, so that you no longer feel threatened and return to your phone.

Thalamic nuclei are comprised of three functionally distinct types: relay, association, and nonspecific (Table 9.1). Relay nuclei transmit information concerning a single system or function (e.g., vision, somatic sensation, cerebellar output) between the thalamus and specific cortical sites. This set of nuclei is mainly found in the ventral tier of the lateral nuclear group. Association nuclei are reciprocally connected to various association cortices and influence activity in those cortical centers (Figure 9.2). Nonspecific nuclei emit widespread cortical projections and may play a role in a diffuse nonspecific arousal system.

The nuclei can be further categorized into five groups: sensory, motor, limbic, multimodal, and intralaminar. Individual nuclei communicate with functionally related cortical sites. Sensory and motor thalamic nuclei compose the relay nuclei and lie in the ventral tier of the lateral nuclear group. The lateral geniculate nucleus (LGN) receives the vast majority of primary retinal ganglion cell axons of

Table 9.1 Functional Divisions of Thalamic Nuclei

Basic Type	Functional Group	Nucleus	Inputs	Outputs	Function
Relay	Sensory	Lateral geniculate	Optic nerve	Primary visual cortex	Vision
		Medial geniculate	Lateral lemniscus; inferior colliculus	Transverse temporal (Heschl's) gyrus	Hearing
		Ventral posterolateral	Medial lemniscus; spinothalamic tract	Primary somatosensory cortex; pain dispersed over cortex	Somatic sensation from the contralateral body
		Ventral posteromedial	Ventral trigeminothalamic tract	Primary somatosensory cortex; pain dispersed over cortex	Somatic sensation from the contralateral face
	Motor	Ventral anterior	Basal nuclei	Frontal motor cortices (premotor cortex)	Initiating and planning movement
		Ventral lateral	Cerebellum; basal nuclei	Primary motor cortex	Motor control and motor learning
Association	Limbic	Anterior	Mammillary bodies; hippocampus	Cingulate gyrus	Alertness, episodic memory, learning, spatial orientation
		Dorsomedial (medial dorsal)	Amygdala; temporal lobe; olfactory system; hypothalamus	Frontal, prefrontal cortex; frontal eye fields	Affective behavior, active memory; decision making, judgment; nonspecific pain perception and arousal
	Multimodal	Pulvinar	Parietal-temporal-occipital association cortex; visual cortex; superior colliculus	Widespread parietal-temporal-occipital association cortex; basal nuclei	Visual perception (dorsal "where" stream), sensory integration, eye movements related to attention
		Lateral posterior (posterolateral)	Visual system inputs	Parietal cortex	Functions closely related to pulvinar
		Lateral dorsal (dorsolateral)	Limbic connections	Cingulate gyrus	Functions closely related to anterior nucleus
Nonspecific	Intralaminar	Reticular	Thalamic nuclei; brainstem reticular formation; globus pallidus externus	No cortical connections; reciprocal intrathalamic connections	GABAergic cells; regulates intrathalamic nuclear activity; affects cognitive and motor functions involving thalamic nuclei
		Intralaminar nuclei Centromedian (centrum medianum)	Frontal motor cortex; sensory pathways; striatum	Frontal lobe; temporal lobe; limbic connections; striatum	Diffuse projection suggests role in nonspecific arousal system; cognitive, limbic, sensory, and motor function

the optic tract. Histologically, the LGN is a six-layered structure, with each layer receiving inputs from only one eye. It consists of parvocellular layers that receive inputs from midget-type retinal ganglion cells (thus the midget cells are also referred to as P-cells). As will be discussed in Chapter 10, circuitry originating from midget cells carries high-resolution, high-acuity visual inputs that contribute to the ventral stream (the "what" stream) in the inferior occipito-temporal cortex. Optic radiations, or the geniculocalcarine tract, carry visual information to the primary visual (striate) cortex in the occipital pole (Figure 9.4). The optic radiations include the dorsal optic radiations that pass posteriorly through parietal and occipital cortices, lateral to the posterior horn of the lateral ventricle, to terminate in the cuneate gyrus; the remaining optic radiations fibers course ventrally, forming Meyer's loop, and pass posteriorly, lateral to the inferior horn of the lateral ventricle to terminate in the lingual gyrus. A lesion of the LGN produces a contralateral homonymous hemianopsia.

The medial geniculate nucleus (MGN) receives its inputs primarily from the inferior colliculus, and processes and relays binaural auditory inputs to the transverse temporal gyrus (of Heschl) in the part of the superior temporal gyrus that extends deeply into the lateral fissure. A lesion of the MGN, as with any central lesion along the auditory pathway, produces a partial hearing loss more prominent contralaterally.

The ventrobasal complex consists of the ventroposterolateral (VPL) and ventroposteromedial (VPM) nuclei. These nuclei are part of the lemniscal system of ascending somatosensory projections whose inputs contribute to conscious sensory experiences. All of the somatic sensory information from the contralateral body and face innervate third-order cells in the VPL and VPM, respectively.

The medial lemniscus and the trigeminal lemniscus (ventral trigeminothalamic tract), as well as the spinothalamic tract carrying nociceptive information from the contralateral body, all terminate on cells in the ventrobasal complex. The VPL nucleus is arranged somatotopically so that cells in the most dorsolateral part of the nucleus represent the caudal-most part of the body; the cervical representation is most medial in the VPL. The VPM lies medial to the VPL so that the neck representation in VPL appears somatotopically adjacent to the representation of the head and face in VPM. Somatotopy is maintained in the thalamocortical projections through the posterior limb of the internal capsule and into the primary somatosensory strip in the postcentral gyrus of the parietal cortex. On first appearance, small hemorrhagic or ischemic strokes in the VPL or VPM nuclei often produce numbness or tingling in the contralateral body or face. Shortly afterward, the paresthesia often progresses into complex, searing pain that is difficult for patients to describe. This comprises the thalamic pain syndrome, or Dejerine–Roussy syndrome, a chronic pain syndrome that is characterized by severe dysesthesia and allodynia (pain perceived from innocuous stimuli) contralateral to the lesion.

Motor thalamic nuclei, ventral anterior (VA) and ventral lateral (VL) nuclei, have been discussed in Chapter 6 in the context of relaying cerebellar and basal nuclear inputs to frontal motor cortices. Dentatothalamic fibers from the contralateral cerebellum innervate the VL nucleus. VL output projects to primary motor and premotor cortex. VA and VL both are innervated by GPi/SNpr basal nuclei output. VA output passes primarily to premotor cortex for planning motor behaviors. Both VA and VL contribute to the motor loop in the basal nuclei.

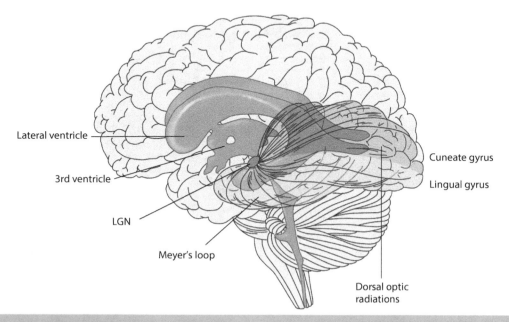

Lateral ventricle

3rd ventricle

LGN

Meyer's loop

Cuneate gyrus

Lingual gyrus

Dorsal optic radiations

FIGURE 9.4

Optic radiations from the lateral geniculate nucleus (LGN) to the primary visual cortex. Dorsal optic radiations pass from the LGN to the cuneate gyrus in the occipital lobe. Meyer's loop swings ventrally before passing posteriorly to synapse in the lingual gyrus. (Image provided by Jamie Graham, 2017.)

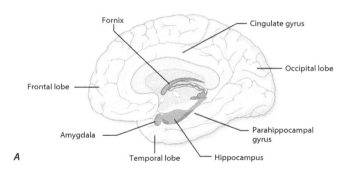

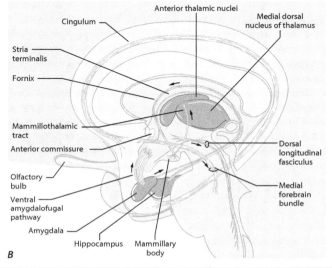

FIGURE 9.5

Sagittal diagram of the limbic system. A. Surface topography of the limbic system and associated prefrontal cortex. **B.** Connections of the limbic structures and their relation to the thalamus, hypothalamus, and midbrain tegmentum. Papez circuit interconnected with the cortical parts of the limbic system, or limbic lobe, with the hippocampus via the fornix, which runs from the hippocampus back to the mammillary bodies, and by tracts from the mammillary bodies to the thalamus and from the thalamus to the cingulate gyrus. (Reproduced from Chapter 25. The Limbic Lobes and the Neurology of Emotion. In: Ropper AH, Samuels MA, Klein JP. eds. Adams & Victor's Principles of Neurology, 10e New York, NY: McGraw-Hill; 2014).

Limbic and multimodal thalamic nuclei make up the association nuclear group (Figure 9.5).

These nuclei, along with the nonspecific nuclei, contribute to a diffuse arousal system. Limbic nuclei include the anterior and the dorsomedial (or medial dorsal) nuclei. Both receive inputs from the limbic loop of the basal nuclei. Their proposed emotional and cognitive functional significance is reinforced by observations

of disturbances in those processes in patients with basal nuclei lesions, such as those with Parkinson's or Huntington's disease (Chapter 8). The anterior nuclear group is one of the principal nuclei along the Papez circuit, originally described as an emotional circuit. Recently, the Papez circuit has been more directly implicated in memory and only minimally related to emotion. The anterior nucleus influences primarily episodic memory (related to events), learning, and spatial orientation. Episodic memory incorporates memories of one's self in temporal, physical, and emotional contexts, as compared to factual memory, which incorporates data only, without context. The mammillary bodies, the most posterior hypothalamic nuclei, receive input from the hippocampal formation through the fornix. Mammillary body output projects to the anterior nucleus via the prominent mammillothalamic tract. Anterior nuclei output innervates the cingulate gyrus, which then contributes to the return circuit to the hippocampus via the cingulum fiber pathway. Lesions in the anterior nuclei, as with lesions in other parts of the Papez circuit, produce a form of declarative memory amnesia that selectively disturbs episodic memory and spatial orientation.

The dorsomedial (or medial dorsal) nucleus (DM) receives input from the amygdala in the temporal lobe and the olfactory cortex, and emits projections to the prefrontal cortex and the hypothalamus. It is involved in affective behavior, decision-making, and judgment. The DM is further implicated in pain processing. Unlike VPL/VPM cortical projections, DM outputs bypass primary somatosensory cortex and directly innervate secondary somatosensory and parietal association cortex, the amygdala, and other limbic system structures. This connectivity demonstrates that (1) the dorsomedial nucleus contribution to pain processing is less precise and less detailed than that relayed through the VPL and VPM nuclei; and (2) nociceptive processing takes place in several cortical and subcortical areas, possibly contributing to the difficulty controlling chronic pain.

Of the multimodal nuclei, the pulvinar is the largest and most posterior. It receives the bulk of its input from the parietal-temporal-occipital association cortex, as well as additional projections from the superior colliculus and visual cortex. Its output projects widely, back to the parietal-temporal-occipital association cortex, and contributes to visual perception along the parietal (dorsal) "where" stream, and sensory integration. The pulvinar also communicates with the basal nuclei and superior colliculus regulating saccadic eye movements and eye movements related to attention. Lesions of the pulvinar in some ways resemble those of the posterior parietal cortex. Patients experience a neglect syndrome in which the contralateral visuospatial world simply ceases to exist in the patient's mental three-dimensional construct.

The other two multimodal nuclei, the lateral posterior (posterolateral) and lateral dorsal (dorsolateral), act in concert with other thalamic nuclei. The lateral posterior nucleus functions with the pulvinar. It also receives inputs from the visual cortex and emits outputs to parietal association cortex to influence visuospatial attention and orientation. The lateral dorsal nucleus acts on the limbic system, along with the anterior nucleus, and may contribute to spatial orientation.

Nonspecific thalamic nuclei include the reticular, midline (centromedian), and intralaminar nuclei. Thalamic reticular nuclei (TRN) have a complex function; however, its output is entirely within the thalamus, with no cortical connectivity. TRN have extensive intrathalamic connections and might be involved in regulating the function of all of the other thalamic nuclei. Intralaminar nuclei, of which the centromedian (centrum medianum) is the largest, are located within the fibers of the internal medullary lamina. Intralaminar nuclei have reciprocal connections with varied sources, including frontal lobe motor areas, the striatum, and other subcortical sites. This set of nuclei appears to have broad outputs and is considered to have a role in a nonspecific arousal system and influence on cognitive, limbic, sensory, and motor function. Degeneration in the intralaminar nuclei has been found in patients with supranuclear palsy and Parkinson's disease, showing the presence of tangles and Lewy bodies similar to the pathology of Parkinson's disease. Also, recent deep brain stimulation therapy inserting electrodes into the intralaminar nuclei has been shown to reduce seizures.

Functional Hypothalamus

Although it is a small brain area, the hypothalamus exerts influence over a formidable array of functions and behaviors, including the expansive category of *homeostasis*, as well as complex behaviors including reproductive and sexual behaviors, circadian rhythms, and emotional responses. It accomplishes these varied functions through broad connectivity with the forebrain and the cerebral cortex, the reticular formation, and the spinal cord, exerting profound control over visceromotor and some somatic motor functions that satisfy the homeostatic and behavioral needs.

Maintaining homeostasis involves the interaction of many different systems. Some theories suggest that the hypothalamus stores certain "set points" that define the metabolic norms for the individual. Set points might be held for blood pressure and vasomotor tone, for body weight, and for water metabolism and electrolyte balance. Hypothalamic output also influences many behaviors. Increased energy demands stimulate feeding behaviors and thirst. Cyclic and episodic functions such as menstruation, pregnancy, and lactation are controlled by hypothalamic control over hormonal production and secretion. Various sexual behaviors are regulated by the hypothalamus, including mating and sexual behaviors, and parenting. Because of its reciprocal cortical, interoceptive, and exteroceptive inputs, and reticular formation circuitry, the hypothalamus compares novel inputs regarding the current conditions of the body with its set points and makes appropriate visceromotor and somatic behavioral changes to return homeostasis (i.e., to return to the set points) or to respond appropriately to the context.

The hypothalamus consists of 11 principal nuclei that can be divided into anatomical zones based on their medial-lateral distribution or by their relationships to recognizable diencephalon landmarks (Figure 9.6). The periventricular zone comprises a thin sheet of cells lining the third ventricle, running from the anterior region posteriorly through the tuberal region. It contains some cells that are loosely distributed throughout the zone plus two more distinct nuclei, the paraventricular and arcuate. External to the periventricular zone is the medial zone, which contains most of the distinct hypothalamic nuclei: supraoptic, anterior, preoptic,

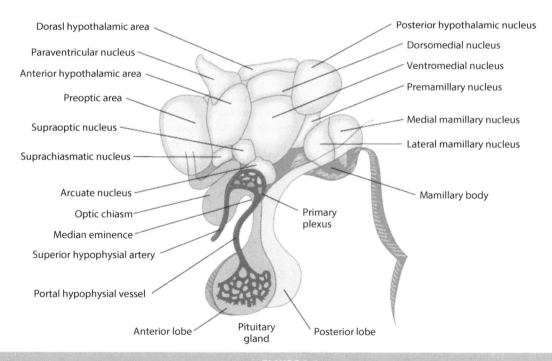

FIGURE 9.6

Human hypothalamus, with a superimposed diagrammatic representation of the portal hypophyseal vessels.
(Reproduced from Lomen-Hoerth C. Nervous System Disorders. In: Hammer GD, McPhee SJ. eds.Pathophysiology of Disease: An Introduction to Clinical Medicine, Seventh Edition New York, NY: McGraw-Hill; 2013).

suprachiasmatic, dorsomedial, ventromedial, posterior, and mammillary nuclei. The lateral zone (lateral hypothalamic area) encompasses an array of loose clusters of cells that are located within the fibers of the medial forebrain bundle.

The anterior (preoptic) region is situated above and anterior to the optic chiasm. It contains the paraventricular, supraoptic, anterior, preoptic, and suprachiasmatic nuclei. The anterior region of the hypothalamus influences parts of the parasympathetic division of the autonomic nervous system. The tuberal region lies above the tuber cinereum and contains the dorsomedial and ventromedial nuclei as well as the arcuate nucleus. The median eminence lies at the base of the tuberal region, where the infundibular stalk emerges to join the posterior pituitary. The median eminence is one of the few brain locations that lack a blood–brain barrier. The posterior (mammillary) region contains the posterior and mammillary nuclei. Posterior regions of the hypothalamus influence sympathetic nervous system function.

A description of individual hypothalamic nuclei function within the body of the text is somewhat ponderous (instead, the information is charted in Table 9.2).

Table 9.2 Hypothalamic Nuclei

Zone	Region	Nucleus	Function	Stimulation/Lesion Presentation	Hormone Release
Periventricular	**Anterior (supraoptic)**	Paraventricular	H_2O regulation; ADH (vasopressin) and oxytocin; also projects to autonomic nuclei in brain stem and spinal cord; cells project axons that release ADH and oxytocin into hypophyseal portal system in the median eminence	Destruction produces diabetes insipidus; loss of oxytocin might be related to social deficiencies associated with autism.	Oxytocin and vasopressin (antidiuretic hormone) to the posterior pituitary; prolactin-releasing hormone, corticotropin-releasing hormone, somatostatin (growth hormone–inhibiting hormone), and thyrotropin-releasing hormone to the anterior pituitary
Medial		Supraoptic	Cells project axons into the posterior pituitary to release vasopressin (ADH)		Oxytocin and vasopressin (antidiuretic hormone) to posterior pituitary
Medial		Anterior	Thermal regulation and heat dissipation; stimulates parasympathetics; contributes to maintaining alertness	Destruction produces hyperthermia.	
Medial		Preoptic	Sexually dimorphic nucleus; release of gonadotropic hormones	It may influence gender, sexual identity and orientation.	Gonadotropin-releasing hormone (aka, luteinizing hormone–releasing hormone) to the anterior pituitary
Medial		Suprachiasmatic	Receives direct retinal inputs; regulates circadian rhythms and sleep	Destruction produces insomnia, narcolepsy.	
Medial	**Tuberal**	Dorsomedial	Regulates feeding bevaviors; influences circadian rhythms especially as relate to regulating body weight	*Stimulation* produces obesity and savage behavior; destruction produces starvation.	
Medial		Ventromedial	Satiety center regulating feeding behavior; also related to social behaviors such as play, male vocalization and marking, female presentation mating behaviors (lordosis)	*Destruction* produces obesity and savage behavior; stimulated by leptin to produce satiety.	
Periventricular		Arcuate	Produces releasing/inhibiting factors; leptin receptors		Prolactin-inhibiting hormone (dopamine) and growth hormone–releasing hormone to the anterior pituitary

(*continued*)

Table 9.2 Hypothalamic Nuclei (*continued*)

Zone	Region	Nucleus	Function	Stimulation/Lesion Presentation	Hormone Release
Medial	**Posterior (mammillary)**	Posterior	Thermal regulation through heat conservation; stimulates sympathetics	Destruction produces poikilothermia.	Vasopressin
Medial		Mammillary	Influences memory and learning through limbic connections from the hippocampus via the fornix; output to anerior thalamic nucleus via mammillothalamic tract	Bilateral destruction produces anterograde amnesia; Korsakoff's syndrome.	
Lateral	Lateral	Lateral	Regulates feeding and drinking, arousal, and cognition	Stimulation induces feeding, inhibited by leptin; destruction produces starvation, also narcolepsy; broad output throughout the nervous system influences various functions, including cognitive functions, sleep/arousal, and homeostasis.	

The ensuing discussion examines nuclei according to a broader scheme including visceromotor, limbic/cognitive, social/sexual, and endocrine (pituitary) function. Visceromotor hypothalamic nuclei initiate behaviors aimed at maintaining homeostasis and energy balance. The limbic/cognitive hypothalamus has components that are part of the Papez circuit and contribute to memory and learning, and others that serve to regulate sleep/wakefulness (arousal), which may have a cyclic component related to circadian rhythms and to general cognition. Nuclei contributing to the social/sexual hypothalamus influence social behaviors as well as reproductive and nonreproductive sexual behaviors. Finally, one of the major hypothalamic functions is the regulation of the pituitary gland (hypophysis); the collection of these nuclei are referred to below as endocrine hypothalamic nuclei. It is noteworthy that many of the hypothalamic nuclei influence more than one of these processes.

Visceromotor hypothalamus

These nuclei are involved primarily with homeostasis, the body's internal regulation of its biochemical and physiological set points. Maintaining homeostasis involves regulating water metabolism and feeding, and dissipating or maintaining body heat to control overall energy levels. The paraventricular nucleus and the supraoptic nucleus are essential in controlling water metabolism. Their cells make vasopressin (also called antidiuretic hormone), which they secrete into the interstitial tissue of the posterior pituitary gland (the neurohypophysis). Vasopressin promotes water retention by increasing renal collecting duct permeability to water, extracting more water and concentrating the urine and returning it to the blood stream. The lateral hypothalamic area also contributes to hydration by stimulating thirst and thus water intake. A lesion of the paraventricular or supraoptic nucleus may produce diabetes insipidus, a characteristic hypothalamic deficit characterized by polydipsia (excessive copious water intake) and polyuria (excessive urination).

Regulating feeding behavior is complex, involving hormones produced outside the nervous system, as well as in several hypothalamic nuclei, that act though receptors in specific sets of hypothalamic neurons. Two significant hormones produced outside the CNS include leptin, produced by adipocytes, and ghrelin, produced by the gastrointestinal system. These two hormones have opposing functions. Ghrelin, which is secreted in anticipation of feeding (hunger), promotes feeding. Leptin signals satiety and suppresses feeding. Erroneous processing of either of these hormones impairs the body's ability to regulate weight. Impaired leptin metabolism leads to hyperphagia (overeating) and obesity, whereas deficiencies in ghrelin metabolism can lead to hypophagia (reduced appetite and eating) that contribute to anorexia and starvation. Hypothalamic areas especially important to weight maintenance include the dorsomedial and ventromedial nuclei. The ventromedial nucleus contains the "satiety center" with neurons possessing leptin receptors that bind the hormone to signal fullness and end the need to eat. Experimental treatments of these nuclei produce striking and opposite effects. Stimulation of the dorsomedial nucleus or destruction of the ventromedial nucleus can lead to starvation, whereas opposite treatments lead to obesity. The lateral hypothalamic area is also involved in regulation of feeding. It contains a population of cells sensitive to leptin that suppress hunger and decrease feeding behaviors. Stimulation of the lateral hypothalamic area increases feeding, whereas its destruction can also produce starvation.

Anterior and posterior hypothalamic areas influence the parasympathetic and sympathetic divisions of the autonomic nervous system, respectively. Activity in the anterior nucleus stimulates parasympathetic vasodilation, sweating, and increased respiration to dissipate body heat. Its destruction can lead to hyperthermia. In contrast, posterior nucleus activity regulates heat conservation through vasoconstriction, piloerection, and shivering. Damage to the posterior nucleus produces poikilothermia, the inability to regulate body temperature.

Limbic/cognitive hypothalamus

The mammillary nuclei influence memory and learning primarily through connections with the hippocampus (via the fornix) and the anterior nucleus of the thalamus (via the mammillothalamic tract). It forms an integral part of the Papez circuit through which information is processed to seat long-term memories and associated learning. The lateral hypothalamic area, through its widespread CNS connectivity, influences cognition, although perhaps not as directly or as obviously as prefrontal or association cortices. Arousal and sleep/wakefulness are often influenced by day–night cycles, or circadian rhythms. The suprachiasmatic nucleus receives direct primary retinal afferent inputs and is integral to maintaining appropriate sleeping and waking activities. The lateral hypothalamic area also contributes to sleep/wakefulness cycling, and injury to either of these nuclei can produce insomnia or a condition called narcolepsy, in which people drop off to sleep at inappropriate times, often when under stress. The dorsomedial nucleus is also affected by circadian rhythms, especially related to timing of feeding. More general arousal is also maintained by the anterior nucleus and the lateral hypothalamic area.

Social/sexual hypothalamus

Appropriate interactions between individuals and among social groups are important factors contributing to the success of many species, including humans. Development of social behaviors begins early in postnatal development and continues for the life of the individual. At some point in their maturation, most people develop sexual identities that contribute to reproductive or nonreproductive interpersonal behaviors. Three hypothalamic nuclei contribute significantly to social and sexual behaviors: the ventromedial, the paraventricular, and the preoptic. The ventromedial nucleus acts relatively early in social development. It stimulates play in young people, which is essential to creating personal identity as well as establishing their place in their social circle. In humans, a degree of playfulness persists throughout life and contributes to overall well-being. It also relates to male vocalization and marking displays, although these behaviors are usually more subtle in humans. The nucleus also influences female presenting behaviors (such as lordosis in animals) that are typically a prelude to reproductive or nonreproductive sexual interactions.

The paraventricular nucleus releases the hormone oxytocin into the neurohypophysis (posterior pituitary gland). This chemical signal has a variety of reproductive and social effects. It is essential for parturition, stimulating uterine contractions and stemming bleeding that results from the infant passing through the birth canal. Later, it influences the let-down reflex, releasing milk for lactation, and it appears to impart maternal bonding. Paraventricular nucleus influences on social behaviors include the drive toward pair bonding. Although it directs maternal and empathetic behaviors in females, it appears to have a significantly different effect on males. Oxytocin reduces feelings of empathy in males. This is postulated to be a survival mechanism, freeing males to hunt and to express aggressive protective behaviors. As oxytocin's effects on social interactions are better understood, an interesting relationship has emerged between inadequate production of oxytocin or oxytocin receptors and autism. One of the hallmarks of autism spectrum disorder is difficulty interpreting and presenting emotions. Recent studies have disclosed mutations in the genes encoding the oxytocin receptor in populations that also display autism-like emotional detachment. In these studies, intraventricular injection of oxytocin improved reciprocal emotional interpretation.

In the 1980s and early 1990s, researchers began to notice differences in the appearance of certain human hypothalamic nuclei

Integration of Systems
Papez Circuit

In 1937, John Papez described a neural circuit involving cortical and subcortical sites that appeared to be related to emotions and emotional behavior. The pathway, called the Papez circuit, included the hippocampus; fornix; mammillary bodies; mammillothalamic tract; anterior thalamic nucleus; and cingulate gyrus and its output fascicle, the cingulum, returning to the hippocampus. The pathway integrates activities of association regions of the cortex, the thalamus, and the hypothalamus, all of which regulate behaviors within the context of emotional self-interest. Subsequent research has failed to fully confirm Papez's original postulate as stated; the orbital and medial prefrontal cortex, ventral basal nuclei, the dorsal medial thalamic nucleus, and the amygdala have been added to the mnemonic system, with the amygdala as the primary nucleus in the circuit. The entire collection of pathways and nuclei has since been named the limbic system. The Papez circuit has survived the dissolution of its role in emotion, and it is now recognized for its involvement in episodic and spatial memory.

Alzheimer's disease (AD) presentation is strongly associated with degeneration of memory, including loss of spatial memory that sometimes results in patients being unable to find their way even in environments that were previously well known. Volumetric studies aimed at demonstrating changes in the volume, cell, and fiber content in the limbic system, as well as studies of glucose metabolism aimed at identifying areas of reduced glucose metabolism that implies functional inactivation, have revealed that these diencephalic regions are affected in AD and may be related to its symptomology.

Images of AD pathology reveal degeneration of medial temporal lobe structures, including the hippocampal formation, and broadening of the ventricles, suggesting cell death and decreased volume in periventricular structures. Recent examination of the brains of AD patients revealed diminished cell number and reduced volume in specific hypothalamic and thalamic nuclei, particularly in the mammillary bodies and the suprachiasmatic nucleus, and neuronal pathology in the supraoptic and paraventricular nuclei. Similar degeneration was noted in the thalamus in the anterior nucleus and the dorsal medial nucleus.

Studies already in Phase I trials have demonstrated that, in some patients, deep brain stimulation in the hypothalamus and fornix have been successful in activating memory circuits, reducing the impaired glucose metabolism in the temporal and parietal lobes, and possibly improving and/or slowing in the rate of cognitive decline without producing serious adverse events. Authors state the urgent need for treatments for the growing population of AD patients as a motivation for this intervention.

based on sex and, of special social significance, between heterosexual and homosexual males. Other studies report similarities in those nuclei between homosexual males and heterosexual females. Since those early studies, more data have emerged in support of the existence of a sexually dimorphic nucleus associated with the preoptic nucleus. These fascinating studies suggest that the sexually dimorphic nucleus in males is larger and has more neurons than in females. Further, the size of the sexually dimorphic nucleus in male-to-female transsexuals is like that of females. Investigation into the influences of the sexually dimorphic component of the preoptic nucleus has led to the concept that sex differing from sexuality, sexual orientation, or gender identification may be a neurodevelopmental issue and not generated by social interactions during postnatal life. It might be incredible to the public of only a few decades ago that now there is widespread acceptance of the dissolution of the "binary" concept of gender.

Endocrine hypothalamus

Endocrine control by the hypothalamus regulates a wide variety of homeostatic, reproductive, and behavioral functions. Regulation occurs through hypothalamic connections with the pituitary, controlling other endocrine glands throughout the body. The pituitary gland, or hypophysis, consists of two distinct portions, the posterior pituitary, or neurohypophysis, and the anterior pituitary, or adenohypophysis. Various hypothalamic nuclei produce releasing or inhibiting hormones (also called releasing or inhibiting factors) that influence anterior and posterior pituitary function. Figure 9.7 provides an overview of the hypothalamic and pituitary hormones that will be discussed.

The pituitary stalk joins the hypothalamus with the posterior pituitary gland. Neurons in the paraventricular and supraoptic nuclei produce two hormones, vasopressin (also called antidiuretic hormone) and oxytocin, that significantly affect water balance and behavior. These hypothalamic neurons emit axons that descend through the pituitary stalk into the posterior pituitary, and secrete their contents directly into interstitial space. The hormones remain stored in the posterior pituitary until plasma volume is reduced or blood osmolality is increased, indicating dehydration. When released, vasopressin increases the permeability of the walls of the renal collecting duct to reabsorb more water and concentrate the urine. Vasopressin also stimulates vasoconstriction to increase blood pressure.

Unlike the tissue of the neurohypophysis, the anterior pituitary is glandular. Releasing or inhibiting hormones (factors) produced in the hypothalamus control secretion from the cells in the anterior pituitary, which then regulates release of trophic or tropic hormones throughout the body. Hypothalamic nuclei neurons secrete the releasing factors into the median eminence. Because its blood–brain barrier is deficient, when the hypothalamic hormones are required, they are mobilized from stores in cells in the median eminence and released directly into hypothalamo–hypophyseal portal circulation. Portal circulation carries into the anterior hypophysis the releasing or inhibiting hormones,

which stimulate or suppress secretion of pituitary hormones into circulation.

Three hypothalamic nuclei secrete different hormones that regulate anterior pituitary hormone release: the paraventricular, preoptic, and arcuate nuclei. In addition to vasopressin and oxytocin to the posterior pituitary, the paraventricular nucleus secretes four releasing/inhibiting factors. First, it secretes corticotropin-releasing hormone, which stimulates release of corticotropin (adrenocorticotropic hormone) from the adrenal gland in response to biological stress. Second, the nucleus produces somatostatin, also known as growth hormone–inhibiting factor. Release of growth hormone stimulates mitosis and is important in children for normal growth, and in adults for tissue maintenance and metabolism. The third paraventricular hormone acting on the anterior pituitary is thyrotropin-releasing hormone, which regulates pituitary control of release of thyroid hormones. These hormones act in nearly all tissues and maintain numerous metabolic functions such as normal development and metabolic

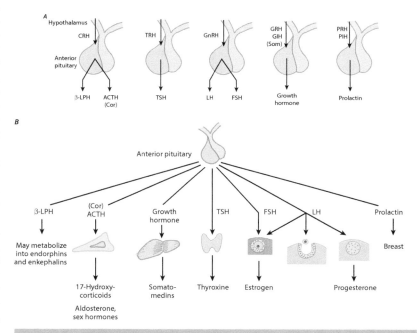

FIGURE 9.7

Hypophyseotropic and anterior pituitary hormones. A. Effects of hypophyseotropic hormones on the secretion of anterior pituitary hormones. CRH = corticotropin-releasing hormone; TRH = thyrotropin-releasing hormone; GnRH = gonadotropin-releasing hormone; GRH = growth hormone-releasing hormone; GIH, also known as somatostatin (Som) = growth hormone-inhibiting hormone; PRH = prolactin-releasing hormone; PIH = prolactin-inhibiting hormone. **B.** Anterior pituitary hormones. ACTH, adrenocorticotropic hormone, also known as corticotropin; TSH = thyroid-stimulating hormone; FSH = follicle-stimulating hormone; LH = luteinizing hormone; β-LPH = beta-lipotropin (may metabolize into endorphins and enkephalins). In women, FSH and LH act in sequence on the ovary to produce growth of the ovarian follicle, ovulation, and formation and maintenance of the corpus luteum. In men, FSH and LH control the functions of the testes. Prolactin stimulates lactation. (Reproduced with permission from Hypothalamic Regulation of Hormonal Functions. In: Barrett KE, et al., eds. *Ganong's Review of Medical Physiology*, 25e New York, NY: McGraw-Hill.)

maintenance. Prolactin-releasing hormone, the final releasing factor produced by the paraventricular nucleus, stimulates the release of the prolactin. Prolactin's best-known role is in the production and release of milk, especially in response to suckling.

The preoptic nucleus produces a releasing hormone of extreme importance in development and function of the reproductive system: gonadotrophin hormone–releasing factor (aka, luteinizing hormone–releasing factor). It acts in the anterior pituitary to release follicle-stimulating hormone and luteinizing hormone. Gonadotrophin hormone–releasing hormone is in low concentration in children, but it is released during puberty and in adolescence. It causes the anterior pituitary to release follicle-stimulating hormone and luteinizing hormone in both males and females. Follicle-stimulating hormone (FSH) and luteinizing hormone (LH) act synergistically to regulate various aspects of reproductive function. Release of FSH produces different responses in males and females; however, in both it regulates the maturation of germ cells that will yield ova or sperm cells. In females, it is released in varying amounts, and with LH, regulates different phases of the menstrual cycle. Although FSH appears to control phases of the cycle, LH concentration spikes to initiate ovulation. Both of these hormones are used medically. Recombinant FSH is administered to women who are undergoing in vitro fertilization treatments to rectify difficulties conceiving. It stimulates overproduction of ova that increases the availability of ova to sperm cells. LH is used in home test kits that indicate ovulation and optimal timing for insemination to conceive. In males, LH is also responsible for producing stable levels of testosterone.

Residing mainly within the periventricular zone in the tuberal region, the arcuate nucleus produces dopamine (in its endocrine role, also referred to as prolactin–inhibiting hormone) into the median eminence for release in the anterior pituitary. This regulates the amount and therefore the effects of prolactin. In addition to its stimulation of lactation, it has been implicated in generating appropriate maternal behaviors. Prolactin levels increase during sexual excitement and orgasm, and may be responsible for feelings of post-coital euphoria. Perhaps less thought provoking, but nonetheless important, prolactin affects hematopoiesis (formation of blood cells) and angiogenesis (formation of new blood vessels) as well as influencing immune system functions. A second hormone released by the arcuate nucleus is growth hormone–releasing hormone, acting as an antagonist to the somatostatin released by the paraventricular nucleus. Growth hormone stimulates cellular mitogenesis essential to development and regeneration. Children with growth hormone deficiencies have slower growth and delayed puberty and often have shorter stature than would be predicted by height of other family members. The anabolic effects of growth hormone are well known for their ability to increase performance in athletes and have been outlawed as PEDs (performance enhancing drugs) by the World Anti-Doping Agency.

Major hypothalamic circuits

Along with the significant connectivity with the pituitary gland, other hypothalamic pathways influence the limbic system and the autonomic nervous system. These connections are largely bidirectional, although the mammillothalamic tract is a one-way pathway connecting the mammillary bodies with the anterior nucleus of the thalamus and constitutes part of the Papez circuit governing memory. Input to the mammillary bodies arrives on the fornix from the hippocampus. The anterior nucleus of the thalamus projects heavily to the cingulate gyrus, and from there, impulses are returned to the hippocampus via the cingulum.

Another set of limbic connections comprises part of the mesolimbic (or reward) circuit and is carried on the medial forebrain bundle, which uses dopamine as its principle neurotransmitter. It contains reciprocal connections with the basal forebrain (structures around the basal nuclei, including the ventral striatum) and the ventral tegmental area in the midbrain. It also projects caudally (receiving reciprocal rostral projections) to reticular formation nuclei in the brainstem, as well as parasympathetic nuclei. Most of these autonomic connections it shares with the dorsal longitudinal fasciculus.

Arising primarily from the paraventricular nucleus, the dorsal longitudinal fasciculus is the main route of autonomic influence exerted by the hypothalamus. It descends through the periaqueductal gray matter and tegmentum of the midbrain, descending through the pons and medulla near the midline in the tegmentum anterior to the fourth ventricle. It accesses reticular nuclei along the pathway, as well as the dorsal motor nucleus of the vagus and nucleus ambiguus. It continues its descent into the spinal cord to innervate preganglionic sympathetic and sympathetic neurons in the lateral horn, which regulate thoracic, abdominal, and pelvic visceral function.

A smaller, less distinct mammillotegmental tract also descends through the brainstem tegmentum to supply parasympathetic nuclei there, including pupillary constriction via the Edinger-Westphal nucleus of cranial nerve III, the oculomotor nerve. Sympathetic control of pupillary dilation is also regulated by the hypothalamus through the hypothalamospinal pathway (Figure 9.8). Along its

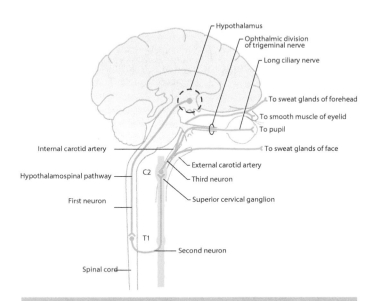

FIGURE 9.8

Hypothalamospinal (oculosympathetic) pathway. This three-neuron pathway projects from the hypothalamus to the ciliospinal center in the lateral horn of T1-3 of the spinal cord, then to the superior cervical (sympathetic) ganglion, and finally to the pupil, the smooth muscle of the eyelids, and the sweat glands of the forehead and face. Interruption of these pathways results in Horner syndrome. (Reproduced with permission from Neuro-Ophthalmic Disorders. In: Aminoff MJ, Greenberg DA, Simon RP. eds. *Clinical Neurology*, 9e New York, NY: McGraw-Hill; 2015).

pathway, this tract innervates the pretectal area in the midbrain and continues caudally to the ciliospinal center in the lateral horn of T1–3 (first through third thoracic spinal cord level). Output from the ciliospinal center projects upward along the sympathetic trunk to the superior cervical ganglion. Postganglionic sympathetic fibers ascend into the head along the carotid artery and its branches, reaching the pupillary dilators in the eye. Horner's syndrome is produced by interruption in this pathway, often with a lateral medullary syndrome or cervical spinal cord injury. It is characterized by the "Horner's triad," meiosis (fixed constricted pupil), ptosis (drooping of the eyelid), and anhydrosis (dry skin as a result of impaired sympathetic innervation of sweat and sebaceous glands). (see Figure 6.23).

Functional Epithalamus

The epithalamus is a small area within the diencephalon with diverse functions, including sleep/wake cycling, limbic system function, arousal, pain and pleasure responses, and some reproductive behaviors. Tumors in the area produce classic clinical findings due to proximity to key vision centers and the third ventricle.

Sleep/wake cycles and circadian rhythm

The epithalamus plays a key role in the sleep/wake cycle through regulation of the hormone melatonin by the pineal gland. Melatonin assists with sleep efficiency and orients each cell of the body to both time of day and season. Axons from retinal ganglion cells carry data related to amplitude and wavelengths of light (rather than images) to the pineal gland via the retinohypothalamic tract. Inputs travel along each optic nerve to the suprachiasmatic nucleus (SCN) of the ipsilateral hypothalamus, lying just above the optic chiasm. The SCN contains the central clock that regulates our 24-hour circadian rhythm. This light stimulus assists with calibrating the SCN daily and directs the pineal gland through a series of sympathetic inhibitory neurons along the retinohypothalamic pathway to reduce melatonin secretion, increasing wakefulness and arousal. Low melatonin levels are seen in sleep disorders associated with aging, disease, and neurodegenerative disorders, such as Alzheimer's. Melatonin is also an antioxidant and may have neuroprotective function as well.

Habenula function

The habenula is an associated limbic structure responsive to the neurotransmitter adenosine triphosphate (ATP), a mediator of the emotional rapid response to pain released at noradrenergic postganglionic sympathetic neurons. ATP inhibitors are being studied for their use in chronic pain management.

Tumors of epithalamus

Tumors in this small area are rare and can be localized by clinical findings with several examples described below. The epithalamus forms the roof of the third ventricle, and a tumor here may interfere with CSF flow by blocking the choroid plexus or cerebral aqueduct, producing hydrocephalus, a serious medical condition that, if left untreated, will be fatal due to tissue compression.

Parinaud's (dorsal midbrain) syndrome occurs when a pineal tumor impacts the vertical gaze centers, located in the most dorsal part of the rostral midbrain reticular formation that mediates conjugate upgaze directed by the third and fourth cranial nerves. The tumor's dorsal, supranuclear location impacts volitional

conjugate upgaze, but it spares reflexive doll's eye upward eye deflection (Chapter 6). Damage from the pineal tumor also partially spares infranuclear (pupillary) reflexes. Concomitant damage to the posterior commissure in the midbrain tectum impairs consensual pupillary reflexes to changing light intensity; however, it spares accommodation reflexes—pupillary diameter and lens shape changes related to changing focal distance. Clinically, in addition to upgaze paralysis, the patient will have retracted eyelids and a pseudo–Argyll Robertson pupil (partially dilated pupils, about 6 mm, that react poorly to light and better to accommodation: nearlight dissociation).

Pineal gland influence on sexual development is inferred from observations of prepubescent children with pineal tumors. The tumors appear to impair normal sexual development, which depends on low levels of melatonin to properly time onset of puberty. Pineal gland lesions that increase secretion of melatonin retard onset of puberty; those that destroy the pineal gland and abolish melatonin release stimulate precocious puberty in both boys and girls.

Functional Subthalamus

The subthalamus is located ventral to the thalamus, lateral to the hypothalamus. This structure functions as a component of the basal nuclei (Chapter 7), with a role in sustaining rhythmic movements. By driving (exciting) tonic activity in GPi/SNpr basal nuclei output neurons, the subthalamus sustains the resting inhibitory output modulating VA/VL motor thalamus activation of frontal motor cortex. Loss of this inhibition is problematic when rhythmic motions become uncontrollable such as in essential tremor or advanced Parkinson's disease.

Bilateral stimulation of the subthalamic nuclei is the most common and effective current treatment for advanced Parkinson's disease. Deep brain stimulation (DBS) alleviates profound motor symptoms seen in PD no longer responding to dopamine and dopamine agonists. Surgeons implant a thin wire electrode through a hole in the cranium, placing the tip at the subthalamic nucleus. The electrode is connected, through insulated wire implanted in a subcutaneous tunnel under the scalp, neck, and shoulder, to a neurostimulator placed in the chest wall. The neurostimulator functions like a battery pack and can be easily turned on or off with a remote device placed over the neurostimulator. This DBS system reduces tremor by stimulating neural activity in the subthalamic nucleus, thereby restoring the resting inhibitory output for more normal motion.

IV CENTRAL EVENTS DURING NOCICEPTION

Nociception involves the transduction of damaging, or potentially damaging, stimuli to the CNS. The stimulus itself is not "painful"; rather, it is simply a form of energy applied to the sensory ending. It does not produce a sensation of pain until it has ascended to the cortex. Behavioral responses elicited by nociception and subsequent pain perception can be useful, providing a warning to prevent further harm, such as preventing a second instance of touching a hot surface or protecting an injured body part. Conversely, because pain also activates cognitive central circuitry, we can suppress behavioral responses to pain when necessary for survival, typically under extreme duress, such as when a lost camper hikes miles on a fractured ankle, without pain, until rescued.

Ascending Nociceptive Pathway

This complex pathway incorporates peripheral sensors and an early reflexive feedback loop at the local spinal cord level (Chapter 5), along with central processing. High-threshold mechanical nociceptors (HTMs) are free nerve endings covered only with a thin basal lamina produced by the investing Schwann cells. HTMs are supplied by small-diameter, thinly myelinated Aδ or unmyelinated C-fiber axons and respond to damaging or potentially damaging mechanical distortion of tissues. Subsets of nociceptors are also responsive to damaging heat or cold, or to the chemicals released from traumatized tissue.

In 1965, Melzak and Wall published a seminal paper describing gating (permitting or inhibiting) transmission of nociceptive inputs in the spinal cord. This was called the gate control theory, offering a clear and eloquent explanation that influenced all subsequent pain research for decades. Modern methodology has identified specific HTMs, of which little was known at the time of the original publication, as well as pre- and postsynaptic axo–axonal synapses in the substantia gelatinosa (second-order targets of primary afferent nociceptors) that influence throughput of noxious information.

Nociceptive responses occur in two phases: primary and secondary hyperalgesia (Figure 9.9). Primary hyperalgesia is activated by damage of the Aδ free nerve endings in the area of acute trauma, which evokes sharp, pricking pain. Primary hyperalgesia is carried mainly on the spinothalamic pathway, conducted to specific thalamic nuclei, then to the cerebral cortex for conscious interpretation of type and intensity of the damaging stimulus. Due to the high degree of somatotopic specificity in the VPL and VPM thalamic nuclei, as well as in the primary somatosensory cortex, primary hyperalgesia is well localized; that is, the person can precisely identify where the injury is. Spinothalamic input to the dorsomedial thalamic nucleus projects more diffusely to the cortex. Combined with the spatial separation of different ascending nociceptive pathways (Chapter 5), this organization might, in part, account for the difficulty managing chronic pain.

C-fiber nociceptors are also damaged with the injury. This activates an antidromic impulse that is carried back down the axon to the injury site. At the site, C-fiber endings release neuroactive peptides, such as substance P and calcitonin gene–related peptide (CGRP) into the tissue. Substance P causes degranulation of mast cells and releases histamine into the area, and CGRP is a potent vasodilator, making the walls of the local capillaries "leaky." Tissue extravasation, causing edema and hematoma, and hyperalgesia are hallmarks of the axon response and neurogenic inflammation, which produces the dull, burning pain of secondary hyperalgesia. Traumatized tissue releases additional chemicals such as ATP, bradykinin, H+, and serotonin. These chemicals produce a widespread subthreshold depolarization of the local nociceptive endings in the periphery. In the spinal cord, central C fibers synapse on 2-degree neurons in the substantia gelatinosa in the dorsal horn and are activated by intensely damaging or repetitive 1-degree afferent nociceptive input, reducing threshold and prolonging responses. This phenomenon, called windup, increases spontaneous firing and elevates neuronal responses resulting in hyperalgesia and allodynia. Elevated sensitivity and response to noxious input at the spinal level can affect the conversion of neuropathic pain (from tissue damage) into persistent neurogenic pain (from central sensitization).

Descending Pain Modulation

Ascending nociceptive pathways not only directly innervate the thalamus via the spinothalamic pathway, they also project to other brainstem and diencephalon structures. Brainstem reticular formation receives nociceptive input via spinoreticular fibers; the periaqueductal gray, via spinomedullary fibers; and the hypothalamus, from the spinohypothalamic pathway. The insula, amygdala, primary motor, and somatosensory, posterior parietal, and prefrontal cortexes are also activated by thalamocortical and hypothalamocortical circuits. Cortical structures are covered in more detail in Chapter 10.

Information processing in the hypothalamus, with its extensive cortical and thalamic interactions, initiates a descending pain

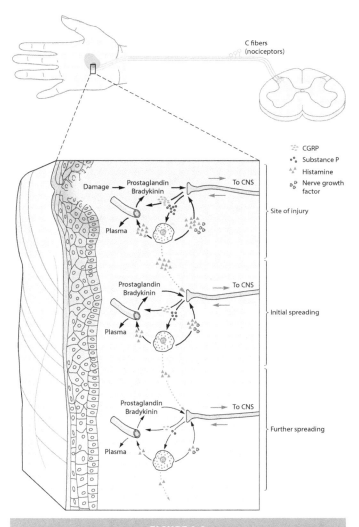

FIGURE 9.9

Neurogenic inflammation. Tissue injury causes the release of bradykinin and the activation of cyclooxygenases, which in turn leads to the generation of prostaglandins and other mediators, such as K+ and H+. Bradykinins and prostaglandins activate and sensitize neurons. Substance P and CGRP, released in retrograde fashion from free nerve endings, dilate local blood vessels. Substance P has also been shown to cause fluid and protein to extravasate from vessels and to trigger the release of histamine from mast cells. (Reproduced with permission from Pain. In: Kandel ER, et al, eds. Principles of Neural Science, Fifth Editon New York, NY: McGraw-Hill; 2012).

modulation circuit (Figure 9.10). The pathway descends to the periaqueductal gray, where it activates endorphinergic cells, which project axons caudally to synapse in the brainstem reticular formation. Populations of cells in the raphe nucleus express serotonin, and cells in the pontine reticular formation express norepinephrine. Both of these sites emit fiber systems that descend to innervate local circuit neurons in the dorsal horn. Inhibitory enkephalinergic dorsal horn cells presynaptically inhibit transmission from primary nociceptors, and postsynaptically inhibit second-order spinal cord nociceptive cell output, effectively closing the gate on nociceptive throughput and preventing pain perception.

With its connectivity with the thalamus and hypothalamus, nociceptive information is also processed in the limbic system. Reciprocal circuits back to the posterior hypothalamic nucleus activate descending brainstem and spinal pathways that elicit sympathetic responses and general arousal. Significant pain can promote the formation of lasting memories through limbic connections to the amygdala, seen in conditioned responses including post-traumatic stress disorder (PTSD).

V   RESPONSE TO INJURY

Central post-stroke pain (CPSP), formerly known as thalamic pain syndrome or Dejerine–Roussy syndrome, typically results from stroke in the VPL/VPM thalamic nuclei. Pathological sensory experiences occur contralateral to the lesion in the areas represented within the damaged area. Commonly, patients report loss of sensation or tingling in the affected areas. Abnormal sensation progresses to the perception of pain that is out of proportion to the stimulus, described as burning, lacerating, squeezing, scalding, or freezing, often triggered by clothing or other normally innocuous touch stimuli. Allodynia, dysesthesia, and hyperalgesia can significantly impair activities of daily living and the overall quality of life in these patients. Therapies for sufferers of chronic thalamic pain include drugs with central effects or local analgesics, surgical ablation of affected thalamic areas, or deep brain stimulation of somatosensory thalamus and periventricular gray region. Because it can produce psychological effects, many patients are referred to management programs to control chronic

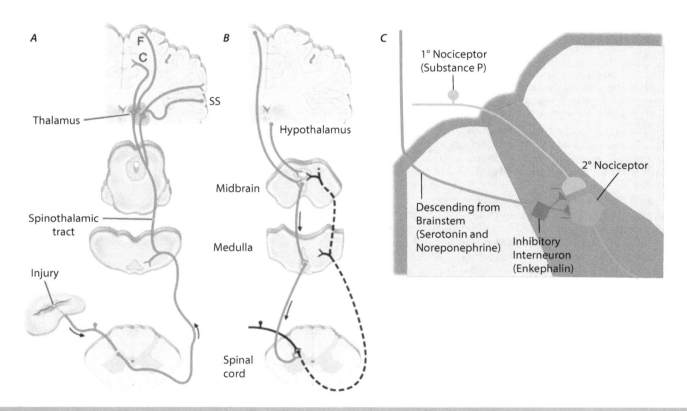

FIGURE 9.10

Pain transmission and modulatory pathways. A. Transmission system for nociceptive messages. Noxious stimuli activate the sensitive peripheral ending of the primary afferent nociceptor by the process of transduction. The message is then transmitted over the peripheral nerve to the spinal cord, where it synapses with cells of origin of the major ascending pain pathway, the spinothalamic tract. The message is relayed in the thalamus to the anterior cingulate (C), frontal insular (F), and somatosensory cortex (SS). **B.** Pain-modulation network. Inputs from frontal cortex and hypothalamus activate cells in the midbrain that control spinal pain-transmission cells via cells in the medulla. **C.** Enlarged dorsal horn. Primary nociceptive afferent axons synapse on second order ells in the substantia gelatinosa in the dorsal horn. Descending axons from the brainstem reticular formation using excitatory serotonin and norepinephrine as neurotransmitters synapse on enkephalinergic interneurons. Enkephalin pre- and post-synaptically inhibits throughput of nociceptive information (**A, B,** Reproduced with permission from Rathmell JP, Fields HL. Pain: Pathophysiology and Management. In: Kasper D, et al, eds. Harrison's Principles of Internal Medicine, 19e New York, NY: McGraw-Hill; 2016; **C,** Image provided by Tony Mosconi, 2017).

> Neuroplasticity
EMDR—Treatment for
Post-Trauma
> Neuroplasticity
EMDR—Treatment for
Post-Trauma
Thalamic function is essential for integrating perception, somatosensation, memory, and cognition when processing experiences. Unfortunately, in some people thalamic function decreases after trauma, a hallmark of post-traumatic stress disorder (PTSD), which produces nervous system malfunction.

Sensory memories become fragmented; including olfactory, taste, visual, and body sensations. Additionally, people experience cognitive distortions of episodic memory, excessive self-blame and shame as well as states of hyperemotion. This prevents integration of a complete memory of the event into consciousness, and instead, thoughts of the trauma produce a series of disjointed sensory

experiences accompanied by negative emotions.

Use of eye movement desensitization and reprocessing (EMDR) is proposed to facilitate repair of this disrupted function by increasing activation of the lateral thalamic nuclei. EMDR is a therapeutic technique developed in 1987 to treat anxiety and PTSD. It uses bilateral stimulation to induce visual smooth pursuit motions as part of a process to

reduce symptoms of anxiety. These left–right eye motions are similar to rapid eye movements that occur when dreaming, hypothesized to incorporate recent events and integrate them into semantic memory. Reprocessing is most effective when the client is distracted by this process of bilateral stimulation so that rather than react in fear, he can choose a different emotional response under the guidance of a therapist.

---

pain. Unfortunately, CPSP is refractory to most treatments, and the prognosis for recovery is poor.

Hypothalamic disease can have a wide variety of detrimental effects. Dysfunction produces diabetes insipidus (impaired water metabolism), causing polydipsia and polyuria, as well as hyper or hypophagia, poikilothermia, gastrointestinal disorders, and labile blood pressure. Additional cognitive effects include depression, drowsiness and fatigue, and irritability. Tumors and stroke can interrupt pituitary gland function, resulting in a reduction of hormonal secretion. Effects can also include reduced or retarded growth, reduction in libido or sexual dysfunction, fatigue, and hypothyroidism. These deficits are typically treated with hormone replacement therapy.

Hypothalamic injury caused by malnutrition, specifically a lack of thiamine (B1), often from chronic alcoholism, causes a disorder called Korsakoff's syndrome. Loss of cells in the mammillary bodies impairs recent memory, learning, and in some patients compels the patient to "confabulate," or to make up events to account for missing time. Confabulation is not lying, and patients actually believe their accounts. Heavy doses of vitamin B1 and better nutrition frequently resolves or reduces the symptoms in early stages of the disease. Patients with chronic alcohol abuse and severe symptoms have a poor prognosis, with comorbid sensory and motor problems.

Deep Brain Simulation (DBS)

Research regarding optimal electrode placement and stimulation parameters is providing hope to millions of people globally, as the procedure is becoming more common. During early stages, many people avoid medication and are unwilling to consider treatments that carry risk of side effects. However, as motor symptoms increase in middle stages, many become willing to consider alternative and higher-risk procedures, particularly when involved in honest and open dialogue with health care providers regarding treatment options. DBS is a complex medical procedure that carries risks, including surgical complications, and also produces unintended cognitive, psychiatric, autonomic, and language effects in certain patients. International clinical research to optimize this effective, if flawed, intervention is also expanding scientific understanding of subthalamic nuclei function, particularly their role in non-motor function. For example, sudomotor dysfunction, most often hyperhidrosis, is extremely common and can be alleviated by subthalamic DBS. Chronic stimulation of the bilateral subthalamic nuclei is producing cognitive changes in some

Frontiers in Research
Deep Brain Stimulation and
Parkinson's Disease
Parkinson's disease is a progressive neurological condition that produces well-known motor and poorly understood non-motor changes that progress over time through early, middle, and late stages, ending in death due to complications from immobility, difficulty swallowing, or respiratory dysfunction. Non-motor changes in neuropsychiatric behavior changes and cognition, sensory disorders, sleep disturbance, and autonomic nervous system failure begin prior to motor disturbances of resting tremor, rigidity, bradykinesia, and postural instability.

Drug therapy during early stages combines levodopa (L-dopa), a precursor to dopamine that can cross the blood–brain barrier, with dopamine agonists to reduce disease-based movement problems. However, over time these effects decline,

and negative side effects, including dyskinesias and psychosis, are common after chronic use. During middle phases of the disease, motor impairments become quite severe, limiting ability to walk, speak, and function independently. Surgical interventions such as pallidotomy and deep brain stimulation, although risky, are more effective than medications to manage increasing motor symptoms of rigidity, tremor, and bradykinesia. In pallidotomy, the neurosurgeon inserts a probe into the globus pallidus, creating a scar and thus inactivating that region, a procedure rarely done since the advent of deep brain stimulation. Placement of stimulators (DBS) in either the subthalamic nuclei or the globus pallidus internus, starting in the 1990s, showed promising early results, with tremendous reduction in motor symptoms exceeding levodopa response.

people, with the exact mechanisms hypothesized to be due to overstimulation of limbic and association area pathways hypothesized to be involved in cognition. In several small studies, changes in the basal ganglia-thalamus-dorsal prefrontal cortex circuitry are noted in patients receiving chronic DBS. Additionally, subtle changes in language include reduction in verbal fluency.

> CASE 9 DISCUSSION: Alzeheimer's Disease

Norma's condition worsened the year leading up to Georg's death, due to stress and increasing inactivity as her loving husband and sole caregiver became ill. Georg soon passed away, and his death impacted Norma's cognitive function significantly. Although she did not recognize her own daughter, she was not rescued from her grief. Every morning she woke crying, remembering her husband was gone.

Her daughter and son-in-law decided to care for her at that time and moved her to their home in California. Their first order of business was to get Norma evaluated and on the right track. She had regressed to a very passive and dependent role during Georg's long illness, and she had been falling recently and had lost weight, becoming frail and shaky when walking. At age 95, she was in fairly good health otherwise. They found a general medicine physician who specialized in geriatrics with a holistic approach. Each visit he spoke directly to Norma regarding her concerns and took his time to answer all their questions, which put the whole family at ease.

They soon had an interprofessional care team including a neurologist, social worker, home health physical therapist, and nurse. Norma's physician was open to discussing new treatments or supplements supported by the growing research in the field of Alzheimer's disease and neuroplasticity. The neurologist prescribed donepezil HCl, an acetylcholinesterase inhibitor, to augment the function of the remaining cholinergic cells within her brain. Nursing recommendations from the home visit included removing tripping hazards and ensuring the environment was safe, with items such as grab bars in the bathroom. The physical therapist developed a strengthening and balance program and, as Norma became stronger, taught the family a maintenance program that allowed Norma to resume daily walks in the neighborhood. Resources provided by the social worker included referral to a Council on Aging program at the local senior center, which offered socialization, light exercise, brain-stimulating games, and midday meals.

Her son-in-law (a former special education teacher) worked on her long-term and short-term memory with flash cards, puzzles, playing cards, personal and household items, name recognition, and conversation. They replaced Norma's salty, processed diet with organic fruits and vegetables, and her appetite improved—she put on about 5 pounds over the next four years. She did enjoy the addition of regular daily hugs and light massage, which helped her body and spirit.

Norma's passions included music and faith. They had her piano shipped from Seattle, and slowly she started to play again. At first she was hesitant, and then as her functioning improved, she played more. Once she became stronger, she never missed Sunday services and also became a regular at Wednesday morning meetings. She was the oldest member and was treated very specially as a result.

Norma's cognitive impairments remained mild for almost 10 years. Most people meeting her for the first time could not tell, as she developed social skills to hide her deficits, through avoidance, automatic phrases, joking, or flirting. She believed she was a useful member of society and often spoke of going back to work and using her master's degree in music.

REFERENCES

Acosta-Cabronero J, Williams GB, Pengas G, Nestor P. Absolute diffusivities define the landscape of white matter degeneration in Alzheimer's disease. *Brain.* 2010;133:529–539.

Arendt T, Brückner MK, Morawski M, Jäger C, Gertz H-J. Early neurone loss in Alzheimer's disease: cortical or subcortical? *Acta Neuropathologica Communications.* 2015;3:10.

Balaban CD. Neural substrates linking balance control and anxiety. *Physiol Behav.* 2002;77:469–475.

Balabana CD, Thayer JF. Neurological bases for balance-anxiety links. *Anxiety Disorders.* 2001;15:53–79.

Balami JS, Chen RL, Buchan AM. Stroke syndromes and clinical management. *Q J Med.* 2013;106:607–615.

Baloyannis SJ, Mavroudis I, Mitilineos D, Baloyannis IS, Costa VG. The hypothalamus in Alzheimer's disease: a Golgi and electron microscope study. *Am J Alzheimer's Dis Other Demen.* 2015 Aug;30(5): 478–487.

Bao A, Swaab DF. Sexual differentiation of the human brain: relation to gender identity, sexual orientation and neuropsychiatric disorders. *Front Neuroendocrinol.* 2011;32:214–226.

Basiago A, Binder DK. Effects of deep brain stimulation on autonomic function. *Brain Sci.* 2016;6(33):1–9.

Benarroch EE. Suprachiasmatic nucleus and melatonin: reciprocal interactions and clinical correlations. *Neurology.* 2008, Aug 19;71(8): 594–598.

Ben-Jonathan N, Hnasko R. Dopamine as a prolactin (PRL) inhibitor. *Endocrine Reviews.* 2001 Dec;22(6):724–763.

Bergmann U. The neurobiology of EMDR: exploring the thalamus and neural integration. *Journal of EMDR Practice and Research.* 2008;2(4):300–314.

Berridge KC, Kringelbach ML. Pleasure systems in the brain. *Neuron.* 2015, May 6;86(3):646–664.

Bole-Feysot C, Goffin V, Edery M, Binart N, Kelly PA. Prolactin (PRL) and its receptor: actions, signal transduction pathways and phenotypes observed in PRL receptor knockout mice. *Endocrine Reviews.* 1998;19(3):225–268.

Bourgeais L, Monconduit L, Villanueva L, Bernard JF. Parabrachial internal lateral neurons convey nociceptive messages from the deep laminas of the dorsal horn to the intralaminar thalamus. *J of Neuroscience.* 2001 March;21(6):2159–2165.

Braak H, Braak E. Alzheimer's disease affects limbic nuclei of the thalamus. *Acta Neuropathologica.* 1991 Feb;81(3):261–268.

Caldwell HK, Young WS. *Oxytocin and vasopressin: genetics and behavioral implications.* Berlin, Heidelberg: Springer-Verlag; 2006.

Coubard O. An integrative model for the neural mechanism of eye movement desensitization and reprocessing (EMDR). *Frontiers in Behavioral Neuroscience.* 2016 Apr;10(52):1–17.

Cozac V, Ehrensperger MM, Gschwandtner U, et al. Older candidates for subthalamic deep brain stimulation in Parkinson's disease have a higher incidence of psychiatric serious adverse events. *Frontiers in Aging Neuroscience.* 2016 June;8(132):1–5.

Dal Bello Haas V. A framework of rehabilitation for neurodegenerative diseases: following care and maximizing quality of life. *Neurology Report.* 2002;26(3):115–129.

Daou I, Beaudry H, Ase AR, et al. Optogenetic silencing of Nav1.8-positive afferents alleviates inflammatory and neuropathic pain. *eNeuro.* 2016 Jan/Feb;3(1):1–12.

Elias CF, Aschkenasi C, Lee C, et al. Leptin differentially regulates NPY and POMC neurons projecting to the lateral hypothalamic area. *Neuron.* 1999 Aug;23:775–786.

Guo C, Sun L, Chen X, Zhang D. Oxidative stress, mitochondrial damage and neurodegenerative diseases. *Neural Regeneration Research.* 2013;8(21):2003–2014.

Hagenston A, Simonetti M. Neuronal calcium signaling in chronic pain. *Cell and Tissue Research.* 2014;357(2):407–426.

Han S, Soleiman MT, Soden ME, Zweifel LS, Palmiter RD. Elucidating an affective pain circuit that creates a threat memory. *Cell.* 2015 July;162:363–374.

Henry JL, Lalloo C, Yashpal K. Central poststroke pain: an abstruse outcome. *Pain Res Manage.* 2008;13(1):41–49.

Herrero JF, Laird JMA, Lopez-Garcia JA. Wind-up of spinal cord neurones and pain sensation: much ado about something? *Prog Neurobiol.* 2000;61:169–203.

Jacob S, Brune CW, Carter CS, Leventhal BL, Lord C, Cook EH. Association of the oxytocin receptor gene (OXTR) in Caucasian children and adolescents with autism. *Neurosci Lett.* 2007, April 24;417(1):6–9.

Jankowski MM, Ronnqvist KC, Tsanov M, et al. Anterior thalamus in memory and navigation. *Frontiers in Systems Neuroscience.* 2013 Aug;7(45):1–12.

de Jong LW, van der Hiele K, Veer IM, et al. Strongly reduced volumes of putamen and thalamus in Alzheimer's disease: an MRI study. *Brain.* 2008;131:3277–3285.

Kleiner-Fisman G, Herzog J, Fisman DN, et al. Subthalamic nucleus deep brain stimulation: summary and meta-analysis of outcomes. *Move Disord.* 2006;21(S14):S290–S304.

Kurrasch D, Cheung C, Lee FY, Tran PV, Hata K, Ingraham HA. The neonatal ventromedial hypothalamus transcriptome reveals novel markers with spatially distinct patterning. *J Neurosci.* 2007 Dec;27(50):13624–13634.

Lanuza E, Nader K, Ledoux J. Unconditioned stimulus pathways to the amygdala: Effects of posterior thalamic and cortical lesions on fear conditioning. *Neuroscience.* 2004;125(2):305–315.

Laxton AW, Tang-Wai DF, McAndrews MP, et al. A phase I trial of deep brain stimulation of memory circuits in Alzheimer's disease. *Ann Neurol.* 2010;68:521–534.

Lazarus L, Ling N, Guillemin R. B-Lipotropin as a prohormone for the morphinomimetic peptides endorphins and enkephalins. *Proc Natl Acad Sci USA.* 1976 June;73(6):2156–2159.

Le Tissier PR, Hodson DJ, Lafont C, Fontanaud P, Schaeffer M, Mollard P. Anterior pituitary cell networks. *Front Neuroendocrinol.* 2012;33:252–266.

Levay S. A difference in hypothalamic structure between heterosexual and homosexual men. *Science.* 1991 Aug;253:1034–1036.

Li J, Hu Z, de Lecea L. The hypocretins/orexins: integrators of multiple physiological functions. *British J of Pharmacology.* 2014;171: 332–350.

Lking Jayes FC, Britt JH, Esbenshade KL. Role of gonadotropin-releasing hormone pulse frequency in differential regulation of gonadotropins in the gilt. *Biol Reprod.* 1997;56:1012–1019.

Lucas BK, Ormandy CJ, Binart N, Bridges RS, Kelly PA. Null mutation of the prolactin receptor gene produces a defect in maternal behavior. *Endocrinology.* 1998;139(10):4102–4107.

Maclean PD. Contrasting functions of limbic and neocortical systems of the brain and their relevance to psychophysiological aspects of medicine. *Am J Med.* 1958;25(4):611–626.

Mendell LM. Constructing and deconstructing the gate theory of pain. *Pain.* 2014 Feb;155(2):210–216.

Mestre TA, Lang AE, Okun MS. Factors influencing the outcome of deep brain stimulation: placebo, nocebo, lessebo, and lesion effects. *Mov Disord.* 2016 Mar;31(3):290–296.

Mullur R, Liu Y, Brent GA. Thyroid hormone regulation of metabolism. *Physiol Rev.* 2014;94:355–382.

Nielsen MS, Barton SD, Hatasaka HH, Stanford JB. Comparison of several one-step home urinary luteinizing hormone detection test kits to OvuQuick. *Fertil Steril.* 2001 Aug;76(2):384–387.

Nielsen S, Chou C, Marples D, Christensen EI, Kishore B, Knepper MA. Vasopressin increases water permeability of kidney collecting duct by inducing translocation of aquaporin-CD water channels to plasma membrane. *Proc Natl Acad. Sci USA.* 1995;92:1013–1017.

Nishio Y, Hashimoto M, Ishii K, Mori E. Neuroanatomy of a neurobehavioral disturbance in the left anterior thalamic infarction. *J Neurol Neurosurg Psychiatry.* 2011;82:1195–1200.

Rogers SL, Friedhoff LT. Pharmacokinetic and pharmacodynamic profile of donepezil HCl following single oral doses. *Br J Clin Psychol.* 1998;46(Suppl 1):1–6.

Schallmo MP, Kassel MT, Weisenbach SL, et al. A new semantic list learning task to probe functioning of the Papez circuit. *J Clin Exp Neuropsychol.* 2015;37(8):816–833.

Shah A, Jhawar SS, Goel A. Analysis of the anatomy of the Papez circuit and adjoining limbic system by fiber dissection techniques. *J Clin Neurosci.* 2012 Feb;19(2):289–298.

Standaert DG, Lee VMY, Greenberg BD, Lowery DE, Trojanowskit JQ. Molecular features of hypothalamic plaques in Alzheimer's disease. *Am J of Pathology.* 1991 Sep;139(3):681–691.

Sterrenburg MD, Veltman-Verhulst SM, Eijkemans MJC, et al. Clinical outcomes in relation to the daily dose of recombinant follicle stimulating hormone for ovarian stimulation in in vitro fertilization in presumed normal responders younger than 39 years: a meta-analysis. *Hum Reprod Update.* 2011;17(2):184–196.

Sutherland RJ, Whishaw IQ, Kolb BJ. Contributions of cingulate cortex to two forms of spatial learning and memory of neuroscience. *J Neuroscience.* June 1988;8(8):1863–1872.

Swaab DF, Chung WCJ, Kruijver FPM, Hofman MA, Ishunina TA. Structural and functional sex differences in the human hypothalamus. *Horm Behav.* 2001;40:93–98.

Takakusaki K. Neurophysiology of gait: from the spinal cord to the frontal lobe. *Mov Disord.* 2013;28(11):1483–1491.

Vann SD. Re-evaluating the role of the mammillary bodies in memory. *Neuropsychologia.* 2010;48:2316–2327.

Vargha-Khadem F. Differential effects of early hippocampal pathology on episodic and semantic memory. *Science.* 1997;277:376–379.

Veinante P, Yalcin I, Barrot M. The amygdala between sensation and affect: a role in pain. *Journal of Molecular Psychiatry.* 2013;1:9.

Walitt B, Čeko M, Gracely JL, Gracely RH. Neuroimaging of central sensitivity syndromes: key insights from the scientific literature. *Current Rheumatology Reviews.* 2016;12(1):55–87.

Weernink MGM, van Til JA, van Vugt JPP, Movig KLL, Groothuis-Oudshoorn CGM, IJzerman MJ. Involving patients in weighting benefits and harms of treatment in Parkinson's disease. *PLoS ONE.* 2016;11(8):e0160771.

Wijesinghe R, Protti DA, Camp AJ. Vestibular interactions in the thalamus. *Frontiers in Neural Circuits.* 2015 Dec;9(79):1–8.

Xie Y, Meng X, Xiao J, Zhang J, Zhang J. Cognitive changes following bilateral deep brain stimulation of subthalamic nucleus in Parkinson's disease: a meta-analysis. *Biomed Res Int.* 2016; Article ID 3596415.

Xu F, Ma W, Huang Y, Qiu Z, Sun L. Deep brain stimulation of pallidal versus subthalamic for patients with Parkinson's disease: a meta-analysis of controlled clinical trials. *Neuropsychiatric Disease and Treatment.* 2016;12:1435–1444.

> **REVIEW QUESTIONS**

1. The thalamic sensory relay neurons include the:
   A. thalamic reticular nuclei.
   B. association nuclear group.
   C. pulvinar.
   D. lateral geniculate nucleus.

2. Somatic sensory information from the contralateral body innervates third-order cells in the:
   A. ventroposterolateral nucleus (VPL) of the thalamus.
   B. ventroposteromedial nucleus (VPM) of the thalamus.
   C. medial geniculate nucleus of the thalamus.
   D. dorsomedial nucleus (DM) of the thalamus.

3. Within the Papez circuit, a lesion of the anterior nuclear group will most likely produce loss of the following:
   A. Ability to control eye motions
   B. Emotion and factual memories
   C. Episodic memory and spatial orientation
   D. Motor control of gait and balance

4. Thalamic dorsomedial nucleus projections bypass the primary somatosensory cortex, with the following consequence:
   A. Pain processing is more precise and detailed than for VPL and VPM.
   B. Pain processing is less precise and detailed than for VPL and VPM.
   C. Pain processing incorporates the reticular formation for nonspecific arousal.
   D. Pain processing is centralized within the temporal association area.

5. These structures regulate water metabolism through secretion of vasopressin.
   A. Paraventricular and supraoptic hypothalamic nuclei
   B. Solitary and parabrachial nuclei
   C. Ventral anterior and ventral lateral nuclei
   D. Reticular and intralaminar nuclei

6. Release of this by the arcuate nucleus stimulates mitosis and is important in adults for tissue maintenance and metabolism.
   A. Somatostatin
   B. Growth hormone–releasing hormone
   C. Oxytocin
   D. Prolactin

7. Every student should know about melatonin secretion, key in our sleep/wake cycle. It is regulated by the pineal gland via this pathway.
   A. The dorsal longitudinal fasciculus to the Edinger-Westphal nucleus
   B. The periaqueductal gray matter pathway to the pineal gland
   C. The retinohypothalamic pathway to the suprachasmatic nucleus
   D. The Papez circuit to the cingulate gyrus

8. Some antihistamine medications used to treat allergic reactions can cause drowsiness. This is because these medications:
   A. shift the biological clock in the suprachiasmatic nucleus to later in the day.
   B. act directly on hypothalamic centers to trigger sleep.
   C. block the central action of histamine, which activates forebrain neurons.
   D. block the actions of the retinal projection to the hypothalamus.

9. Neuropathic pain may convert into persistent neurogenic pain through this process.
   A. Central C fibers are activated by repetitive primary afferent nociceptive input in the dorsal horn.
   B. Thalamic nuclei become desensitized to suppressing touch input.
   C. Primary hyperalgesia triggers release of substance P at the injury site, which produces allodynia.
   D. Secondary hyperalgesia is inhibited by bradykinin release.

10. Central post-stroke pain is typically caused by damage to the following:
    A. VA and VL thalamic nuclei
    B. Hypothalamus and reticular nuclei
    C. The Papez circuit
    D. VPL/VPM thalamic nuclei

CHAPTER 10

Cerebral Cortex

Tony Mosconi, Victoria Graham, and Maryke Neiberg

> **CASE 10** Hemorrhagic Stroke

Dr. T. stood in the den, pointing with his cane to the tin soldier collection. Walking was slow since the hemorrhagic stroke, due to the residual weakness in his trunk and right side. His voice soft and his right hand stiff and shaky from nearly two hours of speaking, he carefully pointed out the impressive collection of tiny figurines, displayed in cases of his own design and construction.

The doctor and his wife of 54 years were just getting ready for bed that night, nearly two years ago, when he collapsed, unresponsive. Paramedics took them to UCLA Medical Center, where Dr. T. remained active as a director, researcher, and educator. During the first few hours, as his wife and their children waited, he underwent first a CT to rule out trauma or a tumor, and then an MRI to establish the amount of tissue damage. The team consulted and decided an emergency craniotomy was indicated, to reduce cerebral damage from the edema. In the days that followed, he began to move his left side, and he was able to take his wife's hand, but his right arm and leg remained weak, and his speech was limited. He could speak haltingly, using only a couple words at a time for most communication except for one topic.

When his health care team came to discuss his plan of care, he resorted to old, deeply ingrained communication skills honed over decades as a

physician and fellow team member. He remained fluent in medical jargon and was able to discuss and participate in medical decisions. Over the years, he had treated thousands of patients, and nearly 150 new patients each month, in his role overseeing coronary care. This exposure proved valuable during his post-stroke recovery. "Phlegmasia cerulea dolens," he stated, slowly for emphasis. He had recalled the words and was able to say them clearly and distinctly to his physicians. It was a rare and potentially fatal condition he had seen in patients who reported horrific pain. "My cardiologist immediately took action and started treatment," he recalls. "I recognized the symptoms in myself, particularly the pain, worse than any I'd ever experienced, worse than any fractures, or even passing a kidney stone."

Phlegmasia cerulean dolens is a rare type of vein thrombosis involving deep veins and their tributaries. Severe, acute cyanosis and swelling is due to the nearly complete blockage of the venous system, creating the blue color and pain that give the condition its name. It is potentially fatal, with a high risk of pulmonary embolism and, when capillaries are blocked, even gangrene. Treatment of the condition consists of anticoagulation and surgical thrombectomy. Dr. T. responded to the treatment and was fortunate to have no gangrene or permanent damage to his legs

from the condition. He made steady progress after the medical team treated his thrombosis, and moved to the inpatient rehabilitation unit for ongoing care. This type of coordinated care is effective, with improved outcomes such as discharge home to independence and self-care. After a few weeks, Dr. T. transferred home for outpatient therapy and to figure out the next step in his life with his wife, Sandy.

"Have you seen the German film *Wings of the Dove*?" he asked. "It was a film about angels who come down to earth, and one decides to stay." He nodded to his wife. "When our daughter first saw it, we both agreed: Mom!"

Growing up in Minnesota, Sandy and Dr. T. attended the same school. "I was from the wrong side of the tracks," Sandy smiled, "He was very smart and appeared to be confident—"

"Cocky," he interjected, smiling back.

In high school, he finally asked her to a Friday night dance, and she brought along a friend. In the retelling, Dr. T. could still recall the friend's first and last names. After high school, Dr. T. and Sandy attended different universities and tried living separate lives, but the pull was strong, and they married when he was in graduate school. Sandy gave birth to their first child while he was in medical school.

I ▌ OVERVIEW OF KEY CONCEPTS

So far, most of our cortical structure discussion has been confined to primary sensory and motor areas, with little discussion of higher cortical functions. Primary cerebral cortex regions comprise a relatively low proportion of the total cortical area. The simplistic modular model of cortical function implied by our brief references to cortical function falls short of the actual complexity of human cognition. Individual cortical areas are inextricably linked with others to create systems that interact to create intellect, emotion, and, ultimately, behavior. The capabilities afforded to us by the evolution of our spectacular neocortex permitted Michelangelo to sculpt the *Pieta*, aeronautical engineers to build the space shuttle, and authors to attempt to write the Great American Novel; and the brain remains the only organ capable of analyzing itself.

An enormous volume of sensory information arrives at primary sensory cortices, yet actual "perception" has yet to emerge. This is apparent in conditions such as cortical blindness, where the physiological function from the retina to primary visual cortex remains largely intact. Without further processing, however, there is no perception of an object, no context or memory or emotion possible. To affect the deeper aspects of the human experience, other regions, called association cortices, contain circuitry that interprets and assesses incoming internal and external stimuli, and generates appropriate behavioral responses. This chapter focuses on those regions of the cerebral cortex that are the sites of sensory integration and the sources of instruction to the motor systems that allow us to engage in goal-oriented behaviors. Complex cognitive processing, such as memory and learning, provides the underpinnings of rehabilitative success, and understanding the neurologic processes for motivation and cognition is essential in neurologic rehabilitation, for only the engaged, motivated patient will fully participate and improve with therapeutic interventions.

One of the most striking features of the human nervous system is the remarkably convoluted cerebral cortex, with gyri and sulci vastly increasing the overall surface area to several hundred cm². The majority of this area is neocortex, with six distinct cellular layers, each with specific sources of inputs and targets of outputs. Although a mere 2–4 mm in thickness, the cortex process an almost inconceivable volume of information that produces complex human thought and behavior.

The case study in Chapter 1 described the injury to the prefrontal cortex of Phineas Gage and his remarkable resilience to such a grave trauma. At the time, there were two schools of thought on brain function. One purported that functions were distributed over the cortex and that every portion of the brain served a single function. The other contended that the cortex acted more as a widespread neural network in which various regions cooperated to achieve its broad range of functions. Interestingly, both groups proclaimed that Gage's survival, function, and eventual decline, with cognitive impairment in evidence through progressively deteriorating appropriateness of behavior, as proof of their theory. Results of recent examination of cortical function, including modern tract tracing (e.g., diffusion tensor imaging), lesion, electrophysiological methods, and the development of powerful tools aimed at exposing cognitive malfunction, seem to suggest that both and neither of the 19th-century groups was correct, and the more likely answer lies in a collaboration of both systems.

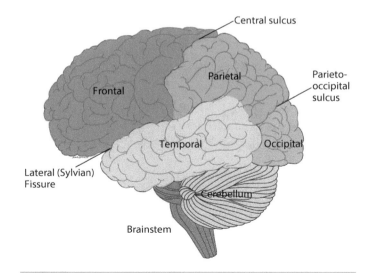

FIGURE 10.1

Lobes of the cerebrum. Frontal, parietal, temporal, and occipital lobes of the cerebrum and their boundaries. (Image provided by Jamie Graham, 2017).

The four lobes of the cerebrum are well known: frontal, parietal, temporal, and occipital (Figure 10.1). Often the limbic system is referred to as the limbic lobe. Within each of the lobes, there are areas of great specificity in connectivity and function. Early understanding of cortical function and specialization were based on examination of autopsy tissue from several patients with comparable behaviors and symptoms, with remarkable accuracy supported by recent technological advancements. Modern tract tracing analyses have revealed extensive connectivity among the lobes and support some aspects of the distributed processing hypothesis.

The practice of phrenology, using topographical anatomy of the skull to infer underlying brain anatomy and predict behavioral variations, shown to be spurious in its conclusions, provided the impetus for more regimented and analytical studies of the cerebral cortex. Among the so-called findings of phrenology, differences were noted in the brains of males and females. Phrenology contended that the female brain was smaller and less complex than that of males. These contentions were influenced by cultural and societal norms of the time. Ongoing research conclusively demonstrating significant sexual dimorphism in the human cerebrum continues to impact our cultural narrative.

II ▌ STRUCTURE OF THE CEREBRAL CORTEX

The human cerebral neocortex is the culmination of the development of our brain. It contains a large amount of nervous tissue: gray matter in a thin ribbon on the surface, and deeper white matter providing extensive communication among the functionally distinct cortical and subcortical cellular areas. Because it processes such an enormous volume and variety of information, the cerebrum is highly organized, with different areas serving specific functions. Subsequent sections in this chapter explore features of this

Table 10.1 Main Cortical Gyri and Their Primary Functions

Lobe	Gyrus	Cortical Area	Brodmann's Area	Function
Frontal	Precentral	Primary motor cortex	4	Descending control of contralateral movement
	Superior frontal	Supplementary motor cortex	6	Gross movements
	Middle frontal	Frontal eye field	8	Contralateral horizontal eye deviation
	Inferior frontal	Broca's area	44	Motor speech area
	Prefrontal	Prefrontal	10	Judgement, planning
Parietal	Postcentral	Primary somatosensory cortex	3,1,2	Somatic sensation from contralateral body and face
	Superior parietal lobule		7	Stereognosis
	Inferior parietal lobule		40	Awareness of self in space
Temporal	Superior temporal gyrus	Transverse temporal gyrus	41,42	Primary auditory cortex
	Parahippocampal gyrus	Hippopcampal formation	25	Limbic system
	Fusiform gyrus		37	Facial recognition
Occipital	Cuneate gyrus	Primary visual cortex	17	Contralateral lower visual quadrant
	Lingual gyrus			Contralateral upper visual quadrant

organization and discuss why the concept of specification of function is being modified by the development of noninvasive imaging techniques that are revealing a much more elaborate interconnectedness among the cortical areas.

Gyrification

As described in Chapter 4, the cortical surface is convoluted, forming gyri, or ridges, named for their position in the lobe, separated by deep grooves called sulci. Resultant gyrification substantially increases cortical area and volume within the rigid confines of the cranium. Many gyri, or portions of gyri, have been correlated with specific functions, particularly in relation to motor and sensory functions, for example, primary motor cortex, primary somatosensory cortex, and primary visual cortex. More complex executive and cognitive functions appear to be more widely dispersed, but still localized within regions of the cortex, with extensive interconnectivity among the regions, as shown in Figure 10.1 and Table 10.1.

Cortical Layering

The thin layer of cerebral gray matter is not a homogeneous cellular plane. Instead, it is arranged into lamina, each making specific afferent and efferent connections. In 1909, Korbinian Brodmann published an opus work describing 52 cytoarchitectonic (cellular architecture) regions in the cortex, based purely on histological differences in cell types and distribution densities in the cortical layers. Characteristic patterns of layering were found in different cortical areas, from which Brodmann inferred different functions. Subsequent analyses supported many of his original deductions. Recently, however, with the advent of modern methods such as multielectrode electrophysiology and sophisticated imaging techniques including functional MRI, some researchers are developing

more detailed and complex topographic-functional maps. This is certainly an important development in neuroscience in light of the immense increase in the volume of information on cortical circuitry and functional modularity.

Still, his map was so influential that Brodmann's areas remain widely used in teaching and research (Figure 10.2). Among the most referenced Brodmann areas are those for sensory processing, movement, and vision processing. The primary somatosensory cortex (S1) areas include 3a, 3b, 1, and 2, area 5 (somatosensory association cortex), and area 40, the secondary somatosensory (S2) cortex. The primary motor cortex (M1) was identified as area 4, and the premotor cortex as area 6. The visual cortex has a particularly striking cytoarchitecture with prominent striations. It was labeled area 17, with areas 18 and 19 forming visual association cortices. We identify several other prominent areas by Brodmann's numbering throughout the rest of this chapter.

Cell types

Among the cell types Brodmann described in the cortex are spiny and smooth stellate cells and pyramidal cells of varying size. Stellate cells are small, star-shaped neurons with multiple dendrites forming extensive local circuits. Spiny stellate cells are predominantly (not exclusively) excitatory, and smooth stellate cells are inhibitory. Stellate cells are most prevalent in the input layers of sensory cortices, and about 20% are smooth.

Pyramidal cells are the main excitatory cell type in the cerebral cortex, with broad-based cell bodies emitting several basal dendrites that distribute horizontally, an apical dendrite that ascends through the layers, and a single descending axon. Average pyramidal cell soma diameters average ~20 μm, up to ~100 μm for Betz cells, which contribute axons to the corticospinal tract. Pyramidal cells are common in output cortical layers; Betz cells feature prominently in layer V in the primary motor cortex.

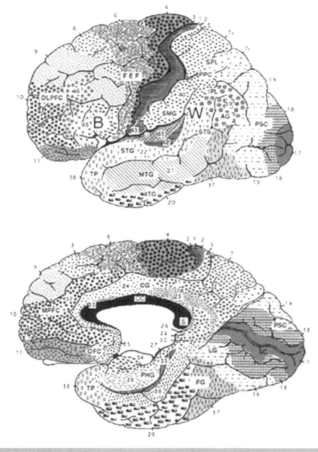

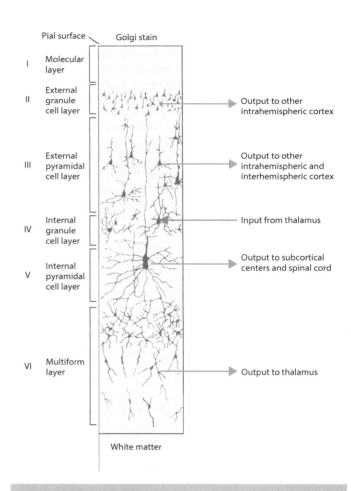

FIGURE 10.2

Brodmann's areas. Lateral (top) and medial (bottom) views of the cerebral hemispheres. The numbers refer to the Brodmann cytoarchitectonic designations. Area 17 corresponds to the primary visual cortex; 41–42, to the primary auditory cortex; 1–3, to the primary somatosensory cortex; and 4, to the primary motor cortex. The rest of the cerebral cortex contains association areas: AG, angular gyrus; B, Broca's area; CC, corpus callosum; CG, cingulate gyrus; DLPFC, dorsolateral prefrontal cortex; FEF, frontal eye fields (premotor cortex); FG, fusiform gyrus; IPL, inferior parietal lobule; ITG, inferior temporal gyrus; LG, lingual gyrus; MPFC, medial prefrontal cortex; MTG, middle temporal gyrus; OFC, orbitofrontal cortex; PHG, parahippocampal gyrus; PPC, posterior parietal cortex; PSC, peristriate cortex; SC, striate cortex; SMG, supramarginal gyrus; SPL, superior parietal lobule; STG, superior temporal gyrus; STS, superior temporal sulcus; TP, temporopolar cortex; W, Wernicke's area. (Reproduced with permission from Mesulam M. Aphasia, Memory Loss, and Other Focal Cerebral Disorders. In: Kasper D, et al, eds. *Harrison's Principles of Internal Medicine*, 19e New York, NY: McGraw-Hill; 2014.)

Cortical laminae

Most of the cerebral cortex is neocortex, with a six-layered anatomy, distinguishable from the allocortex, with only three or four layers. Neocortical laminae are labeled layers I–VI, from superficial to deep (Figure 10.3). Layer IV is called the internal granular

FIGURE 10.3

Structure of the cerebral cortex. The cortical layers are indicated by the numbers. Golgi stain shows neuronal cell bodies and dendrites, Nissl stain shows cell bodies, and Weigert myelin sheath stain shows myelinated nerve fibers. (Modified from Ranson SW, Clark SL. *The Anatomy of the Nervous System*, 10th ed. St. Louis, MO: Saunders; 1959.)

cell layer, so called because it is densely populated with small stellate cells. Layers I–III are the supragranular layers; layers V–VI are infragranular layers.

Supragranular layers I–III are the main targets for ascending inputs from deeper layers (vertical), and for cortico-cortical (horizontal) connections from ipsilateral and contralateral hemispheres. Layer I, the molecular layer, contains few neurons and numerous glial cells. It contains branches of the apical dendrites ascending from layers II, III, and V, and axons from other cortical sites, as well as a substantial projection from the thalamus. This thalamic connectivity appears to contribute to feedback circuitry affecting learning and attention.

Layer II, the external granular layer, and layer III, the external pyramidal layer, are the sources of cortico-cortical output. Layer II contributes projections deeply to contribute to local circuits within deeper layers, and longer projections providing communication among the lobes within the hemisphere. Layer III emits short axons that project locally to layers V and VI, longer projecting axons that synapse in other lobes within the hemisphere, and a large population of axons that crosses through the corpus callosum and the anterior commissure to synapses in the contralateral hemisphere.

In primary sensory cortices, layer IV, the internal granular layer, is well developed and densely populated with stellate cells that are the primary targets of projections from the thalamic relay nuclei; layer IV is virtually nonexistent in motor cortices (the so-called agranular cortex). Although there is a great synaptic density in layer IV, only ~4% arise from thalamocortical axons. The broad dendritic array of the stellate cells receives the apical dendrites of layer V cells and basal dendrites of layer III pyramidal cells, as well as axons from other cortical and subcortical centers. Nearly 80% of layer IV stellate cell local circuit connections are excitatory, suggesting that they might amplify incoming signals for further processing in extragranular layers.

Infragranular layers V–VI contain cells whose axons exit the cortex. Layer V contains many large pyramidal cells and is the principle source of basal nuclear, brainstem, and spinal outputs. Located in layer V are the giant Betz cells that emit axons contributing to the corticospinal tract. Apical dendrites of layer V cells synapse with cells from layers II and III to integrate local and distant circuitry. Layer VI is a multiform layer containing neurons of varied morphologies; its major output returns to the thalamus.

Columnar Organization and the Cortical Module

Early development of the cerebral cortex is highlighted by its unique inside-out temporal sequence, with later-born neurons migrating upward, perpendicular to the cortical surface, passing through established cell layers. Radial glial cells, bipolar cells with elongated processes that span the thickness of the developing cortex, guide this process. These radial glial cell bodies lie deep in the developing cortex near the proliferative ventricular zone lining the expanding ventricles. Asymmetrical mitoses produce a second radial glial cell and either a neuron or a progenitor cell that can form either astrocytes or oligodendrocytes. The processes emerging from the radial glia and extending to the cortical surface provide scaffolds for newborn neurons to follow in their ascent through the cortex. Newborn neurons migrate along their parent radial glial fiber or on nearby glial fibers, forming a column of related cells and creating cortical modules in the developing cerebral cortex. Increases in cortical volume are accomplished by adding more columnar modules rather than by increasing cortical thickness.

Cortical Modules and Mapping the Somatosensory Body

The primary somatosensory cortex (SI) contains a complete map of the contralateral body, constructed from inputs from cutaneous and deep sensory receptors. Activity can be recorded from cells within a specific cortical module when its peripheral receptive field is stimulated. Imagine Michelangelo's great fresco painting *The Creation of Adam* on the ceiling of the Sistine Chapel. Adam reaches out with his left second digit (index finger). When Adam finally touches the finger of the Creator, it will activate his ascending dorsal column-medial lemniscal pathway, innervating second-order neurons in the ipsilateral dorsal column nuclei, then third-order cells in his contralateral ventral posterolateral thalamic nucleus. Thalamocortical projections to S1 are extremely precise, initiating activity only in the cells within the corresponding cortical column for that specific digit. Extrapolating from the details above, there is a column of sister cells representing a spot on Adam's contralateral second digit.

Extremely precise point-to-point somatotopy in S1 is demonstrated by observing that the skin on the fingertip is represented adjacent to the representation of the skin of the proximal second digit, and the columns that represent the third digit are adjacent to those representing the second digit. The extreme precision of this point-to-point arrangement contributes to the high degree of accuracy in localizing the source of the stimulus, so Adam is fully aware of which finger he has extended. Peripheral receptive fields with especially dense innervation, such as the fingertips or the lips, are represented in a disproportionally large area in the contralateral somatosensory cortex. Sparsely innervated peripheral receptive fields, such as the torso or the legs, have smaller cortical representations. In 1937, Penfeld and Bouldrey described this relationship electrophysiologically (cited in Griggs, 1988). Rather than presenting the usual exhaustive verbal description of the complex cortical representation, they commissioned the artist Mrs. H. P. Cantlie to draw a figure with its body size proportional to its density of innervation.

Mrs. Cantlie's original homunculus ("little man") combined motor and sensory data to present a human figure with grotesquely enlarged hands, lips, and face, and absurdly reduced shoulder, trunk, and legs. In 1950, at the behest of Penfeld and Rasmussen, Mrs. Cantlie modified the presentation of her homunculus so that motor and sensory homunculi were presented on left and right sides of a coronal section through primary motor and somatosensory cortices. This image revealed remarkable similarities between the motor and sensory homunculi. Although the value of this innovative presentation cannot be overstated, modern mapping studies reveal more detail and functional somatotopy. Further, some intrinsic implications can be confusing to novice students of neuroanatomy, such as the common lack of distinction between precentral and postcentral gyri and subsequent misinterpretation of the locations of M1 and S1. Minor revisions are made in Figure 10.4 to increase the precision and simplify the localization of the homunculus in cortical areas.

Minicolumns

Within each column in layer IV of the primary somatosensory cortex (S1) lie several smaller units called minicolumns (Figure 10.5). Vertical differentiation among embryonic neuron means that the cells within a minicolumn are developmental sisters. Functional connectivity of these cells is driven from the sensory neurons in the periphery, through the second-order nuclear cells and the tertiary thalamic neurons projecting to precisely positioned cortical cells. The activated sensory endings in the periphery have specific functional adaptation patterns. Progressively higher-order synapses activate neurons with the same adaptation characteristics all the way to the cortical neurons in minicolumns in S1. Recall from Chapter 3 that there are sensory endings that respond with slowly adapting responses and others with rapidly adapting responses. Within the second digit representation in S1 are partially overlapping groups of cells that respond with discrete adaptation responses. Cell groups with slowly adapting responses are adjacent to cells with rapidly adapting patterns, both representing the spot on digit two. This implies that some features of the initial encoding of the tactile stimulus remain discrete through the entire skin-to-cortex pathway.

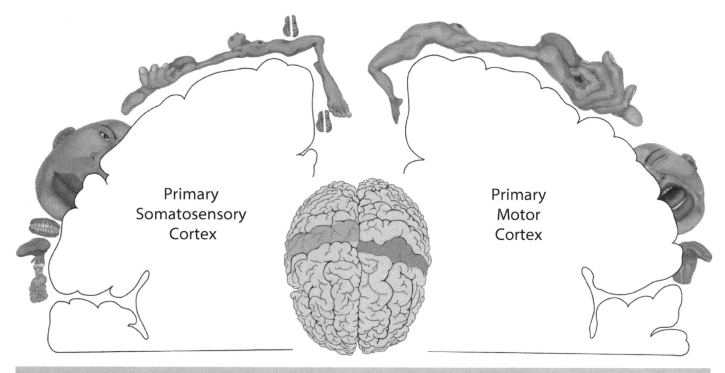

Primary
Somatosensory
Cortex

Primary
Motor
Cortex

FIGURE 10.4

Homunculus revision. The famous somatosensory and motor homunculi as drawn by Mrs. Cantile based on Penfield and Rasmussen's work, with modifications based on new research as well as corrections for accuracy. (Image provided by Jamie Graham, 2017.)

An example would help here. It is back to the point that we do not have perception in the primary somatosensory cortex.

Topography of the Cerebral Cortex

The surface of the cerebral cortex is highly convoluted to present the familiar grooved appearance that is so delicious to zombies. The second trimester sees the elaboration of three of the most prominent sulci that separate the cerebral lobes. Early in the second trimester, after the 12th gestational week, the longitudinal fissure appears, separating the left and right hemispheres. Within the limits of individual and functional variation, the division into lobes and the appearance of gyri and sulci are symmetrical between hemispheres and have a similar anatomy among the human population. Around week 17, the large lateral (Sylvian) fissure begins to form a separation between the temporal lobe below from the frontal and parietal lobes above. In week 21, the central sulcus forms, a prominent superior-inferior groove, separating the frontal lobe anteriorly from the parietal lobe posteriorly. These three deep grooves parcellate the cerebrum and serve to orient the student for detailed identification.

Lobes of the cerebral cortex

The cerebral cortex is divided into lobes, named by the bones that cover each: the frontal, parietal, temporal, and occipital lobes.

The insular cortex, often referred to as a fifth lobe, lies buried beneath the frontal, parietal, and temporal lobes (Figure 10.6).

Frontal lobe: Lying anterior to the central sulcus, the frontal lobe contains the motor regions of the cortex. Vertically oriented parallel to the central sulcus, the precentral gyrus comprises the primary motor cortex (Brodmann area 4). It forms a strip of cortex ascending from the lateral fissure to the anterior part of the paracentral lobule in the medial aspect of the brain. The somatotopy in the primary motor strip has the foot and lower extremity located in the paracentral lobule; the shoulder near the superior margin of the longitudinal fissure; the hand occupying a large portion of the lateral part of the precentral gyrus; and the face represented inferiorly in the strip above the lateral fissure.

Frontal motor cortices extend forward in the frontal lobe beyond the primary motor strip. Brodmann area 6 is a large area anterior to the precentral gyrus. It consists of several portions that include the premotor cortex occupying most of the lateral portion of the posterior frontal lobe; the supplementary motor area lying superiorly in the posterior part of the superior frontal gyrus, the frontal eye field (Brodmann area 8), which, in humans, lies in the posterior part of the middle frontal gyrus near the precentral gyrus; and Broca's area (Brodmann areas 44, 45) lying in the posterior part of the inferior frontal gyrus just anterior to the face representation in the primary motor cortex. Injury to Broca's area can

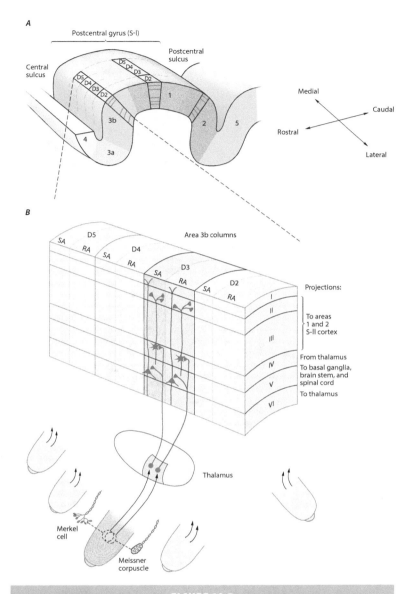

A

Postcentral gyrus (S-I)

Postcentral
sulcus

Central
sulcus

D5
D4 D3
D5 D4 D3 D2
D4 D3 D2
D2 1

Medial

Caudal

3b

2 5

Rostral

4

Lateral

3a

B

SA D5 Area 3b columns

SA RA SA D4

RA SA D3

RA SA D2

RA SA RA

Projections:

I

II

To areas
1 and 2
S-II cortex

III

From thalamus

IV

To basal ganglia,
brain stem, and
spinal cord

V

To thalamus

VI

Thalamus

Merkel
cell

Meissner
corpuscle

FIGURE 10.5

Minicolumns. Smaller units within layer IV of S1 with highly organized and differentiated sensory cells that maintain specific orientation based on peripheral location and adaptation pattern. This allows the initial encoding to be maintained throughout the skin to cortex pathway. (Reproduced from Kandel ER, Schwartz JH, Jessell TM. *Principles of Neural Science*, 4th ed. New York, McGraw-Hill, 2000.)

produce motor aphasia. Beyond the frontal motor cortices, the prefrontal cortex occupies much of the frontal lobe to its anterior pole (Brodmann areas 9, 10, 11, 12, 46, and 47).

Parietal lobe: The postcentral gyrus houses the primary somatosensory cortex (SI) which consists of four separate Brodmann areas, 3a, 3b, 1, and 2, from anterior to posterior, extending from posterior part of the paracentral lobule in the medial aspect of the brain to the lateral fissure. Somatotopy is generally the same as that found

in the primary motor cortex: foot most medially in the posterior paracentral lobule, and face most lateral, adjacent to the lateral fissure. All four of the Brodmann areas comprising the S1 form parallel vertical strips, and in each strip the complete contralateral body and face are represented with identical somatotopy.

A large portion of the parietal lobe, referred to generally as posterior parietal cortex or parietal association cortex, lies behind the primary somatosensory strip. Much of the processing that takes place in the posterior parietal cortex involves integration of somatosensory information into a complete egocentric spatiotemporal construction of the entire body, with output to motor areas guiding behavior. The second somatosensory cortex (S2) receives inputs from all parts of SI. It is found in the supramarginal gyrus (Brodmann area 40) above the lateral fissure posterior to the face representation in SI. Posterior to and associated with S2 and Wernicke's area (Brodmann area 22) in the temporal lobe lies the angular gyrus (Brodmann area 39). All three of these areas are involved with language processing, and injury can lead to sensory aphasia. The superior parietal lobule (Brodmann areas 5, 7) lies behind the upper and medial parts of the postcentral gyrus, continuing into the medial aspect of the hemisphere. Its posterior margin borders the occipital lobe. The separation between the two lobes is inconspicuous on the lateral surface of the brain, but the parieto-occipital sulcus prominently divides the lobes on the medial aspect.

Occipital lobe: The occipital lobe includes the visual cortex. In the medial view, the parieto-occipital sulcus separates the occipital lobe from the parietal and temporal lobes. Within the occipital lobe, a deep calcarine sulcus divides the cuneate gyrus above from the lingual gyrus below. Brodmann areas include areas 17, 18, and 19. Area 17, the primary visual cortex, lines the calcarine sulcus on its upper and lower lips. It has a striking anatomy with an extremely large and prominent layer IV, called the stripe of Gennari, in which there are numerous horizontally oriented myelinated axons contributing to the name *striate cortex*. Areas 18 and 19, visual association cortices, extend upward into the cuneate gyrus and downward into the lingual gyrus. The three visual areas are arranged in parallel strips when viewed from the medial brain surface, and as three concentric circles, area 17 central, when viewed from the occipital pole.

Temporal lobe: The fusiform gyrus (Brodmann area 37) crosses from the occipital lobe into the temporal lobe. It lies below the lingual gyrus posteriorly and extends anteriorly into the temporal lobe between the inferior temporal gyrus laterally and the hippocampal gyrus medially, terminating near the anterior temporal pole on the lower lip of the lateral fissure. It is an important visual association cortical area specifically related to facial recognition and to the visual association cortex in area 19.

In addition to visual association, the temporal lobe contains several other functionally distinct regions. A horizontal shelf on the superior temporal gyrus, extending deeply within the lateral fissure, called the transverse temporal gyrus (Heschl's gyrus), contains the primary auditory cortex, area 22. Intimately related to the primary auditory cortex both anatomically and functionally, Wernicke's area

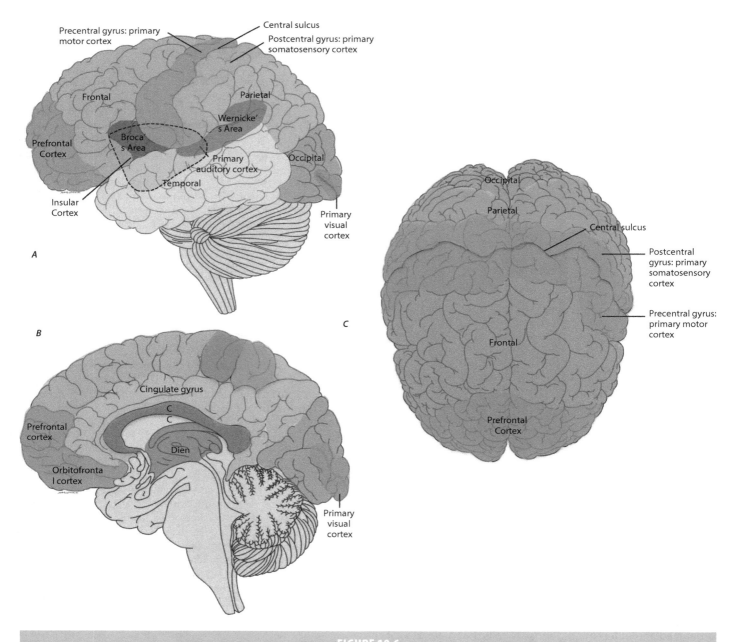

FIGURE 10.6

Lobes of the cerebral cortex. The cerebral cortex is divided into lobes, named by the bones that cover each: the frontal, parietal, temporal, and occipital lobes. The insular cortex (area shaded on image), often referred to as a fifth lobe, lies buried beneath the frontal, parietal, and temporal lobes. (Image provided by Jamie Graham and Tony Mosconi, 2017.)

is contained within the posterior part of the superior temporal gyrus behind the primary auditory cortex in the transverse temporal gyrus. Many descriptions also include within Wernicke's area portions of the adjacent occipital and parietal lobes: the angular gyrus, area 39; and the supramarginal gyrus, area 40.

The inferior medial part of the temporal lobe contains the parahippocampus, area 34, and associated entorhinal cortex (area 28). The hippocampal formation within the parahippocampal gyrus is related to the limbic system and is involved in the circuitry that establishes declarative memories. It is part of Papez's circuit (Chapter 9), connected to the hypothalamic mammillary bodies through the fornix, a fiber bundle that arches forward along the inferior margin of the septum pellucidum. The bulge on the most medial portion in the temporal cortex, the uncus, contains the amygdaloid nucleus, a center related to emotional responses and fear conditioning.

Insular cortex: The insular cortex (areas 13, 14) is a six-layered neocortex deeply situated in the lateral fissure, covered by portions

Before a person can establish his overall sense of self at any instant, the interoceptive and exteroceptive conditions must be ranked, for example, from mild irritation to agonizing pain. Each condition is given in a subjective place along a sensory gradient based on its qualitative physical and emotional significance on the "self." This grading of sensory status occurs in the middle insular region.

The anterior insular cortex is extensively and reciprocally connected with sensorimotor, limbic, and association cortices. Thus it is in a position to integrate emotional and behavioral processing of internal and external stimuli, subjectively rated, into a "sentient self." The sum of all feelings at any moment produces a continuous cognitive construction of self. Functional MRI studies have found significant activity in the anterior insula, along with the anterior cingulate cortex, when subjects were presented stimuli that generated emotional responses. This subjective interpretation can be extremely complex. Consider the person who experiences what most would consider agonizing pain, but for that person is accompanied by sexual arousal.

In cases of insular dysfunction, particularly from middle cerebral artery injury, patients with autism spectrum disorders, frontotemporal dementia (frontotemporal neurocognitive disorder), or advanced Alzheimer's disease present loss of emotional awareness (alexithymia). In schizophrenia also, the volume of the insula is significantly reduced and appears to be related to features of schizophrenia, such as delusions, where the subjective self is dissociated from objective reality.

Limbic system (lobe): The limbic system is an extensive interactive network of cortical and subcortical structures that are involved in complex functions, such as learning and memory, behavioral, autonomic, and endocrine responses to emotional or stressful conditions, and affective behaviors such as addiction, arousal, and motivation. It is called the limbic lobe because it is composed of a rim ("limbus") of structures around the corpus callosum between cortical and subcortical areas (Figure 10.8).

Early studies by Papez described an "emotional circuit"—Papez's emotional circuit—which included the hippocampus, connected with the mammillary bodies in the hypothalamus through the fornix; the anterior nucleus of the thalamus via the mammillothalamic tract; the cingulate gyrus; and the cingulum fiber bundle completing the circuit by returning to the hippocampus. Papez's eponymous circuit described not only cortical processing for the generation of emotions but also, due to hypothalamic connections, a means of generating the physiological changes attendant to strong emotions.

Subsequent studies by Klüver and Bucy contributed to the expansion of Papez's circuit to include additional temporal lobe structures such as the amygdala and adjacent cortical areas. Bilateral temporal lobe lesions in monkeys generated a complex syndrome of altered affective behaviors that included the inability to identify objects visually (visual agnosia); behaviors suggestive of obsessive psychological demand for and responses to external stimuli (tendencies to examine objects intensely by putting them in the mouth or smelling them; compulsive attendance to objects within their vision and grasp, known as hypermetamorphosis); suppression or flattening of emotional behavior, including loss of fear; and altered sexual behavior.

The limbic system now is recognized to include additional cortical and subcortical regions, such as the parahippocampal gyrus

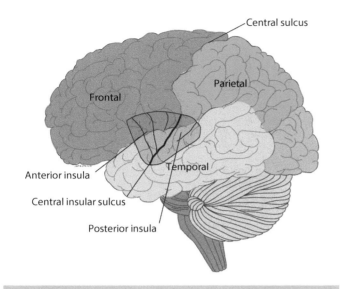

FIGURE 10.7

Projection of insular cortex. Anterior and posterior insular regions are separated by the central insular sulcus, a ventral continuation of the central sulcus. (Image provided by Jamie Graham and Tony Mosconi, 2017.)

of the frontal, parietal, and temporal lobes (Figure 10.7). In fact, the insula cannot be seen without widely opening the lateral fissure. For many years, the insular cortex (insula) was virtually ignored in the neuroscientific literature; however, many more recent studies, including electrophysiological analyses of patients undergoing surgery for intractable epilepsy as well as patient presentations after insular stroke, have revealed a complex set of connections and a broad set of functions for this enigmatic region.

The insula can be divided functionally into anterior and posterior portions, but is also further subdivided on the basis of topographical anatomy. A continuation of the central sulcus, separating frontal and parietal cortical lobes, continues onto the insula as the central insular sulcus that divides the anterior and posterior portions. Posterior insula contains anterior and posterior long gyri. The larger anterior portion contains (from posterior to anterior) the posterior, middle, and anterior short gyri, and the accessory gyrus. The insular apex is directed ventrally. Several recent studies have described a posterior-to-anterior processing of a large volume of different types of inputs that are ultimately related to the homeostatic construction of a sensorimotor, autonomic, and emotional "self."

Many older studies referred to the insula as the gustatory-olfactory cortex, and indeed there is input from those systems to the insula. In addition, posterior insula is a prime target for most of the sensations detected from interoceptive and exteroceptive receptors. These inputs have been described as "affective bodily feelings" and include somatic sensations, including primary and secondary hyperalgesic pain perception; and visceral sensations of fullness, cramps, illness and nausea, hunger, and thirst. Processing of this information generates motivated behaviors aimed at satisfying energy needs and conservation related to maintenance of homeostasis. It also may be the basis of such maladaptive behaviors as fear-avoidance seen in people with chronic pain or chronic vertigo.

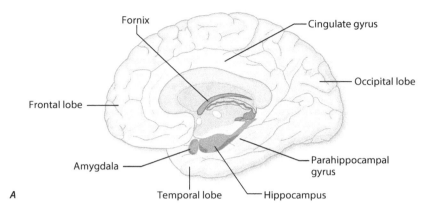

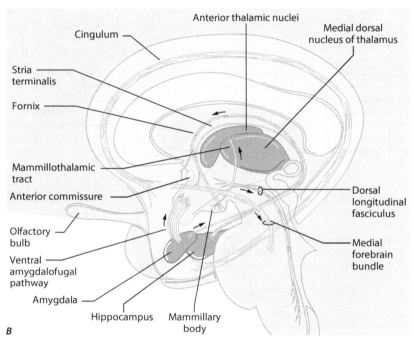

FIGURE 10.8

Limbic system with Papez's circuit. Sagittal diagram of the limbic system. **A.** Surface topography of the limbic system and associated prefrontal cortex. **B.** Connections of the limbic structures and their relation to the thalamus, hypothalamus, and midbrain tegmentum. The cortical parts of the limbic system, or limbic lobe, are interconnected by a septohypothalamic–mesencephalic bundle ending in the hippocampus, and the fornix, which runs from the hippocampus back to the mammillary bodies, and by tracts from the mammillary bodies to the thalamus and from the thalamus to the cingulate gyrus. The Papez circuit is the internal component of this system. (Reproduced from Kandel ER, Schwartz JH, Jessell TM. *Principles of Neural Science*, 4th ed. New York, McGraw-Hill, 2000.)

and the entorhinal cortex around the hippocampus, which are related to learning and memory; the insular cortex, which integrates sensory experiences into a "sentient self"; and the prefrontal cortical areas, including the orbital frontal cortex and the anterior cingulate cortex that mediate complex functions such as decision making, cognition, emotion, and executive control. The olfactory cortex also contributes to the emotional circuitry, which explains why odors can elicit strong emotional responses, even after years. The amygdala is found in the anterior end of the temporal lobes but is often considered with subcortical structures. Its influence contributes to behavioral changes in

response to stress, including learned behaviors based on reward or punishment, and fear conditioning. Connections to midbrain limbic centers, including the serotoninergic cells in the midbrain raphe nucleus, and dopaminergic cells in the ventral tegmental area, provide inputs for these two neurotransmitter systems, both of which are known to influence mood, attention, and motivation.

Identification of numerous "limbic" structures has aided in studies of memory learning and motivated behavior, intelligence, and personality. Unfortunately, lesion studies attempting to ablate particular parts of the system have produced widely varied results.

This argues that any one of the limbic structures alone cannot be ascribed complete responsibility for a process. Instead, the whole system acts to integrate the vast array of influences that contribute to the complexities of human psychology.

Cortical White Matter

CNS pathways, tracts, fasciculi, and funiculi all refer to the densely packed myelinated axons comprising the white matter. Although it is the activity of neurons to receive, process, integrate, and activate to perform the myriad functions of the brain, without the connectivity afforded by the axons in the white matter, neurons would remain isolated, and those complex functions could not occur. White matter axons are the information conducting structures carrying action potential impulses from neuron to neuron in the CNS.

For a long time, white matter was considered to be of little functional significance beyond, perhaps, acting as channels for flow of animal spirits outward from the brain for motor activities, or inward for sensory function. Development of fixation, microscopy, and dissection revealed that white matter was composed of fine threads connecting cortical regions with subcortical. In one of the great neuroscientific historical ironies, Gall and Spurzheim, originators of the pseudoscientific principle of phrenology, were early pioneers of white matter tract dissection. Phrenology purported the existence of well-developed cortical organs wherein resided regulation of specialized functions. Their meticulous dissections demonstrated white matter connections among these organs. They described callosal projections connecting the two hemispheres, association tracts consisting of short (arcuate or U-shaped) fibers connecting adjacent gyri; long intrahemispheric fasciculi connecting lobes; and projection systems, including ascending and descending pathways providing communication between the cerebral cortex and subcortical brainstem and spinal cord regions. These systems still form an organizing framework for discussing CNS white matter.

As with many neuroanatomical discoveries, greater detail concerning the function of white matter tracts came from animal studies of lesioned brains and from autopsied brains of patients with well defined pathologies. The commonly recognized observation that injury to the left side of the brain produced paresis in the right side of the body was found to be related to the decussation of projection fibers in the pyramid. Soon it was found that symptoms of multiple sclerosis were correlated with regions of damaged white matter caused by degenerative demyelination. Even more recently, immunohistological and molecular studies have revealed collections of pathological amyloid plaques in axons of patients with Alzheimer's disease. With concerns over the effects of even minor, asymptomatic traumatic brain injuries (concussions), particularly newsworthy among elite athletes and children, diffuse damage to even small populations of axons has been shown to have potentially debilitating long-term effects.

Among the most impressive innovations in studying white matter tracts has been the development of diffusion tensor imaging (DTI), a modification of magnetic resonance imaging (Figure 10.9). DTI takes advantage of the tendency of water to diffuse from fiber bundles along the long axis of the fibers, to reveal substantial detail about the origins, trajectories, and targets of fasciculi. Although the complex mathematical and probabilistic calculations that go into DTI are far beyond the scope of this text, the spectacular figures and information derived from DTI have contributed greatly to our understanding of cerebral circuitry in normal and pathological systems.

White matter fascicles can be grouped into association, projection, and callosal. Among each group are some particularly relevant examples. Short (arcuate or U-shaped) fibers connecting adjacent gyri arise from layers II–III and contribute to local processing circuitry. These small fiber bundles can be seen just beneath the gray

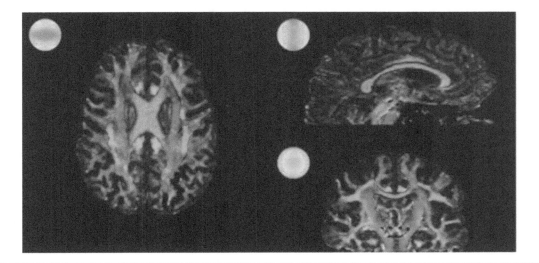

FIGURE 10.9

Diffusion tensor imaging. Diffusion tensor image of white matter in the normal human brain with isotropic resolution (2 mm). This three-dimensional data was acquired in about 16 minutes using diffusion-weighted echo planar acquisition. The direction of diffusion is indicated by the reference color sphere in each image. The image on the left shows a transverse slice though the top of the corpus callosum (red "X" in the center of the brain). The upper-right image is a midsagittal plane (note the corpus callosum in red) and the lower-right image is from a coronal plane centered in the anterior-posterior direction. (Reproduced with permission from Geyer JD, et al. Chapter 2. Neuroimaging in the Management of Neurological Disease. In: Carney PR, Geyer JD. eds. Pediatric Practice: Neurology New York, NY: McGraw-Hill; 2010.)

matter ribbon curving around the sulci. These tiny filaments are easily damaged with even mild head injuries. Chronic traumatic encephalopathy (CTE) is a neuropathology that has received extensive recent examination because of the high-profile tragic outcomes among several professional athletes. CTE can be demonstrated using labeled antibodies against tau proteins, revealing early deposition in damaged axons at the gray-white interface in the depths of the cortical sulci.

Long intrahemispheric fasciculi, arising mainly from cortical layer III, provide communication among the lobes within the hemisphere. These fibers form bands extending between specific cortical areas and have been identified by DTI and confirmed with autopsy dissection. One of the most prominent is the superior longitudinal fasciculus (SLF). The SLF is composed of several subcomponents, each of which joins specific sites. The nomenclature is somewhat disputed, so it will serve this text to discuss the SLF as a single structure with multiple connections. Sensorimotor integration contributing to executive motor control is served by fibers that extend from the superior parietal cortex and supramarginal cortex rostrally to the premotor ventral premotor and prefrontal regions in the superior frontal lobe. A substantial portion of the SLF contributes to speech processing and production. The arcuate fasciculus extends from the caudal part of the superior temporal gyrus around the posterior end of the lateral fissure and continues rostrally with the fibers from the angular gyrus to the lateral portion of the prefrontal cortex; these comprise part of the circuitry related to production of speech. This relationship is emphasized by the observation of interhemispheric asymmetry. In most people, the SLF is significantly larger in the left hemisphere.

The inferior longitudinal fasciculus (ILF) provides communication between the occipital lobe and the inferior temporal lobe. The designation has been reevaluated in humans, being replaced by the term *occipitotemporal system*. This system includes fibers of the traditionally described ILF, which lesion studies suggest is associated with the "what" stream and visual agnosia and prosopagnosia, as well as fibers providing communication between visual association cortex with anterior and medial temporal cortex. These fibers are distinct from another large association bundle in the area, the optic radiations (geniculocalcarine tract), carrying visual input from the lateral geniculate nucleus to the primary visual cortex.

The cingulum is a smaller fiber tract within the cingulate gyrus. Its fibers pass to the entorhinal cortex and adjacent parahippocampal gyrus and contribute to the limbic system circuitry.

The major projection fascicles have been discussed at some length in the text. The most prominent descending projection pathway comprises the motor pathways to the brainstem (the corticobulbar tract) and to the spinal cord (the corticospinal tract). Long ascending pathways of primary importance include the dorsal column-medial lemniscus and the spinothalamic tracts. Remarkable images have been produced showing the CST extending from frontal motor cortex downward through the brainstem, decussating at the caudal end of the pyramids, and descending through the lateral funiculus in the spinal cord. Similarly, the ascending somatosensory pathways have been shown as they terminate in the thalamus. CST, CBT, thalamocortical, and corticothalamic pathways contribute to a dense fiber cup, the internal capsule, convex medially toward the thalamus, with its concavity filled with the lentiform nuclei. The extension of fibers between the cortex and the internal capsule forms the corona radiate.

The largest white matter bundle in the brain is the corpus callosum (CC), and it is the most prominent decussating band. The CC provides interhemispheric connections between corresponding regions. The CC is a large curving structure in the core of the brain. It lies just beneath the cingulate gyrus and arches over the diencephalon. In sagittal section, the CC has a slightly expanded posterior portion called the splenium, which blends anteriorly with the body. The CC curves at its most rostral extent, forming the genu. The small rostrum folds under the genu. At least five portions of the CC have been described. The rostrum and genu provide communication between prefrontal and orbitofrontal cortices of each hemisphere. Anterior in the body region, fibers connect the two premotor and supplementary motor areas. The posterior body connects primary motor areas. The narrow area between the body and the splenium, the isthmus, connects the primary somatosensory areas. Finally, the splenium connects the parietal and temporal lobes as well as the visual cortex. It is again ironic that the description of somatotopy within the corpus callosum initially made by Gall and Spurzheim was met with derision, yet their observations have been supported by ensuing study.

III FUNCTIONAL PROCESSING IN SENSORY, MOTOR, AND ASSOCIATION CORTICES

We experience our lives at the level of the cerebral cortex. Imagine you are standing on a cliff overlooking the ocean. You can smell the salt water, hear the sound of waves, and feel the warm wind on your face. In the cerebral cortex, the physical properties of peripheral stimuli, such as low- or high-energy skin distortion, light wavelengths in the visible spectrum, and sound waves between 20 and 20,000 Hz, are integrated to generate an experience, or perception. It is also the center wherein the conceptualization, planning, and direction for goal-oriented behaviors take place. It is, of course, also where the consciousness resides, which integrates all of our experiences, perceptions, memories, and emotions.

As in the rest of the body, the metabolic demands of the cerebral cortex are meticulously monitored and rigorously controlled. To this end, when the body evolves processes that are efficient and effective, it makes use of those processes wherever possible. This replication of processes is observed in the brain, and an example discussed below is surround inhibition in the somatosensory system, which resembles a process within the visual system. The physiological goal of surround inhibition is to amplify the responses in activated cells while suppressing responses in surrounding or adjacent cells for increased contrast between activated and non-activated circuits.

Central Processing in the Somatosensory System

In earlier chapters, we discussed the anatomical and physiological characteristics of a variety of sensory endings in the peripheral nervous system (Section III) and the ascending pathways that carry encoded information concerning stimuli applied to the sensory endings all the way to the primary somatosensory cortex (SI) in the postcentral gyrus of the parietal lobe (Section V). Primary afferent endings are distributed in the skin and deep tissues. Each type of ending displays specific adaptation patterns of action potential firing. Each ending also has an area of tactile sensitivity, or receptive field, that is related to its morphological characteristics. Tiny Meissner's corpuscles have small punctate receptive fields, whereas large Ruffini endings have relatively vast receptive fields.

In combination, these distinctly different and specific adaptation patterns and receptive field characteristics provide elegant encoding of the subtle complexities of a stimulus. Each ending type encodes different physical characteristics of a stimulus, including the force, velocity, or frequency of the applied stimulus, among other features. Further, spatiotemporal serial activation of endings can confer information about the direction and speed of a moving stimulus.

As previously detailed, sensory information is conveyed rostrally through several synaptic centers, including second-order cells in the ipsilateral spinal cord and brainstem; tertiary cells in the ventroposterolateral and ventroposteromedial nuclei somatosensory nuclei in the thalamus; and higher level neurons in the SI cortex. A collection of primary afferent endings in the periphery project centrally to a second-order neuron, which now has its own larger receptive field. At each ascending level, higher-order cells' receptive fields are constructed of the aggregate of receptive fields from inputs from the lower level (Figure 10.10). At each successively higher level, cells process a broader set of physical characteristics of the stimulus, derived from the different types of input from the variety of sensory endings. It is important to keep in mind that throughout the subcortical pathway, there is no "perception" of the stimulus, but rather the cells receive more detail, and more data, regarding the original stimulus.

Localizing stimuli

When sensory stimuli are applied to the endings in the peripheral receptive field, such as when the skin is distorted, the primary afferent neurons in the center of the receptive field are most strongly activated. Endings in the area surrounding the central site are also activated, although to a lesser extent. This produces an activation pattern defined by a curve, with maximal activation centrally, dropping off with distance from the center. This information is relayed to second higher-order neurons in the brainstem that suppress activity of cells in their adjacent or surrounding receptive fields. The overall effect is to increase the contrast between the active center

and suppressed surround inputs. With higher degree of contrast between activated and inactivated cells comes increased precision in localizing the peripheral stimulus. Center-surround processing is a common functional feature in sensory systems, including the visual system, and generates greater acuity in the final perceptual experience.

At each successively higher synaptic level, neurons have larger receptive fields created by combining smaller fields of lower-order inputs. The higher-order neurons respond with similar adaptation characteristics as their inputs. Local circuitry processes the inputs so that the information is more integrated with other related ascending inputs from the cell's receptive field. Segregation, with local communication, persists all the way up to the level of minicolumnar organization in the primary somatosensory cortex (SI), as described above.

The SI is composed of four parallel areas—3a, 3b, 1, and 2—comprising the somatosensory strip in the postcentral gyrus. A complete homunculus is recapitulated (reconstructed) in all four areas in the somatosensory strip. Each area receives inputs related to different modalities of sensation from the ventroposterolateral and ventroposteromedial somatosensory thalamic nuclei. Areas 3b and 1 receive fine-grained low-threshold mechanoreceptor cutaneous input about surface textures; area 3a receives proprioceptive input (see qualification of this percept below); and area 2 receives input regarding surface contour and shape. Even this far along the somatosensory pathway, the brain has not yet produced the experience of a sensory perception. These SI areas themselves are still integrating and collating the physical characteristics of the peripheral stimulus.

SI areas communicate with each other and generate output to the second somatosensory area (S2, Brodmann area 40) residing above the lateral fissure, posterior to the face representation in SI, and to the superior part of the posterior parietal lobule (Brodmann areas 5 and 7), behind the upper and medial parts of the postcentral gyrus, continuing into the medial aspect of the hemisphere. These

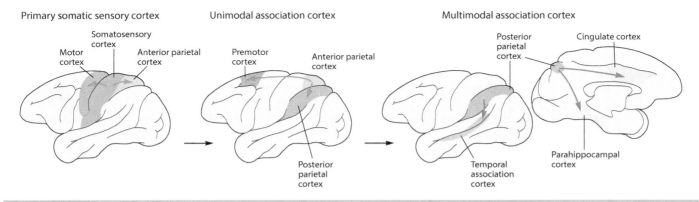

Primary somatic sensory cortex — Unimodal association cortex — Multimodal association cortex

Motor cortex · Somatosensory cortex · Anterior parietal cortex · Premotor cortex · Anterior parietal cortex · Posterior parietal cortex · Posterior parietal cortex · Cingulate cortex · Temporal association cortex · Parahippocampal cortex

FIGURE 10.10

Central sensory processing. The processing of sensory information in the cerebral cortex begins with primary sensory areas, continues in unimodal association areas, and is completed in multimodal association areas. Sensory systems also communicate with portions of the motor cortex. For example, the primary somatosensory cortex projects to the motor area in the frontal lobe and to the somatosensory association area in the parietal cortex. The somatosensory association area, in turn, projects to higher-order somatosensory association areas and to the premotor cortex. Information from different sensory systems converges in the multimodal association areas, which include the parahippocampal, temporal association, and cingulate cortices. (Reproduced with permission from The Functional Organization of Perception and Movement. In: Kandel ER, et al, eds. *Principles of Neural Science*, Fifth Editon New York, NY: McGraw-Hill; 2012.)

areas also receive inputs from widespread cortical centers such as the visual system, the prefrontal cortex, and the limbic system, giving broad context for interpreting the somatic sensation, emotion, and memory, and selecting appropriate behavioral responses, into a rich fully realized experience. At each successively higher synaptic center, the information becomes increasingly abstract and farther removed from the generic physical characteristics encoded by sensory endings in response to the original stimulus.

Consider this example. Your skin is lightly stimulated. This stimulation continues along a spatiotemporal gradient progressing distally along the skin of your forearm, initially recorded in primary afferent endings located within the skin. At successively higher levels along the somatosensory pathway, the information from those receptors is combined and integrated to include data related to the force, direction, and duration of the cutaneous stimulus. High-level processing now includes visual input: the stimulus is a spider walking down your arm. You are reminded of a story about a girl who was bitten by a brown recluse spider and lost her limb. The thought of losing a limb frightens you terribly, engaging emotional fear circuitry carried in the limbic system. Panicky, you brush the harmless barn spider off your arm, suppressing a scream through frontal lobe executive function.

This integrative process of data collection and contextual perception allows you to choose behavior that is both eloquent and highly contextual. This process begins with you initially registering generic physical energies by receptors in the skin, then combining more detailed data regarding the features of the stimulus over time. Additional sensory information upon visually inspecting the stimulus is added to the data, along with integrating memories and emotional context. Thus, your behavioral response completes the complex, but practically instantaneous, process of experiencing a sensory perception.

In the periphery, noxious stimuli are encoded and then relayed through the dorsal horn, brainstem nuclei, and thalamus, to the SI cortex. Processing of nociceptor input happens in the same way as for low-threshold mechanoreception, with cells at each level maintaining the same physiological response characteristics as the original sensory endings. Current hypotheses contend that there is little alteration in the information carried on the ascending spinothalamic tract axons prior to arriving at SI. Thinly myelinated Aδ inputs innervate somatotopically appropriate SI areas, and, like mechanoreceptive inputs, this information is translated to resolve accurate localization and stimulus characteristics associated with the fast, pricking pain of primary hyperalgesia. Cortical processing of C-fiber inputs does not follow the pattern described for myelinated nociceptors.

Dorsal horn laminae I and V receive input from myelinated nociceptors, and lamina V receives from Aδ and C-fiber polymodal nociceptors as well as from non-nociceptive Aβ fibers. Nonnociceptive and myelinated nociceptive inputs from spinal levels innervate cells in thalamic VPL nucleus via the dorsal column-medial lemniscus spinothalamic pathways, and from the thalamus to somatotopically distinct areas 3b and 1 in SI. Areas 3b and 1 are considered be the initial site of nociceptive processing of location and characterization of the stimulus. Some nociceptors, including a preponderance of unmyelinated C fibers that innervate cells in the dorsal horn substantia gelatinosa (laminae II-III), project instead to ventromedial nucleus of the hypothalamus, which projects to the insula (and into cingulate and prefrontal cortices) and to area 3a

in SI. Cells in a large area in 3a are activated by noxious peripheral stimuli and are sensitized with damaged tissue. There is also a suppression of the strict somatotopic response to noxious stimuli with 3a activation. These observations support the role of 3a, with its dense C fiber input, in the prolonged, burning, but poorly localized pain of secondary hyperalgesia.

Ultimately, processing of noxious stimuli appears to occur in SI through interactions of areas 3b and 1 with 3a to encode location, physical characteristics, intensity, and ongoing condition of the damaged tissue. Connections include the hypothalamus, which activates sympathetic responses, and the insula, cingulate, and prefrontal cortices, which engage emotional and memory circuitry, to regulate behavioral responses, long-term conditioning, and descending modulation of pain.

Neuropathic Pain

Pain is the most common reason that most people seek medical attention. Reports also indicate that over 95 million people, an estimated 30.7% of the US population, experience chronic pain. There is some suggestion that this contributes to the epidemic increase in opioid misuse. Clearly chronic pain is a serious concern for therapists, and an understanding of the underlying mechanism is essential when providing care to this population. Recall that pain is not experienced at the site of trauma; the actual experience occurs in the cerebral cortex. At the site of injury, endings encode damaging stimuli. Prolonged or severe damage can lead to hyperexcitability in neurons in the afferent pathway and can produce neuronal death through cytotoxicity that can generate aberrant sensations such as allodynia, dysesthesia, and hyperalgesia, or chronic neuropathic pain.

Ascending nociceptive information is carried on the anterolateral system: the spinothalamic tract for direct thalamic connectivity and precise localization and characterization (intensity, direction of movement, quality) of the damaging stimulus. Activation of the spinohypothalamic tract and thalamic connections elicit responses to pain, such as sympathetic changes and increased states of arousal. These circuits also engage limbic circuits that make the experiences deeply emotional and memorable. Spinoreticular and spinomedullary tracts informing brainstem reticular centers project to cortical centers that contribute to emotional and behavioral responses to pain that can produce long-lasting aversion or phobias.

In the primary somatosensory cortex, the representation of the injured peripheral region expands to include a larger portion of the cortex than normal for improved self-care and avoidance of further injury and protection. Normally, as nociceptive pain resolves over time, territorial expansion withdraws to normal dimensions. In chronic pain, or neuropathic pain, this process appears to be disrupted, and pain is experienced long after the initial cause is resolved.

Cerebral plasticity is recognized as one of the integral changes that underlie transformation of nociceptive (peripheral) pain into neuropathic (central) pain. A novel hypothesis has been developed recently to explain this maladaptive process that can turn temporary, nociceptive pain into chronic neuropathic pain. Researchers speculate that chronic pain is a learned response that outlasts the acute or subacute painful condition. Some spinothalamic projections bypass the ventroposteromedial and ventroposterolateral thalamic nuclei, synapsing in the dorsomedial nucleus and the hypothalamus. Circuits involving the hypothalamus activate sympathetic physiological and behavioral responses. The dorsomedial nucleus connects widely in the cortex, including with the amygdala, insula, cingulate, and prefrontal cortices. Acute pain induces reflex and behavioral responses critical to survival; however, the complex and extensive activation of emotional and cognitive circuits drives memory deep into the individual's self-awareness. This generates a sometimes lifelong fear-conditioned response to painful or even perceived potentially painful situations. Such fearful reactions often complicate therapies aimed at relieving the pain-producing conditions. Therapists need to consider not only the physical complications but also the psychological impediments to acceptance of, and compliance with, treatments.

Central processing in the visual system

Information processing in the primary visual cortex (area 17), or striate cortex, is among the most complex systems in the sensory brain. Posterior to the optic chiasm, the optic tracts contain axons from both retinae and carry the binocular representation of the contralateral visual hemisphere. Retinal ganglion cell axons terminate in one of four regions in the brain (Figure 10.11) (see Chapter 6). The majority of retinal ganglion cell axons are involved with visual perception and continue within the optic tract to the lateral geniculate nucleus (LGN) in the thalamus for processing and relay to the primary visual cortex. Not all of the retinal ganglion cell axons in the optic tract are involved in processing visual information. Some axons project to the superior colliculus, where the inputs contribute to the creation

of a conceptual three-dimensional visual space required for coordinated head and neck movement, and for directing eye movement in response to visual stimuli. Additional axons project to pretectal areas in the midbrain and are associated with autonomic control of pupillary reflexes. Finally, a few axons project to the diencephalon to the supraoptic nucleus of the hypothalamus and the pineal gland for control of diurnal rhythm and hormonal cycling.

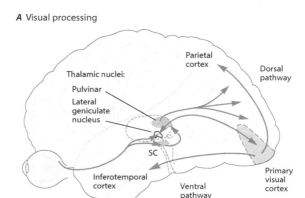

A Visual processing

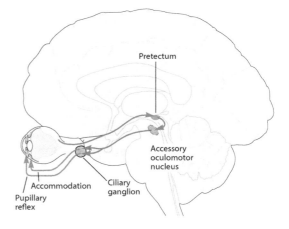

B Pupillary reflex and accommodation

FIGURE 10.11

Pathways for visual processing, pupillary reflex and accommodation, and control of eye position. A. Visual processing. The eye sends information first to thalamic nuclei, including the lateral geniculate nucleus and pulvinar, and from there to cortical areas. Cortical projections go forward from the primary visual cortex to areas in the parietal lobe (the dorsal pathway, which is concerned with visually guided movement) and areas in the temporal lobe (the ventral pathway, which is concerned with object recognition). The pulvinar also serves as a relay between cortical areas to supplement their direct connections. **B.** Pupillary reflex and accommodation. Light signals are relayed through the midbrain pretectum, to preganglionic parasympathetic neurons in the Edinger-Westphal nucleus, and out through the parasympathetic outflow of the oculomotor nerve to the ciliary ganglion. Postganglionic neurons innervate the smooth muscle of the pupillary sphincter, as well as the muscles controlling the lens. **C.** Eye movement. Information from the retina is sent to the superior colliculus (SC) directly along the optic nerve and indirectly through the geniculostriate pathway to cortical areas (primary visual cortex, posterior parietal cortex, and frontal eye fields) that project back to the superior colliculus. The colliculus projects to the pons (PPRF), which then sends control signals to oculomotor nuclei, including the abducens nucleus, which controls lateral movement of the eyes. (FEF, frontal eye field; LGN, lateral geniculate nucleus; PPRF, paramedian pontine reticular formation.) (Reproduced with permission from The Constructive Nature of Visual Processing. In: Kandel ER, et al., eds. *Principles of Neural Science*, Fifth Editon New York, NY: McGraw-Hill; 2012).

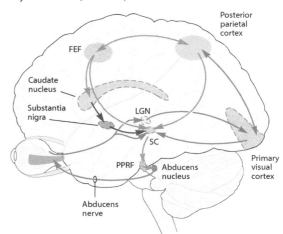

C Eye movement (horizontal)

Lateral geniculate nucleus

Associated with the pathway for visual perception, proper, the LGN is stratified into six cellular layers (Figure 10.12). The cell bodies of the LGN can be differentiated by their size and position.

Smaller cells form the upper four parvocellular layers, and the largest cells form the deepest two, or most ventral, magnocellular layers. The smallest cells are interspersed between the parvocellular and magnocellular layers (i.e., interlaminar neurons) and represent the koniocellular neurons. Neurons in the parvocellular layers (p-LGN cells) receive synapses from P-retinal ganglion cell (midget cell) axons. They have small center-surround receptive fields and are color-sensitive cells most sensitive to contrasts that allow shape and form discrimination. Magnocellular layers receive and process the M-retinal ganglion cell (parasol cell) input. The m-LGN cells behave like M-retinal cells, with large center-surround receptive fields. These also carry color information. Magnocellular-LGN cells are more sensitive to movement of stimuli and have the largest receptive fields. Koniocellular neurons receive inputs relaying information about color. Koniocellular LGN neurons, k-LGN, are more like P-retinal ganglion cells but are more sensitive to color than p-LGN cells.

The LGN receives input from both eyes via the optic tract. The ipsilateral eye synapses in layers 2, 3, and 5, and the contralateral fibers synapse in layers 1, 2, and 6. Each layer contains a perfect representation (retinotopic organization) of the visual field, and within each of the layers the same portions of the visual fields are aligned. Each neuron corresponds to stimulation of one eye only. Each LGN contains the representation of the contralateral visual hemisphere.

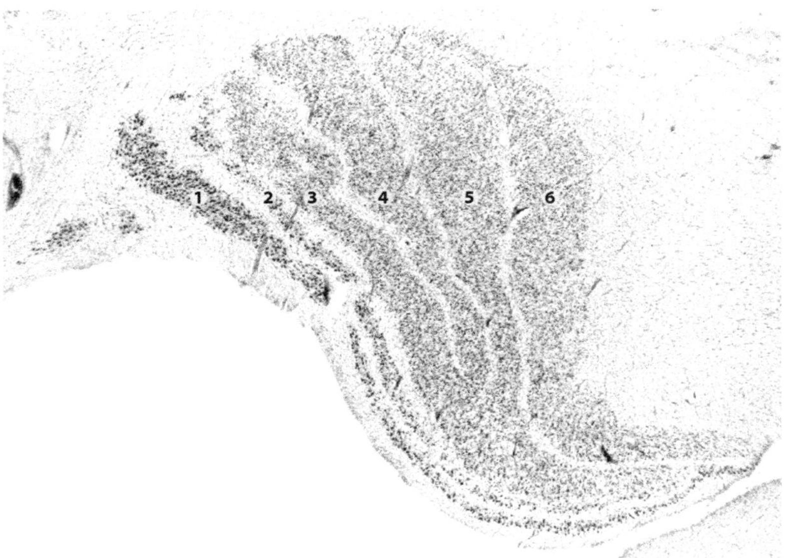

FIGURE 10.12

Lateral geniculate nucleus. The lateral geniculate nucleus is an example of a complex nucleus. The nucleus is shown in a Nissl-stained coronal section of the right hemisphere of a human brain. Axons from different types of neurons in the retina terminate in different layers (1–6) of the nucleus. In addition, each layer receives input from only one eye. (Reproduced with permission from The Organization of the Central Nervous System. In: Kandel ER, Schwartz JH, Jessell TM, Siegelbaum SA, Hudspeth AJ, Mack S. eds. Principles of Neural Science, Fifth Editon New York, NY: McGraw-Hill; 2012).

From the LGN, the optic radiations fan out, passing through the temporal, parietal, and occipital lobes. The radiations course around the inferior temporal horn of the lateral ventricle. Comprising the white matter extending toward the primary visual cortex in the occipital lobe. The inferior radiations form a loop that courses ventrally through the temporal lobe, known as Meyer's loop, conveying information about the contralateral superior visual quadrant. Lesions at this location result in superior quadrant visual field loss from both eyes on the same side, a contralateral superior homonymous quadrantanopia, known as a "pie-in-the-sky" deficit.

The dorsal (superior) optic radiations pass posteriorly and represent the contralateral inferior visual field quadrant. A lesion in the dorsal optic radiations causes an inferior homonymous quadrantanopia, known as a "pie-on-the-floor" deficit. Nasal fibers carrying information from the temporal visual field of each eye connect to the medial aspects of the contralateral lateral geniculate nuclei. Lateral portions of the LGN receive the lower retinal fibers, and superior retinal fibers head for the medial aspect. The hilium of the LGN receives the macular fibers.

Optic radiations project to the primary visual cortex (V1), Brodmann's area 17, located on either side of the calcarine fissure in the occipital lobe. Dorsal optic radiations project to the superior bank of the calcarine fissure, and the fibers of Meyer's loop project to the inferior bank. Lesions in either of these areas also lead to contralateral lower or upper quadrantanopia, respectively. Located above the calcarine fissure is the cuneus (wedge), or cuneate gyrus; and below is the lingua (tongue), or the lingual gyrus.

The fovea is represented near the occipital pole and is disproportionately represented in the visual cortex, taking up as much as 50% of the space.

Most of the LGN axons terminate in the V1. Its characteristic striated appearance can be identified with Nissl stain. Most of the input arrives in layer IV, and the axon collaterals of the myelinated fibers give the striate cortex its characteristic pale appearance, known as the stripe of Genari. Layer IV is organized such that the input is discretely monocular despite the fact that half of the fibers decussate at the optic chiasm. Like the LGN, the V1 is also retinotopically organized, divided into a columnar cortex with six layers and several sublayers. Each of these alternating columns is 1 millimeter wide, and they are known as ocular dominance columns. Ocular dominance columns can be readily identified histologically due to the high levels of the metabolic enzyme cytochrome oxidase. Cortical layers II and III in the ocular dominance columns contain wavelength (color)–sensitive neurons.

The k-LGN, p-LGN, and m-LGN cells send information to neurons within V1 and then to extra striate cortex (areas 18 and 19) for additional processing. In layers II and III the V1 blob cells, named for their appearance when they were stained for cytochrome oxidase, are found in clusters and resemble k-LGN cells. They process color sensitive, monocular input, and they have small concentric receptive fields. The blob cells process information for color perception, color discrimination, and learning and memory of colored objects.

Interblob cells are found in clusters around blob cells. They process P-stream information, are binocular, have elongated receptive fields, exhibit ocular dominance, and have orientation and location specificity. Some interblob cells are sensitive specifically to movement, and others are sensitive to the direction of movement.

The receptive fields of the input layers of the visual cortex represent mainly on-center and off-surround cells. Mixing and blending with fibers from the other eye in layers above and below layer IV, mediated by cortical interneurons, is critical for depth perception. This process of blending ensures that there is always dominance by one eye. Just as ocular dominance columns segregate information from the two eyes to ensure binocular vision and dominance, orientation columns exist to facilitate appreciation of orientation of an object. The orientation column of the primary visual cortex is organized in a pinwheel shape in the tops of the columns. Intersection of dominance and orientation columns are known as hypercolumns. Additional columns exist with specific functions, such as direction sensitivity and spatial frequency.

Neurons project from Area 17 to the higher-order extrastriate visual areas that encircle the V1 cortex. The extrastriate cortex is divided in to V2, V3, and V4. Each of these areas contains a partial or complete representation of the retina. In turn, areas 18 and 19 receive input from the lateral posterior and pulvinar thalamic nuclei. The function of the pulvinar is to establish the relevance of visual stimuli. Damage to the extrastriate cortex does not cause loss of vision as does damage to the striate cortex. It leads to higher-order visual perceptual deficits such as the inability to recognize objects, colors, and movement. Bilateral damage to the fusiform gyrus (area 37) in the inferior temporal gyrus causes inability to recognize faces, known as prosopagnosia.

Two-stream visual processing

The visual system gathers and processes light waves until the stimulus produces the experience we call sight. Information originating in the retina is extracted for detailed inspection, analysis, and identification, and also must be transformed into a three-dimensional, egocentric visual coordinate system that provides spatiotemporal context for all of our behavior. To accomplish these two divergent tasks, visual input to V1 and V2 is processed along a dorsal pathway into the parietal, temporal, and frontal cortices; the ventral pathway projects into the temporal lobe (Figure 10.13). The presence of these separate pathways has been confirmed by functional MRI.

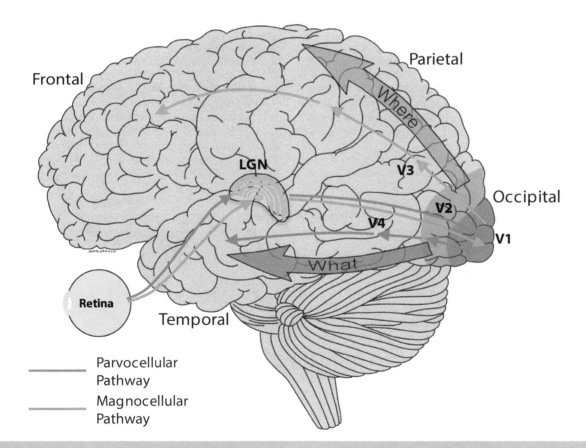

Frontal · Parietal · LGN · V3 · Where · Occipital · V4 · V2 · V1 · Retina · What · Temporal

_____ Parvocellular Pathway

_____ Magnocellular Pathway

FIGURE 10.13

Dorsal and ventral streams. Retinal ganglion cells input to the lateral geniculate nucleus (LGN) very specifically. Midget cell project to the parvocellular region of the LGN, while parasol cells project to magnocellular LGN layers. LGN output projects to the primary visual cortex (V1) in the occipital lobe, and from there to V2. Parvocellular and magnocellular pathways diverge as they exit V2. Dorsal projections project to V3 and from there into the parietal cortex, comprising the dorsal, or "Where" stream. Parvocellular projections pass through V4 en route to the temporal lobe, and comprise the ventral, "What" stream. (Image provided by Jamie Graham and Tony Mosconi, 2017)

Information processed in dorsal versus ventral streams is also different, and consignment into one or the other of the visual streams is determined by which retinal ganglion cell (RGC) type is the source of the input. Information necessary to dorsal stream function is derived from cells with high light sensitivity and the ability to detect movement through space; parasol RGCs (M-RGCs) receive a large volume of input, amplifying light and recording movement. Ventral stream processing extracts fine detail from the perceived object and requires inputs with high spatial resolution and acuity; midget RGCs (P-RGCs) receive discrete inputs and convey color information. The dorsal stream carries information about the egocentric three-dimensional schema from the occipital lobe through the parietal and into the frontal cortex. The ventral stream carries detailed visual information into the temporal lobe.

The dorsal ("where") stream

The dorsal stream is referred to as the "where" stream because it encodes the individual's egocentric three-dimensional personal space and informs behaviors by setting a physical "starting point" and site of ongoing monitoring. It carries forward spatial information that is primarily derived from parasol-type RGCs and passed through the magnocellular layers of the LGN. Input to V1 is processed and sent to V2. From V2, the dorsal stream projects to V3 visual association cortex. From there, spatial information is processed rostrally through parieto-temporo-occipital cortex and into the posterior parietal cortex. Some fibers project all the way into the frontal lobe. The information carried by the dorsal stream encodes velocity and direction of motion of an object and is used to guide tracking eye movements. The dorsal stream is critical for the information that leads to control of skilled actions, such as visual guidance of movements toward an object in space (e.g., shaping the hand to grip a cup).

Lesions of the posterior parietal cortex interrupt the dorsal stream and cause difficulty with visuospatial orientation, motion detection, and guidance of visual tracking eye movements. Patients with focal parietal lesions confirmed by MRI showed impaired perception of horizontal and vertical axes, poor length and distance discrimination, orientation discrimination deficit, and difficulty with position matching. Anterior parietal damage is associated with impaired perception of axes and angles, and posterior parietal damage is associated with impaired perception of position. The affected person has difficulty perceiving motion and reports seeing an object moving with "ratchets," or jumps. The person may also have difficulty using visual information to control saccades, reach for objects (optic ataxia), or judge distance. With their eyes closed, patients with dorsal stream damage also fail to identify objects by their tactile characteristics, a deficit called astereognosis (or rarer, one-sided loss of stereognosis is called tactile agnosia). They often can describe the object's features, but not identify it or discuss its function.

Large areas of damage in the posterior parietal cortex and superior temporal cortex may produce a neglect syndrome, also known as visual inattention. Visual inattention is characterized by a loss of awareness of a visual field, without a frank visual field loss. The structures carrying spatial input to the brain are present and functional; only the dorsal stream circuit is impaired, and there is a loss of perception. A patient with neglect may have normal findings with formal visual field testing in the clinic. Symptoms of neglect can be impressive. Patients typically disregard objects, people, and events that occur within the neglected space. In extreme cases, patients even disavow their own limbs. They do respond with withdrawal of a limb subjected to noxious stimulus, even while denying the perception of pain.

Neglect occurs contralateral to the parietal lobe injury. The right parietal cortex is dominant in establishing spatial coordinates, and the left is involved with speech and language production (Figure 10.14). The right parietal cortex attends to inputs from both the right and left visual fields, and the left parietal cortex attends only to inputs from the right field. Injury to the left posterior

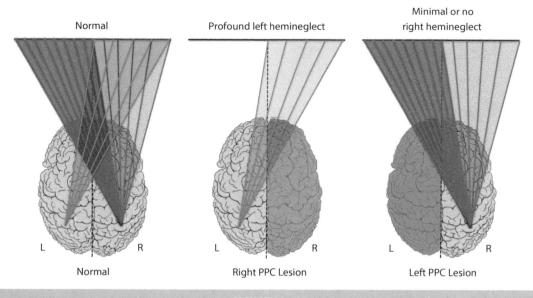

Normal   Profound left hemineglect   Minimal or no right hemineglect

L   R   L   R   L   R

Normal   Right PPC Lesion   Left PPC Lesion

FIGURE 10.14

Asymmetrical spatial representation in parietal cortex. Under normal conditions, both left (L) and right (R) posterior parietal cortices (PPC) maintain representation of three-dimensional space. There is little or no neglect with a left PPC lesion because the right visual hemisphere is also represented in the right PPC. (Image provided by Jamie Graham and Tony Mosconi, 2017.)

parietal cortex, therefore, does not produce contralateral hemineglect because its space is also represented in the right cortex.

The angular gyrus is located along the dorsal stream. It receives visual input related to language and passes it along to Wernicke's area. Because of its relationship with the dorsal stream, the angular gyrus is involved with spatial cognition, and it is involved in establishing left–right direction. It is also related to mathematical processing, especially in the left hemisphere. A lesion of the angular gyrus can produce Gerstmann syndrome, its deficits indicating angular gyrus function: left–right disorientation, acalculia (cannot perform arithmetic), finger agnosia (cannot distinguish among one's own fingers), and agraphia (inability to write).

The ventral ("what") stream

High-resolution information encoding details including color and shape is processed for object representation and form recognition along the ventral "what" stream. Incoming P-pathway axons innervate V1 and V2. The pathway next engages the V4 visual association cortex, then projects forward along the inferior portion of the temporal lobe. The ventral stream information interacts with cognitive processing, including memory, emotion, and fear, and is essential for "processing object quality," meaning recognizing and identifying objects and people, as well as interpreting their significance and purpose, based on characteristics of the object within emotional and experiential context. This circuitry is associated with storage of long-term memory and is critical for visual perception. V2 in particular, is associated with object recognition memory.

Research has suggested that there is little cross talk between the ventral and dorsal streams. It may be that the two streams developed to enable processing within the dorsal stream information that occurs in the background and without interference with the ventral stream, while other aspects of perception, processed by the ventral stream, is allowed to reach consciousness. Others have recently suggested that there is more interstream communication than previously observed. Interactive circuits show increasing activity when the precision demands of the movement are high.

The processing of information within the two streams occurs hierarchically. Each successive processing stage (synaptic level) adds a layer of complexity to the ultimate visual perception. As observed in the somatosensory system, at each successive synapse the information being processed is more abstract and farther removed from the physical properties of light waves activating retinal photoreceptors. Higher-order cell populations engage in specific perceptual functions, such as detecting virtual contours of figures, differentiation based on color and form, motion, and global motion. With each feed forward, there is also a feedback mechanism further mediating perception.

Damage to the ventral stream causes deficits in complex visual perception tasks (visual agnosia), attention, and learning/memory. The fusiform gyrus (Brodmann area 20) is an elongated gyrus coursing from the inferior occipitotemporal cortex anteriorly to the end of the temporal lobe. Its cells are directly related to facial recognition, identifying the person based on familiar, in-context details about individual facial features. Injury to the fusiform gyrus produces a condition called prosopagnosia, face blindness.

Central Processing in the Gustatory System

Three different cranial nerves (VII, IX, and X) deliver information from the sensory organs responsible for taste (taste buds) located on the tongue, soft palate, pharynx, and larynx to the rostral solitary

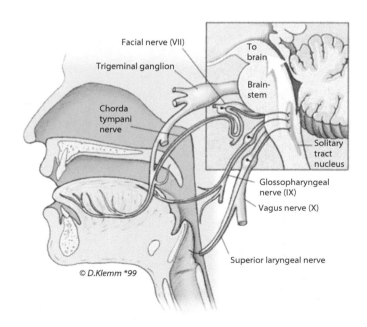

© D.Klemm *99

FIGURE 10.15

Cranial nerves that mediate taste. Schematic of the cranial nerves (CNs) that mediate taste function, including the chorda tympani nerve (CN VII), the glossopharyngeal nerve (CN IX), and the vagus nerve (CN X). (Copyright David Klemm, Faculty and Curriculum Support [FACS], Georgetown University Medical Center; used with permission).

nucleus in the brainstem (Figure 10.15). Taste has developed to guide consumptive behaviors. Taste cravings specific to nutritional deficiencies are examples of health-maintaining plasticity demonstrated within this complex system; sweet tastes drive the selection of energy-rich foods, and bitter tastes direct us to avoid poisonous foods. In fact, in the animal world, an evolutionary solution among many insects hoping to avoid becoming dinner is to become a bitter-tasting bug. In humans, gustatory pleasure and taste preferences are highly individualized, based on central processing, and shaped by personal experience, cultural norms, and ongoing plasticity. Modern molecular studies of taste are revealing new information on the complexity of central gustatory processing. They are also guiding the more recent development of processed food designed for maximum consumption without satiety.

Taste perception begins in chemoreceptors in the taste buds in the mouth. A taste bud contains approximately 200 sensory cells, each innervated by unmyelinated nerve endings that project via the cranial nerves to the rostral gustatory segment of the nucleus solitarius within the medulla. Projections to adjacent nuclei serve visceral reflex functions such as salivation and swallowing. An ill-defined pathway ascends through the pontine parabrachial nucleus to the primary taste cortex in the inferior-most portion of the postcentral gyrus. Cognitive identification and appreciation of taste is most likely generated in the anterior insula. Cells within the uncus, located within the inferior medial temporal lobe, integrate sensory information from olfactory, somatosensory (texture), and visual systems for flavor perception, ranging from pleasure to disgust. Information for autonomic function, such as salivating or retching, is carried to the hypothalamus, and pathways to the basal forebrain integrate emotional responses via the limbic system.

Central Processing in the Auditory System

Consider for a moment how many ways we use auditory information in our daily lives. From the simple startle response to a loud noise, to raising our voice in a crowd, to high-level decisions providing real-time adjustments during complex movements such as playing violin in a symphony orchestra, sound provides meaningful information to inform our behavior. These varied uses necessitate multiple pathways for central processing. It is beyond the scope of this text to cover every pathway in detail, but a few examples are provided for the practicing clinician.

Representations of sounds are maintained in the same relationships as they travel to the cortex for processing through tonotopic organization. Due to the anatomy of the basement membrane in the cochlea, high-frequency sounds stimulate hairs at the base of the cochlea, whereas low frequency sounds stimulate the apex. These action potentials are maintained separately along their journey up the cochlear nerve, with higher frequencies carried on the outer portion of the nerve. This precise organization is maintained throughout the entire pathway for sound discrimination.

The cochlear nerve ascends to the ipsilateral cochlear nucleus, with fibers continuing rostrally through several different pathways. Most fibers cross in the trapezoid body to the contralateral superior olive. Fibers from the superior olive, as well as uncrossed ipsilateral fibers, travel in the lateral lemniscus to the inferior colliculus of the midbrain, and then up to the medial geniculate body in the thalamus. The primary auditory cortex, where sound is processed, is in the superior temporal gyrus, also known as Heschl's gyrus

(Brodmann areas 41 and 42) (Figure 10.16). Neurons in Heschl's gyrus are also tonotopically organized.

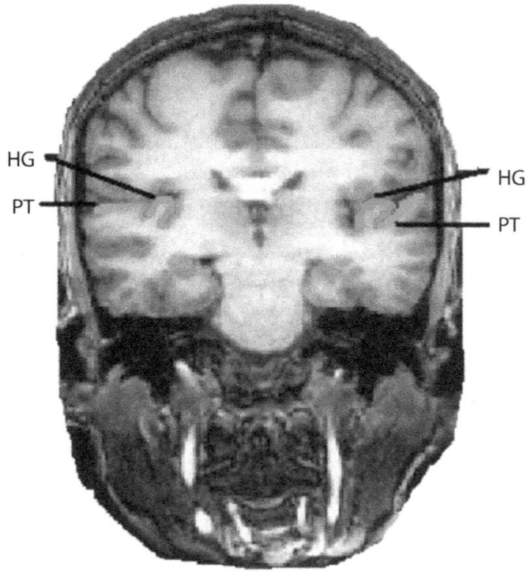

Sound is processed binaurally at every level, from the superior olive up to the cortex. Redundancy in the system provided by dual pathways (one from each ear in the periphery) allows for efficient sound localization and auditory discrimination. Acoustic encoding in tonotopically constrained central pathways organizes auditory inputs so that sound information can be integrated for meaningful interpretation and analysis. Higher level processing such as directing attention allows us to distinguish among competing acoustic stimuli, such as the ability to selectively listen to one instrument played within a symphony, or eavesdrop on a conversation in a crowded restaurant.

Therefore, a lesion anywhere along the ascending pathway will not produce complete deafness, but rather partial hearing loss, more prominent contralateral to the lesion. Partial hearing loss may include such features as inability to hear specific tones or inability to localize sounds in space. The clinical consequence of this complex pathway is that localizing the anatomic source of hearing impairment after CNS damage may be difficult with peripheral acuity testing, such as an audiogram measuring ability to perceive different sound frequencies and volumes.

The result is lateral specialization of processing, with language in the left auditory cortex, and music processing primarily in the right temporal lobe. Language interpretation and production is closely related to auditory processing, and so damage to the left hemisphere typically produces deficits in language processing as well as language expression. Disease or injury to the central auditory pathway rarely causes complete loss of hearing, but rather produces complex and subtle impairments of processing. One example is disrupted use of sound for self-monitoring vocal volume among people with Parkinson's disease.

Central Processing in the Vestibular System

As with hearing, the vestibular sensory apparatus is bilateral. This system of paired sets of receptors localizes movement and position of the head with astounding accuracy and speed. Each inner ear has three semicircular canals and two otolith organs, containing specialized hair cells that detect head motion and position. Changes of varying velocity and magnitude are encoded as proportionally altered afferent discharges. The resulting afferent signal is carried along the vestibular nerve through the internal auditory canal to the brainstem at the pontomedullary junction. From there the input travels to the vestibular nuclei to influence motor output, or onto the cerebellum for further sensorimotor processing.

The vestibular nuclei give rise to pathways to the spine, the nuclei governing the eye muscles, the thalamus, and the cerebellum, for coordination of eye and head movement, to perceive spatial orientation and maintain posture and balance, to modulate blood pressure, and to influence the reticular activating system and the emetic pathway (Figure 10.17).

Subcortical processing

The role of the cerebellum in processing vestibular sensory information is covered in detail in Section VII. A brief discussion is provided here prior to review the role of central subcortical processing in normal function. The primary role of the cerebellum is to monitor sensory information in real time to modify motor output to produce smooth, efficient motion. Although the vestibular reflexes may function without cerebellar input, they become

FIGURE 10.16

Heschl's gyrus. Magnetic resonance image showing Heschl's gyrus (HG, red) and planum temporal (PT, blue) within the upper part of the temporal lobe. (Reproduced, from Oertel-Knöchel V, Linden DEJ. *Neuroscientist* 2011, 17: 457.)

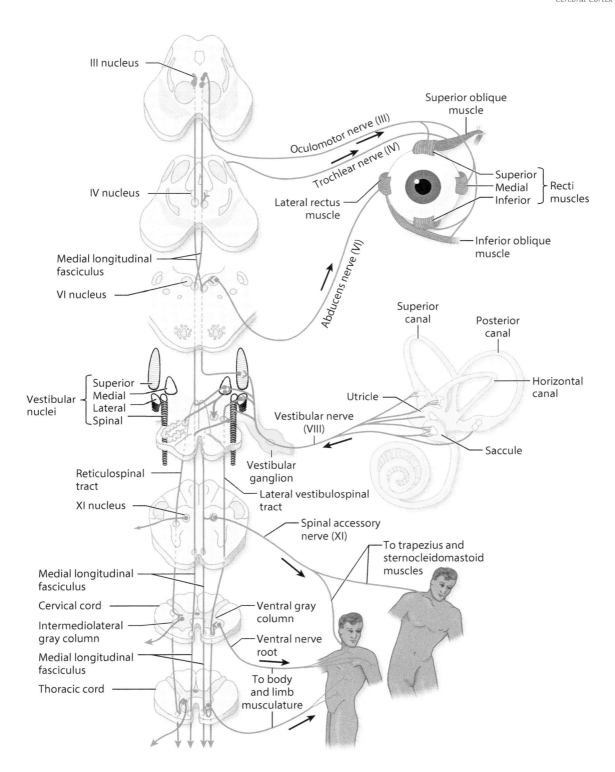

FIGURE 10.17

Vestibular nuclei and pathways. The vestibular reflex pathways. (Reproduced with permission from Chapter 15. Deafness, Dizziness, and Disorders of Equilibrium. In: Ropper AH, et al, eds. *Adams & Victor's Principles of Neurology*, 10e New York, NY: McGraw-Hill; 2014).

uncalibrated and ineffectual with cerebellar damage (Figure 10.18). Various lobes (zones) of the cerebellum adapt the gain of the vestibuloocular reflex (VOR), adjust the duration of VOR responses, and process otolith organ input. The vermis (medial zone) plays a role in vestibulospinal reflex (VSR) function, as lesions in this area produce severe truncal and gait ataxia.

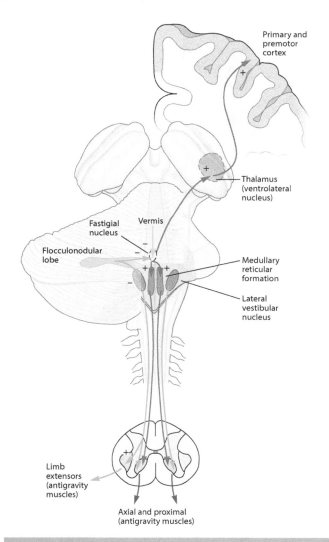

Vestibulocerebellum. The vestibulocerebellum and the vermis control proximal muscles and limb extensors. The vestibulocerebellum (flocculonodular lobe) receives input from the vestibular labyrinth and projects directly to the vestibular nuclei. The vermis receives input from the neck and trunk, the vestibular labyrinth, and retinal and extraocular muscles. Its output is focused on the ventromedial descending systems of the brain stem, mainly the reticulospinal and vestibulospinal tracts and the corticospinal fibers acting on medial motor neurons. The oculomotor connections of the vestibular nuclei have been omitted for clarity. (Reproduced with permission from *The Cerebellum*. In: Kandel ER, et al, eds. *Principles of Neural Science*, Fifth Editon New York, NY: McGraw-Hill; 2012.).

VOR and VSR activate midline (axial) and proximal appendicular muscles. The VOR also communicates extensively with the extraocular eye muscle motor nuclei to drive compensatory eye movement in the direction opposite head movement (Figure 10.19). The interconnections occur through axons passing bilaterally in the medial longitudinal fasciculus. The VSR engages descending vestibular projections to drive muscular contractions associated with maintaining head and neck position, as well as body posture, in response to changes in activity in the labyrinthine receptors. These responses activate synergistic muscle groups in the neck and along the spinal cord for subtle changes in position. Also, with rapid and large-scale positional displacements, as when tripping, the descending vestibulomotor pathways coordinate with the reticulospinal pathways to activate a righting reflex to "catch" oneself before falling.

The descending extrapyramidal pathways related to the vestibular system are the medial and lateral vestibulospinal tracts (VST). Each tract arises primarily from the correspondingly named vestibular nucleus, and each is influenced by cerebellar efferent input. The medial VST descends in the company of the tectospinal tract and the medial longitudinal fasciculus. These pathways regulate head and neck positioning related to external visual and auditory stimuli, and affect balance and postural control relative to those movements. The lateral VST descends through lumbar levels and contributes to activity in postural antigravity muscle contraction.

Some vestibular output contributes to local medullary circuitry involving emetic (vomiting) centers. The main nucleus associated with emesis is the area postrema located caudally in the floor of the fourth ventricle. Area postrema is one of the seven CNS areas that lacks a blood-brain barrier (Chapter 2), and therefore is well situated to detect toxins in the blood and evoke a physiological response aimed at ridding the body of the noxious material. The specific area involved in eliciting vomiting is called the chemoreceptor trigger zone, which includes circuitry that integrates the solitary nucleus and vagal afferents and efferents. Chemosensory and vestibular information is coordinated with the area postrema and nearby somatic and autonomic centers to stimulate the cascade of events that result in expulsion of stomach contents.

Vestibular system outputs to the chemoreceptor trigger zone in the area postrema employ the neurotransmitters—dopamine, histamine, and serotonin—which induce vomiting. Some argue that activation of the vestibular system through disparate visual and labyrinthine stimuli (as with motion sickness) dumps the neurotransmitters into the area postrema, mimicking poisoning and eliciting vomiting.

Cortical processing

Unlike other sensory systems, there is no single "primary vestibular cortex"; all vestibular functions rely on integration with somatosensory and visual inputs to complete the three-dimensional spatial conception of self in space and self-motion through that space. Several sites are involved in integration of vestibular information, and each comprises a multisensory center, processing visual and somatosensory input as well, for conscious subjective perception of orientation and motion within an egocentric three-dimensional coordinate system. Much of the available data for localizing the vestibular cortex has been acquired from studies using monkeys. Recently, however, fMRI and positron emission tomography (PET scanning) have discovered correlations in the human cortex.

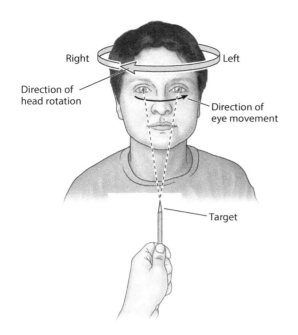 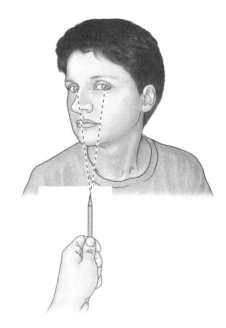

FIGURE 10.19

The vestibuloocular reflex. See text for explanation. (Reproduced with permission from The Vestibular System and Eye Movements. In: Martin J. *Neuroanatomy Text and Atlas,* 4th ed. New York: McGraw-Hill Education, 2012.)

The site most prominently activated by vestibular simulation lies in the parieto-insular vestibular cortex (PIVC) that includes the posterior insula and surrounding inferior parietal and frontal regions (Figure 10.7). Additional multisensory areas include the superior temporal cortex and the temporoparietal junction. All of these sites also emit corticofugal (leaving the cortex) fibers that form reciprocal inhibitory feedback connections between the PIVC and the visual cortex. Other PIVC projections return to the vestibular nuclei, also likely for feedback regulation, or descend with CST fibers to sensory portions of the spinal cord, possibly influencing reflexive postural adjustments. Activity in the PIVC is notably right-hemisphere dominant.

Multisensory information is normally integrated at the cortical level to produce an accurate perception of verticality, a foundational orientation for movement, for interpreting movement, and contributes to an overall sense of "well-being" through activation of intrinsic insular circuitry. Lesions damaging structures in the middle cerebral artery territory, but not with damage in the vascular beds of the anterior or posterior cerebral arteries, produce perceptions of "tilt" away from vertical and promote movements aimed at correcting orientation; they can also generate feelings of self- or object-motion. Visual coordinates describe the surrounding environment in three dimensions; somatosensory inputs fix the self within those coordinates creating an egocentric personal space; and vestibular inputs encode position and movement within the space.

When the sensory systems are properly functioning, the integration of inputs creates a framework for navigating through three-dimensional space with precision and safety. "Sensory reweighting" allows the brain to select or prioritize attention to the system providing the most accurate and reliable sensory information.

For example, recall that the vestibular cortex (PIVC) is intimately interconnected with visual cortex, and synchronous activation and integration of the reciprocal inhibitory feedback circuits are required to generate a three-dimensional orientation of verticality and of movement. During acceleration, the dominant stimulus is through vestibular activation, and the PIVC inhibits the visual cortex to suppress excessive activation of vestibuloocular reflexes that would produce oscillopsia, rapid eye movements that can create the sensation of blurring or jumping of the visual image. Perceiving self-motion is visually dominant, and parieto-occipital projections suppress PIVC output.

Impaired cortical processing Central lesions and normal aging create vestibular dysfunction that can be studied to identify the central pathway and role of cortical processing in normal function. With age, there are fewer hair cells in otolith organs and semicircular ampullae, with reduced sensitivity to gravity and acceleration. Reduced input from the peripheral labyrinth can impair VOR, VCR, and VSR responses, increasing likelihood for falls. Many seniors experience frequent falls due to what was previously called vestibular hypofunction, based on the belief that the peripheral vestibular system was low functioning, because VOR and VSR were diminished upon clinical testing. Elegant studies using caloric testing among subjects from this population, however, determined that the peripheral mechanisms were intact and in communication with cerebellar and cortical areas. Loss of cortical vestibular integration reduces the capacity to evaluate vertical and movement, thus reducing vestibular reflexes and increasing the likelihood of falls. This condition is now called vestibular neglect from the loss of ability to perceive vestibular stimuli.

Although vision is typically the dominant sense in normally sighted individuals, an overdependence on vision in the presence of erroneous information can be problematic. Attending excessively to visual input can produce feelings of vertigo in this population, causing visual-vestibular vertical mismatch. Vestibular neglect occurs when the multisensory cortical areas fail to integrate vestibular input and reduce or abolish vestibular feedback projections to the visual cortex and caudally to the vestibular nuclei. This overreliance on visual information produces increased postural sway and dizziness. Delayed VSR activation to vestibular stimuli results in failure to respond rapidly enough to prevent a fall. An effective therapeutic intervention is visual motion desensitization training using optokinetic stimulation to decrease reliance on visual data and improve integration of vestibular and other sensory information.

IV CENTRAL PROCESSING OF SOMATIC MOTOR FUNCTION

An eight-year-old violin prodigy springs onto the stage and skips toward his seat with his instrument. Because he is only eight, it isn't surprising that his shoelace is untied, and he trips. He catches himself before he falls, rescuing his instrument and his dignity, then resumes on his way to the seat and gives a brilliant rendition of Vivaldi's *The Four Seasons*. In this short vignette, we wonder what motor function performed by this young man is more impressive: catching himself before falling and righting his balance and posture completely without thought, or exhibiting magnificent dexterity as he performed a complex musical score.

Frontal Motor Cortex

Our motor systems are intricately interconnected both anatomically and functionally, and it is the cooperation between automatic reflexive movements and volitional, deliberate movements that allowed Antonio Stradivari to build a $16 million violin, or Simone Biles to perform a triple-twisting Yurchenko on the women's vault to win Olympic gold. For these purposes, we have developed descending cortical, brainstem, and spinal cord pathways that mediate the range of movements from pure monosynaptic reflex arcs to dexterous bilateral multijoint movements. Spinal reflexes have been discussed in Chapter 5, and the brainstem pathways, including the reticulospinal, vestibulospinal, and tectospinal tracts in Chapters 5, 6, and 7. These systems maintain muscle tone and response throughout movement, maintain axial posture, respond to rapid changes in the center of gravity of the body or position of the head, and orient the head and body in response to external stimuli. Their functions are conducted without conscious control. In fact, for many of these behaviors, conscious control would take too long for the movements to, for example, save the boy from falling, or help Simone stick her landing. The cerebellum receives unconscious proprioceptive input to make ongoing subtle changes to motor activity, but the movements are planned, initiated, and directed in the motor cortices present in the frontal cortex.

Primary motor cortex

Motor control centers are concentrated in several areas in the frontal lobe, collectively referred to as the frontal motor cortex (Figure 10.20). Primary motor cortex (Brodmann's area 4) is identified by a thick layer V containing pyramidal neurons varying in size from small cells less than 20 μm in diameter to giant Betz cells of

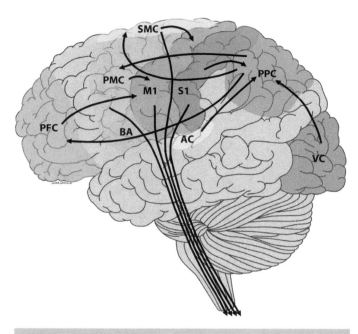

Primary motor cortex. Movement is directed by output from the primary motor cortex (M1). Spatial coordinates are maintained in the posterior parietal cortex (PPC), which has received sensory inputs from the primary somatosensory cortex (S1), visual cortex (VC), and auditory cortex (AC). PPC output innervates the prefrontal cortex (PFC), as well as premotor (PMC) and supplementary motor cortex (SMC). PFC, PMC, and SMC contribute to the highest hierarchical level, and instruct M1 output. PMC, SMC, M1, and S1 all emit axons that descend through brainstem and spinal levels. Arrows illustrate the direction of information flow. BA, Broca's area. (Image provided by Jamie Graham and Tony Mosconi, 2017.)

nearly 100 μm. Layer V motor neurons are referred to as upper motor neurons, in contrast to α-motor neurons in the ventral horn, called lower motor neurons. Remarkably, some upper motor neurons have axons that can exceed 1 meter in length. Primary motor cortex emits the axons of the CST and CBT. These are the developmentally newest motor pathways, and they control our very precise, finely controlled "fractional" movements present in the distal limbs, particularly in the hands, and in the face. Axons in the lateral CST descend into the contralateral spinal cord and monosynaptically innervate α-motor neurons in the lateral part of the ventral horn that supply muscles in the distal extremities (Chapter 5). Axons in the ventral CST are largely uncrossed, comprising around 5–10% of all CST fibers, and descend in the ventromedial spinal cord. These axons innervate neurons in the medial part of the ventral horn that, through collaterals and interneurons, bilaterally supply axial and proximal girdle muscles. CBT fibers innervate motor cranial nuclei providing volitional innervation to muscles derived from somatic or branchial arch tissues (CNs III, IV, V, VI, VII, IX, X, XI, and XII). An additional small contingent of axons descends with the CST arising from the layer V cells in the primary somatosensory cortex, synapsing on local circuit neurons, possibly modulating proprioceptive or mechanoreceptive input.

Early electrophysiological experiments revealed that stimulating the surface of the cortical motor strip along a medial to lateral course elicits movements consecutively in body parts progressing from legs to face, generating a homunculus resembling that in SI, complete with disproportionately large hand and face representations. Lower extremity representation is found in the anterior part of the paracentral gyrus on the medial surface of the brain. Progressing laterally along the motor strip, the body is represented from caudal to rostral, with the motor innervation to the face, lips, tongue, and larynx found most laterally, above the lateral fissure. The hand representation is located in a sharply curving structure called the knob or "omega sign" region. Lesions in this structure correlate with motor impairment in the contralateral hand. This peculiar shape is useful in positively identifying the precentral gyrus. Long-time violinists are known to have a prominent knob, and Einstein had one as well; he was an accomplished violinist.

SI cortex somatotopy possesses an extremely precise point-to-point correspondence between the peripheral receptive field and its central representation. Overlapping cutaneous territories, for example, are minimal and confined to slight blending at contiguous borders. Enhanced microstimulation techniques stimulating or recording from single cells in the motor cortex have demonstrated that individual muscles are represented by neurons in more than one noncontiguous location and in combination with numerous other groups of muscles. It has been proposed that activation of this widespread array engages synergistic muscle contraction aimed at producing movements rather than producing contraction in a particular muscle. Further, antagonistic, or competing, movements are simultaneously suppressed.

Consider again reaching for a beverage. Contraction of shoulder muscles provides a stable foundation for extension of the elbow. As the arm extends, the wrist rotates in the direction that aligns the hand with the target vessel, and the fingers curl into a shape appropriate for grasping. Cells of the individual muscles of the digits are interspersed among and overlap extensively with those supplying muscles of the shoulder, arm, and forearm. Possibly this organization provides a mechanism for activation of synergistic muscle groups that efficiently produces complex movements that answer a specific need, such as grasping a glass. Each cell representing a muscle, and each group of muscles in a synergistic group, cannot function in isolation; therefore orchestration of movements requires extensive connections through local cortical circuitry.

Premotor cortex

Frontal motor cortex comprises much more than Brodmann's area 4. Anterior to the primary motor cortex is an extensive portion of the frontal lobe called the premotor cortex, area 6. It extends from the medial surface of the posterior part of the frontal lobe (the anterior part of the paracentral lobule) laterally down to the lateral fissure. Its medial-most portion is the supplementary motor cortex, and at its lateral-most end, just above the lateral fissure is Broca's area (areas 44, 45) governing the movements associated with speech. Also associated with premotor cortex is the frontal eye field (area 8) lying anterior to the primary motor cortex, described in Chapter 6. Prefrontal cortex exerts significant influence over output from motor cortices and therefore over behavior. Another small contribution to the motor cortices is the cingulate motor area (area 24) lying in the superior part of the cingulate gyrus adjacent to the

supplementary motor cortex. Its association with limbic structures may affect emotional aspects of behavior.

Premotor cortex receives extensive sensory association inputs from posterior parietal association cortex, which it integrates into a plan of action that it emits to the spinal cord either directly or through reciprocal connections with the primary motor cortex. About 30% of the axons descending in the CST arise from the premotor cortex. Some of these synapse directly onto spinal cord motor neurons, but most synapse on local circuit interneurons. The posterior parietal cortex integrates sensory input from somatosensory, visual, and auditory cortices to construct a body schema, a three-dimensional representation of the body, with all of its parts registered in relation to each other and to the surrounding sensory world. The spatiotemporal construct is used to establish context for selecting, planning, and initiating movement aimed at accomplishing a motor task. It is continually updated throughout movement, monitoring the changing position of the body and its parts in the surrounding (peripersonal) space.

Elucidation of the extensive connectivity and complex function of the premotor cortex has arisen primarily from studies of nonhuman primates. Extension of these studies in humans has confirmed much of this data. More recently, lesion studies and high-resolution imaging analyses continue to support the generalization of the principle findings to humans.

Ventral premotor cortex: Modern descriptions state that the premotor cortex is composed of dorsal and ventral portions, each of which contains a rostral and caudal subcompartment. These individual portions have related but specialized functions in producing movement. The caudal part of the dorsal premotor cortex (often called PMDc) is involved in certain aspects of planning and executing reaching behaviors, particularly under visual guidance. Cells are directionally sensitive, firing best when reaching in a favored direction. PMDr (the rostral portion of the dorsal premotor cortex) is related to learning arbitrary rules concerning movement. For example, PMDc is active as monkeys learn to raise their arm to receive a tasty reward, or a student learns to raise her hand to be excused to the restroom. PMDr lies in proximity to the frontal eye field, and there appear to be connections that allow eye movement to modulate PMDr activity. Connectivity between the posterior parietal cortex and the caudal ventral premotor area (PMVc) engages cells in the PMVc in response to somatosensory, visual, and auditory stimuli, especially stimuli within peripersonal space. There is some suggestion that this system developed as a protective mechanism so that motor responses can be made quickly in response to potentially dangerous contact. PMVr is engaged with modifying hand position during grip and in directing the hand toward the face (as when eating). It is active as the hand forms, grasps, and grips an object, and orients the object toward the mouth. Stimulation of PMVr always produces hand-to-mouth movements and the accompanying movements that turn the head to align with the approaching hand as the mouth opens.

In 1996, Rixollatti and colleagues discovered a special set of neurons that were active when a monkey performed a behavior and when it watched another monkey or the experimenter perform the behavior. They called these mirror neurons, and since their original reporting, mirror neurons have been discovered in humans in the supplementary motor area, the primary somatosensory cortex, and the inferior parietal cortex. Observing human infant eye tracking movements suggests that the mirror neuron system is established before 12 months of age and may underlie imitative learning. Further speculation argues that the mirror neuron system is essential for the development of human social behavior and empathy. The concept of behavioral alignment, or behavioral mirroring, is fundamental to cooperative and communal human society.

Additional practical features about PMC function can be gleaned from patient presentation after lesions. Recall our beverage management example in Chapter 5. The shape of the hand begins to change into a conformation appropriate for the grip on the glass. Its shape and the amount of force exerted to grasp the glass are different for a tiny teacup versus a beer stein, and for an empty vessel compared to a full one. If the premotor cortex is damaged, patients experience difficulty selecting appropriate movements, and their errors affect timing and sequencing of movements. This impaired motor condition is called apraxia, and its appearance distinguishes PMC lesions from lesions in primary motor cortex and the subsequent upper motor neuron syndrome.

Motor impairments seem to be associated with interruption of the communication between the body schema and the planning and execution of movement rather than faulty comprehension of coordination. Apraxia affects long-established behaviors such as picking up a glass, and patients are unable to even pantomime common actions such as combing their hair or brushing their teeth. Visually guided, conceptualized, or instructed movements are impacted; however, automatic behaviors are spared, with PMC

lesions producing apraxia. A therapist might ask a patient to touch his nose with his right hand, and the patient would fail to produce the proper sequence, force, and speed of movements to accomplish the simple task. Moments later, the patient might distractedly reach up and scratch his nose with his right hand.

Dorsal premotor cortex: Dorsal portions of the premotor cortex (PMD) mediate selection of movements like the PMV does, but the influence of the PMD is greater when performing internally driven movements (self-selected, chosen movements) or with motor sequences performed from memory. Internally driven movements contrast with externally driven movements, or movements directed by sensory cues, as the movements discussed above in relation to the PMV. Cells in the PMD fire 1–2 seconds before initiation of internally driven movements, suggesting that the PMD is involved with the selection and planning of self-selected behaviors. Lesions in the PMD diminish self-initiated (spontaneous) movements but spare goal-oriented (externally driven) movements.

Supplementary motor area

Supplementary motor area (area 6) is situated in the medial surface of the premotor cortex. Although inconclusive, evidence suggests that the supplementary motor area may be related to bimanual complex movements. Transcranial stimulation, PET, and fMRI studies demonstrate that the supplementary motor area is active when conducting complex, externally driven movement plans, and appears to direct distal finely controlled movements bilaterally. The number of errors was increased during execution of precisely timed movements from memory.

Motor Hierarchy

Motor control encompasses multiple levels, including cortical processing to select, plan, and initiate movement. Subcortical and brainstem circuitry integrates sensory input with motor output, constantly monitoring and refining the spatiotemporal conditions of the body schema. At the spinal level, where the motor plan is executed, sensory input is received, and reflexes, coordination, and patterned movement sequences are carried out. This arrangement constitutes what has become known as the motor hierarchy (Figure 10.21).

In the cortex, the highest level in the motor hierarchy, sensory areas generate a three-dimensional context for subsequent movement. Somatosensory, visual, and auditory inputs, all arising from peripheral receptors, are processed along with memories and emotional affects from limbic circuitry, to construct the self in time and space. This information establishes the starting conditions

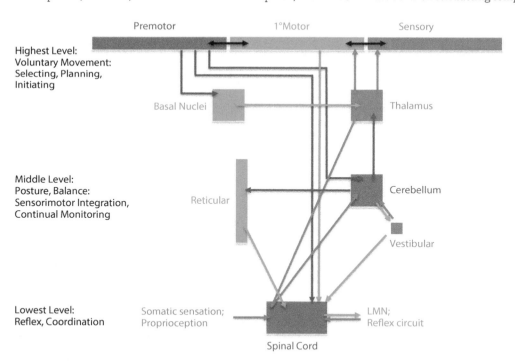

Highest Level:
Voluntary Movement:
Selecting, Planning,
Initiating

Middle Level:
Posture, Balance:
Sensorimotor Integration,
Continual Monitoring

Lowest Level:
Reflex, Coordination

Premotor · 1°Motor · Sensory

Basal Nuclei · Thalamus · Reticular · Cerebellum · Vestibular · Somatic sensation; Proprioception · LMN; Reflex circuit · Spinal Cord

FIGURE 10.21

The motor hierarchy. The highest level in the motor hierarchy is involved in movement selection, planning and initiation, and includes primary, premotor and supplementary cortices, basal nuclei and thalamus. Middle level structures regulate balance, posture, and sensorimotor integration through continual monitoring of movement. These include cerebellum, vestibular nuclei, and reticular formation. The lowest level, the spinal cord, emits motor axons and receives sensory input to regulate volitional and reflexive movements. (Image provided by Tony Mosconi, 2017.)

for generating volitional movements. The sensory association areas project to prefrontal cortex for integration of spatiotemporal readiness with selection of appropriate responses to internal or external conditions. Sensory and cognitive information projected to the premotor and supplementary motor areas develops the motor plan. Outputs to the cerebellum rectify the plan to ongoing sensorimotor conditions, and outputs to the basal nuclei refine and select the precise series of muscle contractions required to accomplish the motor goal. The primary motor cortex emits the perfected motor signal in the corticospinal/corticobulbar pathways to the lower motor neurons in the brainstem and spinal cord for ultimate expression in skeletal muscle contraction.

Brainstem centers are activated. These include the extrapyramidal systems: vestibulospinal, reticulospinal, and tectospinal tracts. The extrapyramidal pathways regulate balance, posture, and head and neck movement to direct the eyes. All of these functions are conducted mainly unconsciously. Some of the actions, such as righting reflexes, cannot be processed through the cerebral cortex because that delay could be catastrophic.

The lowest hierarchical level is the spinal cord (brainstem sensorimotor nuclei as well). At this level, CST axons monosynaptically activate α-motor neurons, the lower motor neurons that emit axons contributing to peripheral nerves that synapse on muscle fibers to produce twitch. Proprioceptors contribute a returning sensory limb to regulate muscle reflexes, including establishing muscle tone and signaling readiness for contraction. Somatic sensation, in addition to proprioception, is received in the spinal cord dorsal horn. What input is not engaged in local reflex circuits can be directed to the cerebellum on spinocerebellar pathways and processed at the unconscious level in the cerebellum to be reintegrated in the constantly evolving motor plan. Other sensory inputs are directed to the thalamus and somatosensory cortex for conscious sensory appreciation. This information is reintegrated in the sensory cortices and once again contributes to the modification of the motor signal.

Lesions in structures at the different levels in the motor hierarchy produce predictable and characteristic deficits. Primary motor cortex lesions produce contralateral deficits in fine motor control ranging from mild paresis to spasticity, clonus, hypertonicity, and hyperreflexia associated with the upper motor neuron syndrome. Damage in premotor and supplementary areas, as well as injuries in the posterior parietal cortex, produce various forms of apraxia. Basal nuclei lesions produce mainly contralateral deficits, although pure unilateral lesions are not the norm. Deficits from lesions in the basal nuclei produce resting tremors—uncontrolled (hyperkinetic) movement when none is desired. Other basal nuclei, when injured, produce hypokinetic or bradykinetic motor presentations (Parkinson's disease and other types of parkinsonism). Cerebellar lesions, on the other hand, produce ipsilateral signs, including ataxia (failure of coordinated muscle contraction), intention tremors, and hypotonia. Impairment of the brainstem extrapyramidal systems can have wide-ranging motor consequences. Impairments of balance are common, as is the loss of reflexes related to maintaining or regaining balance, diminished ability to react to sensory stimuli in peripersonal space, and possibly vertigo and dizziness. Deficiencies in eye movements and speech can also occur. Because upper motor neuron axons contribute lateral and ventral CST fascicles in the spinal cord, lesions there can also produce an upper motor neuron syndrome. Damage to lower motor neurons in the ventral horn, such as with poliomyelitis or amyotrophic lateral sclerosis, or damage to their peripheral

projections in the ventral roots, spinal nerves, and peripheral nerves, produce weakness or flaccid paralysis and reduction or abolition of reflexes and muscle tone. Recognizing the characteristic presentations produced by damage anywhere in the sensorimotor system, in order to make a differential diagnosis, is now an indispensible weapon in the arsenal of the doctor of physical therapy.

Motor Learning

Motor learning refers to development and modification of CNS circuits that integrate sensory and motor function to increase the efficiency, accuracy, and effectiveness of behaviors. Simple behaviors, such as reaching, are typically learned quickly with basic feedback sensory return. Learning complex skills, such as neurosurgery, requires extensive and intensive practice with tactile, visual, and cognitive feedback to modify and perfect multijoint, multistage movements for specialized function.

The circuitry for developing skilled behavior involves virtually all of the previous systems reviewed in this text, engaging a frontoparietal-striatal-cerebellar circuitry. Sensory input, especially tactile, vestibular, and visual, is assessed and assimilated into a three-dimensional spatial construct within which movement occurs. Conscious sensory inputs are processed through thalamus to primary sensory cortices and assessed further in association cortices such as the visual association cortex and posterior parietal cortex. Unconscious sensory input is processed in the cerebellum. The cerebellum acts as a difference engine, continually comparing the plan with the execution throughout the behavior. Basal nuclei also continually refine the motor output to limit errant movements and perfect the behavior. With increasing intensity of concentration (attention) and repetition, the spatial coordinates become more precise and refined and coordination of all of the individual movements and the sequence of complex motor behavior is perfected.

Motor learning loop

Recall the motor learning loop directed by output from the lateral zone (posterior lobe) cerebellar cortex. The brainstem circuit begins with output from the dentate nucleus projecting to the contralateral red nucleus. Red nucleus fibers descend to innervate the ipsilateral inferior olivary nucleus. Cells in that nucleus, comprising climbing fiber cerebellar inputs, decussate and enter the contralateral (original) cerebellum through the inferior cerebellar peduncle. When learning a new task, climbing fibers regulate (suppress) the excitatory effects of mossy fibers (mainly cortico-ponto-cerebellar inputs) on the Purkinje cells. Purkinje cells are inhibitory (regulatory) over the dentate nucleus neurons. Thus, when learning a new task, cerebellar output is freed (disinhibited), increasing the excitation of the contralateral thalamus and increasing overall movement. Motor learning requires repeated attempts (increased movement) to refine the execution of the task. As the behavior is perfected, the climbing fiber regulation of mossy fiber input is reduced; thus movements are curtailed, and only the appropriate ones are permitted.

Successful motor learning next integrates this cerebellar activity during task performance with activation of direct and indirect pathways through the basal nuclei. The direct pathway is said to increase movement, and the indirect pathway decreases movement. As we discussed previously (Chapter 8), both the direct and indirect pathways are concomitantly active. When learning a task, concurrent with the increase in cerebellar output promoting movement,

> **> Neuroplasticity**
> **Cortical adaptation in utero**
> We now appreciate how plastic our entire nervous system can be, from the period of intense pruning during infancy to the ability of even an older brain to learn and adapt to new challenges. A rare presentation of cerebral palsy in a young girl born with only one functioning hemisphere demonstrates exceptional embryonic plasticity. This patient had a congenital disruption in brain development during or before the seventh week of gestation, precluding the growth of her entire right hemisphere.
>
> One would expect her to have severe impairments due to the presence of only the left diencephalon and telencephalon, which did produce contralateral hemiparesis at birth. However, surprisingly, her visual field was nearly intact bilaterally. This information is normally carried on cranial nerve II from each eye, crossing at the optic chiasm to the contralateral lateral geniculate (LGN) of the thalamus, then finally areas V1–V3 in the occipital lobe for processing. Loss of the right diencephalon and cortex so early in her development set the stage for dramatic neuroplasticity.
>
> Functional MRI of her thalamus and cortex, combined with mapping of her visual fields with campimetry, allows the complexity of her neuroplastic response to be understood. During normal embryologic development, the cranial nerves grow from the eye to cross at the optic chiasm, in response to genetic cues. Decussation at the optic chiasm is a dance, with encoding at the retina setting the stage for the partnership and guiding molecular coding of the associated hemisphere, calling the nerve fibers to the proper location.
>
> In the instance of this patient, all the optic nerve fibers traveled to the left LGN, which was able to expand its role and provide retinotopic maps for both eyes. Finally, the cortical regions for visual perception had to be completely remapped to allow for precise function without confusion caused by the extra data. This neuroplasticity was reinforced after birth, as she began using this newly formed pathway for vision. Truly our capacity for neuroplasticity is expansive, and brings continued hope for neurorehabilitation.

the direct pathway effects are ascendant and the indirect pathway is subordinate, permitting freer movement. As the task is perfected, activity in the indirect pathway has greater effect. Movements are restricted to only the best motions that accomplish the behavior perfectly. Cerebellar, basal nuclear, and cortical circuitry is never disengaged, and with sensorimotor integration, behaviors can be developed, refined, and perfected to best accomplish motor goals.

As described, the posterior parietal cortex, in which temporospatial coordinates are constructed and maintained, emits profuse projections to the prefrontal cortex, to be integrated into controlled, appropriate, goal-oriented responses. Activity in the premotor cortex plans for and initiates the movement, innervating the primary motor cortex for projection to the spinal cord for regulated execution of the orderly sequence of muscle contractions. Supplementary motor cortex further contributes to refined complex bilateral hand movements.

To facilitate motor learning, complex movements are broken down into shorter sequences in a process referred to as chunking. Chunking dissects a long sequence of tiny subtle motions into fewer, more manageable sets of movements. Once the brain develops a successful solution to a problem, rather than devise many different approaches to address diverse conditions, it repeatedly employs the successful strategy; thus the brain chunks information to facilitate learning in numerous other situations, including memorizing, reading, and learning to speak.

Motor learning affects neuroplastic expansion of sensorimotor representations of body structures involved in the behavior. Increases in the area in the primary motor cortex have been well documented, as has expansion in premotor and supplementary motor cortical representations. These alterations, in combination with the identification of a movement map in primary motor cortex, may underlie the chunking of complex behaviors facilitating motor learning.

One final consideration related to motor learning after nervous system injury relates to the broad range of cortical centers involved in making coordinated movements. Because associative and cognitive centers are recruited for making appropriate, regulated movements, it is frequently difficult for patients after traumatic brain injury to perform two simultaneous behaviors. It is often necessary to determine whether gait anomalies are due to injury to cortical centers or to subcortical injuries involving, for example, the cerebellum or spinal cord. One easy test of dual task function is to walk with the patient and to try to carry on a conversation. Some patients tend to stop when they talk and cease to converse when walking. This is referred to as cortical gait and confidently diagnoses cortical impairment of gait over injury to the cerebellum, basal nuclei, or the spinal cord.

V ASSOCIATION AND COGNITION

By some accounts, nearly 80% of the human cerebral cortex is association cortex, and association cortices are by far best developed in primates. Most of the discussion so far in this text has centered on primary sensory and motor areas. Each sensory modality has its own primary cortical area, but as has been discussed, experiences are not actually derived in primary cortices. It is not until the data regarding the stimulus have been integrated within the greater experiential/memorial/emotional context that the sensation is experienced.

Sensory information passes from the bottom upward, originating in the periphery, ascending through the brainstem to the primary sensory cortices, then to the association cortices for experience. Each of the sensory cortices has specific association cortical areas that integrate the information delivered by its own sensory pathways, for example, secondary somatosensory cortex and visual association cortex. From the sensory association cortices, information is further processed in higher-order association cortical areas. Motor systems, in contrast, are organized from the top down. Association cortices integrating the sensory schema with the motor plan project to the primary motor cortex, then down to the spinal level and out to the periphery.

Parietal, temporal, and frontal cortices contain most of the higher-order association areas. Parietal association cortex processes internal and external sensory stimuli to create the body's spatiotemporal schema. Temporal association cortex identifies the specific features and significance of these stimuli. Frontal association cortex selects and plans appropriate responses to the stimuli. Visual association cortex selectively emphasizes visual inputs.

Two thalamic nuclei, the pulvinar and the dorsomedial (DM) nuclei, do not communicate directly with primary or secondary cortices. The pulvinar is in reciprocal communication with the temporal association areas, and the DM with frontal areas. Cortico-cortical inputs provide additional inputs to association areas, including intra- and interhemispheric projections. Thus, higher order association cortices process information that has already been processed in other cortical areas. Subcortical inputs from the midbrain and more caudal brainstem reticular formations introduce specific neurotransmitter circuits that are related to learning, motivation, and arousal, and, when impaired, lead to psychiatric disorders such as ADHD, depression, and addiction.

Lesions in Association Cortices

As is often the case, the functions of cortical areas can be deduced from the effects presented by patients with specifically identified lesions. Modern technology permits this type of examination in real-time rather than from autopsy. Damage to the parietal cortex can be expected to impair aspects of spatial representation. Because of extensive visual input to the construction of the body schema, these deficits often appear as deficits of attention. The condition resulting from parietal lobe injury, especially affecting the inferior parietal lobule, is called a neglect syndrome, often specified as visual neglect. Patients are unable to attend to objects, events, or even to portions of themselves in the affected space. They may even fail to identify a part of their own body in the neglected space, often vigorously denying it as their own. They might deny that they have perceived a noxious stimulus while actually withdrawing from it. In these patients, the sensorimotor functions remain intact; it is the processing of the information into experience that is impaired. It is notable that the neglect syndrome is nearly always associated with right parietal cortex lesions. This is because the right parietal cortex is dominant in establishing the body schema, whereas the left hemisphere function is dominant in language processing. Injury to the right parietal lobe abolishes spatial input from the left space, but with injury to the left parietal lobe, spatial coordinates remain intact in the right cortex and are spared.

The temporal association cortex processes visual information with memory. Injuries to the temporal association cortex produce deficits of recognition. Patients are unable to recognize and identify objects, people, or complex scenes in their visual field. The condition is called visual agnosia, the inability to interpret visual inputs, even while patients retain the ability to describe details of the scene. The impairments result from an interruption in processing along the ventral "what" stream. Visual agnosia appears in a variety of types and can result in the inability to perceive movement (akinetopsia), apperceptive visual agnosia (inability to identify shapes and to distinguish visual inputs), or associative visual agnosia (ability to describe shapes, but not to identify them). One particularly distressing type of agnosia is face blindness, prosopagnosia. Patients with lesions in the fusiform gyrus (primarily in the right hemisphere) are unable to recognize faces, even those of their loved ones or their own face. Patients often attempt to hide their impairment, learning to identify people by specific characteristics such as their sex, hair or eye color, notable gait, or clothing. Failing to recognize friends or mistakenly addressing strangers causes some people profound embarrassment and isolation.

The frontal association cortex, especially the prefrontal cortex, is perhaps the most significant area for creating one's "personality." Among even association cortices, the frontal area is best developed. Its functions are broad, affecting a person's character, decision making, self-control, and responses appropriate to conditions. In the case presented in Chapter 1, Phineas Gage suffered a devastating injury damaging his prefrontal cortices. After his physical recovery, his friends described the once mild-mannered, hard-working Gage as "no longer Gage." His personality devolved from polite and respectable to vulgar and irascible. He acted out without restraint, made increasingly poor decisions, became bumptious, and made unrealistic grandiose plans. In 1935, A. Egas Moniz performed the first frontal lobotomy, a Nobel Prize–winning medical approach to cure intractable psychiatric disturbances. It involved detaching the prefrontal cortex by alcohol injection (later by using an orbitoclast, a metal rod inserted through the roof of the orbit, used to sever prefrontal fiber connections) to ameliorate the most severe presentations. Lobotomy did improve the behaviors, but, tragically, with elimination of prefrontal association cortical circuitry, patients eventually came to behave "as mental invalids and drooling zombies." Fortunately, in the early 1950s, Thorazine was developed as a noninvasive "pharmacological lobotomy," and frontal lobotomies are now extremely rare.

Cognition

Every moment we are bombarded with waves of stimuli competing for our attention, requiring continual assessment and reassessment, and instigating behavioral responses. Our experiences influence our decisions and inform our responses. The effects of our responses are catalogued and incorporated into our personal body of knowledge, our memories, to be retrieved as necessary. The term *cognition*, vague though it is, encompasses our knowledge, our ability to extrapolate and deduce novel information from previous information, to access that knowledge to direct future behavior, our thoughts. Cognition is complex and remains poorly defined and understood. Still, cognition has become part of the common jargon of neuroscientists exploring the way external and internal stimuli are identified, interpreted in the spatiotemporal context, and ranked on their significance in order to make appropriate behavioral responses. As this text is designed for the future health care clinician, in this section, we limit the discussion of cognition to human behavior and performance in rehabilitation settings after nervous system damage. Although it is now possible to measure some neural aspects of the cognitive process in real time with imaging technology, the main method for describing and measuring cognition in the clinical setting is through observation of behavior. A discussion of cognition is facilitated by dividing it into three parts: attention, memory, and learning.

Attention

Life in the modern human world is vastly complex, filled not only with a constant barrage of external stimuli, lights, sounds, tactile and olfactory assaults, but also by a multitude of internal cues concerning energy or metabolic needs (hunger or thirst), discomfort, or pain. These concerns are processed in higher-order centers to produce emotional responses such as anticipation, dread, excitement, and love, which cause physiological changes that are reprocessed as new internal stimuli. The insistent recursion of this description is

Frontiers in Research
Robotics

Robots are machines designed to perform complex tasks. Their use in rehabilitation is promising; however, the high cost during these early stages of development makes them prohibitive for most people, as does their typically large size and added weight. The ability of robots to read data mimics our own body's ability to receive and contextually analyze incoming sensory information. These data can be programmed for use by a robot to trigger a response, such as stabilizing the knee when a predetermined amount of weight is loaded through a robotic knee joint. Therapists are abile to program the robot to make a proportional response, which is particularly helpful in recreating the highly specific range of normal human motion. Additionally, much of neurologic rehabilitation depends upon cortical activation to drive neuroplasticity after central nervous system damage. A cortically triggered robot could become a foundation for neurologic rehabilitation in the very near future. To this end, researchers are developing sophisticated technology for rehabilitation, and testing results with animal models of CNS damage and in humans after acquired brain injury.

One novel application of multiple technologies by Nicolelis and colleagues in Brazil is showing exciting early results among patients with spinal cord injury. The study originally sought to determine the value of a brain–machine interface to improve walking in a population of chronic spinal cord–injured individuals. This research focused on people who had sustained complete spinal cord injury (with no sacral nerve function) years previously. It has long been considered that this population is stable and no longer capable of neurologic recovery, so any changes are unlikely to be due to spontaneous recovery. This population has also been shown to be responsive to intensive locomotor training, with improved ability to function despite absence of neurological improvement in sensation or voluntary muscle contraction below the level of injury. These patients have a great need for better rehabilitation programs to maximize their recovery.

The study incorporated several factors that brilliantly recreate normal movement: cognitively directed motion, specific and realistic sensory feedback during movement, and task-specific gait training in an upright posture. This was possible due to thoughtful application of modern technology, with subjects first working with virtual reality headsets showing an avatar of first-person perspective during leg motion; they could look down at their legs and see them move. Brain mapping during this process created an individual pattern that was then programmed into a robotic gait trainer that used the patients' brain waves to generate a robotic-assisted walking pattern. Additional sensory feedback was provided in real time, providing normally expected information such as the sensation of weight bearing on the ground. This information was sent to the subjects' arms, as leg sensation had been lost. After a year of training, every single subject had changes in sensation and volitional motor control below the level of injury. Most noteworthy and life changing was the improvement in bowel and bladder control, which was completely absent at the start of the study. This study fundamentally changes our understanding of recovery after central nervous system damage, influencing the field of neurorehabilitation as powerfully as the discoveries of central pattern generators in the spinal cord and the process of neuroplasticity in normal development and recovery.

---

dizzying. How, then, is a person to focus on the imperatives and disregard the incidentals? Fortunately, we can selectively process relevant information at the expense of irrelevant in a complex behavior called attention. Clinically, attention is measured behaviorally by noting a patient's ability to sustain focus on a task during brief screening tests. More complex attentional testing is sometimes necessary, such as screening for sports-related concussion. Attention requires each individual to process sensory information at several levels and is described in three parts: alerting, orienting, and executive functioning. Alerting, as the name implies, is a network for maintaining a general level of responsiveness. The orienting network controls the process of selection, including distractor suppression and noise reduction. Finally the executive network acts at the level of post-sensory representation, and is engaged when there is competition among stimuli.

Attention can be categorized as sustained or alternating. Sustained attention, also called vigilance, is the ability to maintain focus over a long period, attending to an observation or task until it is completed. Sustained focus underlies activities such as learning and building motor skills. Alternating attention allows the movement of focus between different stimuli that require different routes of central processing. Contrary to the opinions of a vast majority of teenage drivers, it is not possible to "multitask" driving, eating, talking, and texting. Neuroscience now recognizes this as impossible. The behavior that appears to be competently accomplishing several things at the same time is actually alternating attention switching among brief bouts of attention on the diverse acts. Too often, under these circumstances, the ultimate failure of the overlapping behaviors ends up involving insurance companies and prolonged periods of loss of driving privileges. Although many people are able to drive and carry on a conversation with a passenger in the car without significant degradation of performance, the ability to safely alternate attention becomes increasingly more challenging the more complex or abstract the additional task. When mobile phones became widely available, more people began driving and speaking on the phone. The original increase in accidents under these conditions was initially assumed to be due to the dual task challenge of using motor skills to drive concurrent with verbal and manual skills to use the phone, so it became illegal to drive and use the phone unless it was hands-free. However, this did not reduce the accident rates significantly, and after more research it was discovered that the task was too abstract (for example, one maintains a mental image of the person on the other side of the phone), thus making the cognitive demand too high.

There is currently an increasing effort to map the neural pathways for attention. Our previous discussion about the influence exerted by the rostral reticular formation (the reticular activating system) illustrated that neural processing of attention extends beyond the cortex. Brainstem modulatory systems project to the posterior parietal cortex, the neural substrate for sensory integration and visuospatial attention. Prefrontal cortex, in conjunction with fast and slow visual processing mediated in the angular gyrus in the posterior parietal cortex, is also central to alternating attention, and lesions in the prefrontal cortex severely impair the ability to rapidly switch behaviors. Damage to the pulvinar, which has reciprocal connections with the visual cortex, impairs attention to visual cues. Clearly, as with most higher-order cortical functions, control of attention is multifactorial and still in need of elucidation of basic circuitry and patterns of cortical activation.

Memory

Attention directs our perception toward those objects, events, and conditions that are of significance to our existence, prehistorically to our very survival. Information garnered by focused attention is encoded and stored in our memory for retrieval at a later time. It is our memory that enables us to learn language, recognize members of our family, and maintain personal continuity over our lifetime; it gives us our identity. Some loss of memory is common as we age. However, pathological memory loss, as with Alzheimer's disease or amnesia, produces tragic changes in relationships, as patients lose their ability to recognize family and friends, and ultimately lose their own identity.

As complex as memory is, it is not surprising that there are several types of memory and multiple cortical areas dedicated to the function. Sensory memory relates to the acquisition of the data that are to be incorporated into the individual's body of knowledge. Sensory association cortices maintain this information, effectively passing it along to short-term memory (STM) for consolidation into long-term memory (LTM).

STM is initiated when incoming information reaches the hippocampal formation and is relayed to the prefrontal cortex. The acquisition of the incoming information is directed by attention to the internal and external stimuli. The total volume of information that can be managed by the STM system is limited. It was originally described as the "magic seven, plus or minus 2," meaning that seven items could be held in STM before it was either processed into LTM or lost. The "magic number" has more recently been downgraded to about four. To increase this number and hasten information acquisition, people chunk related information. Chunking is an effective way to increase overall speed and volume of information processing and was already described with motor learning. The duration for which STM can store information is limited, lasting no longer than ~20 seconds; thus the information processed in STM relates to those items about which the individual is currently thinking.

Often considered synonymous with STM, working memory is similarly limited in volume and duration of retention. The major difference between working and short-term memory is in what is done with the information. STM briefly stores items, whereas the information in working memory is manipulated. Processing information through working memory guides decision making. Studies have shown that working memory is processed in the dorsolateral prefrontal cortex. Spatial tasks engage the right cortex while verbal and object information is processed in working memory in the left hemisphere.

STM is initially processed in the hippocampal formation. The hippocampus, within the inferior medial temporal lobe, is essential for consolidation of short-term memories into long-term storage. Incoming sensory inputs arrive partially processed through circuits in the basal nuclei, thalamus, and cortex. Association cortices input to the hippocampus, and the information then enters Papez's circuit.

The fornix carries the information to the mammillary bodies in the hypothalamus. Mammillary body output projects to the anterior nucleus via the prominent mammillothalamic tract. Anterior nuclei output innervates the cingulate gyrus that then contributes to the return circuit to the hippocampus via the cingulum fiber pathway. One additional function of the hippocampus is to then distribute information in LTM to various cortical centers.

Once in LTM, different types of information are processed in different cortical and subcortical areas. Unlike STM, memories in LTM persist, sometimes over a lifetime. Elderly persons can remember events from their childhood. Storage of LTM has long been associated with changes in synaptic function. Unconscious rehearsal through Papez's circuit, mainly taking place during sleep, seats the information deeply in the individual's body of knowledge by establishing new synapses and, through synaptic plasticity, by modifying presynaptic neurotransmitter release and postsynaptic receptor density and distribution to increase the facility of firing at the synapse, thus making the circuit more stable through repeated activity. This process is referred to as Hebbian learning and described colloquially by the phrase "neurons that fire together wire together." More recent studies have contradicted this concept based on observations that all synapses function essentially the same way and that they turn over rapidly and constantly. Synapses established during learning will disappear, yet the memory persists. The new theory argues that, in addition to synaptic plasticity, LTMs are seated through changes in the nucleus and altered protein manufacture.

Whatever the mechanism, information stored in LTM is associated with stable and (sometimes) permanent changes in circuitry in several cortical sites. LTM can be described as either nondeclarative or declarative. Nondeclarative memories are not accessed through conscious recall; instead, the memories are incorporated into ingrained behaviors, as with playing a learned piece of music on a piano. This type of memory is learned over time by repetition until the individual movements are virtually automatic. Nondeclarative memory is often referred to as implicit memory, and it is unconsciously recovered from previous experience with the task. One does not consciously remember all of the movements associated with riding a bike; after learning how, one simply jumps on and rides. Implicit memory is also known as procedural memory. The movements are coded by the cerebellum and basal nuclei and are representations of motor learning.

Declarative memory can be accessed consciously and includes information regarding facts, events, and recollection that can be described verbally. Again, there are different categories of declarative memory: semantic and episodic (sometimes equated with autobiographical). Semantic memory includes facts and concepts that are part of the individual's common body of knowledge; colors, numbers, state capitals, and other facts garnered over their lifetime, but not associated with any experiential context. This is more complex than it might seem on the surface. Semantic memory is integrated into general cognition so that when hearing the word *dog*, for example, one can recognize both a border collie and a miniature pincer as dogs (Figure 10.22). Additionally, one can recognize a painting or cartoon as a dog and even recognize it as a portrait of a specific dog. This carries over to the ability to recognize an abstract dog on a sign. To carry the example further, one can extrapolate the term *dog* to recognize a hot dog.

Episodic memory incorporates autobiographical memories of people, places, and events in temporal, physical, and emotional

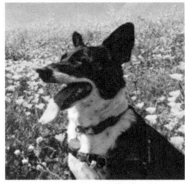
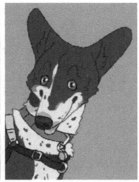
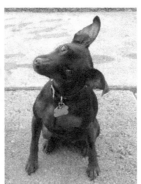

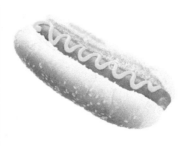

FIGURE 10.22

Semantic memory. Semantic memory allows us to generalize the word dog, and enables us to recognize a dog in multiple contexts. (Images are public domain, except sketch of Salem by Jamie Graham, photos of authors' dogs, Salem and Toby, 2017.)

acetylcholinergic neurons there and throughout the cerebral cortex. Frontotemporal lobar degeneration is related to cell loss in the frontal and temporal cortices. It presents as loss of autobiographical memory and dementia. Parkinson's disease, with its progressive degeneration of basal nuclei, particularly the substantia nigra pars compacta, impairs working and spatial memory.

Bilateral injury to the temporal cortex produces a profound loss of the ability to seat most new long-term memories. The celebrated case of the patient known for decades as H.M., after his death identified as Henry Molaison, was tremendously influential to elucidation of mechanisms of memory. He had bilateral temporal lobe resection to ameliorate debilitating seizures possibly produced by a head injury when he was a child. Although his seizures were controlled, H.M. was institutionalized because he developed a severe case of anterograde amnesia. Anterograde amnesia is the loss of ability to seat new LTM, compared with retrograde amnesia, where the patient is unable to recall events and people from their past. H.M. retained his memories of his life before the surgery but was evermore unable to establish new memories. He met his physicians for the first time every time they visited. His procedural memories and working memory remained intact. In fact, he was able to learn and improve in certain simple tasks, but every time he was tested, he insisted that it was the first time he attempted the task. His case reinforced the notion that the temporal lobe was essential for memory consolidation but that LTM episodic memory, working memory, and procedural memory were processed in different cortical areas. Henry Molaison's contribution to cognitive neuroscience cannot be overestimated.

Learning

Memory underpins learning, forming the basic body of knowledge for the individual. We learn, in great part, through practice (especially for motor behaviors) and rehearsal. Demonstration of learning is through changes in physical or intellectual behavior. We apply the new knowledge to new scenarios, and the application differentiates learning from remembering. Our patients may remember to lock the brakes on their wheelchair after repetition and practice, but we only consider the behavior learned when they can transfer this information to a new surface or integrate the behavior without being reminded.

context. This type of memory can also be used to mentally place one's self into situations in the past, to project oneself into the future, or even insert oneself into imaginary or fanciful circumstances. Episodic memory, therefore, is central to various theories of the mind. Emotional aspects of the events can also drive episodic learning, such as persistent fear of dogs after being bitten as a child.

Separate but related cortical areas are involved in processing STM and consolidating LTM (Figure 10.23). We have previously mentioned that procedural memories rely on processing through the basal nuclei and cerebellum, and these are seated deeply so that they do not depend on conscious recall to be activated. Also, input of information to STM passes first through temporal lobe structures, including the hippocampal formation, and reverberated through Papez's circuit. Consolidation of STM into LTM also relies on circuitry through the prefrontal cortex, and working memory more specifically in the dorsolateral prefrontal areas. In addition to housing the hippocampus, the temporal lobe processes a number of types of declarative memory. Its association with the visuotemporal "what" stream, the temporal lobe, is essential for recognition and associated with episodic (autobiographical) memory. In the anterior pole of the temporal lobe, the amygdala processes emotionally charged items or events. The dog bite elicits fear; recollection of the first kiss stirs feelings of nostalgia and a certain pleasure; recalling the loss of a loved one evokes grief.

Ascribing specific functions to these separate areas largely has been the result of analyses of patients with lesions that produced identifiable memory perturbations. Alzheimer's disease is well known to affect the hippocampal formation, with significant loss of

VI CORTICAL PROCESSING OF LANGUAGE

Arguably, human language is one of our most significant evolutionary and social developments. Our language is open ended, unlike those of nonhuman animals, employing a finite number of sounds (or symbols or gestures) to express a nearly infinite scope of concrete and abstract; factual and fanciful; past, present, and predictive

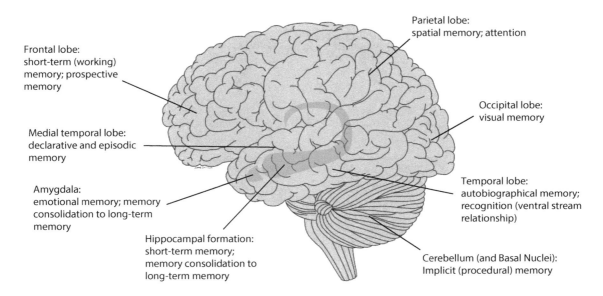

FIGURE 10.23

Cortical memory areas. Brain areas concerned with encoding long-term memories. (Image provided by Jamie Graham and Tony Mosconi, 2017.)

communication. Also, unlike nonhuman species, our language is culturally specific rather than species specific. English speakers are able to learn the languages of Italians or Germans or Japanese, and each uses similar, albeit arbitrary, syntactical and grammatical rules. Examination of the development of language has spanned the investigational gamut from paleontology to creationism. Clearly this discussion is beyond the bounds of this text; however, here we examine the neural mechanisms underlying the processing and production of language in humans, and we emphasize the generation of spoken language, as well as the most common impairments of speech production and language comprehension seen clinically.

Historical Models of Speech Production

Speech has long been considered to be a product of activity in the dominant hemisphere. By most accounts, more than 95% of right-handed people and over 70% of left-handers are left-brain dominant. Since the end of the 19th century, three structures in the left hemisphere were historically recognized to comprise the speech centers, mainly on the basis of postmortem examination of the brains of individuals with characteristic post-injury speech deficits. Broca described a locus in the posterior part of the inferior frontal gyrus (Broca's area; areas 44 and 45) as the site of injury in people with poor articulation, poor repetition, difficulty "finding the right words," and difficulty producing fluid speech. Patients instead offered only the content words, without verbal embellishment, called telegraphic speech. A patient might say, "Drove, car, store, food," for "I drove in my car to the grocery store to buy food for dinner." Comprehension is usually relatively good compared to the difficulties with verbal expression. This condition has come to be called Broca's aphasia, although some of the difficulties presented are related to apraxia of speech, difficulty producing the movements required for speech.

Wernicke identified patients whose speech difficulties were related to the inability to comprehend speech. His patients had relatively fluent speech, but their speech was littered with sound and word substitutions that rendered it unintelligible. Although their thought processes were generally intact, they could not understand what was being communicated to them, through speech, writing, or gestures, and also did not appreciate that their speech lacked meaning. Wernicke's postmortem examinations revealed common damage to an area in the posterior part of the superior temporal gyrus, since called Wernicke's area (area 22); and the deficit, Wernicke's aphasia.

The major circuit connecting the anterior region, Broca's area, with the posterior region, Wernicke's area, is the arcuate fasciculus, forming a conspicuous inferior part of the superior longitudinal fasciculus. Small lesions of the arcuate fasciculus can produce conduction aphasia. People with conduction aphasia have relatively good auditory comprehension and good motor speech production, with difficulty repeating phrases, especially complex ones; they display frequent errors in spontaneous speech such as phonemic paraphasia (for example, replacing *tapewriter* for *typewriter*). Transpositions in sentences and use of neologisms are called jargon aphasia or "word salad." These are sometimes humorous, as with those of the famous Oxford fellow and preacher, William Spooner, who once told a lazy student, "You have tasted a whole worm." Patients with conduction aphasia are aware of their errors but have difficulty preventing them while speaking. Of note, this behavior, paraphasia, is common among neurologically intact people under duress, such as when upset, tired, or anxious.

Current Models of Speech

Modern speech theories have largely abandoned the idea of control by those three structures, in favor of a network of areas with broader inclusion of expanded territories and subcortical centers. Current opinions no longer rely on information gleaned from postmortem anatomical correlation with patient presentation. Instead,

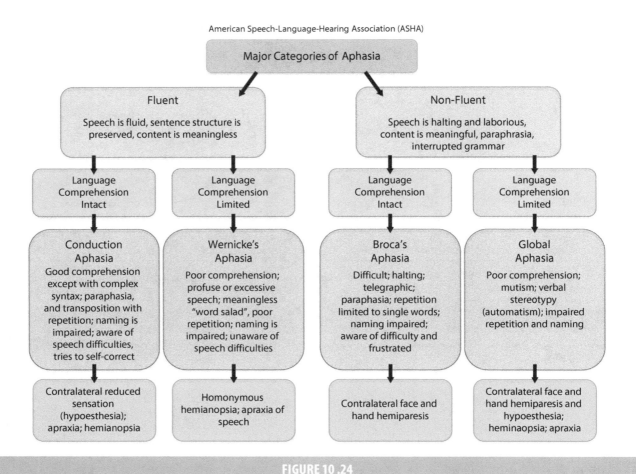

American Speech-Language-Hearing Association (ASHA)

Major Categories of Aphasia

Fluent

Speech is fluid, sentence structure is preserved, content is meaningless

Non-Fluent

Speech is halting and laborious, content is meaningful, paraphrasia, interrupted grammar

Language Comprehension Intact

Language Comprehension Limited

Language Comprehension Intact

Language Comprehension Limited

Conduction Aphasia

Good comprehension except with complex syntax; paraphasia, and transposition with repetition; naming is impaired; aware of speech difficulties, tries to self-correct

Wernicke's Aphasia

Poor comprehension; profuse or excessive speech; meaningless "word salad", poor repetition; naming is impaired; unaware of speech difficulties

Broca's Aphasia

Difficult; halting; telegraphic; paraphasia; repetition limited to single words; naming impaired; aware of difficulty and frustrated

Global Aphasia

Poor comprehension; mutism; verbal stereotypy (automatism); impaired repetition and naming

Contralateral reduced sensation (hypoesthesia); apraxia; hemianopsia

Homonymous hemianopsia; apraxia of speech

Contralateral face and hand hemiparesis

Contralateral face and hand hemiparesis and hypoesthesia; heminaopsia; apraxia

FIGURE 10.24

Classification of aphasia. Guidelines for categorizing aphasia (Modified from the American Speech-Language-Hearing Association, 2017; http://www.asha.org).

they are based on methods of examination not available to Broca or Wernicke, such as MRI, diffusion tensor MRI, fMRI, and transcranial magnetic stimulation (TMS), which are noninvasive and performed on living subjects. Speech language production difficulties, called aphasia, may be categorized into fluent and nonfluent types (Figure 10.24). These types are further divided clinically by amount of language comprehension into fluent conductive and Wernicke's aphasia, or nonfluent Broca's and global aphasia.

Broca's area still comprises a significant part of the anterior cortical speech center (Figure 10.25). Anatomically, Broca's area is situated in proximity to the face, tongue, and larynx representation in the primary motor cortex, structures that clearly are related to producing verbal sounds. Neuroimaging studies support an expanded role for Broca's area to include production of meaningful gestures related to or accompanying speech. This could explain why patients who use sign language for communication have difficulties after injuring Broca's area. Increased detail from imaging and TMS studies suggest that Broca's area is not involved in the actual production of speech sounds. Rather, it acts as a center for integration of the sensorimotor and cognitive network serving speech production. This may explain why some studies have found Broca's area to be quiescent during or prior to articulation, and a lesion specifically confined to Broca's area fails to produce an expressive aphasia.

The motor-speech region is now expanded to include the insula, premotor, and supplementary motor areas, and part of the middle frontal and inferior precentral gyri. Lesions to the insula can result in apraxia of speech (difficulty making the sounds of speech not due to muscular malfunction) and aphasia. The symptoms are even more severe when the damage expands to injure more of these cortical areas surrounding Broca's area. Some researchers suggest the term *Broca's territory* to include all of these anterior structures, and injury to them is collectively referred to as anterior or motor aphasia.

Posterior cortical sites surrounding Wernicke's area (suggesting the name *Wernicke's territory*), related to sensory processing of information related to speech, have also been enlarged to extend around the posterior end of the lateral fissure, including the supramarginal gyrus and the angular gyrus, extending to include middle and inferior temporal lobe regions. These latter two centers together form Geschwind's territory, named for the man who first predicted their relationship to speech. Some researchers are promoting the term *Wernicke's territory* to include the greater area surrounding area 22.

The traditional role assigned to Wernicke's area is receptive (sensory) speech, understanding the words and gestures associated with language. It lies in close proximity to primary and association auditory cortices, and in relationship with visual cortices, Wernicke's

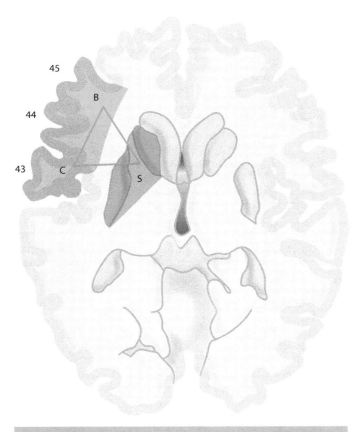

FIGURE 10.25

Cerebral structures concerned with language output and articulation. Broca's area; pre- and postcentral gyri; striatum. Areas 43, 44, and 45 are Brodmann cytoarchitectonic areas. A lesion in any one of the components of this output network (B, C, or S) can produce a mild and transient Broca's aphasia. Large lesions, damaging all three components, produce severe, persistent Broca's aphasia with sparse, labored, agrammatic speech but well-preserved comprehension. (Used with permission from Dr. Andrew Kertesz.)

area is optimally situated to receive and integrate sensory inputs from various forms of language and to integrate them into the ability to generate coherent responses through speech, writing, or gestures.

Analyses using TMS over Wernicke's area in the dominant hemisphere have demonstrated its function at the level of individual word resolution. In linguistics, "ambiguous" words, words that have many meanings when related out of context, have both dominant and subordinate meanings. For example, the dominant (most frequently associated) meaning of the ambiguous word *pitcher* would be "container." Its subordinate meaning would be to "mound," referring to the sport of baseball. Wernicke's area in the dominant hemisphere processes and selects dominant meanings for words, in contrast to the selection of subordinate meanings in the homologous region in the contralateral, nondominant cortex. Injury to the dominant hemisphere produces more severe deficits in receptive speech; lesions to the contralateral side produce more

subtle language difficulties, such as inability to comprehend jokes, metaphors, or double entendre.

The inferior temporal lobe is related to processing language in terms of integrating auditory input within a broader scheme of semantic comprehension, converting the sensory input into experiential and verbal context. In this way, the visual "what" stream is integrated into the sensory processing of language, providing a mechanism that could underlie the inability to name objects (anomia) or faces (prosopagnosia) with lesions in the inferior occipitotemporal cortex. A two-pathway hypothesis for language processing reminiscent of the dorsal and ventral visual streams has recently emerged that takes into account both the expanded array of involved cortical structures and the greater anatomical and functional detail of the arcuate fasciculus described by diffusion tensor MRI.

The arcuate fasciculus provides reciprocal communication between Broca's and Wernicke's areas. It is a prominent part of the superior longitudinal fasciculus, extending from the temporal lobe, around the posterior end of the lateral fissure, and passing anteriorly into the frontal lobe. Diffusion tensor MRI tractography suggests that this dorsal portion conforms to the classical description of the direct connections, between premotor cortices around Broca's territory and the superior temporal cortices around Wernicke's territory, made by the arcuate fasciculus. This pathway coordinates sensorimotor construction of language articulation: the selection of appropriate words and the generation of appropriate sounds to make those words.

A second, indirect portion of the arcuate fasciculus passes parallel and lateral to the direct fibers. This contribution consists of anterior and posterior portions. The anterior segment provides communication between the frontoparietal areas around Broca's territory with the inferior parietal cortex (Geschwind's territory). The posterior segment connects the inferior parietal cortex with Wernicke's territory. Indirect circuitry, through communication with higher-level association cortices, integrates language comprehension with the circuits that produce semantic expression.

Including Geschwind's territory into the language circuitry seems intuitive when examining the functions and anatomical disposition of its component supramarginal and angular gyri. These two areas integrate somatosensory and visual inputs into the auditory and semantic comprehension circuits. The ability to interpret the symbols of language through visual (letters on a page) or tactile (Braille dot patterns) recognition of characters, or auditory (spoken alphabet), can be explained through these connections. Lesions of the supramarginal and angular gyri create difficulties in writing (dysgraphia/agraphia), often including difficulties reading or understanding speech (aphasias), difficulty with mathematics (dyscalculia/acalculia), finger agnosia, and left–right disorientation. This cluster of symptoms is called Gerstmann syndrome, and it is often the result of a stroke in the parieto-occipito-temporal junction.

VII   RESPONSE TO INJURY

The study of neuroscience is essential for practicing clinicians. In a professional program, future coursework will cover clinical application of this material in greater detail, along with practical lab-based techniques for examination and treatment. The next section offers a brief overview of CNS response to injury. We present only a sample of the numerous ways the brain can suffer damage.

Acquired Brain Injury

Acquired brain injury includes all nontraumatic brain injuries caused by tumor (neoplasm), excess CSF and increased intracranial pressure (hydrocephalus), and hemorrhagic or ischemic stroke. Conversely, traumatic brain injury is caused by an external force that, either directly (for example, a blow to the head) or indirectly (as with a whiplash injury) damages delicate nervous tissue inside the cranial vault. Neoplasms and cerebral palsy are described below; both hemorrhagic and ischemic strokes were previously described in Chapter 2, Vascular Supply of the Central Nervous System, and are briefly reviewed next.

Stroke

Stroke is one of the leading causes of death after heart disease and cancer. A stroke describes an ischemic or hemorrhagic event by which the brain is transiently or permanently affected by lack of oxygen and nutrients. This usually occurs when a blood vessel is obstructed by a clot or bursts (Figure 10.26). The FAST acronym (facial drooping, arm weakness, speech difficulties, and time to call 911) is used to recognize the onset of stroke and get treatment immediately.

An ischemic infarction (an area of tissue death due to lack of oxygen) is the most common type of stroke. About 85% of strokes are ischemic. Ischemic stroke is usually as a result of cerebrovascular disease and associated with interference with the hemodynamic flow of blood by emboli. Disorders of the heart such as atrial fibrillation, ischemic heart disease, heart valve disease, and infective endocarditis are contributors to a smaller percentage of ischemic strokes.

Symptoms of ischemic stroke are variable and depend on the location and extent of the lesion (Figure 10.27). Occlusion of the middle cerebral artery presents with contralateral mono- or hemiparesis, contralateral hemisensory defect, and may include transient monocular blindness of a defect in vision, usually a contralateral hemianopsia. If the insult occurs on the dominant side (Broca's or Wernicke's area) it may be associated with aphasia. Occlusion of the anterior cerebral artery is associated with contralateral motor and sensory deficits, but also affects cognition and gait apraxia.

Ischemic strokes of the vertebrobasilar system are usually associated with severe vertigo, nausea, and headache. The vertigo typically lasts only for a few minutes. A small branch of the anterior inferior cerebellar artery supplies the inner ear, and sudden hearing loss is characteristic of vertebrobasilar involvement. Other signs and symptoms include ataxia, nystagmus, decreased pain and temperature discrimination, and diplopia due to gaze palsies, the extent of the ocular involvement determined by the location of the lesion.

Ischemic events are classified according to the time course and the outcome of the event. A transient ischemic attack (TIA) describes the temporary reduction of blood flow, creating fully reversible and focal neurological deficits. TIAs are sometimes called ministrokes. The onset is very fast and symptoms of the TIA usually lasts about 2–15 minutes. Symptoms may present as temporary numbness of the arm or one side of the face and difficulty speaking or reading. A TIA may cause a temporary, painless loss of vision. Known as amaurosis fugax, TIAs are considered to be a warning of impending stroke and should always be further investigated.

The second classification of ischemic stroke is that of reversible neurological deficit. This describes an area with focal ischemia that improves within 72 hours. The third classification describes the cerebral infarction, with stereotypical deficits of a more permanent nature.

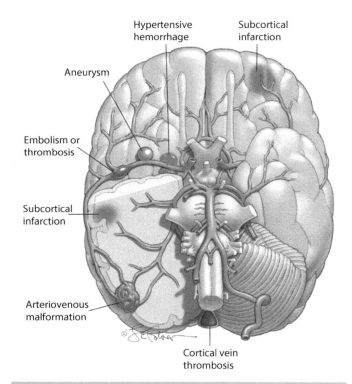

FIGURE 10.26

Types of strokes. Illustrations of a brain showing various types of strokes seen in pregnancy: (1) subcortical infarction (preeclampsia), (2) hypertensive hemorrhage, (3) aneurysm, (4) embolism or thrombosis in middle cerebral artery, (5) arteriovenous malformation, and (6) cortical vein thrombosis. (Reproduced with permission from Neurological Disorders. In: Cunningham F, et al, eds. *Williams Obstetrics*, Twenty-Fourth Edition New York, NY: McGraw-Hill; 2013).

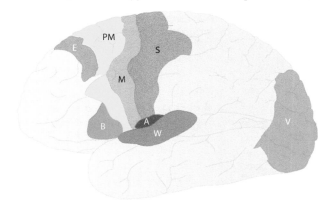

FIGURE 10.27

Symptoms of ischemic stroke. Brain areas commonly resulting in stroke syndrome deficits: E is frontal eye field, PM is premotor, M is primary motor, S is primary sensory, V is visual, B is Broca's, W is Wernicke's, and A is primary auditory. (Reproduced with permission from Jacobson FL, Hsu L. Neurologic Imaging. In: McKean SC, et al, eds. *Principles and Practice of Hospital Medicine*, 2e New York, NY: McGraw-Hill, 2017).

Hemorrhagic stroke is associated with intracerebral or subarachnoid hemorrhage; about 15% of strokes are due to this type of injury. This type of stroke has a higher mortality rate than ischemic stroke. The blood creates swelling and increased pressure in the brain. The risk factors for hemorrhagic stroke include smoking, hypertension, oral contraceptives, alcohol, pregnancy, and drug abuse. Further complications of hemorrhagic stroke include rebleeding and cerebral ischemia as a result of the degrading blood cells.

Intracerebral hemorrhage occurs when a blood vessel bursts in brain tissue, and is associated with uncontrolled high blood pressure. A genetic arteriovenous malformation in the brain may start to bleed.

Subarachnoid hemorrhage is most commonly caused by a ruptured aneurysm but may also be caused by an arteriovenous malformation. The most common location for aneurysms is at the distal internal carotid and the middle cerebral artery. About 4% of people have unruptured aneurysms smaller than 12 mm, and they are just slightly more prevalent in men. Rupture of an aneurysm is associated with very severe headache, nausea and vomiting, and neck pain or stiffness. Additional causes of hemorrhagic events include trauma, anticoagulants, and coagulation disorders.

Neoplasms

A mass is considered anything that takes up space in the brain or spinal cord, which may include a tumor, blood, or even cerebral spinal fluid. A neoplasm ("new growth") is abnormal tissue growth that creates a mass, called a tumor. Tumors are named for tissue of origin (for example astrocytoma, as seen in Figure 10.28), anatomical location, and benign (noncancerous) or malignant progression. Brain tumors may be primary, arising from brain tissue (Figure 10.29); or secondary, metastatic (spreading) from a tumor located in other tissues (Figure 10.30). The World Health Organization grades brain tumor prognosis in four tiers based on the presence or absence of certain properties indicating

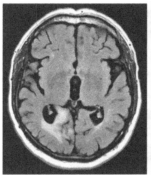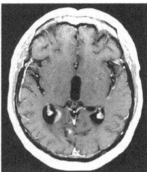

FIGURE 10.29

Primary central nervous system neoplasm. Primary central nervous system lymphoma. Left: Axial T2-FLAIR MRI showing hyperintensity in the right periatrial white matter, without mass effect. Right: Contrast-enhanced MRI reveals two foci of nodular parenchymal enhancement. (Reproduced with permission from Intracranial Neoplasms and Paraneoplastic Disorders. In: Ropper AH, et al, eds. *Adams and Victor's Principles of Neurology*, 11eNew York, NY: McGraw-Hill; 2015).

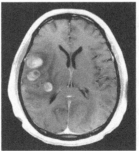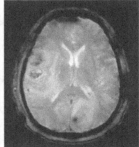

FIGURE 10.30

Metastatic neoplasm in brain. Contrast-enhanced MRI (left) showing multiple metastases from renal cell carcinoma. Note the extensive hypointense edema surrounding each lesion. The right image is a gradient echo MRI in which blood products appear hypointense (dark). This sequence can aid in detection of small or nonenhancing hemorrhagic metastases, such as the lesion in the left occipital lobe. (Reproduced with permission from Intracranial Neoplasms and Paraneoplastic Disorders. In: Ropper AH, et al, eds. *Adams and Victor's Principles of Neurology*, 11eNew York, NY: McGraw-Hill; 2015).

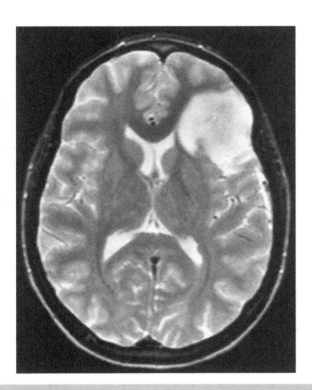

FIGURE 10.28

Tumor named for tissue of origin. Astrocytoma of the left frontal lobe; the T2-weighted MRI shows an infiltrating tumor with minimal mass effect and mild edema. The degree of contrast enhancement is variable but most often less than glioblastoma. (Reproduced with permission from Intracranial Neoplasms and Paraneoplastic Disorders. In: Ropper AH, et al, eds. *Adams and Victor's Principles of Neurology*, 11eNew York, NY: McGraw-Hill; 2015).

carcinogenesis. These include signs of abnormal cell nuclei (nuclear atypia), mitosis (cell division, excessive when related to cancerous growth), endothelial proliferation (supporting angiogenesis for tumor growth), and finally, necrosis (a form of cell death more common in cancer cells due to their resistance to apoptosis).

Clinically the most common (up to 90% incidence) early signs of neoplasm are due to increased intracranial pressure. These include mild, generalized symptoms: headache, nausea, and fatigue. More frank signs include visual changes due to papilledema (optic disc swelling), vomiting, and cognitive changes, as well as seizure activity due to abnormal cellular metabolism. Other clinical manifestations depend on function of the involved tissues. Treatment to limit pressure on nervous tissue may include surgical resection, targeted tissue destruction via radiation therapy, and chemotherapy to destroy rapidly dividing tissues.

Recurrence of cancer, even after aggressive treatment, remains common. Discovery of cancer stem cells that lie dormant for years, then switch on and cause neoplasm, has led to new treatments. Cancer stem cells are both chemoresistant and radioresistant due to their enhanced ability to repair DNA, up-regulated cell cycle control mechanisms, increased free-radical scavengers, and other enhanced cell survival mechanisms. New therapies target cancer stem cells when dormant (or quiescent), using chemoquiesent drugs and designer drugs individualized to each patient.

Cerebral palsy

Cerebral palsy (CP) is a motor disturbance caused by damage to the motor cortex (less commonly affecting the cerebellum) pre- or postnatally, either from abnormal fetal development or an acquired brain injury in early infancy. Clinical signs become apparent during infancy or early childhood, commonly presenting as movement impairment, altered (usually increased) muscle tone, and developmental delay (Figure 10.31). CP is the primary cause of childhood disability; however, its magnitude varies from mild to severe and can include sensory loss, communication disorders, and other concomitant medical conditions based on the type and amount of nervous system damage. There is not a single cause of CP; many conditions such as genetic disorders, maternal infections, or fetal trauma can cause abnormal brain development. Low birth weight or prematurity is linked to an increased risk of CP, as are multiple births or complications during delivery, such as breech positioning. Higher rates of CP are linked to postnatal presence of a low Apgar score (a quick assessment performed at 1 and 5 minutes after delivery, assessing the infant's skin color, breathing, heart rate, muscle tone, and reflexes), small head circumference, or conditions such as severe jaundice. CP is not progressive, and most children with CP have good potential to improve and respond well to therapies that promote neuroplasticity, enhance development, and accommodate impairments (Figure 10.32).

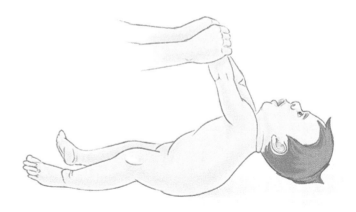

FIGURE 10.31

Head lag in cerebral palsy. Many children with cerebral palsy of all types will show early head lag when pulled to sit; as they age the LE and UE may show increased tone (spasticity) pulling the arms and legs into flexion but the head may still lag behind the shoulders. (Reproduced with permission from Carney PR, & Geyer JD (Eds). *Pediatric Practice: Neurology*. New York, NY: McGraw-Hill; 2010).

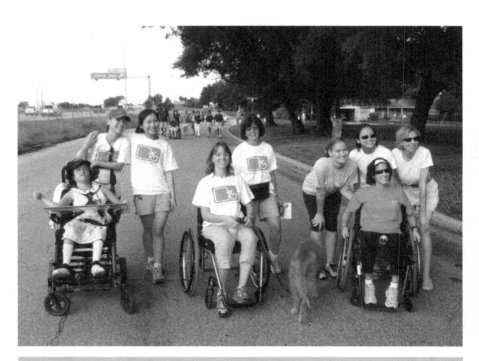

FIGURE 10.32

Thriving after cerebral palsy. Dr. Woodard, daughter Anika, and dog Nikki are part of a team of University of South Florida (USF) medical students, faculty, and family who participated in a "wheel-a-thon" to raise money for Tampa's first fully accessible playground. Teaching medical students the therapeutic value of sports and recreation for people with disabilities is an important aspect of the USF curriculum. (Reproduced with permission from Chapter 6. Social Justice. In: Usatine RP, Smith MA, Chumley HS, Mayeaux EJ, Jr.. eds. *The Color Atlas of Family Medicine*, 2e New York, NY: McGraw-Hill, 2013).

Traumatic Brain Injury

Traumatic brain injury (TBI) is defined as an insult to the brain caused by external physical force (Figure 10.33). It might produce diminished or altered states of consciousness as well as impaired cognition or physical function. TBI is the leading cause of injury-related death, and among those who survive, 70% have permanent loss of function, placing a burden on families and society. TBI may be from either open or closed head injury (Table 10.2). Closed head injury creates forces that damage neurologic structures. Mechanisms include impact loading, or contact with an object, and impulsive loading, such as whiplash, which sets the head in motion without direct impact upon the skull. Further differentiation of the disruptive mechanisms includes the type and direction of the load, which includes acceleration/deceleration, translational (anterior/posterior or lateral), and rotationally directed forces. Understanding the force as it relates to brain anatomy assists in diagnosing neurological structures likely to be involved, as well as predicts outcome.

Damage after TBI is either primary or secondary. Primary TBI involves damage at the tissue level (including white matter shearing, contusion, edema, and hematomas) or cellular level (such as leaky ion channels or microporation of cell membranes). Secondary damage after TBI involves a complex cascade of neurochemical changes in which cellular disruption leads directly to further cell death via apoptosis and necrosis. Medical diagnosis of TBI is based on clinical findings using anatomic imaging via noncontrast CT to visualize bone fractures, lumbar puncture to determine whether there are blood or blood byproducts in the CSF, and MRI diffusion tensor imaging to visualize the condition of long white matter tracts. In severe cases of TBI with poor prognosis, evoked potential and electroencephalogram tests are used to determine status of electrical activity in the brain.

Traumatic brain injury is further described as hemorrhagic and nonhemorrhagic. There are four types of intracranial hemorrhage and four types of nonhemorrhagic brain injury. Several examples of hemorrhagic and non-hemorrhagic brain injury are shown in Figure 10.34.

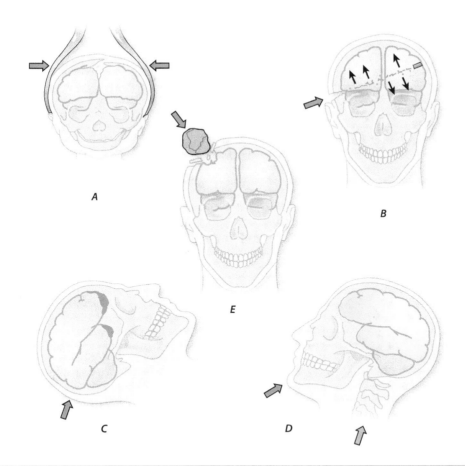

FIGURE 10.33

Mechanisms of external cranial injury producing traumatic brain injury. Mechanisms of craniocerebral injury. *A.* Cranium distorted by forceps (birth injury). *B.* Gunshot wound of the brain. *C.* Falls (also traffic accidents). *D.* Blows on the chin ("punch-drunk"). *E.* Injury to skull and brain by falling objects. (Reproduced with permission from Intracranial Neoplasms and Paraneoplastic Disorders. In: Ropper AH, et al, eds. *Adams and Victor's Principles of Neurology*, 11e New York, NY: McGraw-Hill; 2015).

Table 10.2 Traumatic Brain Injury Categorization

	Type	Definition
Head Injury	Open	Opening of the dura mater
	Closed	Skull and dura mater remain intact
Tissue Damage	Primary	Direct brain insult; damage from mechnical stress in tissue (white matter shearing, contusion, edema, disruption of cell membranes)
	Secondary	Induced by chemical and electrical changes in tissue brought on by direct damage to tissue; apoptosis or necrosis
Vascular Damage	Hemorrhagic	Can be epidural, subdural, subarachnoid, and intracerebral; signs include headache, drowsiness, nausea, vomiting, confusion, and seizure
	Non-hemorrhagic	Can be diffuse axonal injury, concussion, chronic traumatic encephalopathy, and whiplash associated disorder

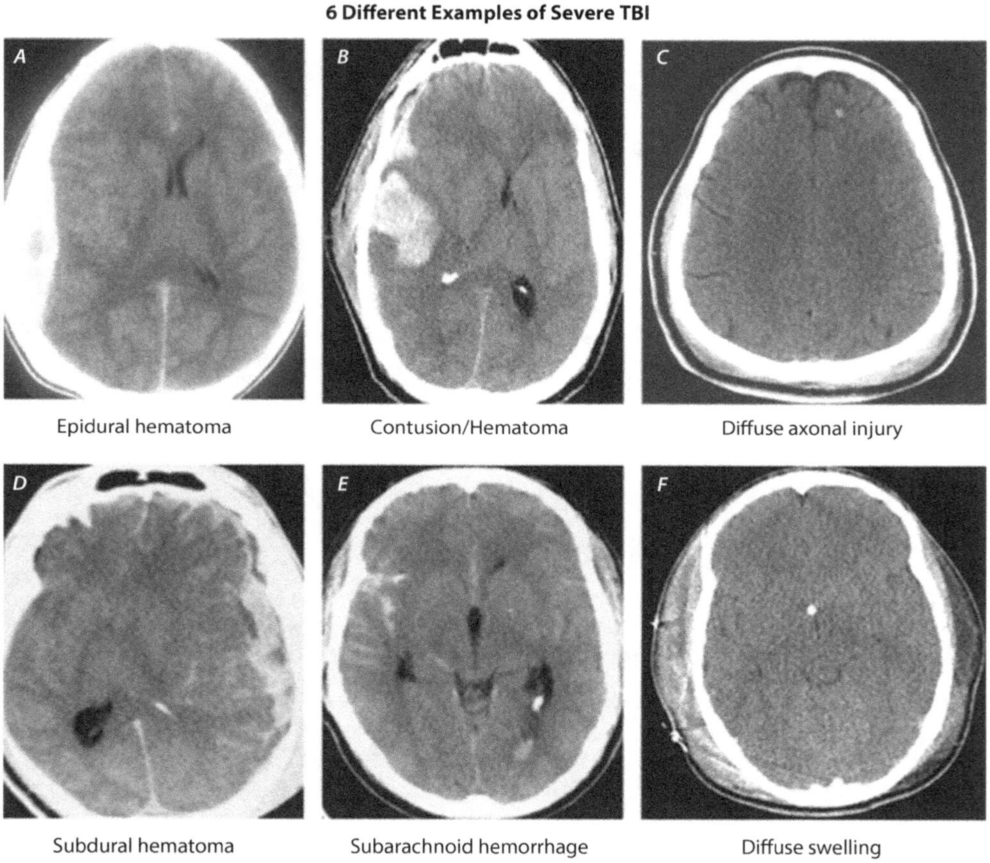

6 Different Examples of Severe TBI

Epidural hematoma

Contusion/Hematoma

Diffuse axonal injury

Subdural hematoma

Subarachnoid hemorrhage

Diffuse swelling

FIGURE 10.34

Six different examples of severe traumatic brain injury (TBI). Blood appears white in this T2 Weighted CT scan of six different traumatic brain injuries. *A.* Epidural hematoma; note the lens-shaped bleeding due to intact cranial suture lines. *B.* Contusion/hematoma producing bleeding into cranial tissue. *C.* Diffuse axonal injury shows in CT as areas of small white spots. *D.* Subdural hematoma, bleeding crosses suture lines, but does not extend into cortical tissue or ventricles. *E.* Subarachnoid hemorrhage showing blood extending into ventricles. *F.* Diffuse swelling with global pressure on delicate brain tissue due to pressure from all directions within the cranial vault. (Used with permission of Alisa Gean, MD, University of California, San Francisco.)

Anatomic descriptions for hemorrhagic brain injury include epidural, subdural, subarachnoid, and intracerebral. Clinical findings include headache, drowsiness, nausea, vomiting, confusion, and seizure. Nonhemorrhagic TBI includes diffuse axonal injury, concussion, chronic traumatic encephalopathy, and whiplash-associated disorder. These conditions vary in severity of clinical findings and easily may be missed in examination; early diagnosis is only possible if one recognizes the neurological commonality of diffuse clinical findings, such as fatigue, headache, visual disturbance, mild memory loss, and vertigo, which may begin immediately or even after many years post TBI. Making diagnosis even more difficult are biases among health care providers, who may misattribute these often vague and seemingly unrelated symptoms, which delays diagnosis and treatment. Further, nonhemorrhagic TBI increases risk of depression and anxiety, conditions that impair cognition and also increase risk for prolonged recovery.

Acute medical management after TBI seeks to minimize complications from primary damage such as infection and to reduce secondary damage. Pharmacological interventions include neuromuscular blockades to create temporary paralysis, and medications for neuroprotection. Treatments to prevent seizures remain ineffective. Blood sugar must be tightly managed, as excessive glucose is cytotoxic. Surgical intervention, such as decompressive craniotomy, may be performed to relieve pressure caused by ongoing uncontrolled bleeding. Other medical interventions during early treatment of TBI include avoiding hyperthermia, which may cause metabolic disturbances; closely measuring intracranial pressure; mechanical ventilation and supplemental oxygen to maintain cerebral tissue perfusion; and close monitoring of caloric intake via intravenous feeding, as nutritional demands increase during tissue healing.

Concussion. Concussion is the most frequently observed traumatic brain injury (TBI). Concussion is referred to as a mild TBI that may or may not produce a temporary loss of consciousness that resolves spontaneously. Among the most common signs of a concussion are headache, feeling as if "in a fog," emotional lability, and depression. Effects are usually cleared within a few weeks but can last months or years, emphatically indicating that fallacy in the term *mild TBI*; all of them can become life-altering injuries. Concussions are brain injuries caused by direct impact on the skull and brain, violent shaking of the head, or "whiplash" injury. Rapid linear deceleration of the skull meets the inertia of brain mass within the boney chamber, and the brain impacts the inside of the skull. Many types of trauma cause concussions, such as falls or automobile accidents (more common in adults), or "headbanging" or domestic abuse (more common in younger people), and the effects of concussions have become widely recognized among battlefield war veterans.

Neuropathologies from concussion are widespread rather than focal. They include damage to small blood vessels, which complicates recovery by limiting both the available oxygen and glucose, as well as reducing the brain's capacity to remove cytotoxins from the area of damage during the healing process. If these small veins continue to flow unabated, a subdural hematoma might form. Diffuse axonal injury appears across the cerebral cortex, its underlying white matter, and in subcortical sites such as the midbrain. Areas most susceptible are at locations where rotational forces are concentrated, such as in the depths of sulci and in the junction between

the diencephalon and midbrain. Expression of axonal pathology is often delayed so that the signs of diffuse axonal injury are not immediately observed. Patients return to home, work, or back to the field before their brains have healed. Because they frequently go undiagnosed, mortality in these patients can occur some hours or weeks after the event. Diffusion tensor imaging now offers the ability to inspect the condition of the long fiber pathways in real time, no longer relying on postmortem examination.

Chronic traumatic encephalopathy. In 2005, former NFL player Mike Webster, a four-time Super Bowl champion with the Pittsburgh Steelers and NFL Hall of Fame inductee, died of heart failure in a Pittsburgh hospital at the age of 50. "Life after football" for him and his family wasn't what it was cracked up to be. Soon after retirement, Mike began to have memory losses and inability to concentrate or make smart decisions. He became abusive and violent. His family lost their house, finally ending his marriage. Mike Webster was well known to every football fan in Pittsburgh, and soon there were comments on his rumpled, dirty appearance. He slept in his truck or under bridges off and on. He frequently was lost and could not find his home, became more paranoid and disoriented, and later developed profound dementia. Dr. Bennett Omalu (subject of the feature film *Concussion*, Columbia Pictures, 2015) and his colleagues in the Department of Pathology at the University of Pittsburgh received the brain of the icon. They assayed the tissue and discovered distinctive pathological features including tau-immunoreactive neurofibrillary tangles, astrocytic tangles, and spindle-shaped and threadlike neurites throughout the brain. This pathology defined behavioral and cognitive deficits attributable to a specific identified mechanism: repeated blows to the head. Tens of thousands of tiny subclinical concussions combined to claim "Iron Mike" Webster.

The condition is called chronic traumatic encephalopathy (CTE), originally termed *dementia pugilistica* ("punch drunk") syndrome because it was seen in boxers who had taken too many head shots over their careers. Similarly, in previous wars, soldiers subjected to concussive explosions were said to be "shell shocked." For patients with CTE, speech is slurred, and conversation is confused and disjointed; these patients can become violent, lethargic, depressed, or bipolar. Frequently they walk with a drunken gait. Common causes include recurrent sports-related trauma, multiple car accidents, or abuse. Brains affected by CTE are, in many ways, similar to those of patients with Alzheimer's disease (AD). In both, the frontal, parietal, and temporal cortices are atrophied, as are the mammillary bodies and the medial temporal lobe. Characteristically, hippocampal degeneration is prominent. The lateral and third ventricles are usually distended from loss of cells in surrounding nuclei and loss of white matter in the hemispheres.

Beyond the obvious etiology of CTE, two other differences distinguish CTE from AD. First, AD is a cerebral degenerative disorder unrelated to external trauma and presents little brainstem pathology. AD forebrain cellular damage includes the familiar neurofibrillary tangles and amyloid plaques in neurons and interstitial tissues mainly in frontal, temporal, and parietal cortices. Second, because CTE is the result of repeated blows to the head, cortical and subcortical tissues are subjected to linear and rotational forces that shear axons at sites where the forces are concentrated. The midbrain is positioned at the junction between the forebrain and the brainstem and subject to damage to the long pathways between the forebrain and the brainstem, produced by rotational forces. Another less intuitive site of torque when the brain is forcefully displaced is in the depths of the sulci, where subtle twists in the cortex are focused. In the regions where axon damage is concentrated, sulcal depths and midbrain CST, cellular changes appear and include expression of tau-immunoreactive protein, which is proposed to initiate a cellular death cascade.

Athletes, especially at highly competitive and elite levels, want to play more than they are worried about getting hurt. Most are deceptive about their injuries to keep from being pulled from the game. The next day or next week, they are still hiding symptoms from the team medical staff, coaches, teammates, and even families. New concussion protocols are being established commonly, and players, coaches, and physician opinions are no longer sufficient to send a player back into the game. Reliable, rapid tests are being refined so that player injury can be more objectively assessed. One such test was developed with the knowledge that patients with concussions have visual impairments, referred to as convergence insufficiency, that cause slow or poorly controlled tracking, impaired saccades, and blurred vision. The King-Devick [K-D] test tests for visual, attention, and cognitive deficits associated with concussion. On the sideline, a medical professional uses an app to test how well and fast a subject can name numbers presented on a changing screen. The K-D test has been shown to be over 85% accurate in identifying concussion.

Recognizing, assessing, and dealing with the aftermath of concussions has received a burst of public scrutiny because of the impact on youth sports and on the billion-dollar professional sports industries. It is now apparent that, with repeated subclinical concussions (*mild* TBIs), the brain accumulates frequent small injuries that do not fully recover between events and produce widespread pathological changes that might not manifest permanent psychological or behavioral changes for hours to days, even years after participation in the contact sport ends.

Whiplash associated disorder. Whiplash was a diagnosis first used in the 1920s to describe the back-and-forth head motion during a car accident. Whiplash injuries were understood to be localized to the cervical spine, and described by a 5-point scale to grade injury severity according to presence of clinical findings, from mild injuries producing no pain or physical signs, to the most severe injuries accompanied by fracture or spinal cord injury. The most common injury is grade II, which is spinal pain and musculoskeletal injury with no obvious nervous system injury or fracture (Figure 10.35). This categorization, however, is inadequate to describe the complex cervical spine injury that produces neck pain and loss of mobility, due to ligamentous and joint capsule injury. Damage to the cervical disc and spinal nerve roots are common sources of radicular and chronic pain. Injury severity did not always correlate with patient report, and the diagnosis was often challenged within the legal system as exaggerated or even fraudulent.

Further complicating this diagnosis were reports that patients subjected even to fairly mild whiplash forces often reported a constellation of additional symptoms, including chronic pain with sensory hypersensitivity, visual disturbance, vertigo, post traumatic stress disorder (PTSD), and even mild cognitive changes. This spectrum of effects reinforces the fact that a "whiplash" is, in fact, a supraspinal nervous system TBI. Thus the term *whiplash-associated disorder* (WAD) is now commonly used to describe these "associated" symptoms, legitimizing a far greater scope to the appreciation of the range of neurological deficits produced by the violent head movements.

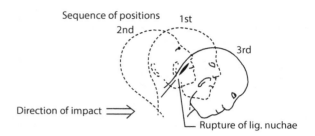

FIGURE 10.35

Whiplash. Extension injury (whiplash) of the cervical spine. Violent force from behind produces rapid translation between three sequential positions and may cause damage to the delicate local nervous and musculoskeletal tissues; if severe enough, this may injure the strong ligamentum nuchae. (Reproduced with permission from The Spine, Pelvis, and Extremities. In: LeBlond RF, et al, eds. *DeGowin's Diagnostic Examination*, 10e New York, NY: McGraw-Hill, 2014).

VIII THERAPIES AFTER INJURY OR DISEASE

Evidence-based clinical practice continues to change neurorehabilitation, challenging old beliefs and outdated practice models with new research and technology, expanding our therapeutic reach. Two approaches to physical therapy, mirror therapy and constraint-induced movement therapy (CIMT), function by driving cortical plasticity to promote movement and suppress fear-conditioned protective behaviors.

Mirror Therapy

In humans, fMRI, TMS, and electroencephalographic studies have described a dispersed system of cells, mirror cells, that responds to observing (or visualizing) directed behaviors, that includes premotor cortex, including supplementary motor cortex and ventral premotor area, S1, and sensory association cortices, including inferior parietal cortex, angular gyrus, and fusiform gyrus, Wernicke's area, and Broca's area. Different parts of the system are activated appropriate to the behavior that is being presented (mirrored). If the behavior is without purpose, mirror neurons are not activated, but mirror neurons can be activated by watching directed behaviors that are functionally similar movements ("salience matters"). Some suggestion has been made that the mirror system evolved to maintain some activity in the injured circuitry while the brain repairs itself, rather than leaving the cells in prolonged quiescence ("use it or lose it"). Therapies that engage the mirror system replace lost somatic and proprioceptive inputs with visual, and enhance remodeling by maintaining activity in the denervated cortex.

Mirror therapy (Neuroplasticity Box, Chapter 1) is shown to promote cortical remapping, likely by activating the mirror cell system. Activating mirror cells might unmask quiescent synaptic connections that are weakened from disuse. Originally used to relieve phantom pain experienced by most people with limb loss, mirror therapy is now used commonly across many patient populations, including patients with reduced hand function after acquired brain injury, chronic pain, and chronic regional pain syndrome. Cortical areas that contribute to descending sensorimotor

Integration of Systems
Evolution of Neurorehabilitation

The field of neurological rehabilitation is fairly new, developing in the United States of America only over the past 100 years. Just as the nervous system functions in an integrated fashion, neurological rehabilitation is best delivered within an interprofessional model. The ideal rehabilitation center incorporates many different types of therapy, including respiratory, recreational, music, art, and even animals (Figure 10.36). The professions forming the cornerstone of neurologic rehabilitation are occupational therapy, physical therapy, and speech therapy. The profession of speech, language, and pathology (SLP) developed from the field of elocution (public speaking) and expanded in the 19th century in response to Broca's and Wernicke's discoveries of specific areas in the brain for speech and language. Early practitioners were primarily lay people who were considered gifted orators. The American Speech Society was formed in 1925.

Occupational therapy (OT) developed as a field for occupational retraining of blind soldiers in the United Kingdom in World War I. Soldiers exposed to mustard gas, a chemical agent released by German soldiers, had acute loss of vision. The OT profession (Figure 10.37) specialized in the occupational retraining of these men and later expanded to include other forms of occupational therapy, with a traditional emphasis on function of the upper extremity, particularly the hand, as well

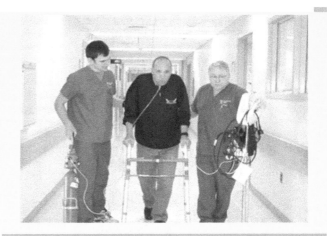

FIGURE 10.36

Collaborative care models. Physical therapy has long been incorporated into acute care. Image shows collaborative gait training with both Respiratory Therapist and Physical Therapist of a patient after Coronary Artery Bypass Graft in 1990, using equipment that is basically unchanged today. A regular walking schedule is an important component of pulmonary rehabilitation. Walking distance is increased progressively, and oxygen supplementation often is used in a patient who desaturates with exercise. (Reproduced with permission from Cruz ES, Bharara A, Bharara N. Pulmonary Rehabilitation. In: Maitin IB, Cruz E. eds. *CURRENT Diagnosis & Treatment: Physical Medicine & Rehabilitation New York*, NY: McGraw-Hill; 2014).

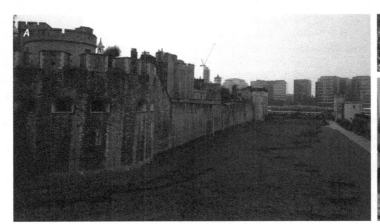
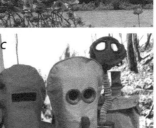

FIGURE 10.37

The First World War. *A.* In this beautiful art installation commemorating the 100 year anniversary of the war, red flowers spill over the Tower of London and onto the grounds below. ***B.*** Each of the 888,246 British military deaths during World War I is represented by one red ceramic poppy. ***C.*** Gas masks used by soldiers to protect against sulfur (mustard) gas, named for its smell. Unfortunately the mask was ineffective against the sulfur droplets that remain on skin and other surfaces; this first use of chemical weapons produced horribly painful, rarely fatal burns. During and after the war the country was overwhelmed by soldiers recovering from blindness, disfigurement and loss of limb, necessitating rehabilitation in the form of occupational therapy. (Images provided by Jamie Graham and Tony Mosconi, 2017).

as academics, vocational training, and psychiatric adjustment after injury.

Finally, physical therapy (PT) expanded into the large profession we have today in response to the polio epidemics of the early 20th century. Millions of people, overwhelmingly children, were acutely debilitated with "infantile paralysis." We now know that this was due to a poliovirus attack on anterior horn cells, causing cell death and the characteristic lower motor neuron presentations of flaccid paralysis, hypotonia, and hyporeflexia, but without sensory loss. Effects could be seen in both spinal and cranial nerves, with the worst cases requiring negative-pressure breathing machines, called "iron lungs" (Figure 10.38). As with many diseases, funding was essential to finding a cure, and having a celebrity advocate in the case of polio was quite helpful in lending support and financing for resources and research. The most notable was President Franklin Delano Roosevelt, who managed to hide the extent of his paralysis and disability from the public. Nevertheless, he was a powerful advocate, and with his support the March of Dimes to Cure Infantile Paralysis began as a publicly funded program. Average Americans were encouraged to send in their spare change (a dime) to help find a cure for this terrible disease. In addition to research, the funds were used to start the first educational programs for physical therapy, as well as to open community rehabilitation hospitals that focused on neurological rehabilitation.

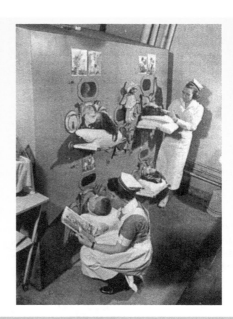

FIGURE 10.38

Polio epidemic. Young patients with respiratory paralysis from polio, being treated in an "iron lung." (Photograph by Hansel Mieth, courtesy Time Life Pictures, Getty Images, 1938.)

feedback projections to the limb are lost, with failure to regulate muscle contraction and pain transmission, resulting in searing pain and perceived dyskinesia in the amputated limb. Mirror therapy interjects visual feedback to convince the brain that the limb is in good condition and reduce motor output. Modern fMRI, TMS, and electroencephalographic studies have demonstrated activity in the mirror cell system during mirror therapy, and its use to treat paresis or paralysis after acquired brain injury offers a promising adjunct to traditional functionally based therapies.

An additional value of mirror therapy in treating chronic pain conditions is its ability to convey a highly desired subjective experience: movement without pain. Chronic pain trains the brain to expect that movement will hurt, and so promotes protective behavior or causes patients to cease moving entirely. This type of fear conditioning is quite pervasive and often persists even after the original source of pain is removed. The patient only has to imagine moving the painful body part to experience the pain. He or she becomes a "pain athlete" through rigorous and repetitive practice ("repetition matters"), reinforcing this self-limiting thought pattern. In such patients, seeing the reflection of their injured limb looking healthy and moving freely can help break the fear conditioning and encourage movement, and engagement of the mirror neurons supports activity in the denervated cortical areas, promoting plastic remodeling.

Constraint-Induced Movement Therapy (CIMT)

As mentioned above, regions of the cortex can become quiescent after injury. With time, the neuronal circuitry atrophies, and

valuable cortical area is lost. Forcing the patient to use the impaired limb in preference to the healthy one also forces the damaged cortex to maintain activity. Most people with hemiparesis use their paretic leg, even poorly, to stand and walk; however, there is less need to use the paretic arm. Many people find ways to function with only one arm. Learned non-use, similar to pain fear conditioning, is reinforced behaviorally and at a cellular level with dendritic pruning and withdrawal. It becomes a stubborn challenge to rehabilitation, particularly in upper extremity function. Members of one group tested whether preventing use of the healthy arm would drive improvement in movement of their impaired limb. The scientists produced unilateral cortical lesions that produced upper extremity paresis in monkeys, then restrained their intact arm. These industrious monkeys achieved spectacular functional return in their newly paralyzed arm. Brain histology demonstrated huge lesions, which should have produced the stereotypical paralysis. They concluded that "forced use" drove neuroplastic changes, creating new pathways for motor control.

Translating this exciting discovery to a human rehabilitation model has been challenging. Ethical considerations, along with human qualities regarding motivation and frustration tolerance, required a softer approach. The term *forced use* has been replaced with a more accurate and emotionally palatable term, *constraint-induced movement therapy* (CIMT). Successful CIMT requires patient and family involvement as well as certain minimum criteria, including partial motion of the paretic arm, adequate balance to remain safe without use of the intact arm, and cognitive ability to understand the ultimate goal and tolerate the inevitable frustration. Patients receiving CIMT wear a mitt over their healthy hand for several hours daily while they practice behaviors requiring them to use the other hand. The treatment is intensive and repetitive to forcefully drive the formation of alternate synaptic pathways to achieve their desired goals. These behavioral changes are sustained, along with neuroplastic changes seen on imaging, including expanded motor cortical representation of the paretic hand, and they encourage the use of CIMT among appropriate patient populations.

> ## CASE 10 DISCUSSION: Resources for Ideal Recovery

Dr. T. made excellent progress in the months since his stroke, and this was due to many factors. He began with a robust nervous system, partially due to genetics in the form of normal fetal development. His childhood was filled with loving support and enrichment that encouraged learning and curiosity. As the male child of a practicing physician, he had strong self-efficacy, the belief in his own ability to succeed, due to daily exposure to his father's career, combined with social and cultural support toward that career path. A lifetime of cognitive neuroplastic growth from his medical practice, complex hobbies, a strong work ethic, and secure, loving social ties strengthened his central nervous system, providing an ideal neurologic foundation for recovery after damage. Finally, he had the benefit of quality health care, offered without delay and continuing throughout the recovery process.

The patient cases in the preceding chapters chronicle successful recovery from often devastating neurologic damage. These stories of triumph over adversity share common themes, of neuroplastic strength, environmental support through emotional and cognitive enrichment, and timely access to quality medical care and rehabilitation. As future practicing clinicians, you will have the profound honor to assist in this process and the obligation to continue your studies as new information becomes available. The field of neuroscience is constantly changing because of tremendous global efforts of basic science and clinical research. Equally valuable is the knowledge that patients are at the center of the process, and they require information and support for ideal recovery. Patient and family education is known to improve outcomes and adherence to ideal care plans and to increase self-efficacy. The psycho-emotional components of care, including peer support, behavioral modification, and psychotherapy to cope with the inevitable cost of loss that often comes with neurological disease or injury, are also critical components to successful rehabilitation. Ideal clinical practice incorporates all these resources into collaborative, patient-focused care, providing our patients the best chance of living fuller, more satisfying lives.

REFERENCES

Acharya S, Shukla S. Mirror neurons: enigma of the metaphysical modular brain. *J Nat Sci Biol Med.* 2012 Jul;3(2):118–124.

Agnew ZK, Brownsett S, Woodhead Z, de Boissezon X. A step forward for mirror neurons? Investigating the functional link between action execution and action observation in limb apraxia. *J Neurosci.* 2008 Jul 30;28(31):7726–7727.

Ahn S, Lee SK. Diffusion tensor imaging: exploring the motor networks and clinical applications. *Korean J Radiol.* 2011 Nov–Dec;12(6):651–661.

American Speech-Language-Hearing Association Task Force on Central Auditory Processing Consensus Development. Central auditory processing: current status of research and implications for clinical practice. *Am. J. Audiol.* 1996;5(2):41–54.

Amunts K, Zilles K. Architectonic Mapping of the human brain beyond Brodmann. *Neuron.* 2015 Dec 16;88(6):1086–1107.

Apkarian AV, Baliki MN, Geha PY. Towards a theory of chronic pain. *Prog Neurobiol.* 2009 Feb;87(2):81–97.

Ariani G, Wurm MF, Lingnau A. Decoding internally and externally driven movement. *Plans. J Neurosci.* 2015 Oct 21; 35(42):14160–14171.

Baddeley A. Working memory. *Curr Biol.* 2010 Feb 23; 20(4): R136–R140.

Balcer L, Galetta K, Galetta S, Leong D, Liu M, Ventura R. The King-Devick test of rapid number naming for concussion detection: meta-analysis and systematic review of the literature. *Concussion.* 2015 Sept 15; 1(2): 2056–3299.

Bennett IJ, Madden DJ. Disconnected aging: cerebral white matter integrity and age-related differences in cognition. *Neuroscience.* 2014 Sep 12; 276: 187–205.

Bertolini G, Wicki A, Baumann CR, Straumann D, Palla A. Impaired tilt perception in Parkinson's disease: a central vestibular integration failure. *PLoS One.* 2015 Apr 15;10(4):e0124253.

Bigler ED. Distinguished Neuropsychologist Award Lecture 1999. The lesion(s) in traumatic brain injury: implications for clinical neuropsychology. *Arch Clin Neuropsychol.* 2001 Feb;16(2):95–131.

Bodegård A, Geyer S, Grefkes C, Zilles K, Roland PE. Hierarchical processing of tactile shape in the human brain. *Neuron.* 2001 Aug 2.;31(2):317–328.

Borsook D, Becerra L, Fishman S, et al. Acute plasticity in the human somatosensory cortex following amputation. *Neuroreport.* 1998 Apr 20;9(6):1013–1017.

Brandt T, Dieterich M. The vestibular cortex. Its locations, functions, and disorders. *Ann N Y Acad Sci.* 1999 May 28; 871: 293–312.

Buchsbaum BR, Baldo J, Okada K, Berman KF, Dronkers N, D'Esposito M, Hickok G. Conduction aphasia, sensory-motor integration, and phonological short-term memory—an aggregate analysis of lesion and fMRI data. *Brain Lang.* 2011 Dec;119(3):119–128.

Budson A, Cantu R, Gavett B, et al. Chronic traumatic encephalopathy in athletes: progressive tauopathy following repetitive head injury. *J Neuropathol Exp Neurol.* 2009 July;68(7):709–735.

Burkhalter A, Bernardo KL. Organization of corticocortical connections in human visual cortex. *Proc Natl Acad Sci USA.* 1989 Feb;86(3):1071–1075.

Capaday C, Ethier C, Van Vreeswijk C, Darling WG. On the functional organization and operational principles of the motor cortex. *Front Neural Circuits*. 2013 Apr 18;7:66.

Caria A, de Falco S. Anterior insular cortex regulation in autism spectrum disorders. *Front Behav Neurosci*. 2015 Mar 6;9:38.

Catani M, Jones DK, ffytche DH. Perisylvian language networks of the human brain. *Ann Neurol*. 2005 Jan;57(1):8–16.

Catani M, Jones DK, Donato R, Ffytche DH. Occipito-temporal connections in the human brain. *Brain*. 2003 Sep;126(Pt 9):2093–2107.

Cattaneo L, Rizzolatti G. The mirror neuron system. *Arch Neurol*. 2009 May;66(5):557–560.

Chiarovano E, Vidal PP, Magnani C, Lamas G, Curthoys IS, de Waele C. Absence of rotation perception during warm water caloric irrigation in some seniors with postural instability. *Front Neurol*. 2016 Jan 25;7:4.

Chinellato E, Del Pobil AP. The neuroscience of vision-based grasping: a functional review for computational modeling and bio-inspired robotics. *J Integr Neurosci*. 2009 Jun;8(2):223–254.

Cieslak M, Ingham RJ, Ingham JC, Grafton ST. Anomalous white matter morphology in adults who stutter. *J Speech Lang Hear Res*. 2015 Apr;58(2):268–277.

Cisek P, Kalaska JF. Neural correlates of reaching decisions in dorsal premotor cortex: specification of multiple direction choices and final selection of action. *Neuron*. 2005 Mar 3;45(5):801–814.

Conrad J. et al. P35. Neglect and vestibular failure – Spatial or attentional deficit? *Clinical Neurophysiology*. 2015 Aug;126(8):e113–e114.

Corkin S. What's new with the amnesic patient H.M.? *Nat Rev Neurosci*. 2002 Feb;3(2):153–160.

Corkin S, Amaral DG, González RG, Johnson KA, Hyman BT. H. M.'s medial temporal lobe lesion: findings from magnetic resonance imaging. *J Neurosci*. 1997 May 15;17(10):3964–3979.

Craig AD. The sentient self. *Brain Struct Funct*. 2010 Jun; 214(5–6): 563–577.

Crichton P. Penfield's homunculus. *J Neurol Neurosurg Psychiatry*. 1994 Apr; 57(4): 525. Erratum in *J Neurol Neurosurg Psychiatry*. 1994 Jun; 57(6): 772.

Cummins AJ. The physiology of symptoms: III. Nausea and vomiting. *Am J Dig Dis*. 1958;3(10):710–721.

Dayan E, Cohen LG. Neuroplasticity subserving motor skill learning. *Neuron*. 2011 Nov 3;72(3):443–454.

de Jong LW, van der Hiele K, Veer IM, et al. Strongly reduced volumes of putamen and thalamus in Alzheimer's disease: an MRI study. *Brain*. 2008 Dec;131(Pt 12):3277–3285.

de Oliveira FF, Correia Marin Sde M, Ferreira Bertolucci PH. Communicating with the non-dominant hemisphere: implications for neurological rehabilitation. *Neural Regen Res*. 2013 May 5;8(13):1236–1246.

de Oliveira FF, Damasceno BP. A topographic study on the evaluation of speech and language in the acute phase of a first stroke. *Arq Neuropsiquiatr*. 2011 Oct;69(5):790–798.

Dennis BD, Bawor M, Paul J, et al. The impact of chronic pain on opiod addiction treatment: a systematic review protocol. *Sytematic Reviews*. 2015;4:49.

Diamond A. Executive functions. *Annu Rev Psychol*. 2013;64:135–168.

Diedrichsen J, Kornysheva K. Motor skill learning between selection and execution. *Trends Cogn Sci*. 2015 Apr;19(4):227–233.

Donati AR, Shokur S, Morya E, et al. Long-term training with a brain-machine interface-based gait protocol induces partial neurological recovery in paraplegic patients. *Sci Rep*. 2016 Aug 1;6:30383.

Dotto L. Sleep stages, memory and learning. *CMAJ*. 1996 Apr 15;154(8): 1193–1196.

DuPrey KM, Webner D, Lyons A, Kucuk CH, Ellis JT, Cronholm PF. Convergence insufficiency identifies athletes at risk of prolonged recovery from sport-related concussion. *Am J Sports Med*. 2017 May 1;363546517705640.

Flinker A, Korzeniewska A, Shestyuk AY, et al. Redefining the role of Broca's area in speech. *Proc Natl Acad Sci USA*. 2015 Mar 3;112(9):2871–2875.

Fogassi L, Gallese V, Fadiga L, Luppino G, Matelli M, Rizzolatti G. Coding of peripersonal space in inferior premotor cortex (area F4). *J Neurophysiol*. 1996 Jul;76(1):141–157.

Gaetz M. The neurophysiology of brain injury. *Clin Neurophysiol*. 2004 Jan;115(1):4–18.

Gerstmann J. Syndrome of finger agnosia, disorientation for right and left, agraphia and acalculia. *Ninety-Fifth Annual Meeting of the American Psychiatric Association*. Chicago, May 11, 1939.

Gilaie-Dotan S. Visual motion serves but is not under the purview of the dorsal pathway. *Neuropsychologia*. 2016 Aug;89:378–392.

Gong G, He Y, Concha L, et al. Mapping anatomical connectivity patterns of human cerebral cortex using in vivo diffusion tensor imaging tractography. *Cereb Cortex*. 2009 Mar;19(3):524–536.

Goodale MA, Milner AD. Separate visual pathways for perception and action. *Trends Neurosci*. 1992 Jan;15(1):20–25.

Grafton ST, Hamilton AF. Evidence for a distributed hierarchy of action representation in the brain. *Hum Mov Sci*. 2007 Aug;26(4):590–616.

Graziano MS, Aflalo TN. Mapping behavioral repertoire onto the cortex. *Neuron*. 2007 Oct 25;56(2):239–251.

Graziano MS, Taylor CS, Moore T. Complex movements evoked by microstimulation of precentral cortex. *Neuron*. 2002 May 30;34(5):841–851.

Griggs RA. Who is Mrs. Cantlie and why are they doing these terrible things to her homunculi? *Teaching of Psychology*. 1988;15(2):105–106.

Gross RG, Grossman M. Update on apraxia. *Curr Neurol Neurosci Rep*. 2008 Nov;8(6):490–496.

Gu X, Hof PR, Friston KJ, Fan J. Anterior insular cortex and emotional awareness. *J Comp Neurol*. 2013 Oct 15;521(15):3371–3388.

Hamilton AF. Reflecting on the mirror neuron system in autism: a systematic review of current theories. *Dev Cogn Neurosci*. 2013 Jan;3:91–105.

Harpaz Y, Levkovitz Y, Lavidor M. Lexical ambiguity resolution in Wernicke's area and its right homologue. *Cortex*. 2009 Oct;45(9):1097–1103.

Hasson U, Frith CD. Mirroring and beyond: Coupled dynamics as a generalized framework for modelling social interactions. *Philos Trans R Soc Lond B Biol Sci*. 2016 May 5;371(1693).

Hauser MD, Chomsky N, Fitch WT. The faculty of language: what is it, who has it, and how did it evolve? *Science*. 2002 Nov 22;298(5598):1569–1579.

Holle D, Schulte-Steinberg B, Wurthmann S, et al. Persistent Postural-Perceptual Dizziness: A matter of higher, central dysfunction? *PLoS One*. 2015 Nov 16;10(11):e0142468.

Horikawa T, Kamitani Y. Generic decoding of seen and imagined objects using hierarchical visual features. *Nat Commun*. 2017 May 22;8:15037.

Hubel DH, Wiesel TN. Shape and arrangement of columns in cat's striate cortex. *J Physiol*. 1963 Mar;165:559–568.

Hülsdünker T, Mierau A, Strüder HK. Higher balance task demands are associated with an increase in individual alpha peak frequency. *Front Hum Neurosci*. 2016 Jan 6;9:695.

Jerger J, Chmiel R, Wilson N, Luchi R. Hearing impairment in older adults: new concepts. *J Am Geriatr Soc*. 1995;43(8):928–935.

Johannes CB, Le TK, Zhou X, Johnston JA, Dworkin RH. The prevalence of chronic pain in United States adults: results of an Internet-based survey. *J Pain*. 2010 Nov;11(11):1230–1239.

Jutzeler CR, Curt A, Kramer JL. Relationship between chronic pain and brain reorganization after deafferentation: a systematic review of functional MRI findings. *Neuroimage Clin*. 2015 Oct 3;9:599–606.

Kamali A, Flanders AE, Brody J, Hunter JV, Hasan KM. Tracing superior longitudinal fasciculus connectivity in the human brain using high resolution diffusion tensor tractography. *Brain Struct Funct*. 2014 Jan;219(1):269–281.

Karnath HO, Dieterich M. Spatial neglect—a vestibular disorder? *Brain*. 2006 Feb;129(Pt 2):293–305.

Katzung BG, Trevor AJ. Introduction to the pharmacology of CNS drugs. *Basic & Clinical Pharmacology*, 13e; Figure 21-3. 2015.

Kell CA, von Kriegstein K, Rösler A, Kleinschmidt A, Laufs H. The sensory cortical representation of the human penis: revisiting somatotopy in the male homunculus. *J Neurosci*. 2005 Jun 22;25(25):5984–5987.

Kerr AL, Steuer EL, Pochtarev V, Swain RA. Angiogenesis but not neurogenesis is critical for normal learning and memory acquisition. *Neuroscience.* 2010 Nov 24;171(1):214–226.

Kitamura T, Ogawa SK, Roy DS, et al. Engrams and circuits crucial for systems consolidation of a memory. *Science.* 2017 Apr 7;356(6333):73–78.

Kohler E, Keysers C, Umiltà MA, Fogassi L, Gallese V, Rizzolatti G. Hearing sounds, understanding actions: action representation in mirror neurons. *Science.* 2002 Aug 2;297(5582):846–848.

Kozasa EH, Sato JR, Lacerda SS, et al. Meditation training increases brain efficiency in an attention task. *Neuroimage.* 2012 Jan 2;59(1):745–749.

Krauzlis RJ. Recasting the smooth pursuit eye movement system. *J Neurophysiol.* 2004 Feb;91(2):591–603.

Lees-Haley PR, Green P, Rohling ML, Fox DD, Allen LM 3rd. The lesion(s) in traumatic brain injury: implications for clinical neuropsychology. *Arch Clin Neuropsychol.* 2003 Aug;18(6):585–594.

Lemon CH. It's all a matter of taste: gustatory processing and ingestive decisions. *Mo Med.* 2010 Jul–Aug;107(4):247–251.

Lemon CH, Katz DB. The neural processing of taste. *BMC Neurosci.* 2007 Sep 18;8(Suppl 3):S5.

Liu Y, Lin W, Liu C, et al. Memory consolidation reconfigures neural pathways involved in the suppression of emotional memories. *Nat Commun.* 2016 Nov 29;7:13375.

Makris N, Kennedy DN, McInerney S, et al. Segmentation of subcomponents within the superior longitudinal fascicle in humans: a quantitative, in vivo, DT-MRI study. *Cereb Cortex.* 2005 Jun;15(6):854–869.

Mansour AR, Farmer MA, Baliki MN, Apkarian AV. Chronic pain: the role of learning and brain plasticity. *Restor Neurol Neurosci.* 2014;32(1):129–139.

McKee AC, Cantu RC, Nowinski CJ, et al. Chronic traumatic encephalopathy in athletes: progressive tauopathy after repetitive head injury. *J Neuropathol Exp Neurol.* 2009 Jul;68(7):709–735.

Miller AD, Leslie RA. The area postrema and vomiting. *Front Neuroendocrinol.* 1994 Dec;15(4):301–320.

Minaeian A, Patel A, Essa B, Goddeau RP Jr, Moonis M, Henninger N. Emergency department length of stay and outcome after ischemic stroke. *J Stroke Cerebrovasc Dis.* 2017 May 24. pii: S1052-3057(17)30214-8.

Mitchell DE, Della Santina CC, Cullen KE. Plasticity within excitatory and inhibitory pathways of the vestibulo-spinal circuitry guides changes in motor performance. *Sci Rep.* 2017 Apr 12;7(1):853.

Molina-Luna K, Buitrago MM, Hertler B, et al. Cortical stimulation mapping using epidurally implanted thin-film microelectrode arrays. *J Neurosci Methods.* 2007 Mar 30;161(1):118–125.

Mountcastle V. The columnar organization of the neocortex. *Brain.* 1997;120:701–722.

Mori S, Oishi K, Faria AV. White matter atlases based on diffusion tensor imaging. *Curr Opin Neurol.* 2009 Aug;22(4):362–369.

Morgane PJ, Galler JR, Mokler DJ. A review of systems and networks of the limbic forebrain/limbic midbrain. *Prog Neurobiol.* 2005 Feb;75(2):143–160.

Moxon KA, Oliviero A, Aguilar J, Foffani G. Cortical reorganization after spinal cord injury: always for good? *Neuroscience.* 2014 Dec 26;283:78–94.

Naranjo EN, Cleworth TW, Allum JH, et al. Vestibulo-spinal and vestibulo-ocular reflexes are modulated when standing with increased postural threat. *J Neurophysiol.* 2016 Feb 1;115(2):833–842.

Nishio Y, Hashimoto M, Ishii K, Mori E. Neuroanatomy of a neurobehavioral disturbance in the left anterior thalamic infarction. *J Neurol Neurosurg Psychiatry.* 2011 Nov;82(11):1195–1200.

Omalu BI, DeKosky ST, Hamilton RL, et al. Chronic traumatic encephalopathy in a national football league player: Part II. *Neurosurgery.* 2006 Nov;59(5):1086–1092; discussion 1092–3.

Omalu BI, DeKosky ST, Minster RL, Kamboh MI, Hamilton RL, Wecht CH. Chronic traumatic encephalopathy in a National Football League player. *Neurosurgery.* 2005 Jul;57(1): 128–134; discussion 128–34.

Ostry DJ, Romo R. Tactile shape processing. *Neuron.* 2001 Aug 2;31(2):173–174.

Pierrot-Deseilligny C, Milea D, Müri RM. Eye movement control by the cerebral cortex. *Curr Opin Neurol.* 2004 Feb;17(1):17–25.

Pieters T, Majerus B. The introduction of chlorpromazine in Belgium and the Netherlands (1951–1968); tango between old and new treatment features. *Stud Hist Philos Biol Biomed Sci.* 2011 Dec;42(4):443–452.

Pons TP, Garraghty PE, Friedman DP, Mishkin M. Physiological evidence for serial processing in somatosensory cortex. *Science.* 1987 Jul 24;237(4813):417–420.

Pouget P. The cortex is in overall control of "voluntary" eye movement. *Eye (Lond).* 2015 Feb;29(2):241–245.

Prudente CN, Stilla R, Buetefisch CM, et al. Neural substrates for head movements in humans: a functional magnetic resonance imaging study. *J Neurosci.* 2015 Jun 17;35(24):9163–9172.

Qiu A, Mori S, Miller MI. Diffusion tensor imaging for understanding brain development in early life. *Annu Rev Psychol.* 2015 Jan 3;66:853–876.

Rakic P. The radial edifice of cortical architecture: From neuronal silhouettes to genetic engineering. *Brain Res Rev.* 2007 Oct;55(2):204–219.

Ramachandran VS. Mirror neurons and imitation learning as the driving force behind the great leap forward in human evolution. *Edge Foundation.* 2017 Jan 16.

Ramachandran VS, Hubbard EM. Hearing colors, tasting shapes. *Sci Am.* 2003 May;288(5):52–59.

Ramachandran VS, Hubbard EM. Psychophysical investigations into the neural basis of synaesthesia. *Proc Biol Sci.* 2001 May 7;268(1470):979–983.

Rauchs G, Desgranges B, Foret J, Eustache F. The relationships between memory systems and sleep stages. *J Sleep Res.* 2005 Jun;14(2):123–140.

Rimkus Cde M, Junqueira Tde F, Callegaro D, Otaduy MC, Leite Cda C. Segmented corpus callosum diffusivity correlates with the Expanded Disability Status Scale score in the early stages of relapsing-remitting multiple sclerosis. *Clinics (Sao Paulo).* 2013;68(8):1115–1120.

Rivara CB, Sherwood CC, Bouras C, Hof PR. Stereologic characterization and spatial distribution patterns of Betz cells in the human primary motor cortex. *Anat Rec A Discov Mol Cell Evol Biol.* 2003 Feb;270(2):137–151.

Rizzolatti G, Craighero L. The mirror-neuron system. *Annu Rev Neurosci.* 2004;27:169–192.

Rossi AF, Pessoa L, Desimone R, Ungerleider LG. The prefrontal cortex and the executive control of attention. *Exp Brain Res.* 2009 Jan;192(3):489–497.

Rubio-Garrido P, Pérez-de-Manzo F, Porrero C, Galazo MJ, Clascá F. Thalamic input to distal apical dendrites in neocortical layer 1 is massive and highly convergent. *Cereb Cortex.* 2009 Oct;19(10): 2380–2395.

Saur D, Kreher BW, Schnell S, et al. Ventral and dorsal pathways for language. *Proc Natl Acad Sci USA.* 2008 Nov 18;105(46):18035–18040.

Scoville WB, Milner B. Loss of recent memory after bilateral hippocampal lesions. 1957. *J Neuropsychiatry Clin Neurosci.* 2000 Winter;12(1):103–113.

Scholz J, Klein MC, Behrens TE, Johansen-Berg H. Training induces changes in white-matter architecture. *Nat Neurosci.* 2009 Nov;12(11):1370–1371.

Schmahmann JD, Pandya DN. Cerebral white matter—historical evolution of facts and notions concerning the organization of the fiber pathways of the brain. *J Hist Neurosci.* 2007 Jul–Sep;16(3):237–267.

Shallo-Hoffmann J, Bronstein AM. Visual motion detection in patients with absent vestibular function. *Vision Res.* 2003 Jun;43(14):1589–1594.

Sharma R, Hicks S, Berna CM, Kennard C, Talbot K, Turner MR. Oculomotor dysfunction in amyotrophic lateral sclerosis: a comprehensive review. *Arch Neurol.* 2011 Jul;68(7):857–861.

Shinder ME, Newlands SD. Sensory convergence in the parieto-insular vestibular cortex. *J Neurophysiol.* 2014 Jun 15;111(12):2445–2464.

Shipp S. Structure and function of the cerebral cortex. *Curr Biol.* 2007 Jun 19;17(12):R443–R449.

Shu SY, Wu YM, Bao XM, Leonard B. Interactions among memory-related centers in the brain. *J Neurosci Res.* 2003 Mar 1;71(5):609–616.

Shura RD, Hurley RA, Taber KH. Insular cortex: structural and functional neuroanatomy. *J Neuropsychiatry Clin Neurosci.* 2014 Fall;26(4): 276–282.

Squire LR, Stark CE, Clark RE. The medial temporal lobe. *Annu Rev Neurosci.* 2004;27:279–306.

Simons JS, Garrison JR, Johnson MK. Brain mechanisms of reality monitoring. *Trends Cogn Sci.* 2017 Jun;21(6):462–473.

Standaert DG, Lee VM, Greenberg BD, Lowery DE, Trojanowski JQ. Molecular features of hypothalamic plaques in Alzheimer's disease. *Am J Pathol.* 1991 Sep;139(3):681–691.

Sutherland RJ, Whishaw IQ, Kolb B. Contributions of cingulate cortex to two forms of spatial learning and memory. *J Neurosci.* 1988 Jun;8(6):1863–1872.

Taber KH, Warden DL, Hurley RA. Blast-related traumatic brain injury: what is known? *J Neuropsychiatry Clin Neurosci.* 2006 Spring;18(2): 141–145.

Tan SY, Yip A. António Egas Moniz (1874–1955): Lobotomy pioneer and Nobel laureate. *Singapore Med J.* 2014 Apr;55(4):175–176.

Tarczy-Hornoch K, Martin KA, Jack JJ, Stratford KJ. Synaptic interactions between smooth and spiny neurones in layer 4 of cat visual cortex in vitro. *J Physiol.* 1998 Apr 15;508(Pt 2):351–363.

Thaler D, Chen YC, Nixon PD, Stern CE, Passingham RE. The functions of the medial premotor cortex. I. Simple learned movements. *Exp Brain Res.* 1995;102(3):445–460.

Thier P, Ilg UJ. The neural basis of smooth-pursuit eye movements. *Curr Opin Neurobiol.* 2005 Dec;15(6):645–652.

Trettenbrein PC. The demise of the synapse as the locus of memory: a looming paradigm shift? *Front Syst Neurosci.* 2016 Nov 17;10:88.

Vallar G. Spatial neglect, Balint-Homes' and Gerstmann's syndrome, and other spatial disorders. *CNS Spectr.* 2007 Jul;12(7):527–536.

Van Ombergen A, Lubeck AJ, Van Rompaey V, et al. The effect of optokinetic stimulation on perceptual and postural symptoms in visual vestibular mismatch patients. *PLoS One.* 2016 Apr 29;11(4):e0154528.

van Polanen V, Davare M. Interactions between dorsal and ventral streams for controlling skilled grasp. *Neuropsychologia.* 2015 Dec;79(Pt B):186–191.

Vysetti S, Shinde S, Chaudhry S, Subramoney K. Phlegmasia cerulea dolens—a rare, life-threatening condition. *Scientific World Journal.* 2009 Oct 14;9:1105–1106.

Wakana S, Jiang H, Nagae-Poetscher LM, van Zijl PC, Mori S. Fiber tract-based atlas of human white matter anatomy. *Radiology.* 2004 Jan;230(1):77–87.

Ward Z. Letter to the editor: reexamining Penfield's homunculus. *J Hist Neurosci.* 2014; 23(2): 198–203.

Williams JH, Whiten A, Suddendorf T, Perrett DI. Imitation, mirror neurons and autism. *Neurosci Biobehav Rev.* 2001 Jun;25(4):287–295.

Woolsey TA, van der Loos H. 1970. The structural organization of layer IV in the somatosensory region (S I) of mouse cerebral cortex. *Brain Res.* 2016 Nov 15;1651:121.

Yousry TA, Schmid UD, Alkadhi H, et al. Localization of the motor hand area to a knob on the precentral gyrus. A new landmark. *Brain.* 1997 Jan;120(Pt 1):141–157.

Zaidi FH, Hull JT, Peirson SN, et al. Short-wavelength light sensitivity of circadian, pupillary, and visual awareness in humans lacking an outer retina. *Curr Biol.* 2007 Dec 18;17(24):2122–2128.

Zhuo M. Cortical plasticity as a new endpoint measurement for chronic pain. *Mol Pain.* 2011 Jul 28;7:54.

> **REVIEW QUESTIONS**

1. Brodmann's areas were originally defined by the following:
   A. Different cellular types and density in cortical layers
   B. Speed of nerve conduction within the corpus callosum
   C. Presence or absence of sulci and gyri in the outer cortical layers
   D. Topographical variations in the skull that imply underlying brain anatomy

2. The following statement best describes the six layers of the cortex:
   A. The deepest granular layers are the main targets for ascending input from the ipsilateral and contralateral cortex.
   B. Layers are numbered from superficial to deep, and contain different cell types that give each layer a different look and function.
   C. Layers are numbered by quantity of stellate cells that project from the thalamus to the neocortex.
   D. Only the deepest layers contain glial cells for repair and maintenance due to high risk of injury in these areas.

3. Ocular dominance, the dominance of one eye over the other, occurs for the following functions:
   A. Tear production and coordination of extraocular muscle function
   B. Light perception and blink reflex
   C. Binocular vision and orientation of objects in space
   D. Input for both sleep and wake cycles

4. Cortical motor control incorporates the following information for selection, planning, and producing motion:
   A. Information from area S1 for complex, distal, bimanual control
   B. Outputs to the dorsal columns for precise muscle contraction
   C. Visual, somatosensory, vestibular, and auditory information
   D. Afferent input from corticospinal and corticobulbar tracts

5. The somatosensory homunculus demonstrates:
   A. general mapping of sensory receptors in area S1.
   B. precise location of sensory receptors in area S2.
   C. mapping of motor and sensory information in areas M1 and S1.
   D. proportional representation of sensory mapping in area S1.

6. Central processing of vestibular information is best described as:
   A. occurring primarily within the vestibular cortex in the temporal lobe.
   B. integrating visual and somatosensory information for accurate interpretation.
   C. subservient to somatosensory input, such as pressure and vibration.
   D. dominant over vision and proprioception in normally sighted individuals.

7. Pain is experienced within the cortex in the following
   sequence:
   A. Dorsal horn, spinal cord nuclei, thalamus, S1 cortex
   B. Skin receptor, ventral horn, limbic lobe, thalamus, S1
       cortex
   C. Ventral horn, dorsal column, thalamus, lamina V
   D. Dorsal horn, lamina V, brainstem nuclei, S1 cortex

8. Cognition is adversely affected by cortical injury,
   including:
   A. damage to the parietal lobe, which changes the patient's
       behavioral responses and personality.
   B. damage to the frontal lone, which impairs spatial coordi-
       nation and attention.
   C. damage to the temporal lobe, which impairs processing
       visual inputs into memory.
   D. damage to the occipital lobe, which impairs the consoli-
       dation of short-term memory to long-term memory.

9. Speech production deficits are divided into several broad
   categories, including:
   A. fluent and nonfluent aphasia.
   B. Graham's and Mosconi's aphasia.
   C. cognitive and prosodic aphasia.
   D. temporal and motor aphasia.

10. Ideal rehabilitation after acquired brain injury requires
    knowledge of which of the following?
    A. Neuroplasticity principles, neurologic response to injury,
        potential medical complications
    B. Factors that influence patient participation, such as past
        experiences and ongoing social and emotional support
    C. Detailed principles of neuroanatomy and neuroscience
        to localize damage and address functional and behav-
        ioral consequences
    D. An effective rehabilitation provider will integrate all the
        information described above as well as new research for
        best clinical practice.

Cranial Nerve Testing

Victoria Graham, Maryke Neiberg, and Tony Mosconi

Clinical testing of cranial nerves is quick and yields valuable information. Formal assessment of cranial nerve function is important for clinical diagnosis as well as tracking therapeutic progress after nervous system damage. Injury produces classic presentations based on the laterality of the lesion and the anatomic distribution of long pathways and CN nuclei at the injury site, allowing for precise localization of the damage based on clinical findings. Clinical assessment of cranial nerve function requires practice and a solid understanding of what is normal. A thorough examination includes observation for facial or postural asymmetry, and listening for difficulty with speech. These initial observations inform the selection of specific follow up questions regarding difficulty with basic function including vision, hearing, balance, eating, and speech production.

 HOW TO TEST CN I, THE OLFACTORY NERVE

Cranial nerve I is responsible for the sense of smell. Each nostril detects odors independently and connects directly to the forebrain. Loss of CN I function may be one of the earliest sign of Alzheimer's or Parkinson's disease; periodic, in-office testing is advised.

Observation

There is no directly observable behavior of olfactory dysfunction. The patient may have reduced appetite or decreased enjoyment of meals, which may lead to weight loss or signs such as baggy clothing.

Screening

Ask whether loss of smell is present or if food tastes different than it did in the past. A history of smoking may confound the diagnosis; ask about smoking habits as part of the comprehensive history.

Examination

Test patency of the nostrils, listening for a clear passage while inhaling. Close a nostril and test the smell discrimination of each olfactory bulb by asking the patient to identify or name (if communication allows) scents such as vanilla versus citrus, or coffee versus chocolate.

 HOW TO TEST CN II, THE OPTIC NERVE

Observation

Note behaviors such as bumping into or avoiding objects. Observe for squinting or an eye turn.

Screening

Inquire about blurry or dim vision. Ask about difficulty with peripheral vision such as bumping or walking into objects. Inquire about difficulty driving at night or during dusk. Ask about ease of reading and use of computer or tablet.

Examination

Evaluate visual acuity, contrast sensitivity, and visual fields as appropriate and critical to appropriate diagnosis.

Visual acuity

Measure the Snellen visual acuity of each eye at 20 feet (far) and at 16 inches (near), indicating function of the central (foveal) vision at distance (Figure A.1) and at near. Repeat the measurement, using a pinhole. If acuity improves to 20/30 or better, the patient may simply need a new glasses prescription to correct his vision. If the visual acuity does not improve to at least 20/30, it may indicate pathology that should be further investigated.

Central visual field

Utilize an Amsler grid to evaluate central vision. An Amsler grid is a small printed square, divided into a grid, with a dot in the

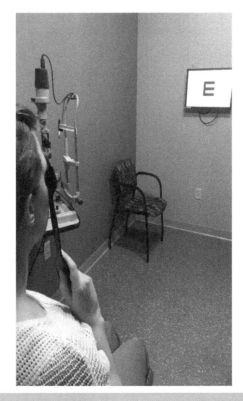

FIGURE A.1

In-office visual acuity measurement of the left eye.

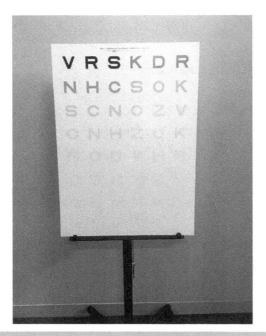

FIGURE A.2

Pelli-Robson contrast sensitivity chart.

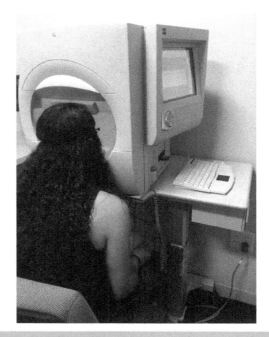

FIGURE A.3

Automated visual field testing.

middle. Each eye is tested individually, and the patient is asked to identify and describe areas of visual loss or distortion while keeping steady fixation on the central dot.

Contrast sensitivity. Contrast sensitivity assesses vision in terms of decreasing increments of contrast and is very effective in demonstrating mild visual loss, or visual loss under dim conditions. A special eye chart with sine waves or contrast sensitivity gratings is used under very specific illumination conditions to determine visual function (Figure A.2).

Peripheral visual fields. Compare each quadrant of the patient's peripheral visual field to the examiner's visual field, and note any abnormalities. Each eye is tested separately. Evaluate the right and left visual field pattern to look for diagnostic patterns of vision loss, such as bitemporal hemianopia. To formally evaluate the visual field, use a threshold visual field device or a visual field perimeter (Figure A.3).

Light perception

Use a bright light source to check the pupils for direct and consensual response. Measure the size of each pupil in bright and dim light (Figure A.4). Look for unequal pupil size, known as anisocoria.

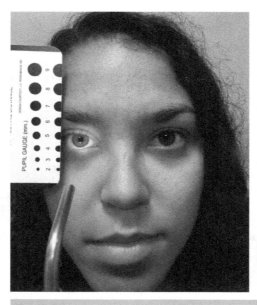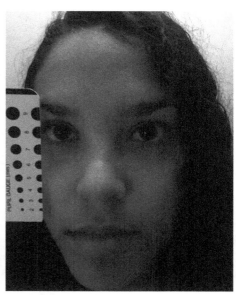

FIGURE A.4

As part of the pupillary evaluation, the size of each of the pupils is measured in bright and dim illumination.

The abnormal pupil could be the dilated or constricted pupil. A small pupil is caused by Horner syndrome or pain, or may be iatrogenic from inadvertent use of miotic eye drops. Adie pupil or CN III palsy causes a large pupil.

Perform the swinging flashlight test to check for an afferent pupillary defect (Figure A.5). During this test, the examiner

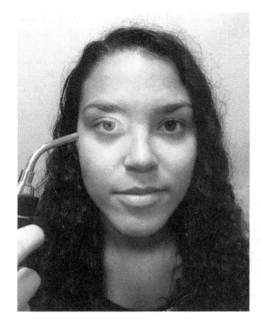 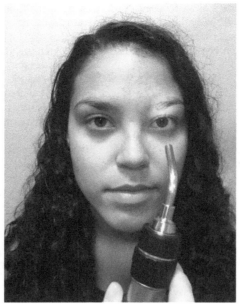

FIGURE A.5

As demonstrated in the images, shining a bright light in either pupil should not alter the size of the pupil. If the pupil constricts or dilates during the swinging flashlight test, an efferent pupillary defect is present. Note how the light is contained during the test to one side of the face only and is not allowed to spill over to the other eye.

instructs the patient to look at a distant target while the examiner illuminates only one pupil at a time with a very bright light for 3 to 4 seconds. The examiner smoothly and rapidly moves the flashlight over to the other eye, without interrupting the constant and even illumination of each of the eyes. This process is repeated, illuminating each eye for 3 to 4 seconds, to observe the pupillary response. If both right and left visual pathways are intact, both pupils should remain the same size, regardless of which eye is illuminated. An abnormal response is present when one pupil dilates or constricts when directly illuminated.

Color vision

Perform color vision screening to evaluate CN II functioning. Color vision testing reflects the condition of the cone cells in the macula. Test each eye separately to detect subtle acquired visual defects. Congenital color vision defects are the same in both eyes.

Direct evaluation of the optic nerve, macula, and retina with ophthalmoscopy is critical. The optic nerve should appear flat and rosy. It should have a small optic cup. Imaging the optic nerve and/or bits with ultrasound or magnetic resonance imaging may be helpful.

HOW TO TEST CN III, THE OCULOMOTOR NERVE

Observation

Observe the patient for a head turn. Observe the direction of each eye, and note the preferred eye. The lid on the affected side may droop (ptosis). If the lid does not droop, the patient might wear an eye patch to alleviate double vision. Lift the lid to observe the direction of the affected eye. The eye will be turned downward and outward. Observe the pupils for anisocoria.

Screening

Ask about the presence of a drooping eyelid. Ask whether lifting the eyelid creates double vision. Ask about double vision while driving.

Inquire whether double vision goes away when one eye is closed or if the lid is dropped. (If the double vision persists, the problem is most likely optical and not neurological.) Ask whether the double vision is constant or intermittent, and if the images are horizontally or vertically apart. Ask about the onset and duration, and about any other focal neurological signs that would qualify the patient for an emergency room visit.

Examination

Examine the pupil size and function. Measure the lid position of each eye.

Study the position and movement of each eye individually. Two muscle pairs are responsible for movement of the eyeball to a particular direction. The inferior obliques and superior recti are elevators, whereas the superior obliques and inferior recti are depressors.

In primary gaze (looking straight ahead at a target), each muscle of the eye forms an angle with the visual axis at which it executes its primary action. The superior rectus and inferior rectus each form a 23-degree angle with the visual axis, and the inferior oblique forms a 51-degree angle, whereas the superior oblique (CN IV) forms a 54-degree angle. Each muscle also has a secondary action and a tertiary action. Secondary positions of gaze are along the horizontal and vertical plane, whereas tertiary actions occur as the eye executes oblique actions (summarized in Table A.1: Extraocular Muscles).

When an ocular muscle receives a signal to contract, an opposite but equal inhibitory impulse is sent to its antagonist so that it might relax and lengthen. This law is known as Sherrington's law of reciprocal innervation and is an important clinical concept.

A small target, like a penlight, is moved slowly in the shape of an H or double H.

To evaluate for underaction or overaction of a muscle, observe the extent of excursion of the eyeball. Diplopia may increase or disappear in a particular gaze. Underaction occurs when the eye moves in the field of the affected muscle. Hering's law states that conjugate (or yoke) muscles receive the same amount of innervation.

Overaction is often easier to observe. Hering's law applies to the levator palpebrae superioris also, and in CN III palsy the unaffected eye may appear to be much wider open than the paretic eye. The eye will be able to abduct due to the functioning CN VI but will be limited in all other fields of gaze.

Cover test

Evaluate the alignment of the eyes using the cover test. Alternately covering and uncovering one eye at a time with a paddle should not elicit much movement from either eye (Figure A.6). Both eyes should remain straight ahead and fixated on the target. In medial rectus palsy, the unaffected nonparetic eye looks straight ahead at the target. The paretic eye is turned outward due to the unopposed action of the lateral rectus in the same eye (refer to Sherrington's law above). When the fixating eye is covered, the paretic eye will take up fixation. To do so, it must go from its outward position. The eyes will alternately take up fixation, moving out to take up the paretic position and turning inward to take up fixation as the paddle is moved from eye to eye.

By the same token, it is possible to identify an inward turn of the eye, such as in lateral rectus (CN VI) palsy. In lateral rectus palsy, the paretic eye is turned inward. The paretic eye takes up fixation if the fixating eye is covered, and moves outward from its resting place. This inward movement confirms an esotropia.

When evaluating CN III palsy with the cover test, the lid should be lifted or taped up. The affected eye will be turned *"down and out"* in an exo-hypotropia. The amount of lid droop, or ptosis, should also be measured. Shine a penlight into the eye at the level of the pupil to create a pupillary reflex. Use a small measuring stick or millimeter rule to measure from the pupillary light reflex to the upper lid. Then measure from the pupillary light reflex downward to the lower lid. Repeat this measurement for each eye, and compare the findings for the two eyes. Express the two measurements as a "fraction." It is easy to determine which eye has the ptosis and if there is an upper lid or lower lid ptosis present.

Record the size of the pupils in dim and bright illumination, looking for a direct and consensual response. In a CN III palsy, the affected pupil may be larger and sluggish to respond to light. CN III carries the parasympathetic efferent fibers to the sphincter pupillae. In addition to evaluating eye movement and ptosis, examine the pupils.

Table A.1: Extraocular Muscles

CN	Muscle	Motion Direction		
		Vertical	**Horizontal**	**Torsion**
III	Medial rectus	—	Adduction	—
VI	Lateral rectus	—	Abduction	—
III	Inferior rectus	Depression	Adduction	Extorsion
IV	Superior oblique	Depression	Abduction	Intorsion
III	Superior rectus	Elevation	Adduction	Intorsion
III	Inferior oblique	Elevation	Abduction	Extorsion

HOW TO TEST CN IV, THE TROCHLEAR NERVE

Screening

Ask the patient about double vision and, if present, to clarify whether it is horizontally or vertically separated, or both.

Observation

Observe the patient's posture for a depressed or elevated head. Look for a head turn or a head tilt. Cranial nerve IV innervates the superior oblique. Its primary function is to extort and depress the eye. In a CN IV palsy, the patient presents with intortion and hypertropia.

FIGURE A.6

Cover test of left eye. The cover test is utilized to determine the presence of an eye turn. *A.* Starting position: observe the left eye. *B.* While covering the right eye, observe for motion of the left, uncovered eye. Covering an eye should not generate any movement of the other eye. The test should be repeated on the other eye to complete the investigation.

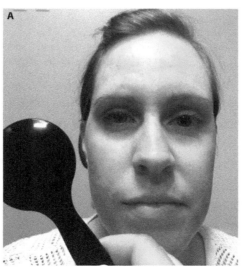
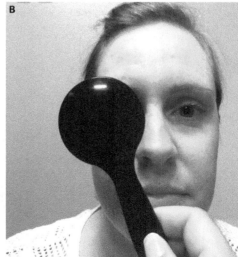

Examination

Use a penlight to evaluate ocular motility. Start directly in front of the patient in primary position, penlight held at 40 cm from the patient. Move the penlight into the cardinal positions of gaze, in the shape of an H. Note any underactions or overactions of the eyes during excursions. Perform the cover test. The affected eye will be elevated and extorted. Cover the normally fixating eye. The paretic eye (which was resting upward) will take up fixation.

Park three-step test to identify the paretic muscle

Step 1: Perform the cover test primary gaze (see Figures A.7 and Figure A.8) to determine whether a hypertropia or hypotropia is present. Step 1 identifies four muscles that may be involved in the hypertropia or hypotropia. The four muscles involved are the elevators of one eye and the depressors of the other eye.

Step 2: Perform the cover test while the patient turns the head to the side but looks at the target to the front. Repeat the cover test

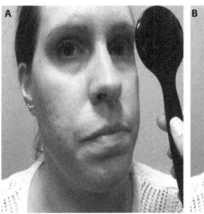 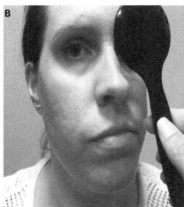 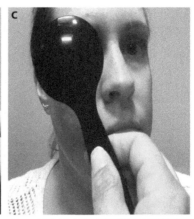

FIGURE A.7

The Park's three-step test. This test is performed to determine the muscle involved in an oblique muscle palsy. Step 1 is performed in primary gaze (see Figure A.8) to determine whether a hypertropia is present. Step 1 identifies four muscles that may be involved: the elevators in one eye and the depressors of the other eye. *A.* Step 2, as illustrated here, has the patient turn his or her head to the side while fixating on a target to the front. The goal is to determine whether the hypertropia is more noticeable in right or left gaze. This step narrows the possibly involved muscles to two from the original four, indicating an abductor in one eye and an adductor in the other. As in step 1, the eye is covered and the uncovered eye is observed for motion. Shown here: *B.* Covering left eye and observing right eye for motion. *C.* Covering right eye and observing left eye for motion.

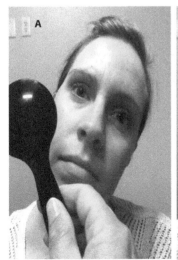 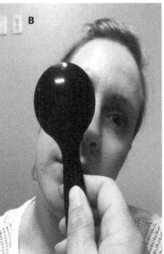 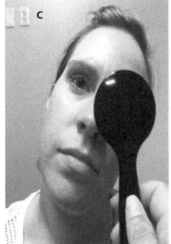 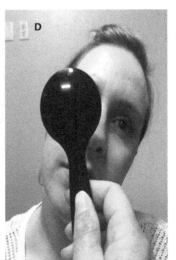

FIGURE A.8

Step 3 of the Park's three-step test evaluates the hypertropia while the head is tilted and determines whether the hypertropia is increased when the head is tilted to the left or right side. This step determines the single muscle involved in torsion of the affected eye. Shown: *A.* Starting position for left head tilt. *B.* Covering right eye and observing for motion of left. *C.* Covering left eye and observing for motion of right eye. *D.* Retesting left eye.

while the patient looks to the other side. The head turn simulates an eye turn but allows the cover test to be performed by the examiner. This step identifies the gaze in which the hyperdeviation or hypodeviation is worse and reduces the number of suspected muscles to two.

Step 3: Perform the cover test while the patient tilts the head to the shoulder, and then repeat for the other shoulder. The direction in which the tilt is worse identifies the muscle affected. This step determines the single muscle involved in torsion of the affected eye.

Step 1 is performed in primary gaze (see Figures A.7 and A.8) to determine whether a hypertropia is present. Step 1 identifies four muscles that may be involved: the elevators in one eye and the depressors of the other eye. Step 2 has the patient turn the head to the side while fixating a target to the front. The goal is to determine whether the hypertropia is more noticeable in the right or left gaze. This step narrows the possibly involved muscles to two from the original four, indicating an abductor in one eye and an adductor in the other. As in step 1, the eye is covered, and the uncovered eye is observed for motion. Step 3 of the Park's three-step test evaluates the hypertropia while the head is tilted and determines whether the hypertropia is increased when the head is tilted to the left or right side. This step determines the single muscle involved in torsion of the affected eye. Finally, ophthalmoscopy will show that the macula sits slightly lower than the optic nerve, because the eye is extorted in addition to being elevated. Typically, the macula and optic nerve are at the same horizontal level.

HOW TO TEST CN V, THE TRIGEMINAL NERVE

Screening

Inquire about sensory loss to the face, difficulty chewing, facial pain, or dry eye.

Observation

Observe for reduced muscle mass around the ipsilateral temporomandibular joint, inability to open or close the mouth, or asymmetrical deviations.

Examination

Sensory testing of the trigeminal nerve is conducted on each of the three divisions separately to localize lesions, whereas motor testing is performed only on the mandibular branch.

Sensory testing

Test sensory function of the nerve by testing each of the three sensory branches for light touch and pinprick sensation (Figures A.9–A.11). The ophthalmic branch is tested at the forehead, the maxillary branch, the cheek, and the mandibular branch at the jawline. The ophthalmic branch also carries the afferent sensory component of the corneal reflex, which can be tested with a light touch at the corner of the eye. Both eyes blink in response to the corneal contact; cranial nerve VII carries the motor signal to the orbicularis oculi muscles. This reflex is typically only tested during coma and may be extinguished in habitual contact lens wearers. All motor efferent function is carried on the mandibular branch to eight nerves primarily involved with mastication. To test muscle function, ask the patient to perform a motion, and note

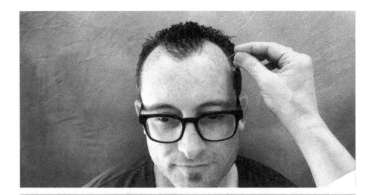

FIGURE A.9

Use a safety pin to test perception of sharp (pinprick) or dull (light touch) sensation in all three sensory areas. Shown: V1 testing of pain sensation using the sharp end of the pin.

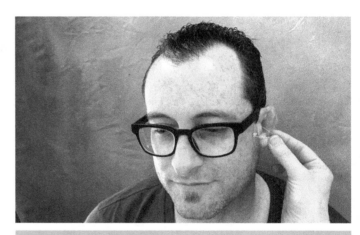

FIGURE A.10

Shown: Testing light touch over area V2 at the cheek. Patient is instructed to indicate either "sharp" or "dull."

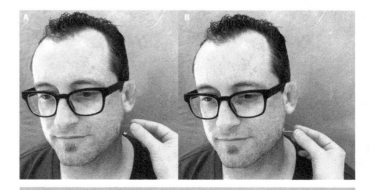

FIGURE A.11

Testing: *A.* pinprick and *B.* light touch over area V3 at jawline.

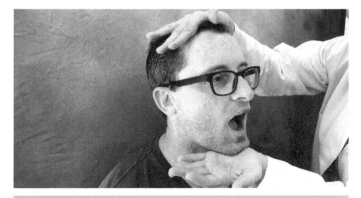

FIGURE A.12

Apply upward force to attempt to close the patient's mouth. Other hand is for counterpressure only, to avoid causing head or neck motion while testing.

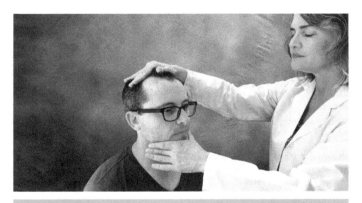

FIGURE A.13

Apply a downward force along the patient's mandible to test strength of mouth closure.

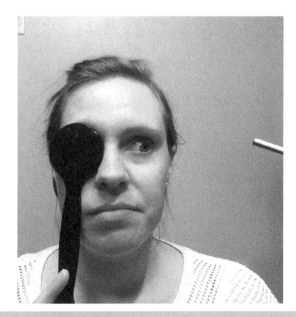

FIGURE A.14

CN VI (abducens nerve) function of the left eye is evaluated by having the patient look at a target to the left, demonstrating abduction of the left lateral rectus muscle. Examining the patient who has both eyes open while looking to the left evaluates left gaze. Left gaze is facilitated by CN VI (abducens nerve) in the left eye and CN III (oculomotor nerve) in the right eye.

To test jaw protrusion produced by the lateral and medial pterygoids, ask the patient to push his jaw forward, and then resist manually. This motion is normally strong and symmetrical.

 HOW TO TEST CN VI, THE ABDUCENS NERVE

Screening

Inquire about double vision and duration, and ask whether the double vision is constant or intermittent. Ask about double vision and whether images are horizontally or vertically apart. Ask about focal neurological signs that qualify the patient for an emergency room visit.

Observation

Observe whether the patient is wearing an eye patch or has a head turn or lid droop. Observe the direction of each eye. With CN VI palsy, the paretic eye will be turned inward to the nose.

Examination

The function of CN VI is to abduct the eye toward the temporal side of the head. Perform the cover test. An affected CN VI leaves the medial rectus unopposed, which will pull the eye toward the nose into esotropia. CN VI plays an important role in voluntary gaze of the eyes to the left or right. Check the eye movements to the sides of both eyes together, and look for an overaction of the unaffected eye in the field of the affected eye function (Figure A.14). This overaction is due to Hering's law, which states that conjugate muscles

any asymmetry and whether he or she has the ability to maintain the motion against manual resistance. Specific motion testing is described below.

Motor testing

Jaw opening is produced by the action of bilateral lateral pterygoids and three suprahyoids: digastric, mylohyoid, and geniohyoid. Ask the patient to open his mouth, noting any deviations. The jaw will deviate on whether it opens toward the weak side because of loss of ipsilateral pterygoid muscle strength. To manually test strength, place the heel of your hand under the patient's chin, and attempt to close the mouth, which will not be possible with normal strength (Figure A.12). The clinician must use caution when applying resistance, as many people have painful temporomandibular joints.

Jaw closure is produced by the masseter, temporalis, and medial pterygoid, and is tested by asking the patient to close her jaw and keep it closed as you attempt to open it forcefully with your hand (Figure A.13). These muscles are normally very strong, and the patient should be able to easily resist your efforts. You can also palpate the large masseter and temporalis muscles as they contract, and compare muscle mass for each side.

receive the same amount of innervation. In a CN VI palsy, the pupils should respond normally. Check the cranial nerves systematically and individually; multiple nerves are often involved with CN VI palsy, in particular CN VII and VIII.

HOW TO TEST CN VII, THE FACIAL NERVE

Screening

Inquire about facial reconstructive surgery or congenital conditions prior to concluding observations or findings are new. Ask whether any changes are noted in ability to smile, eating or drinking, or dry eye. If there is cranial nerve VII loss, the patient may not be aware of lost light touch sensation of the outer ear, tympanic membrane, and external auditory meatus, as well as to soft palate and nasal cavity, so patient education may be indicated for safety. Also, loss of parasympathetic function may impair function of the lacrimal and salivary glands, causing dry eye or difficulty chewing, drinking, and swallowing.

Observation

Look for facial symmetry, particularly during conversation.

Examination

Testing of the facial nerve typically only includes muscles of facial expression, specifically of each branch to localize the lesion. CN VII innervates many structures; a thorough clinician will identify potential functional limitations caused by nerve damage, and address these findings through referral and patient education.

Sensory testing

Use a spoon to place either sugar or salt onto the tip of the patient's tongue, and ask for identification (Figure A.15). Tactile sense to the outer ear and soft palate are rarely tested clinically, as motor findings are easier to observe and quantify.

Motor testing

Test motor function cranial to caudal, beginning with the temporofacial branch, which innervates the muscles of the upper face via temporal, zygomatic, and infraorbital branches. The frontalis and/or bicularis oculi muscles are most commonly tested due to their clearly observable and easily tested motor function.

Frontalis. Sit across from the patient, demonstrating the behavior as you ask the patient to raise the eyebrows. Observe motion, noting each side. If patient is able to produce motion, test strength by placing your thumbs above each eyebrow, and gently press inferiorly, asking the patient to raise the eyebrows and not let you pull them down. Normally the patient should be able to contract against your gentle resistance.

Orbicularis oculi. Ask the patient to open and close both eyes (Figure A.16) and then alter closing them unilaterally (Figure A.17). Observe for depth of closure by noting eyelash length at end of excursion and comparing sides. Normal is complete closure, with no iris visible. Grade strength by comparing speed of excursion between each eye, noting whether one side closes more quickly. Grade partial closure by amount of eye exposed at full excursion: strongest is if iris no longer visible; weaker is if no iris is visible, but a small amount of sclera is visible; weakest is if iris is fully visible

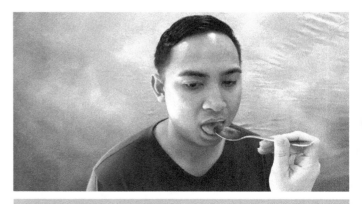

FIGURE A.15

Place sugar or salt on patient's anterior tongue to test taste sensation.

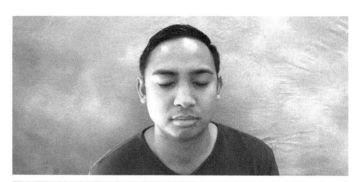

FIGURE A.16

Patient closing both eyes.

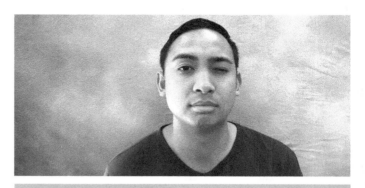

FIGURE A.17

Alternating eye closure.

(Figure A.18). Measure the palpebral aperture, using a millimeter rule, from the corneal reflex produced by a handheld hand held penlight to the upper lid and then from the corneal reflex to the lower lid. Repeat for the other eye (Figure A.19).

Next test several muscles of the lower face innervated by the cervicofacial branch via buccal, mandibular, and cervical nerves.

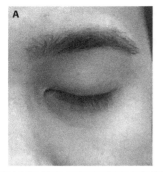 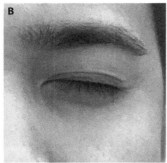 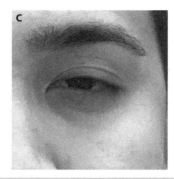 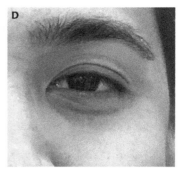

FIGURE A.18

A. Full closure of left eye. Grade partial closure by amount of eye exposed at full excursion. *B.* Strongest partial closure with iris no longer visible, but eye remains partially open. *C.* Weaker partial closure; iris is no longer visible, but small amount of sclera is visible. *D.* Weakest is when iris and sclera are fully visible.

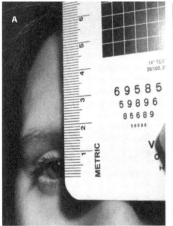 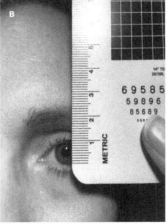

FIGURE A.19

Measure the palpebral aperture, using a millimeter rule, from the corneal reflex produced by a handheld penlight to the upper lid and then from the corneal reflex to the lower lid. The numerator is from the corneal reflex to the upper lid, and the denominator is from the *B.* corneal reflex to the lower lid. Repeat for the other eye. Shown: *A.* Right eye (OD) 1/7 mm, Left eye (OS) 3/7 mm.

Procerus. Ask the patient to wrinkle his nose, noting any flattening of the nasolabial folds. You may also observe this area for associated muscle contractions during other facial motion testing, as subtle weakness may be observed. Test for normal strength by adding resistance: place your thumbs alongside the bridge of the nose, and resist outwardly (Figure A.20). A normal-strength muscle will be able to maintain the nasal creases even with your manual resistance.

Zygomaticus major. Ask the patient to smile broadly, and compare each side for symmetry (Figure A.21). To establish an objective

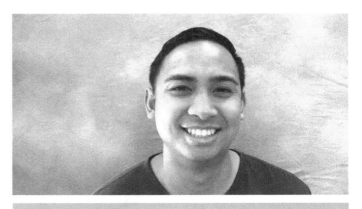

FIGURE A.20

Resist motion of the procerus with lateral pull.

FIGURE A.21

Smile at your patients, and they will usually smile back more naturally than if you ask them to smile. You can also get them to laugh, or you can note facial symmetry during your examination.

baseline for any asymmetry due to weakness, measure each side with a goniometer, noting distance from the central incisor to the corner of the mouth.

Buccinator. Ask the patient to suck in the cheeks, observing and listening for any air loss (Figure A.22). Insert a tongue depressor into the mouth to test strength, with the flat side against the teeth. Push out toward the patient's cheek while contracting the buccinator. A strong muscle will hold against your resistance (Figure A.23).

Orbicularis oris. Ask patient to purse lips, and hold them against the tongue blade (Figure A.24). Observe for complete mouth

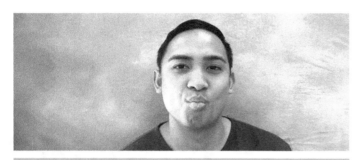

FIGURE A.22

Demonstrating buccinator function bilaterally.

closure and symmetry. Apply resistance toward the oral cavity with the flat side of a tongue blade placed across the upper and lower lips. Normal strength will easily contract and hold resistance against the tongue blade.

◼ HOW TO TEST CN VIII, THE COCHLEAR NERVE

Screening

Ask about hearing loss, tinnitus, or fullness in ears. Inquire about sound differentiation, such as in crowded rooms or high versus low frequencies. To screen for hearing loss, place your hands near the patient's ears, on either side. Alternate rubbing your index finger and thumb together, and ask the patient to tell if the sound is heard on one side more than the other.

Observation

Always screen cochlear CN VIII in the presence of facial CN VII or vestibular CN VIII findings, due to close anatomic proximity in IAC.

Examination

The Rinne and Weber tests are used together to screen for unilateral hearing loss by comparing sound conduction (SC) to air conduction (AC). Abnormal findings may indicate referral for audiometry, and it is important to note that normal results may still miss bilateral

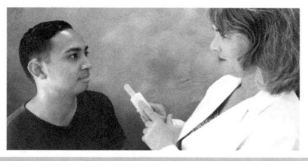
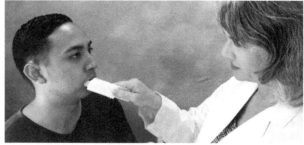

FIGURE A.23

To test buccinator strength, insert sterile tongue blade into the patient's mouth between teeth and cheek. Press outwardly to resist muscle action.

FIGURE A.24

When testing orbicularis oris, it is easiest to purse your own lips and ask patient to mimic you. *A.* Patient demonstrating active motion. *B.* To quantify any weakness, add resistance medially with a tongue blade.

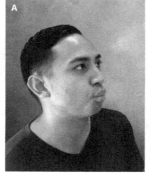
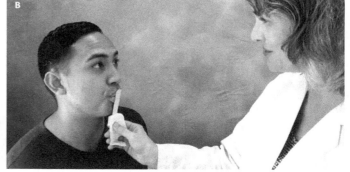

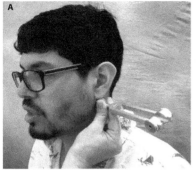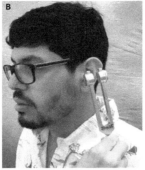
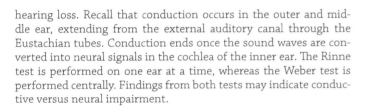

Rinne test. **A.** Strike tuning fork and hold it against the mastoid process. When patient can no longer hear the sound, then **B.** move the tuning fork to just outside the ear. In a normal test, the patient will hear the tuning fork once again.

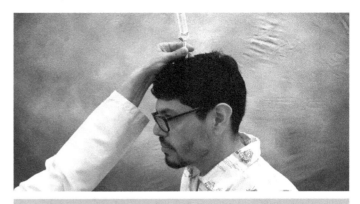

Weber test.

hearing loss. Recall that conduction occurs in the outer and middle ear, extending from the external auditory canal through the Eustachian tubes. Conduction ends once the sound waves are converted into neural signals in the cochlea of the inner ear. The Rinne test is performed on one ear at a time, whereas the Weber test is performed centrally. Findings from both tests may indicate conductive versus neural impairment.

Rinne test

Strike the tuning fork (512 Hz) and then, with it still vibrating, place it against the patient's mastoid process (Figure A.25A). Ask the patient to tell you when the sound is no longer audible, and then move the tuning fork to just outside the external auditory meatus (Figure A.25B). The patient should still be able to hear the sound in a normal test, indicating the same or greater hearing for air conduction as for bone conduction (AC > BC). An abnormal test indicates conductive loss (such as a peripheral blockage), and BC will be greater than AC, which means the patient will not hear the tuning fork in the air as well as when placed against the bone.

Weber test

Strike the tuning fork (256 Hz) and place it on the top of the patient's head at midline (Figure A.26). Ask the patient which side is the loudest; normal findings will be heard equally in each ear. When the sound is perceived louder in one ear, it is described as lateralized to that side. This means that BC > AC during this test, and it indicates normal neural function on that side, as the cochlear basilar membrane detected the sound wave vibrations and sent the neural signal up for auditory processing.

Combining test findings is more complicated and is described in Table A.2. If the person has normal findings for both tests, the patient is unlikely to have ipsilateral hearing loss. If the Rinne test is abnormal (BC > AC) and the Weber test lateralizes to the same ear, then the person is likely to have conductive loss. This is because the louder sound is only coming from the inner ear signals, without any external noise from the environment. If the Rinne test is normal and the Weber test lateralizes to the same intact ear, then the loss is sensorineural because only the intact ear can perceive the sound coming from the vibrating tuning fork.

Table A.2 Rinne and Weber Tests—Interpreting Findings

Weber Test Findings	Weber Test Results	Rationale
Centralized	No ipsilateral hearing loss detected	Both tests normal
Lateralized to the conductive loss side	Conductive loss in lateralized ear	Because the louder sound is only coming from the inner ear signals without any external noise from the environment
Lateralized to the normal hearing side	Sensorineural loss in nonlateralized ear	Because only the intact ear can perceive the sound coming from the vibrating tuning fork

Note: Abnormal findings may indicate referral for audiometry. Normal findings may still miss bilateral hearing loss.

 HOW TO TEST CN VIII, THE VESTIBULAR NERVE

Screening

Ask whether the patient has vertigo (spinning sensation), a feeling of imbalance, or nausea with positional changes. Further determine whether the vertigo is intermittent or constant and associated with hearing loss.

Observation

Acute vestibular loss may cause severe dizziness or vertigo that produces nystagmus or a staggering gait. Dizziness can be divided into four types that include vertigo, presyncope, unsteadiness, and nonspecific dizziness. Interruption of the shared blood supply from the posterior cerebral circulation by infarction in the area of the anterior inferior cerebellar artery (AICA) may both affect hearing and cause transient dizziness. These patients are significantly at risk for stroke. Acute vestibular syndrome (AVS) is typically associated with symptoms such as nausea and/or vomiting and intolerance to head movement that lasts longer than 24 hours. These patients typically present to the emergency room due to the associated symptoms. AVS is usually presumed to be a vestibular neuritis that is viral or post-viral in nature, but central causes of vertigo include multiple sclerosis, and brainstem and cerebellar ischemic stroke. Most vestibular dysfunction presenting to general practice has a subtle clinical presentation only seen with specific testing to elicit responses.

Examination

The head thrust test, also known as the horizontal head impulse test (h-HIT), measures the horizontal semicircular canal VOR. The clinician and patient are seated across from each other (Figure A.27A). Flex the patient's head 30 degrees to ensure cupular stimulation of the canals by bringing them into the horizontal plane (Figure A.27B).

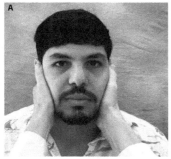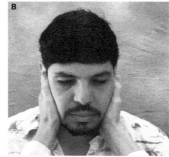

FIGURE A.27

Preparing to perform head thrust maneuver. **A.** Patient seated in front of clinician, who is holding his head steady. **B.** Tilt head down 30 degrees to orient horizontal semicircular canals in the transverse plane.

Ask the patient to maintain focus on your nose as you move the head to one side quickly, approximately 15–25 degrees (Figure A.28). Normal VOR function will trigger eye motion in the opposite direction of head motion, maintaining the precise angle to keep images stable on the fovea. Clinically, the eyes will appear to remain still. An abnormal finding will be eye motion, as the VOR reflex will not accurately move the eyes opposite head motion. Clinically this is commonly seen with VOR reflex hypofunction, during which the patient looks away from the central target (your nose) at the end of the head movement, then quickly makes a corrective eye saccade back to midline. Corrective saccades occur with vestibular hypofunction, because inhibition on the intact side (inhibitory cutoff) is less effective in encoding the amplitude of a head movement than excitation, which has been lost on the hypofunction side.

The HINTS test is a three-part battery of tests that can be used in the emergency room to attempt to rapidly classify AVS as being central or peripheral origin. HINTS is only useful when the vertigo is present longer than 24 hours and constant. Although helpful, an MRI is still the gold standard for differentiating peripheral versus central lesions. As indicated by its acronym, this test has three components: the head impulse test (HI), observation for nystagmus (N), and test of skew deviation (TS).

Performing the HINTS

1. To interpret the results, an abnormal VOR (positive head impulse, HI) in a patient with AVS usually indicates a peripheral lesion of the vestibular system or an AICA infarction, whereas a normal response in a patient with AVS is almost always associated with stroke.
2. To observe for nystagmus, carefully observe the patient's lateral eye movements. A direction-changing nystagmus in lateral gaze most likely has a central etiology.
3. Finally, the alternating cover test can be used to evaluate for a vertical deviation of the eyes. When there is an imbalance of the otolithic inputs, a skew (S) deviation manifests as a vertical imbalance in the eyes.

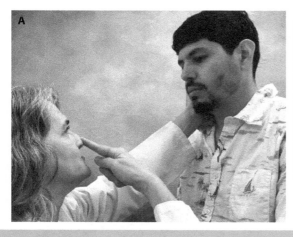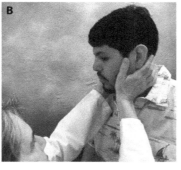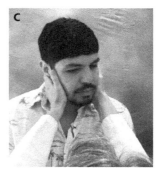

FIGURE A.28

Head thrust maneuver. **A.** Instruct patient to keep looking at your nose while you rapidly turn his head to each side **B.** and **C.**

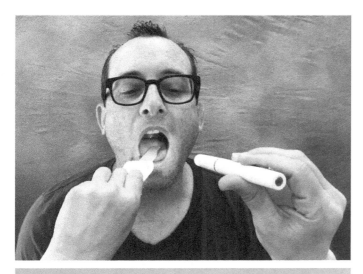

FIGURE A.29

Viewing the back of the throat for palatoglossal arch elevation during phonation.

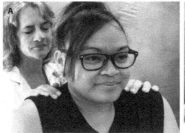 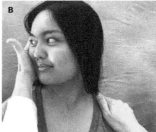

FIGURE A.30

Testing of CN XI. **A.** Patient shrugs shoulders to test strength of upper trapezii, as resistance is added downward. **B.** Testing left sternocleidomastoid muscle, with head rotation to right resisted manually.

 HOW TO TEST CN IX, THE GLOSSOPHARYNGEAL NERVE

Screening

Cranial nerves IX and X are usually evaluated together. Many of their functions overlap; they are both mixed sensory and motor, and both exit from the brain stem side by side, through the jugular foramen, and are often damaged together.

Observation

When viewing the palate, it should appear to have symmetry on each side; the uvula should be centered; and the palate should rise when the patient says "aah."

Examination

When evaluating CN IX, also evaluate CN X to CN XII, and check the pupils for Horner's syndrome. Use a penlight to illuminate the inside of the mouth, and ask the patient to say "aah" while you use the tongue depressor to gently push down the tongue (Figure A.29). Observe the palate; the arch should rise and move posteriorly as the patient says "aah." If needed for testing, gently brushing the palate should create a gag reflex. The gag reflex should be tested on each side of the posterior pharyngeal wall. The gag reflex should only be tested in unconscious patients or those with brainstem pathology or impaired swallowing.

 HOW TO TEST CN X, THE VAGUS NERVE

Observation

There are no separate CN X findings that can be definitively observed. As for CN IX, listen to the patient talk; listen for hoarseness, whispering, or nasal speech. When viewing the palate, it should appear

to have symmetry on each side, and the palatoglossal arches should rise when the patient says "aah."

Screening

Cranial nerves IX and X are usually evaluated together, if needed. Many of their functions overlap; they exit from the brainstem through the jugular foramen, side by side, and are often damaged together.

Examination

Use a penlight to illuminate the inside of the mouth, and ask the patient to say "aah" while you use the tongue depressor to gently push down the tongue (Figure A.29). Observe the palatoglossal arches. They should rise and move posteriorly as the patient says, "aah." Gently brushing the palate should create a gag reflex. If you do need to test the reflex, warn the patient that you will be testing it before you do. The oculocardiac reflex is mediated by the vagus. Applying gentle pressure on the closed eyes should cause the heart rate to slow but, as part of the triad, may also cause nausea and syncope.

 HOW TO TEST CN XI, THE SPINAL ACCESSORY NERVE

Observation

Observe the volume and contour of the sternocleidomastoid muscle. Also observe the shoulder contour, and look for drooping.

Screening

Ask the patient whether there is any weakness or difficulty moving her head or shoulders.

Examination

To test upper trapezius muscles, place your hands on the sides of both of the patient's shoulders and passively elevate them, noting any loss of motion. Allow the shoulders to return to resting, and then ask your patient to repeat the motion. Note any asymmetry or difficulty (Figure A.30A). A strong muscle will be able to move easily

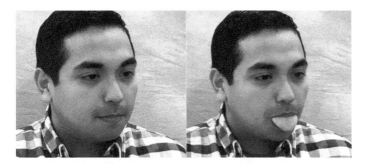

FIGURE A.31

Testing tongue protrusion.

through the motion. To test for normal strength, resist motion by pulling shoulders downward while instructing the patient, "Hold it, and don't let me move you." To evaluate the sternocleidomastoid muscle, ask the patient to rotate the head from side to side. If this is easily accomplished, add manual resistance. Muscles with normal strength can tolerate manual resistance. To test, the examiner pushes gently on the patient's forehead with his or her palm and asks the patient to resist the movement (Figure A.30B). Then the examiner asks the patient to turn the head to the right side, and gently resists this movement to the right, which evaluates the left sternocleidomastoid muscle. The patient is then asked to turn the head to the left, and the examiner repeats the resistance to test the opposite side.

 HOW TO TEST CN XII, THE HYPOGLOSSAL NERVE

Observation

Observe the tongue for lower motor findings of atrophy due to loss of innervation to intrinsic muscles, or fasciculations (small, local involuntary motions caused by spontaneous depolarization of resting muscle tissue).

Screening

Ask the patient whether there is any difficulty eating or drinking.

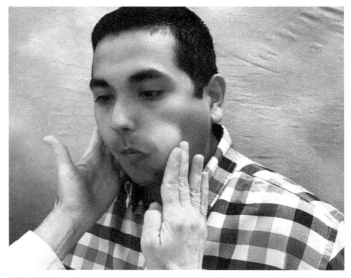

FIGURE A.32

Evaluating muscle function for clearing food in mouth. A normal tongue can easily hold against your manual resistance.

Examination

The tongue should be strong and able to resist significant forces with symmetrical function. Ask the patient to stick out the tongue three times (Figure A.31). A normally functioning genioglossus produces a straight motion without deviation in any direction from the midline. A weak genioglossus causes tongue deviation to the weak side, with protrusion, due to the unopposed pull of the stronger contralateral genioglossus.

To examine other muscle function, use a tongue depressor to push gently on the side of the tongue from each side, asking the patient to resist. Assess the relative strength of the tongue resistance in each direction. Another option is to ask the patient to push the tongue against either cheek forcefully; a normal tongue will be strong enough to resist your push against the cheek on either side (Figure A.32). For all muscles except the genioglossus, weakness produces inability to move toward the impaired side.

Glossary

abducens (VI) nerve: Cranial nerve; axons innervate the lateral rectus muscle.

abducens nucleus: Contains lateral rectus motor neurons and internuclear neurons; located in pons.

accessory cuneate nucleus: Relays somatic sensory information from upper trunk, arm, and neck to the cerebellum; located in medulla.

accessory (XI) nerve: Cranial nerve that innervates the sternocleidomastoid muscle and the upper part of the trapezius muscle.

accessory optic system: Transmits visual information to brain stem nuclei for eye movement control.

accommodation-convergence reaction: A complex response that prepares the eyes for near vision by (1) increasing lens curvature, (2) constricting the pupils, and (3) coordinating convergence of the eyes.

accommodation reflex: Increase in lens curvature that occurs during near vision.

acetylcholine: Neurotransmitter used by motor neurons and neurons in several nuclei, including the basal nucleus and the pedunculopontine nucleus.

acetylcholinesterase: Enzyme that inactivates acetylcholine.

acousticomotor function: Motor behavioral response triggered or controlled by sound such as orienting toward a sound.

adrenergic: Neuron that uses adrenalin as a neurotransmitter or neuromodulator.

adhesion: Union of two surfaces that are normally separate, such as in wound healing or in some pathological process.

afferent: Axons that transmit information toward a particular structure; *afferent* is not synonymous with *sensory*, which means related to processing information from a receptor sheet (e.g., body surface or retina).

airway protective reflex: Closure of the larynx to prevent fluid and food from entering the trachea.

akinesia: Impairment in initiating voluntary movement.

alar plate: Dorsal portion of the neuroepithelium that gives rise to sensory nuclei of the spinal cord and brain stem.

allocortex: Cortex having a variable number of layers, but always fewer than six.

alveus: Thin sheet of myelinated axons covering hippocampal formation; axons of pyramidal neurons in the hippocampus and subiculum.

Alzheimer disease: Presenile dementia.

amacrine cells: Retinal interneuron.

amygdala: Telencephalic structure that plays an essential role in emotions and their behavioral expression; has three component nuclear divisions: basolateral, central, and corticomedial.

amygdaloid nuclear complex: Another name for the amygdala.

anastomosis: A network of interconnected arteries.

aneurysm: An abnormal ballooning of a part of an artery due to weakening of the arterial wall.

angiogram: Radiological image of vasculature.

anosmia: Absence of the sense of smell.

ansa lenticularis: Output pathway of the internal segment of the globus pallidus; axons terminate in the thalamus.

anterior: Toward the abdomen; synonymous with *ventral*.

anterior cerebral artery: Supplies blood to the medial frontal lobes and underlying deep structures.

anterior choroidal artery: Supplies blood to the choroid plexus in the lateral ventricle and several deep structures.

anterior cingulate gyrus: Portion of the cingulate important for emotions; activated while experiencing painful stimuli; a major target of the limbic loop of the basal ganglia.

anterior circulation: Arterial supply provided by the internal carotid artery.

anterior commissure: Tract that interconnects the anterior temporal lobes and olfactory structures on the two sides of the brain.

anterior communicating artery: Interconnects anterior cerebral arteries on the two sides of the brain; part of the circle of Willis.

anterior inferior cerebellar artery (AICA): Supplies the caudal pons and parts of the cerebellum.

anterior limb of the internal capsule: Subcortical tract between the anterior portions of the caudate nucleus and putamen; rostral to the thalamus.

anterior lobe of the pituitary gland: Contains epithelial cells that release hormones for controlling a variety of target glands in the periphery.

anterior nuclei of the thalamus: Receive input from the mammillary bodies and project to the cingulate gyrus.

anterior nucleus of the thalamus: Receives input from the mammillothalamic tract and projects to the cingulate cortex.

anterior olfactory nucleus: Relays information from the olfactory nucleus to other parts of the central nervous system.

anterior perforated substance: Basal forebrain region where branches of the anterior and middle cerebral arteries (lenticulostriate) penetrate and supply deep structures.

anterior spinal arteries: Branches of the vertebral artery that supply the ventral half of the spinal cord; courses within the ventral sulcus of the spinal cord; also receives arterial blood from radicular arteries.

anterior temporal lobes: Involved in emotions, especially during anxiety states.

anterior thalamic nuclei: Participate in aspects of learning and memory; principal target of the mammillary bodies.

anterograde: Away from a neuron's cell body and toward the axon terminal; typically related to the pattern of degeneration (*see* Wallerian degeneration) or axonal transport.

anterograde amnesia: Failure to remember new events.

anterolateral system: Spinal pathways for pain, temperature, and itch; includes spinothalamic, spinomesencephalic (spinotectal), and spinoreticular tracts.

anteroventral cochlear nucleus: Portion of the cochlear nucleus important for sound localization in the horizontal plane; located in the rostral medulla.

antidiuretic hormone: Released by the posterior lobe of the pituitary; acts on the kidney to concentrate urine.

aphasia: Impairment in language; characterized by reduced ability of a person to read, write, or speak their intentions.

apraxia: Inability to perform a movement when asked, even though the person has the physical ability to contract the muscles, is willing to perform the movement, and has already learned to make the movement.

aortic arch: Site of arterial blood pressure sensor.

arachnoid granulations: Unidirectional valves for cerebrospinal fluid to flow from the subarachnoid space to the circulatory system.

arachnoid mater: Middle meningeal layer.

arachnoid villi: *See* arachnoid granulations.

arbor vitae: Appearance of cerebellar white matter on sagittal section.

archicortex: Primitive three-layered cortex; primarily in hippocampal formation.

arcuate nucleus: Hypothalamic nucleus important for control of neuroendocrine function and feeding.

area 3a: Brodmann's cytoarchitectonic area; part of the primary somatic sensory cortex that receives information from muscle receptors; involved in balance sense.

area postrema: Portion of caudal medulla where there is no blood–brain barrier; important for sensing blood-borne toxins and in control of vomiting.

Argyll Robertson pupils: Pupil sign characterized by a small diameter and the pupil being unreactive to light but which gets smaller to accommodation; associated with neurosyphilis.

ascending pathway: Pathway transmitting information from lower levels of the central nervous system to higher levels; typically used to describe somatic sensory pathways of the spinal cord and brain stem.

association cortex: Areas of cortex that serve diverse mental processes but that are not engaged in basic stimulus processing or control of muscle contractions; formally those areas that associate sensory events with motor responses and perform mental processes that intervene between sensory inputs and motor outputs.

associative loop (of basal ganglia): The basal ganglia circuit that receives input primarily from association cortex of the frontal, parietal, and temporal lobes and projects to prefrontal and premotor cortical areas.

astrocytes: Class of glial cell that serves diverse support functions, including axonal guidance during development and helping to maintain the blood–brain barrier.

ataxia: Uncoordinated and highly inaccurate movements; typically associated with cerebellar damage.

athetosis: Slow, writhing involuntary movements.

autism spectrum disorder: A condition presenting with deficits in social interactions, impaired verbal and nonverbal communication, and expression of stereotyped patterns of behavior.

autonomic motor column: Formation of sympathetic and parasympathetic preganglionic neurons into rostrocaudal columns in the spinal cord and brain stem.

autonomic nervous system: Part of peripheral nervous system engaged in the control of body organs; consists of separate sympathetic and parasympathetic divisions.

axial muscles: Muscles located close to the body midline; control neck and back.

axon: Portion of neuron specialized for conducting information encoded in the form of action potentials.

axon terminal: Presynaptic component of the synapse; where neurotransmitters are released.

β-endorphin: An endogenous opiate cleaved from the large peptide proopiomelanocortin; plays a role in opiate analgesia.

Babinski's sign: Extension (also termed dorsiflexion) of the big toe in response to scratching the lateral margin and then the ball of the foot (but not the toes); associated with lesions of the corticospinal system in adults; present normally in children until about two years of age.

ballistic movement: Movement with high initial velocity.

bare nerve endings: Sensitive to noxious and thermal stimuli as well as itch-producing agents.

baroreceptor: Blood pressure receptor.

basal cells: Cells that differentiate to become taste receptor cells; thought to be stem cells.

basal forebrain: Portion of the ventral telencephalon caudal to the frontal lobes; contains the basal nucleus (of Meynert) and structures for emotions and olfaction.

basal ganglia: Telencephalic nuclei with strong interconnections with the cerebral cortex; serve diverse motor, cognitive, and emotional functions.

basal hair cells: Auditory hair cells located near the cochlear base.

basal nucleus (of Meynert): Contains neurons that use acetylcholine as their neurotransmitter and project widely throughout the cerebral cortex; neurons are among the first to degenerate in Alzheimer disease.

basal plate: Portion of the ventral neuroepithelium that gives rise to motor nuclei of the spinal cord and brain stem.

base (midbrain): The most ventral portion of the midbrain; also termed basis pedunculi.

base of the pons: Ventral portion of the pons; contains primarily pontine nuclei and descending cortical axons.

basilar artery: Supplies pons and parts of the cerebellum and midbrain.

basilar membrane: Component of the organ of Corti that oscillates in response to sounds; mechanical displacement of the membrane stimulates auditory hair cells.

basis pedunculi: Ventral portion of the midbrain; contains descending cortical axons.

basket neurons: Inhibitory interneurons of the cerebellar cortex; make dense and strong synaptic connections on cell body of Purkinje neuron.

basolateral nuclei (of the amygdala): Division of amygdala that receives information from sensory systems and cortical association areas.

bed nucleus of the stria terminalis: C-shaped component of the amygdala; related in function to the central nucleus.

benign positional vertigo: Most common form of vertigo, or the sudden sensation of spinning; can be evoked for testing purposes by placement of the head in a particular position and then quickly lying down backwards over a table.

bilateral control: Form of somatic or visceromotor control in which a cranial nerve or spinal motor nucleus receives projections from both sides of the cortex; typically provides a measure of redundancy, so that if one projection becomes damaged, the other projection can provide basic control.

bilateral projection: One structure sends axons to both sides of the central nervous system.

bilateral temporal visual field defect: *See* bitemporal heteronymous hemianopia.

bipolar morphology: Neuron shape characterized by a pair of axon-like processes emerging from opposite sides of a neuron's cell body; bipolar neuron.

bipolar neurons: One of three major morphological types of neuron; characterized by a pair of axon-like processes emerging from opposite sides of the neuron's cell body; most commonly sensory relay neurons.

bitemporal heteronymous hemianopia: Loss of peripheral vision; common with lesions involving the optic chiasm.

blind spot: Blind portion of visual field; corresponds on the retina to the exit point of the optic nerve, where there are no photoreceptors.

blobs: Location of color-sensitive neurons in primary visual cortex; primarily in layers II and III.

blood–brain barrier: Cellular specializations that prevent blood-borne materials from gaining access to the central nervous system.

blood-cerebrospinal fluid barrier: Specializations that prevent blood-borne materials from gaining access to the cerebrospinal fluid.

border zone infarct: Loss of arterial supply at the peripheral borders of the territories supplied by major cerebral vessels.

border zones: Peripheral borders of the territories supplied by major cerebral vessels.

brachium of inferior colliculus: Output pathway from the inferior colliculus to the medial geniculate nucleus.

brachium of superior colliculus: Input pathway to the superior colliculus from the retina.

bradycardia: Slowness of the heartbeat, so that the pulse rate is less than 60 per minute.

bradykinesia: Movement disorder in which movements are slowed or absent.

brain: Cerebral hemispheres, diencephalon, cerebellum, and brain stem.

brain stem: Medulla, pons, and midbrain.

branchial arches: Also known as gill arches; territory of developing head and neck; many cranial nerves develop in association with the branchial arches.

branchiomeric: Derived from the branchial arches.

branchiomeric motor column: Motor neurons that innervate muscles that develop from the branchial arches.

branchiomeric skeletal motor fibers: *See* branchiomeric motor column.

Broca's area: Portion of the inferior frontal lobe important for articulation of speech.

Brodmann's areas: Divisions of the cerebral cortex based on the size and shapes of neurons in the different laminae and their packing densities; named after Korbinian Brodmann, a German neuroanatomist who worked during the late 19th and early 20th centuries.

Brown-Séquard syndrome: Set of signs associated with spinal cord hemisection; include ipsilateral loss of motor functions, ipsilateral loss of mechanical sensations, and contralateral loss of pain, temperature, and itch; all caudal to the lesion.

bulb: Archaic term for medulla and pons; commonly used to describe a cortical projection system (*see* corticobulbar tract).

C-shaped: Description of the shape of many telencephalic structures.

calcarine fissure: Located in the primary visual cortex; occipital lobe.

callosal connections: Connections made by callosal neurons.

callosal neurons: Class of cortical projection neuron.

capillary endothelium: Inner layer of a capillary in brain and spinal cord contributes to the blood brain barrier.

carotid circulation: *See* anterior circulation.

carotid sinus: Blood pressure–sensing organ.

carotid siphon: Segment of the internal carotid artery.

cataplexy: Transient loss of muscle tone without loss of consciousness.

cauda equina: Spinal nerves within the vertebral canal caudal to the last spinal segment.

cauda: Any tail, or taillike structure, or tapering or elongated extremity of an organ or other part.

caudal: Toward the tail or coccyx.

caudal nucleus (of the spinal trigeminal nucleus): Important for facial pain, temperature sense, and itch; located in the caudal medulla; rostral extension of the dorsal horn.

caudal solitary nucleus: Important for viscerosensory function; located in the caudal medulla.

caudate nucleus: Input nucleus of the basal ganglia; comprised of the head, body and tail.

cell body: Where the nucleus is located and from which the axon and dendrites emerge.

cell bridges: *See* striatal cell bridges.

cell stains: Method of revealing neuronal cell bodies; an example is the Nissl stain.

central canal: Portion of the ventricular system located in the spinal cord and caudal medulla.

central nervous system: Division of the nervous system located within the skull and vertebral column.

central nucleus (of the amygdala): Nuclear division of the amygdala important for the visceral expression of emotions, such as changes in blood pressure and gastrointestinal function during anxiety.

central sulcus: Separates frontal and parietal lobes.

central tegmental tract: Contains the ascending gustatory projection from the solitary nucleus to the thalamus and descending axons from the parvocellular red nucleus to the inferior olivary nucleus.

centromedian nucleus: Thalamic diffuse-projecting nucleus with widespread projections to the frontal lobe and striatum.

cephalic flexure: Bend in neuraxis at the level of the midbrain.

cerebellar glomerulus: Basic processing unit of the cerebellum; comprises one mossy fiber axon terminal (presynaptic), and many granule cell dendrites and several Golgi axons (postsynaptic).

cerebellar tentorium: Rigid dural flap dorsal to the cerebellum; separates the cerebellum from the cerebral cortex and defines the posterior fossa.

cerebellopontine angle: Where the cerebellum joins the brain stem.

cerebellothalamic tract: Output pathway from the deep cerebellar nuclei to the thalamus.

cerebellum: Portion of the hindbrain; important for automatic control of movements and thought to play a role in automating many complex sensory and cognitive functions.

cerebral angiography: Radiological technique for imaging brain vasculature.

cerebral aqueduct (of Sylvius): Portion of the ventricular system in the midbrain.

cerebral cortex: Portion of the telencephalon; important for diverse sensory, motor, cognitive, emotional, and integrative functions.

cerebral hemispheres: Major brain division.

cerebral peduncle: Ventral portion of midbrain, formally corresponds to the tegmentum and base.

cerebral segment (of internal carotid artery): Immediately proximal to the bifurcation into the middle and anterior cerebral arteries.

cerebrocerebellum: Comprises the lateral cerebellar cortex and dentate nucleus; important for motor planning.

cerebrospinal fluid: Watery fluid contained within the ventricular system and subarachnoid space.

cervical: Spinal cord segment; there are eight in total.

cervical flexure: Bend in the developing nervous system; located in the midbrain; persists into maturity.

cervical segment (of internal carotid artery): The most proximal portion of the internal carotid; from the carotid bifurcation to the point of entrance to the carotid canal of the skull.

cholinergic: A neuron that uses acetylcholine as its neurotransmitter.

chorda tympani nerve: A branch of cranial nerve VII; carries taste afferents.

chorea: Disordered movement characterized by involuntary rapid and random movements of the limbs and trunk.

choroid epithelium: Cells of the choroid plexus specialized to secrete cerebrospinal fluid.

choroid plexus: Intraventricular organ that contains cells that secrete cerebrospinal fluid.

ciliary ganglion: Peripheral ganglion containing parasympathetic postganglionic neurons.

ciliary muscle: Intraocular muscle that increases lens curvature.

cingulate cortex: Comprises anterior, middle and posterior divisions; diverse behavioral functions, including role in emotional valance and movement control.

cingulate gyrus: C-shaped gyrus on medial brain surface spanning the frontal and parietal lobes; surrounds the corpus callosum.

cingulate motor areas: Premotor cortical area located in the cingulate gyrus.

cingulum: C-shaped tract located within the white matter of the cortex beneath the cingulate gyrus.

circle of Willis: Anastomotic network of arteries on the ventral surface of the diencephalon.

circumventricular organs: A set of eight structures lying near the ventricular surface that do not have a blood–brain barrier.

cisterna magna: The portion of the subarachnoid space, dorsal to the medulla and caudal to the cerebellum, where cerebrospinal fluid pools.

cisterns: Portions of the subarachnoid space where cerebrospinal fluid pools.

Clarke's nucleus: Contains neurons that project to the ipsilateral cerebellum via the dorsal spinocerebellar tract.

claustrum: Telencephalic nucleus located beneath the insular cortex.

climbing fibers: Axons of the inferior olivary nucleus that synapse on Purkinje neurons in the cerebellar cortex; forms one of the strongest excitatory synapses in the central nervous system.

cochlea: Inner ear organ for hearing.

cochlear apex: Portion of the cochlea sensitive to low-frequency tones.

cochlear division (of the vestibulocochlear nerve): Cranial nerve sensitive to sounds.

cochlear nuclei: First relay site for axons of the cochlear division of the vestibulocochlear nerve; located in the medulla.

collateral circulation: Redundant arterial supply for a given structure.

collateral sulcus: Separates the parahippocampal gyrus from more lateral temporal lobe regions.

colliculi: Set of four structures on the dorsal midbrain; superior colliculi are important for saccadic eye movement control, and inferior colliculi are important for hearing.

color columns: Collections of neurons in the primary visual cortex, predominantly located in layers II and III; also termed color blobs.

columnar organization (of the cerebral cortex): Vertical arrays of neurons that serve similar functions.

commissural neurons: Class of cortical neuron that contains an axon that projects to the contralateral cortex via the corpus callosum.

commissure: Tract through which axons cross the midline.

computerized tomography: A technique for producing images of a single plane of tissue.

conditioned taste aversion: Rapid and very robust form of learning in which an individual avoids foods that made it ill.

cone bipolar cells: Class of retinal interneuron that transmits control signals from cone cells to ganglion neurons.

cones: Photoreceptor class sensitive to light wavelength (i.e., color).

constrictor muscles of the iris: Produce pupillary constriction.

contralateral: Relative spatial term related to the opposite side of the body.

contralateral homonymous hemianopia with macular sparing: Visual field defect in which there is a loss of vision in the contralateral visual field but preservation of foveal (or macular) vision; can be produced with visual system lesions affecting a portion of the primary visual cortex.

contralateral homonymous hemianopia: Visual field defect characterized by the loss of sight of the contralateral visual field; can be produced with visual system lesions affecting the optic tract, lateral geniculate nucleus, optic radiations, or primary visual cortex.

constraint: The state of being checked, restricted, or compelled to avoid or perform some action.

convolution: A tortuous irregularity or elevation caused by the infolding of a structure upon itself.

cornea: Transparent avascular portion of the sclera.

corona radiata: Portion of the subcortical white matter superior (or dorsal) to the internal capsule.

coronal: Plane of section or imaging plane; parallel to the coronal suture; equivalent to transverse plane for cerebral hemispheres and diencephalon.

corpus callosum: Commissure connecting the two cerebral hemispheres; contains four major subdivisions Rostrum, genu, body, and splenium.

corpus striatum: Subcortical telencephalic nuclei comprised of the caudate nucleus, putamen, and nucleus accumbens; generally synonymous with the striatum.

cortex: Thin sheet of neuronal cell bodies and afferent and efferent axons.

cortical column: Collection of radially oriented neurons that have similar functions and anatomical connections; basic functional unit of the cerebral cortex.

cortical nucleus (of the amygdala): Receives input from olfactory structures; projects to the hypothalamus via the stria terminalis.

corticobulbar fibers: Axons that originate in the cerebral cortex and project to the brain stem; primarily terminating in the cranial nerve motor nuclei of the pons and medulla; projections to specific nuclei and to the reticular formation usually have more specific terms (e.g., corticoreticular).

corticobulbar tract: Cortical projections that terminate on cranial nerve motor nuclei in the medulla and pons.

cortico-cortical association neurons: Cortical neurons that project axons to cortical areas on the same side.

corticofugal: Leaving the cerebral cortex.

corticomedial nuclei: Nuclei of the amygdala that play a role in visceral motor control.

corticopontine pathway: Descending projection from the cerebral cortex to the pontine nuclei; major input to the cerebrocerebellum.

corticoreticular fibers: Axons that originate from neurons in layer V of the cortex that project to the reticular formation.

cortico-reticulo-spinal pathway: Indirect cortical pathway to the spinal cord via neurons of the reticulospinal tract.

corticospinal tract: Projection from the cerebral cortex to the spinal cord.

cranial and spinal roots: Nerves that enter and exit the spinal cord and brain stem.

cranial nerve II: Optic nerve; contains axons of retinal ganglion cells; major targets are the lateral geniculate nucleus, rostral midbrain, nuclei at the midbrain-diencephalon junction, and hypothalamus.

cranial nerve motor nuclei: Location of motor neurons whose axons are located in the cranial nerves.

cranial nerves: Sensory and motor nerves containing axons that enter and exit the brain stem, diencephalon, and telencephalon; analogous to the spinal nerves.

cribriform plate: Part of the ethmoid bone; contains tiny foramina through which olfactory nerve fibers course from the olfactory epithelium to the olfactory bulb.

crude touch: A nondiscriminative form of tactile sensation that remains after damage to the dorsal column-medial lemniscal pathway or to large-diameter afferent fibers; may be mediated by unmyelinated C-fiber mechanoreceptors.

crus (of the fornix): Posterior portion of fornix where it has a flattened appearance.

cuneate fascicle: Tract containing ascending axons of dorsal root ganglion neurons that innervate the upper trunk (rostral to T6), arm, neck, and back of the head; mediates mechanosensations.

cuneate nucleus: Termination of axons in the cuneate fascicle; neurons project axons to contralateral ventral posterior nucleus of the thalamus; mediates mechanosensations.

cuneocerebellar tract: Pathway from the lateral cuneate nucleus to the cerebellum; courses through the inferior cerebellar peduncle.

cytoarchitecture: Characterization of the morphology of the cerebral cortex based on the density of neuronal cell bodies.

cytochrome oxidase: Mitochondrial enzyme; marker for neuronal metabolism.

declarative memory: Memory such as the conscious recollection of facts.

decussate: Crossing the midline.

decussation: A site where axons cross the midline.

deep brain stimulation (DBS): Use of electrodes to electrically stimulate an area of the brain; most commonly used in the basal ganglia to treat movement disorders.

deep cerebellar nuclei: Sets of nuclei located beneath the cerebellar cortex; fastigial, interposed (comprising the globose and emboliform), and dentate nuclei.

deep cerebral veins: Veins that drain the diencephalon and parts of the brain stem.

Deiters' nucleus: Lateral vestibular nucleus; origin of the lateral vestibulospinal tract.

dendrites: Receptive portion of a neuron.

dentate gyrus: Component of the hippocampal formation; receives input from the entorhinal cortex and contains neurons that project to the hippocampus proper.

dentate nucleus: One of the deep cerebellar nuclei; transmits the output of the lateral cerebellar hemisphere.

depression: A psychiatric disorder characterized by the persistent feeling of hopelessness and dejection; can be associated with poor concentration, lethargy, and sometimes suicidal tendencies.

dermatome: Area of skin innervated by sensory axons within a single dorsal root.

descending motor pathways: Connections between the cerebral cortex or brain stem to the spinal cord; densest to the intermediate zone and ventral horn.

descending pain inhibitory system: Neural circuit for modulating transmission of information about pain from nociceptors, through the dorsal horn, and to the brain stem; primarily originates from serotonergic neurons in the raphe nuclei and noradrenergic neurons in the reticular formation; projects to the spinal cord dorsal horn.

descending projection neurons: Neurons that give rise to descending pathways.

detached retina: Pathological condition in which portions of the retina separate from the pigment epithelium.

diabetes insipidus: Condition in which the kidneys are unable to concentrate urine because of the absence of vasopressin (or antidiuretic hormone); the individual produces copious amounts of urine.

diencephalon: One of the secondary brain vesicles; major brain division in maturity, containing primarily the thalamus and hypothalamus; means "between brain".

diffuse-projecting neurons: Thalamic neurons that project widely to several cortical areas.

diffusion-weighted magnetic resonance imaging: Type of magnetic resonance imaging that can distinguish axonal orientation, especially axons within tracts.

direct path: Pathway through the basal ganglia from the striatum to the internal segment of the globus pallidus; promotes the production of movements.

disinhibition: Removal of inhibition; net effect is similar to excitation.

distal: Situated away from the center of the body, or from the point of origin; specifically applied to the extremity or distant part of a limb or organ.

distal muscles: Muscles that innervate the limbs, especially distal to the elbow; controlled principally by the lateral descending motor pathways.

dopamine: Neurotransmitter.

dopaminergic: Neurons that use dopamine as their neurotransmitter.

dorsal: Close to the back; also termed posterior.

dorsal cochlear nucleus: Auditory relay nucleus located in the pons; receives input from primary auditory receptors and projects to the contralateral inferior colliculus; implicated in vertical localization of sounds.

dorsal column nuclei: Cuneate and gracile nuclei; receive input from mechanoreceptor axons in the dorsal columns.

dorsal column–medial lemniscal system: Tracts, nuclei, and cortical areas collectively involved in mechanosensations (touch, vibration sense, pressure, and limb position sense).

dorsal columns: Located on the dorsal spinal cord surface; contain ascending axons of mechanoreceptors; gracile fascicle (or tract) carries axons that originate from receptors on the leg and lower back, whereas the cuneate tract carries axons that originate from receptors on the upper back, arm, neck, and back of the head.

dorsal cortex (of inferior colliculus): Portion of the surface of the inferior colliculus.

dorsal horn: Laminae I–VI of the spinal gray matter; processes incoming somatic sensory information, especially about pain, temperature, and itch.

dorsal intermediate septum: Separates the cuneate and gracile fascicles.

dorsal longitudinal fasciculus: Pathway to and from the hypothalamus; located in the periventricular and aqueductal gray matter.

dorsal median septum: Divides the dorsal columns into right and left halves.

dorsal motor nucleus of the vagus: Contains parasympathetic preganglionic neurons whose axons course in the vagus nerve (cranial nerve X); located in the medulla.

dorsal raphe nucleus: Located in the rostral pons and caudal midbrain; most neurons in the nucleus use serotonin as their neurotransmitter; projects widely to telencephalic and diencephalic structures.

dorsal root: Spinal sensory root.

dorsal root ganglia: Contains cell bodies of primary sensory neurons that innervate skin and deep tissues of the back of the head, neck, limbs, and trunk.

dorsal spinocerebellar tract: An ipsilateral pathway to the cerebellum; originates in Clarke's nucleus.

dorsolateral prefrontal cortex: Cortical region important for organizing behavior, working memory, and a variety of higher mental processes.

dorsoventral axis: Between the back and abdomen.

dura mater: Outermost and toughest meningeal layer; contains an outer periosteal layer and an inner meningeal layer.

dural sinuses: Channels within the meningeal layer of the dura, through which venous blood and cerebrospinal fluids are returned to the systemic circulation.

dynorphin: Neurotransmitter/neuromodulator.

dysarthria: Poor speech articulation without loss of meaning.

dysphagia: Impairment in ability to swallow.

dysprosody: Speech with a flat, unchanging melody.

ectoderm: Outermost layer of the embryo.

Edinger-Westphal nucleus: Contains parasympathetic preganglionic neurons that innervate smooth muscle in the eye to control pupil diameter and lens curvature.

efferent: Axons transmit information away from a particular structure, efferent is not synonymous with *motor,* which means related to muscle or glandular function.

eighth cranial nerve (VIII): Vestibulocochlear nerve; separate cochlear division for hearing and vestibular division for balance.

electrical synapses: Site of communication between neurons that does not use a neurotransmitter; usually associated with a gap junction, where ions and other small and intermediate-sized molecules can pass.

emboliform nucleus: One of the deep cerebellar nuclei; together with the globose nucleus is termed the interposed nucleus.

encapsulated axon terminals: Specialized tissue surrounding the terminal of certain mechanoreceptors; helps to determine the sensitivity and duration of the response of the receptor to a mechanical stimulus.

endocrine hormones: Biologically active chemicals released by endocrine cells into the blood; regulate metabolism, growth, and other cellular and bodily functions.

endoderm: Innermost layer of the embryo.

endogenous ligand: A protein made in the body that binds to a receptor protein.

endolymph: Fluid that fills most of the membranous labyrinth; resembles intracellular fluid in its ionic constituents; has a high potassium concentration and low sodium concentration.

enkephalin: Neurotransmitter.

enteric nervous system: Nervous system division that controls the functions of the large intestine.

enteroendocrine cells: Specialized cells located in the gastrointestinal tract; ghrelin, which promotes feeding, is secreted by enteroendoendocrine cells in the stomach.

entorhinal cortex: Portion of the medial temporal lobe; major input to the hippocampal formation.

ependymal cells: Epithelial cell type that lines the ventricles.

epiglottis: Pharyngeal structure that, during swallowing, helps to prevent passage of fluids and food into the trachea.

episodic memory: Memory of events that have a specific spatial and temporal context (such as meeting a friend last week).

ethmoid bone: Cranial bone; contains the cribriform plate, through which olfactory sensory axons course en route from the olfactory mucosa to the olfactory bulb.

evaginations: An outpouching of a layer or part, or a protrusion of some part or organ from its normal position.

explicit memory: Conscious recollection of facts; also termed declarative memory.

extended amygdala: Collection of basal forebrain nuclei that share morphological, histochemical, and connection characteristics; includes central nuclei of the amygdala and the bed nucleus of the stria terminalis; participates in reward and substance abuse along with the ventral striatum.

external capsule: White matter region between the putamen and the claustrum; contains primarily cortical association fibers.

external nucleus: Component of the inferior colliculus that participates in ear reflexes in animals, such as when a cat orients its ears to a sound source.

external segment of the globus pallidus: Contains neurons that project to the subthalamic nucleus; part of the indirect basal ganglia path.

extrastriate cortex: Visual cortical areas excluding the primary (or striate) cortex.

extreme capsule: White matter region between the claustrum and insular cortex; contains primarily cortical association fibers.

facial (VII) nerve: Contains axons of motor neurons that innervate muscles of facial expression, as well as the stapedius muscle and part of the digastric muscle; exits from the pontomedullary junction.

facial colliculus: Surface landmark on ventricular (dorsal) surface of the pons; overlies the genu of the facial nerve and the abducens nucleus.

facial motor nucleus: Located in the pons, it contains motor neurons whose axons course within the facial nerve to innervate muscles of facial expression, the posterior belly of the digastric muscle, and the stapedius muscle.

facial nucleus: Contains motor neurons that innervate muscles of facial expression, as well as the stapedius muscle and part of the digastric muscle; located in the pons.

falx cerebri: Dural flap between the two cerebral hemi-spheres; extension of the meningeal layer of the dura.

fastigial nucleus: One of the deep cerebellar nuclei; transmits the output of the vermis to the medial descending motor pathways.

fenestration: The presence of openings in a body part or the creation of openings to allow for viewing of parts.

fenestrated capillaries: Contain pores through which substances can diffuse from within the capillary to surrounding tissue.

fimbria: Portion of the fornix that covers part of the hippocampal formation.

first lumbar vertebra: Marks the approximate location of the caudal end of the spinal cord within the vertebral canal.

fissure: Groove in the cortical surface; more consistent in shape and depth than a sulcus.

flaccid paralysis: Inability to contract a muscle, together with a profound loss of muscle tone.

FLAIR: MRI pulse sequence that suppresses signal related to cerebrospinal fluid; abbreviation for fluid attenuated inversion recovery.

flexure: Bend in the axis of the central nervous system or axis of the embryo.

flocculonodular lobe: Portion of the cerebellar cortex involved in eye movement control and balance.

flocculus: *See* flocculonodular lobe.

floor plate: Ventral surface of the developing central nervous system; key site for organizing the dorsoventral patterning of the spinal cord during development.

folia: Thin folds of the cerebellar cortex.

foramen: A natural opening or passage, especially one into or through a bone.

foramen of Magendie: Opening in the fourth ventricle where cerebrospinal fluid can pass into the subarachnoid space; located on the midline.

foramina of Luschka: Openings in the fourth ventricle where cerebrospinal fluid can pass into the subarachnoid space; located at the lateral recesses of the ventricle.

forebrain: Most rostral primary brain vesicle; divides into the telencephalon and diencephalon.

Forel's field H2: Another name for the lenticular fasciculus; region of the white matter though which axons from the internal segment of the globus pallidus course en route to the thalamus.

form pathway (for vision): Circuit specialized for discriminating features of the shapes of visual stimuli; information in this path is used for object recognition.

fornix: A major output tract from the hippocampal formation.

fourth ventricle: Portion of the ventricular system located in the brain stem; separates medulla and pons from the cerebellum.

fovea: Portion of the retina with the greatest visual acuity, where only cone receptors are located; located in the center of the macula.

fractionate movements: Ability to isolate one movement from another, such as move one finger while keeping the other fingers still.

fractionation (of movement): Ability to move one finger or limb segment independent of the other fingers or limb segments; often termed individuation.

fractured somatotopy: Characteristic of a central sensory or motor representation in which the somatotopic plan is disorganized and a single body part becomes represented at multiple sites.

Friedreich's ataxia: An autosomal recessive disease that results in progressive spinocerebellar ataxia; chromosome 9 mutation; expansion of a GAA trinucleotide repeat within the gene that codes for the mitochondrial protein frataxin.

frontal: Close to the forehead.

frontal association cortex: Major association area located rostral to the premotor cortical regions on the lateral and medial brain surfaces and on the orbital surface.

frontal eye fields: Portion of the lateral frontal lobe important in the control of eye movements.

frontal lobe: One of the lobes of the cerebral hemisphere.

functional localization: Identification of brain regions that participate in particular functions.

functional magnetic resonance imaging (fMRI): A form of magnetic resonance imaging that can monitor blood oxygenation, which correlates with neuronal activity.

functional neuroanatomy: Examines those parts of the nervous system that work together to accomplish a particular task.

GABA: γ-aminobutyric acid; principal inhibitory neurotransmitter in the central nervous system.

gag reflex: Stereotypic contraction of pharyngeal muscles in response to stimulation of the posterior oral cavity; the afferent limb is the glossopharyngeal nerve, and the efferent limb is the vagus nerve primarily.

ganglion: Collections of neuronal cell bodies outside the central nervous system.

ganglion cell layer: Innermost retinal cell layer; contains cell bodies of ganglion cells.

ganglion cells: Retinal projection neurons; axons course in the optic nerve and terminate in the diencephalon and midbrain.

geniculate ganglion: Location of cell bodies of primary sensory neurons that project in the intermediate nerve (cranial nerve VII).

genu: Latin for knee; used to describe structures with an acute bend, such as the corpus callosum and facial nerve.

genu of the internal capsule: Separates the anterior and posterior limbs of the internal capsule.

ghrelin: Protein secreted by enteroendocrine cells of the stomach; promotes food intake.

girdle muscles: Striated muscles that insert proximally and attach on parts of the shoulder or hip.

glial cells: Major cell type in the nervous system; outnumber neurons about 10 to 1; also termed glia.

globose nucleus: Deep cerebellar nucleus; together with the emboliform nucleus comprise the interposed nuclei, which transmit information from the intermediate cerebellar hemisphere.

globus pallidus: Basal ganglia nucleus; comprises distinct internal and external divisions.

glomerulus: Collection of neuronal cell bodies and processes surrounded by glial cells; structures within the glomerulus are physically isolated from surrounding neurons; typically corresponds to a basic functional processing unit.

glossopharyngeal (IX) nerve: Cranial nerve; located in the medulla.

glutamate: Principal excitatory neurotransmitter of neurons in the central nervous system.

Golgi neurons: Inhibitory interneurons of the cerebellar cortex.

Golgi tendon organ (or receptor): Stretch receptors in muscle tendon that signals active muscle force; afferent component of the golgi tendon reflex; distal receptive portion of group Ib axons.

gracile fascicle: Medial component of the dorsal column; transmits mechanoreceptive information from the legs and lower trunk to the ipsilateral gracile nucleus.

gracile nucleus: Target of the axons of the gracile fascicle; transmits information to the contralateral thalamus via the medial lemniscus.

granular layer: Innermost cell layer of the cerebellum; primarily contains granule and Golgi neurons and the axon terminals of mossy fibers.

granule cell: Cerebellar excitatory interneuron; cell of origin of parallel fibers.

granule neurons: The only excitatory interneuron of the cerebellar cortex.

gray matter: Portions of the central nervous system that contain predominantly neuronal cell bodies.

great cerebral vein (of Galen): Major vein; carries venous drainage from the diencephalon and deep telencephalic structures.

gyri: Grooves in the cerebral cortex.

gyrus rectus: Located on the inferior frontal lobe; runs parallel to the olfactory tract.

habenula: Portion of the diencephalon; located lateral and ventral to the pineal gland; part of a circuit with the midbrain medial dopaminergic and the serotonergic systems.

hair cells: Auditory receptor neurons.

hearing: One of the five major senses.

hemiballism: Movement disorder produced by damage to the subthalamic nucleus; characterized by involuntary rapid (ballistic) limb movements.

hemiplegic cerebral palsy: An acquired condition characterized by perinatal damage to brain circuits; commonly affects sensory and motor cortical areas; damage to the corticospinal tract produces motor signs that include spasticity and incoordination.

hemorrhagic stroke: Condition following the rupture of an artery; tissue around the hemorrhage can become damaged because blood leaks out of the artery under high pressure.

Heschl's gyri: Location of primary auditory cortex.

hierarchical organization: Property of neural systems in which individual components comprise distinct functional levels with respect to one another.

higher-order auditory areas: Regions of the temporal lobe that process complex aspects of sounds; major input from lower-order auditory areas (e.g., primary and secondary).

hindbrain: Most caudal portion of the brain; includes the medulla, pons, and cerebellum.

hippocampal formation: Telencephalic structure located primarily within the temporal lobe; comprises the dentate gyrus, hippocampus, and subiculum; involved in learning and memory.

hippocampal sulcus: Separates the dentate gyrus from the subiculum; largely obscured in the mature brain.

hippocampus: Component of the hippocampal formation.

histamine: Neuroactive compound; generally excitatory; important in hypothalamic circuits for regulating sleep and wakefulness.

Hoffmann's sign: Thumb adduction in response to flexion of the distal phalanx of the third digit; an upper limb equivalent of the Babinski sign.

horizontal cells: Retinal interneuron.

horizontal localization of sound: Ability to identify the position of the source of a sound in the horizontal plane.

Horner syndrome: Constellation of neurological signs associated with dysfunction of the sympathetic innervation of the head.

Huntington disease: Genetic autosomal dominant disorder; produces hyperkinetic motor signs.

hydrocephalus: Buildup of cerebrospinal fluid within the brain.

hyperkinetic signs: Set of abnormal involuntary motor behaviors characterized by increased rate of occurrence and inability to control; examples include tremor, tics, chorea, and athetosis.

hypoglossal motor neurons: Innervate intrinsic tongue muscles.

hypoglossal (XII) nerve: Cranial nerve located in the medulla.

hypoglossal nucleus: Location of hypoglossal motor neurons.

hypokinetic signs: Set of abnormal involuntary motor behaviors characterized by decreased rate of occurrence or slowing; examples include bradykinesia (slowing of movements) and failure to initiate a motor behavior in a timely manner.

hypophonia: Soft, breathy voice with reduced modulation of volume and pitch; commonly seen in early Parkinson's disease.

hypothalamic sulcus: Roughly separates the hypothalamus and thalamus on the medial brain surface.

hypothalamus: Major brain division; part of diencephalon.

immunocytochemistry: Process in which antibodies to a particular molecule are used to label that molecule in tissue.

implicit memory: Memory of procedures and actions; also termed nondeclarative memory.

incus: One of the middle ear ossicles (bones); essential for conducting changes in air pressure from the tympanic membrane to the oval window; located between the other two ossicles.

indirect cortical pathways: Motor pathway from the cerebral cortex that synapses first in the brain stem before synapsing on spinal neurons.

indirect path: Pathway through the basal ganglia from the striatum, to the external segment of the globus pallidus, to the subthalamic nucleus, and then to the internal segment of the globus pallidus; functions to retard the production of movements.

infarction: Death of tissue because of cessation of blood flow.

inferior cerebellar peduncle: Predominantly an input pathway to the cerebellum.

inferior colliculus: Located in the caudal midbrain, on its dorsal surface; contains neurons that are part of the ascending auditory pathway.

inferior ganglia: Location of primary somatic sensory cell bodies of vagus and glossopharyngeal nerves that innervate visceral tissues.

inferior oblique muscle: Extraocular muscle that depresses the eye, mostly when the eye is adducted.

inferior olivary nuclear complex: Collection of nuclei in the medulla that give rise to the climbing fibers of the cerebellum; forms the olive, a surface landmark on the ventral medullar surface.

inferior parietal lobule: Located dorsal to the lateral sulcus; important for a variety of higher brain functions, including language and perception.

inferior petrosal sinus: Major dural sinus.

inferior rectus muscle: Extraocular muscle that depresses the eye, especially when eye is abducted.

inferior sagittal sinus: Major dural sinus.

inferior salivatory nuclei: Location of parasympathetic preganglionic neurons that innervate cranial glands.

inferior temporal gyrus: Important in visual form perception.

inferior vestibular nucleus: Receives direct input from the vestibular organs; projects to various brain stem and spinal targets for eye movement control and balance.

infundibular stalk: Interconnects hypothalamus and pituitary gland; also termed the infundibulum.

initial segment: Junction of the neuronal cell body and axon; important site for integration of electrical signals and for initiating action potentials conducted along the axon.

inner hair cells: Principal auditory receptor neuron.

inner nuclear layer: Retinal layer that contains the cell bodies and proximal processes of the retinal interneurons, bipolar, horizontal, and amacrine cells.

inner synaptic (or plexiform) layer: Where synaptic connections between the bipolar cells and the ganglion cells are made.

input nuclei (of basal ganglia): Consisting of the striatum; receive input from cerebral cortex.

in situ: In its place.

insular cortex: Portion of the cerebral cortex buried beneath the frontal, parietal, and temporal lobes; several sensory representations are located there, including those for taste, balance, and pain.

insulin: Hormone secreted by the pancreatic islet cells; can inhibit food intake through hypothalamic circuits.

intention tremor: Slow oscillatory movement of the distal limb as it approaches the endpoint of the movement; results from cerebellar dysfunction or damage.

interaural intensity difference: A mechanism for determining the horizontal location of high-frequency sounds.

interaural time difference: A mechanism for determining the horizontal location of low-frequency sounds.

infratentorial: Beneath the tentorium of the cerebellum.

intermediate hemisphere: Portion of the cerebellar cortex involved in limb and trunk control.

intermediate horn: The lateral intermediate zone of the spinal cord; location of sympathetic preganglionic neurons.

intermediate nerve: Sensory and parasympathetic branch of cranial nerve VII.

intermediate zone: Portion of spinal gray matter located between the dorsal and ventral horns.

intermediolateral cell column: *See* intermediolateral nucleus.

intermediolateral nucleus: Location of sympathetic preganglionic neurons; present from about T1 to about L2.

internal arcuate fibers: Decussating fibers of the dorsal column nuclei.

internal capsule: Location of axons coursing to and from the cerebral cortex; present between the thalamus and parts of the basal ganglia.

internal carotid artery: Major cerebral artery; supplies blood to the cerebral cortex and many deep structures excluding the brain stem and cerebellum.

internal medullary laminae: Bands of white matter that divide the thalamus into several nuclear divisions.

internal segment of the globus pallidus: One of the principal output nuclei of the basal ganglia.

interneurons: Neurons with an axon that remains locally within the nucleus or cortical region where the cell body is located.

internuclear neurons: Neurons located in the abducens nucleus that project to the contralateral oculomotor nucleus to transmit control signals for horizontal saccadic eye movements.

internuclear ophthalmoplegia: Produced by lesion of the medial longitudinal fasciculus between the levels of the abducens and oculomotor nuclei; interrupts axons of internuclear neurons; inability to adduct the ipsilateral eye when looking to the side opposite the lesion.

interpeduncular cistern: Where cerebrospinal fluid collects between the cerebral peduncles.

interpeduncular fossa: Space between the cerebral peduncles.

interpolar nucleus: Component of the spinal trigeminal nucleus; important for facial pain, especially within the mouth and teeth.

interposed nuclei: Deep cerebellar nuclei; comprises the globose and emboliform nuclei.

intersegmental neurons: Spinal interneurons that interconnect neurons in different segments; also termed propriospinal neurons.

interstitial nucleus of Cajal: Involved in eye and head control; located in rostral midbrain; gives rise to a small descending motor pathway.

interstitial nucleus of the MLF: Center for control of vertical eye movements; located in rostral midbrain.

interventricular foramen (of Monro): Conduit through which cerebrospinal fluid and choroid plexus passes from the lateral ventricles to the third ventricle.

interventricular foramina: *See* interventricular foramen.

intracavernous segment: Portion of internal carotid artery as it passes through the cavernous sinus.

intralaminar nuclei: Set of thalamic nuclei that have diffuse cortical projections and may play a role in regulating the level of cortical activity and arousal.

intrapetrosal segment: Portion of the carotid artery as it travels through the petrous bone.

intrasegmental neurons: Local spinal interneurons; their axons remain with the segment of the cell body.

intrinsic nuclei (of basal ganglia): Include the external part of the globus pallidus, part of the ventral pallidum, subthalamic nucleus, substantia nigra pars compacta, ventral tegmental area.

ipsilateral: On the same side; term used relative to a particular landmark or event.

ischemia: Decreased delivery of oxygenated blood to the tissue.

ischemic stroke: Occlusion of an artery that results in downstream cessation of blood flow.

isthmus: Narrow portion of the developing brain stem between the pons and midbrain; in maturity the isthmus is typically included as part of the rostral pons.

itch: Sensory experience produced by histamine.

itch-sensitive receptors: Activation leads to the sensation itch; also termed pruritic receptor.

jaw-jerk (or closure) reflex: Automatic closure of the jaw upon stimulation of muscle spindle afferents in jaw muscles; analogous to the knee-jerk reflex.

jaw proprioception: The ability to sense jaw angle; more commonly used to describe the sensory events signaled by primary sensory neurons whose cell bodies are located within the mesencephalic trigeminal nucleus.

juxtarestiform body: Efferent pathway from the cerebellum to the caudal brain stem; principal location of axons from the fastigial nucleus to vestibular and other brain stem neurons.

knee-jerk reflex: Automatic extension of the leg upon stimulation of the patella tendon; the stimulus stretches muscle spindle receptors in the quadriceps muscle.

Korsakoff syndrome: A form of memory loss in patients with alcoholism or thiamine deficiency; produced by degeneration of the mammillary bodies and parts of the medial thalamus.

lacrimal gland: Tear gland.

lamella: A thin scale, plate, or sublayer, as of bone.

lamina terminalis: Rostral wall of the third ventricle; marks location of most anterior portion of the neural tube.

laminated: Morphological feature in which neuronal cell bodies or axons form discrete layers.

large-diameter axon: Mechanoreceptive sensory axons.

large-diameter fiber entry zone: Site at which large-diameter axons enter the spinal cord; located medial to Lissauer's tract.

laryngeal closure reflex: Automatic contraction of laryngeal adductor muscles to prevent food and fluids from entering the trachea.

lateral cerebellar hemisphere: Cortical component of the cerebrocerebellum; involved primarily in motor planning.

lateral column: Portion of the spinal white matter; contains diverse somatic sensory, cerebellar, and motor control pathways.

lateral corticospinal tract: Pathway in which descending axons for voluntary limb control descend; originates primarily from the motor areas of the frontal lobe.

lateral descending pathways: Motor pathways for controlling limb muscles.

lateral gaze palsy: *See* internuclear ophthalmoplegia.

lateral geniculate nucleus: Thalamic visual relay nucleus.

lateral hypothalamus (or hypothalamic zone): Important for feeding and sleep-wakefulness; orexin-containing neurons are unique to this brain region.

lateral intermediate zone: Portion of spinal gray matter that plays a role in limb muscle control.

lateral lemniscus: Ascending brain stem auditory pathway.

lateral medullary lamina: Band of axons that separates the external segment of the globus pallidus and the putamen.

lateral medullary syndrome: Set of neurological signs associated with occlusion of the posterior inferior cerebellar artery; signs include difficulty in swallowing, vertigo, loss of pain and temperature sense on the ipsilateral face and contralateral limbs and trunk, ataxia, and Horner syndrome.

lateral olfactory stria: Pathway by which axons from the olfactory tract project to the olfactory cortical areas.

lateral posterior nucleus: Thalamic nucleus with projections to the posterior parietal lobe.

lateral rectus muscle: Ocular abductor muscle; moves eye laterally.

lateral reticular nucleus: Precerebellar nucleus; transmits information from the cerebral cortex and spinal cord to the intermediate cerebellum.

lateral septal nucleus: Telencephalic nucleus; part of limbic system.

lateral sulcus: Separates the temporal lobe from the frontal and parietal lobes.

lateral superior olivary nucleus: ontains neurons sensitive to interaural intensity differences; plays role in horizontal localization of high-frequency sounds.

lateral ventral horn: Contains motor neurons that innervate limb muscles.

lateral ventricle: Telencephalic component of the ventricular system; bilaterally paired, with four components (anterior horn, body, atrium, posterior horn, and inferior horn).

lateral vestibular nucleus: Key brain stem nucleus for control of proximal muscles; important in balance; gives rise to the lateral vestibulospinal tract.

lateral vestibulospinal tract: Ipsilateral pathway; component of the medial descending pathways.

laterality: Pertains to one side or the other.

L-dopa: Precursor to dopamine; used in the treatment of Parkinson disease.

lenticular fasciculus: Region of the white matter through which axons from the internal segment of the globus pallidus course en route to the thalamus.

lenticular nucleus: Globus pallidus (both internal and external segments) and putamen.

lenticulostriate arteries: Branches of the middle cerebral artery and anterior cerebral artery that supply deep structures of the cerebral hemispheres, including parts of the internal capsule and basal ganglia; originate from the proximal portions of the arteries.

leptin: Hormone produced by adipocytes in proportion to the amount of body fat; suppresses feeding.

levator palpebrae superioris muscle: Principal eyelid elevator.

limb position sense: Ability to judge the position of one's limbs without using vision.

limbic association cortex: Diverse regions of primarily the frontal and temporal lobes; involved in emotions, learning, and memory.

limbic loop (of basal ganglia): The basal ganglia circuit that receive input from limbic cortical areas, basolateral amygdala, and the hippocampal formation and projects to the orbitofrontal cortex and anterior cingulate cortex.

limbic system: Brain structures and their interconnections that collectively mediate emotions, learning, and memory.

Lissauer's tract: Location of central branches of small-diameter afferent fibers prior to termination in the superficial dorsal horn.

lobe: Major division of the cerebral cortex.

lobule: A division of a lobe.

locus ceruleus: Principal noradrenergic brain stem nucleus; located in the rostral pons.

long circumferential branches: Brain stem arterial branches that supply the most dorsolateral portions; also supply the cerebellum.

longitudinal axis: The head-to-tail (or head-to-coccyx) axis of the nervous system.

lumbar: Spinal cord segment; there are five in total.

lumbar cistern: Space within the vertebral canal where cerebrospinal fluid pools; commonly used for withdrawing cerebrospinal fluid from patients.

lumbar tap: Process of removing cerebrospinal fluid from the lumbar cistern; needle is inserted into the intervertebral space between the third and fourth (or the fourth and fifth) lumbar vertebrae.

M cell: Retinal ganglion neuron with a large dendritic arbor; plays a preferential role in sensing of visual motion; magnocellular.

macroglia: Glial cell class that comprises oligodendrocytes, Schwann cells, astrocytes, and ependymal cells; serve a variety of support and nutritive functions; contrast with microglia.

macula lutea: Portion of the central retina that contains the fovea.

macular region: Portion of the retina surrounding the macula lutea.

macular sparing: Maintenance of vision around the fovea after visual cortex damage that produces a loss of parafoveal and peripheral vision.

magnetic resonance angiography: Application of magnetic resonance imaging to study vasculature by monitoring motion of water molecules in blood vessels.

magnetic resonance imaging: Radiological technique to examine brain structure; uses primarily the water content of tissue to provide a structural image.

magnocellular division (of red nucleus): Component of the red nucleus that contains large neurons that project to the spinal cord as the rubrospinal tract.

magnocellular neurosecretory system: Hypothalamic neurons in the supraoptic and paraventricular nuclei that project their axons to the posterior lobe of the pituitary, where they release oxytocin and vasopressin.

magnocellular visual system: Components of the visual system in the retina, lateral geniculate, and visual cortical areas that originate from M-type ganglion cells; sensitive primarily to moving stimuli.

main (or principal) trigeminal sensory nucleus: Brain stem relay nucleus for mechanosensory information from the face and oral cavity.

malleus: One of the middle ear ossicles (bones); essential for conducting changes in air pressure from the tympanic membrane to the oval window; attaches to the tympanic membrane.

mammillary bodies: Hypothalamic nuclear complex; contains the medial and lateral mammillary nuclei; the mammillary bodies give rise to the mammillothalamic and mammillotegmental tracts.

mammillotegmental tract: Originates from the lateral mammillary nucleus; terminates in the pontine tegmentum.

mammillothalamic tract: Originates from both the medial and lateral mammillary nuclei; terminates in the anterior thalamic nuclei.

mandibular division: Trigeminal sensory nerve root that innervates primarily the lower face and parts of the oral cavity.

marginal zone: Outermost layer of the dorsal horn.

mastication: Chewing.

maxillary division: Trigeminal sensory nerve root that innervates primarily the lips, cheek, and parts of the oral cavity.

mechanoreceptive afferent fibers: Sensory axons that have mechanoreceptive terminals.

mechanoreceptors: Sensory receptors sensitive to mechanical stimulation.

medial descending pathways: Motor pathways for controlling axial and other proximal muscles.

medial dorsal nucleus (of the thalamus): Principal thalamic nucleus projecting to the frontal lobe.

medial forebrain bundle: Pathway that carries functionally diverse brain stem pathways to subcortical nuclei and the cerebral cortex, including the monoaminergic pathways.

medial geniculate nucleus: Thalamic auditory relay nucleus.

medial lemniscus: Brain stem tract that contains axons traveling from the dorsal column nuclei to the thalamus.

medial longitudinal fasciculus: Brain stem tract that contains axons from the vestibular nuclei, extraocular motor nuclei, and various brain stem nuclei; primarily for control of eye movements.

medial mammillary nucleus: Principal nucleus of the mammillary body; projects to the anterior nuclei of the thalamus.

medial medullary lamina: Band of myelinated axons that separates the internal and external segments of the globus pallidus.

medial olfactory stria: Small tract that contains axons from other brain regions that project to the olfactory bulb.

medial orbital gyri: *See* medial orbitofrontal gyri.

medial orbitofrontal gyri: Part of the limbic association cortex.

medial prefrontal cortical areas: Portion of the prefrontal cortex one function of which is object recognition.

medial preoptic area: Portion of the anterior hypothalamus that contains parvocellular neurosecretory neurons; sexually dimorphic.

medial rectus muscle: Extraocular muscle that adducts eye (i.e., moves toward the nose); innervated by the oculomotor nerve (cranial nerve III).

medial septal nucleus: Telencephalic nucleus; important projections to the hippocampal formation; gives rise to cholinergic and GABA-ergic projections.

medial superior olivary nucleus: Contains neurons sensitive to interaural timing differences; plays role in horizontal localization of low-frequency sounds.

medial ventral horn: Contains motor neurons that innervate proximal limb and axial muscles; controlled by the medial descending pathways.

medial vestibular nucleus: Part of the vestibular nuclear complex; gives rise to the medial vestibulospinal tract for head and eye coordination.

medial vestibulospinal tract: Motor pathway for coordinating head and eye movements.

median eminence: Contains the primary capillaries of the hypophyseal portal system; located in the proximal portion of the infundibular stalk; lacks blood–brain barrier.

median raphe nuclei: Located along or close to the brain stem midline; use serotonin as neurotransmitter.

medium spiny neurons: Major class of striatal neuron; projects to the globus pallidus.

medulla: Major brain division; part of hindbrain.

medullary dorsal horn: Extension of dorsal horn into the medulla; also termed caudal nucleus.

Meissner's corpuscle: Mechanoreceptor.

melanin-concentrating hormone: Peptide that affects food intake.

membranous labyrinth: Cavity within which the vestibular apparatus are located; contains endolymph.

meninges: Membranes that cover the central nervous system; comprises dura, arachnoid, and pia.

Merkel's receptor: Mechanoreceptor.

mesencephalic trigeminal nucleus: Contains cell bodies of jaw muscle stretch receptors; only site in the central nervous system that contains cell bodies of sensory receptor neurons; more similar to a ganglion than a nucleus.

mesencephalic trigeminal tract: Contains the axons of jaw muscle stretch receptors.

mesencephalon: Secondary brain vesicle; major brain division; also termed midbrain.

mesocorticolimbic dopaminergic system: Dopaminergic projection to the frontal lobe and ventral striatum; primarily originates from the ventral tegmental area.

mesoderm: Middle layer of the embryo.

mesolimbic dopaminergic system: Originates from the ventral tegmental nucleus; supplies dopamine to nucleus accumbens and parts of frontal lobe; sometimes termed mesocorticolimbic dopaminergic system.

metencephalon: Secondary brain vesicle; gives rise to the pons and cerebellum.

Meyer's loop: Component of the optic radiation from the lateral geniculate nucleus to the occipital lobe that courses through the rostral temporal lobe; axons transmit visual information from the contralateral upper visual field.

microglia: Class of glial cell that subserves a phagocytic or scavenger role; responds to nervous system infection or damage; contrasts with macroglia.

microzones (of cerebellum): Small clusters of Purkinje neurons receive climbing fiber inputs that have similar physiological characteristics, such as processing somatic sensory information from the same body part.

midbrain: Major brain division.

midbrain dopaminergic neurons: Correspond to dopaminergic neurons in the substantia nigra pars compacta and the ventral tegmental area.

midbrain tectum: Region dorsal to the cerebral aqueduct; corresponds to the superior and inferior colliculi.

middle cerebellar peduncle: Major input pathway to the cerebrocerebellum; consists of axons of pontine nuclei.

middle cerebral artery: Supplies blood to the lateral surface of the cerebral cortex and deep structures of the cerebral hemisphere and diencephalon.

middle ear ossicles: Three bones that conduct sound pressure waves from the tympanic membrane to the oval window.

middle temporal gyrus: Located on the lateral temporal lobe; important in higher visual functions, especially object recognition.

midline thalamic nuclei: Diffuse-projecting nuclei; one of its major targets is the hippocampal formation.

midsagittal: Anatomical or imaging plane through the midline that is parallel both to the longitudinal axis of the central nervous system and to the midline, between the dorsal and ventral surfaces.

miosis: Pupillary constriction.

mirror neurons: Discharged when an animal performs a movement or sees movements being performed by another.

mitral cells: Projection neuron of the olfactory bulb.

mixed nerve: Peripheral nerve composed of somatic sensory and motor axons.

modality: Sensory attribute that corresponds to quality (e.g., pain).

molecular layer: Outermost cerebellar layer; contains stellate and basket neurons, Purkinje cell dendrites, climbing fibers, and parallel fibers.

mossy fiber terminal: Enlarged axon terminal; one of the principal components of the cerebellar glomerulus.

mossy fibers: In the cerebellum, major input to the cortex that originates from diverse structures, including the spinal cord and pontine nuclei; in the hippocampus, axon branch of granule cells in the dentate gyrus that synapse on neurons in the CA3 region.

motion pathway (for vision): Circuit specialized for discriminating the speed and direction of moving visual stimuli.

motor cranial nerve nuclei: Contain cell bodies of somatic and branchiomeric motor neurons; nuclei containing parasympathetic preganglionic motor neurons are typically termed autonomic motor nuclei or columns.

motor homunculus: Representation of body musculature in the primary motor cortex; organization is similar to the form of the body.

motor learning: In animals or humans, learning to perform some motor task in response to a given event or stimulus.

motor neurons: Central nervous system neurons that have an axon that projects to the periphery, to synapse on striated muscles (somatic or branchiomeric motor neurons) or autonomic postganglionic neurons and adrenal cells (autonomic motor neurons).

motor unit: A single alpha-motor neuron and all of the muscle fibers that it innervates.

Müller cell: Retinal glial cell that stretches from the outer to the inner limiting membranes; have important structural and metabolic functions.

multipolar neurons: Neurons with a complex dendritic array and a single axon; principal neuron class in the central nervous system.

muscarinic receptors: Membrane proteins that transduce acetylcholine into neuronal depolarization; named for agonist muscarine.

muscle spindle receptor: Stretch receptor in muscle; has efferent sensitivity control.

myelencephalon: Secondary brain vesicle; forms the medulla of the mature brain.

myelin: Fatty substance that contains numerous myelin proteins.

myelin sheath: Covering around peripheral and central axons to speed action potential conduction; formed by Schwann cells in the periphery and oligodendrocytes in the central nervous system.

myelin stains: Methods to reveal the presence of the myelin sheath.

myotatic reflexes: Mechanoreceptors in muscle excite or inhibit motor neurons at short latency with only one or just a few synapses (e.g., the knee-jerk [stretch] reflex).

narcolepsy: Disease in which the patient experiences persistent daytime sleepiness; often associated with cataplexy, which is the transient loss of muscle tone without a loss of consciousness.

nasal hemiretina: Portion of the retina medial to a vertical line that runs through the macula.

nasal mucosal glands: Located in the nasal cavity, secrete mucous, which is rich in glycoproteins; protects the nasal epithelium.

neocortex: Phylogenetically most recent portion of the cerebral cortex; most abundant form of cortex; has six or more layers.

neural crest: Collection of dorsal neural tube cells that migrate peripherally and give rise to all of the neurons whose cell bodies are outside of the central nervous system; also gives rise to Schwann cells and the arachnoid and pial meningeal layers.

neural degeneration: Deterioration in neuron structure and function.

neural groove: Midline region of the neural tube where neurons and glial cells do not proliferate; where the floor plate forms.

neural induction: Process by which a portion of the dorsal ectoderm of the embryo becomes committed to form the nervous system.

neural plate: Dorsal ectoderm region from which the nervous system forms.

neural tube: Embryonic structure that gives rise to the central nervous system; cells in the walls of the neural tube form neurons and glial cells, whereas the cavity within the tube forms the ventricular system.

neuraxis: Principal axis of the central nervous system.

neuroactive compounds: Chemicals that alter neuronal function.

neuroectoderm: Portion of the ectoderm that gives rise to the nervous system; corresponds to the neural plate.

neurohypophysis: Portion of the pituitary that develops from the neuroectoderm; where vasopressin and oxytocin are released into the systemic circulation.

neuromelanin: Polymer of the catecholamine precursor dihydroxyphenylalanine (or dopa), which is contained in the neurons in the pars compacta.

neuromeres: Segments of the developing hindbrain.

neuron: Nerve cell.

neurophysins: Protein that derives from the prohormone that gives rise to oxytocin and vasopressin; coreleased with oxytocin and vasopressin.

neuroplasticity: The brain's ability to reorganize itself by forming new neural connections throughout life.

neurotransmitter: Typically small molecular weight compounds (e.g., glutamate and γ-aminobutyric acid, and acetylcholine) that excite or inhibit neurons.

nigrostriatal dopaminergic system: Originates from the substantia nigra pars compacta and terminates primarily in the dorsal and lateral portions of the putamen and caudate nucleus.

nigrostriatal tract: Pathway in which nigrostriatal axons course.

nociceptors: Somatic sensory receptors that are selectively activated by noxious or damaging stimuli.

nodulus: Portion of the cerebellum critical for vestibular control of eye and head movements.

nondeclarative memory: Memory of procedures and actions.

noradrenalin: Neurotransmitter; also termed norepinephrine.

noradrenergic: Neuron that uses noradrenalin as a neurotransmitter.

notochord: Releases substances important for organizing the ventral neural tube, such as determining whether a developing neuron becomes a motor neuron; located ventral to the developing nervous system.

noxious: Tissue damaging.

noxious stimuli: A tissue-damaging stimulus; can be mechanical, thermal, or in response to various forms of trauma.

nucleus: Collection of neuronal cell bodies within the central nervous system.

nucleus accumbens: Component of the striatum located ventrally and medially; key structure in drug addiction.

nucleus ambiguus: Contains primarily motor neurons that innervate the pharynx and larynx; also contains parasympathetic preganglionic neurons; located in the medulla.

nucleus of the diagonal band of Broca: Cholinergic telencephalic nucleus with diverse cortical projections; located in the basal forebrain.

nucleus of the lateral lemniscus: Auditory projection nucleus; located in the rostral pons.

nucleus of the trapezoid body: Contains inhibitory neurons that receive input from the anteroventral cochlear nucleus and project to the lateral superior olivary nucleus; may participate in shaping the interaural timing sensitivity of neurons in the lateral superior olivary nucleus located in the pons.

nucleus proprius: Contains neurons that process somatic sensory information; corresponds to laminae III–IV of the dorsal horn.

nystagmus: Rhythmical oscillations of the eyeball.

occipital lobe: One of the lobes of the cerebral hemisphere.

occipital somites: Somites from which neck and cranial structures develop.

ocular dominance columns: Clusters of neurons in the primary visual cortex that receive and process information predominantly from either the ipsilateral or the contralateral eye.

oculomotor (III) nerve: Motor cranial nerve; contains axons that innervate the medial rectus, superior rectus, inferior rectus, inferior oblique, and levator palpebrae muscles, as well as axons of parasympathetic preganglionic neurons.

oculomotor loop: Basal ganglia circuit that engages frontal eye movement control areas.

oculomotor nucleus: Contains motor neurons that innervate the medial rectus, superior rectus, inferior rectus, inferior oblique, and levator palpebrae muscles.

odorants: Chemicals that produce odors.

olfactory bulb: Telencephalic structure that receives input from olfactory sensory neurons and projects to the olfactory cortical areas.

olfactory discrimination: Ability to discriminate one odorant from another.

olfactory epithelium: Portion of the olfactory mucosa that contains olfactory sensory neurons.

olfactory (I) nerve: Central branches of olfactory sensory neurons; travels the short distance between the olfactory mucosa, through the cribriform plate, to synapse in the olfactory bulb.

olfactory receptor: Transmembrane protein complex in an olfactory sensory neuron; transduces a particular set of odorants into a neural potential; any given olfactory sensory neurons contains a single (or just a few) olfactory receptor types.

olfactory sulcus: Groove on the inferior frontal lobe surface in which the olfactory bulb and tract course.

olfactory tract: Contains axons that interconnect the olfactory bulb with the other olfactory nuclear regions of the brain.

olfactory tubercle: Region on the ventral brain surface that receives input from the olfactory tract; may play a role in emotions in addition to olfaction.

oligodendrocytes: Class of glial cell that forms the myelin sheath around axons within the central nervous system.

olive: Landmark on ventral surface of the medulla under which the inferior olivary nucleus is located.

olivocochlear bundle: Efferent projection from the inferior olivary nucleus to hair cells in the cochlea.

olivocochlear projection: See olivocochlear bundle.

Onuf's nucleus: Located in sacral spinal cord; contains motor neurons that innervate anal and urethral sphincters.

operculum: Portions of frontal, parietal, and temporal lobes that overlie the insular cortex.

ophthalmic artery: Supplies the eye; can be a pathway for collateral brain circulation after occlusion of the internal carotid artery.

ophthalmic division: Trigeminal sensory nerve root that innervates primarily the upper face.

optic chiasm: Site of decussation of ganglion cell axons from the nasal hemiretinae.

optic disk: Site on retina where ganglion cell axons exit from the eye.

optic (II) nerve: Sensory cranial nerve that contains axons of retinal ganglion cells; major projections are to the lateral geniculate nucleus, superior colliculus, and pretectal nuclei.

optic radiations: Pathway from the lateral geniculate nucleus to the primary visual cortex; forms the lateral wall of the posterior horn of the lateral ventricle.

optic tectum: Also termed the superior colliculus.

optic tract: Retinal ganglion cell axon pathway between the optic chiasm and the lateral geniculate nucleus.

optokinetic reflexes: Ocular reflexes that use visual information; supplements the actions of vestibuloocular reflexes.

oral nucleus: Rostral component of the spinal trigeminal nucleus.

orbitofrontal (or orbital) gyri: Portion of the inferior frontal lobe that contains the orbital gyri; overlie the bony orbits.

orbitofrontal cortex: Part of prefrontal cortex; important for emotion and personality.

orexin: Peptide that is essential for the proper maintenance of the aroused state; loss of orexin is implicated in the sleep disorder narcolepsy; may also participate in feeding; also termed hypocretin.

organ of Corti: Component of the inner ear for transducing sound into neural signals.

organum vasculosum of the lamina terminalis: One of the circumventricular organs; region in which the blood–brain barrier is absent; axons project to magnocellular neurons of the paraventricular nucleus.

orientation column: Cluster of neurons in the primary visual cortex that processes information about the orientation of a visual stimulus.

orthonasal olfaction: When molecules travel from the external environment, through the nostrils (nares), to activate olfactory neurons in the olfactory epithelium.

orthostatic hypotension: Sudden reduction in systemic blood pressure upon standing upright; sometimes termed postural hypotension.

otic ganglion: Contains parasympathetic postganglionic neurons that innervate the parotid gland, which secretes saliva.

otolith organs: The utricle and saccule; sensitive to linear acceleration.

outer hair cells: Class of auditory receptor neurons; may be more important in regulating the sensitivity of the organ of Corti than in auditory signal transduction.

outer nuclear layer: Retinal layer that contains the cell bodies of photoreceptors (rods and cones).

outer synaptic (or plexiform) layer: Retinal layer in which connections are made between photoreceptors and two classes of retinal interneurons (horizontal cells and bipolar neurons).

output nuclei (of basal ganglia): Consisting of the globus pallidus-internal part, part of the ventral pallidum, and the substantia nigra pars reticulata.

oxytocin: Peptide released by magnocellular neurons in the paraventricular and supraoptic nuclei.

P cell: Retinal ganglion neurons with a small dendritic arbor; plays a preferential role in sensing of form and color; parvocellular.

pacinian corpuscle: Rapidly adapting mechanoreceptor sensitive to high-frequency vibration.

pain: Sensation evoked by noxious stimulation.

palate: Arch-shaped portion of the superior oral cavity.

paleocortex: Type of cerebral cortex with fewer than six layers; commonly associated with processing of olfactory stimuli; located on the basal surface of the cerebral hemispheres, in part of the insular cortex, and caudally along the parahippocampal gyrus and retrosplenial cortex.

pallidotomy: Therapeutic lesion of a portion of the globus pallidus to alleviate dyskinesias.

parabrachial nucleus: Transmits viscerosensory information from the solitary nucleus to the diencephalon; located in the rostral pons.

parafascicular nucleus: Thalamic diffuse-projecting nucleus with widespread projections to the frontal lobe and striatum.

parahippocampal gyrus: Located on medial temporal lobe; contains cortical association areas that project to the hippocampal formation.

parallel fibers: Axons of cerebellar granule cells that course along the long axis of the folia; a single parallel fiber makes synapses with many Purkinje cells.

parallel organization: Property of neural systems in which pathways with similar anatomical organizations serve distinct functions.

parallel sensory pathways: Two or more sensory pathways that have similar anatomical projections and overlapping sets of functions.

paramedian arterial branches: Supply the most medial portions of the brain stem; originate primarily from the basilar artery.

paramedian pontine reticular formation: Transmits control signals from the contralateral cerebral cortex to brain stem centers for controlling horizontal saccades; major target of neurons in this structure is the abducens nucleus.

parasagittal: Anatomical or imaging plane off the midline that is parallel both to the longitudinal axis of the central nervous system and to the midline, between the dorsal and ventral surfaces.

parasympathetic nervous system: Component of the autonomic nervous system; originates from the brain stem and the caudal sacral spinal cord.

parasympathetic preganglionic neurons: Autonomic neurons located in the central nervous system; project to parasympathetic postganglionic neurons, which are located in the periphery.

paraterminal gyrus: Located anterior to the rostral wall of the third ventricle and ventral to the rostrum of the corpus callosum.

paraventricular nucleus: Hypothalamic nucleus that contains magnocellular neurosecretory neurons, parvocellular neurosecretory neurons, and descending projection neurons that regulate the functions of the autonomic nervous system.

paravertebral ganglia: Contain sympathetic postganglionic neurons.

parietal lobe: One of the lobes of the cerebral hemisphere.

parietal-temporal-occipital association area: Association cortex at the junction of the parietal, temporal, and occipital lobes; important for linguistics, perception, and other higher brain functions.

parietooccipital sulcus: Separates the parietal and occipital lobes.

Parkinson disease: Results from loss of dopaminergic neurons in the substantia nigra pars compacta; characterized by slowing or absence of movement (bradykinesia) and tremor.

parotid gland: Salivary gland; innervated by axons of the glossopharyngeal (IX) nerve.

parvocellular division (of red nucleus): Component of the red nucleus that contains small neurons that project to the inferior olivary nucleus as the rubroolivary tract.

parvocellular neurosecretory system: Hypothalamic neurons located predominantly in the periventricular zone; neurons project to the median eminence where they make neurovascular contacts with capillaries and release factors into the blood that are carried to the anterior lobe by the portal veins.

parvocellular visual system: Components of the visual system in the retina, lateral geniculate, and visual cortical areas that originate from P-type ganglion cells; sensitive primarily to color, size, and the shapes of stimuli.

peduncles: A large collection of axons.

pedunculopontine nucleus: A pontine nucleus that receives a projection from the internal segment of the globus pallidus; participates in diverse functions, including regulating arousal and movement control; contains cholinergic neurons.

perforant pathway: Projection from the entorhinal cortex to the dentate gyrus.

periamygdaloid cortex: One of the olfactory cortical areas; receives a direct projection from the olfactory tract; located on the rostromedial temporal lobe.

periaqueductal gray matter: Central region of the midbrain that surrounds the cerebral aqueduct; participates in diverse functions, including pain suppression.

periglomerular cell: An inhibitory interneuron in the olfactory bulb that receives input from olfactory sensory neurons and inhibits mitral cells in the same and adjacent glomeruli.

perilymph: Fluid that fills the space between the membranous labyrinth and the temporal bone; resembles extracellular fluid and cerebrospinal fluid.

peripheral autonomic ganglia: Clusters of sympathetic and parasympathetic postganglionic neurons.

peripheral nervous system: Contains the axons of motor neurons, the peripheral axons and cell bodies of dorsal root ganglion neurons, the axon of autonomic preganglionic neurons, and the cell body and axon of autonomic postganglionic neurons.

periventricular nucleus: Contains parvocellular neurosecretory neurons; located in the hypothalamus, beneath the walls of the third ventricle.

periventricular zone: Portion of the hypothalamus that contains most of the parvocellular neurosecretory neurons; located beneath the walls and floor of the third ventricle.

pharynx: The portion of the digestive tube between the esophagus and mouth; the throat.

pheromones: A chemical produced and secreted by an animal that influences the behavior and development of other members of the same species.

pia mater: Inner meningeal layer; adheres closely to the surface of the central nervous system.

pigment epithelium: External to the photoreceptor layer; it serves a phagocytic role during renewal of rod outer segment disks.

pineal gland: Endocrine gland located dorsal to the superior colliculus that is involved in the sleep/wake cycle; secretes melatonin.

pinocytosis: A mechanism by which cells ingest extracellular fluid and its contents.

piriform cortex: One of the olfactory cortical areas; receives a direct projection from the olfactory tract; located on the rostromedial temporal lobe.

pituitary portal circulation: Connects capillary beds of the median eminence and anterior lobe of the pituitary; portal vein.

pons: One of the major brain divisions; Latin for bridge.

pontine cistern: Site of accumulation of cerebrospinal fluid at the pontomedullary junction.

pontine flexure: Bend in the developing nervous system at the pons.

pontine nuclei: Relay information from the ipsilateral cerebral cortex to the contralateral cerebellar cortex and deep nuclei, principally the lateral cerebellar cortex and the dentate nucleus.

pontomedullary junction: Where the pons and medulla join.

pontomedullary reticular formation: Contains diverse motor, sensory, and integrative nuclei; especially important in arousal and visceral and skeletal muscle control.

portal circulation: Contains two capillary beds joined by portal veins; present in the pituitary gland and the liver.

portal veins: Join the two capillary beds of a portal circulation.

positron emission tomography: Functional imaging technique based on the emission of positively charged unstable subatomic particles (positrons); PET.

postcentral gyrus: Important for mechanical sensations, including position sense; located in the parietal lobe.

postcommissural fornix: Principal division of the fornix; contains axons principally from the subiculum that terminate in the mammillary bodies.

posterior: Toward the abdomen.

posterior cerebellar incisure: Shallow groove in the posterior lobe of the cerebellum.

posterior cerebral artery: Supplies portions of the occipital and temporal lobes as well as the diencephalon.

posterior circulation: Arterial supply provided by the vertebral and basilar arteries.

posterior commissure: Interconnects midbrain structures in the two halves of the brain stem; axons that mediate the pupillary light reflex in the nonilluminated eye course within the anterior commissure.

posterior communicating artery: Branch of the internal carotid artery that joins the posterior cerebral arteries; connects the anterior and posterior circulations, thereby providing a pathway for collateral circulation; part of the circle of Willis.

posterior inferior cerebellar artery (PICA): Supplies the dorsolateral medulla and portions of the inferior (posterior) cerebellum.

posterior limb of the internal capsule: Component of the internal capsule that lies lateral to the thalamus; carries axons from various sources including those coursing to and from the primary motor and somatic sensory cortical areas.

posterior lobe of cerebellum: Portion of cerebellar cortex between the anterior and flocculonodular lobes; comprises lobules VI–IX.

posterior lobe (of pituitary gland): Contains axons and terminations of the paraventricular and supraoptic nuclei of the hypothalamus; axon terminations release vasopressin (ADH) and oxytocin at neurovascular contacts with systemic capillaries.

posterior parietal lobe (or cortex): Caudal to the primary somatic sensory cortex; important for proprioception, spatial awareness, attention and visually guided limb and eye movements; part of the where pathway for visual motion and actions.

posterior spinal arteries: Supply blood to the dorsal columns and dorsal horn predominantly.

posterolateral fissure: Separates the posterior and flocculonodular cerebellar lobes.

posteroventral cochlear nucleus: Contributes to a system of connections that regulate hair cell sensitivity.

postganglionic neuron: Autonomic neuron that projects to a peripheral motor target, such as a smooth muscle or a gland.

postsynaptic neuron: Component of a synapse; contacted by a presynaptic neuron.

precentral gyrus: Contains the primary motor cortex and the caudal portion of the premotor cortex; located in the frontal lobe.

precommissural fornix: Small division of the fornix that contains axons primarily from the hippocampus that terminate in the septal nuclei.

prefrontal association cortex: Involved in diverse functions, including thought and working memory.

prefrontal cortex loop: Circuit of the basal ganglia that projects to the prefrontal cortex; involved in higher brain functions, such as thought and working memory.

prefrontal cortex: *See* prefrontal association cortex.

preganglionic neuron: Autonomic neuron located in the central nervous system.

premotor areas: Participate in the planning of movements; located in the frontal lobe, in areas 6, 23, and 24.

premotor cortex: Specific premotor region located in the lateral portion of area 6.

preoccipital notch: Surface landmark that forms part of the boundary between the temporal and occipital lobes on the lateral surface.

preoptic area: Serves diverse functions including the control of sex hormone release from the anterior pituitary gland and regulation of sleep and wakefulness; located in the most rostral part of the hypothalamus.

preoptic sleep center: Hypothalamic center that regulates transition from wakefulness to sleep.

prepositus nucleus: Participates in eye position control; receives abundant inputs from the vestibular nuclei; located in the medulla.

presynaptic neuron: Component of the synapse; transmits information to the postsynaptic neuron.

presynaptic terminal: Axon terminal.

pretectal nuclei: Involved in pupillary light reflex; located in the junction between the midbrain and diencephalon.

prevertebral ganglia: Sympathetic ganglia that lie along the vertebral column.

primary auditory cortex: First cortical processing site for auditory information; located in the transverse temporal gyri (of Heschl) in the temporal lobe; corresponds to cytoarchitectonic area 41.

primary fissure: Separates the anterior and posterior lobes of the cerebellum.

primary motor cortex: Contains neurons that participate in the control of limb and trunk movements; contains neurons that synapse directly on motor neurons; consists of area 4.

primary olfactory cortex: Defined as the target areas of olfactory tract axons; located in the rostromedial temporal lobe and the basal surface of the frontal lobes; corresponds to the paleocortex.

primary olfactory neurons: Transduce odorant molecules into neural signals; located within the olfactory epithelium.

primary sensory (or afferent) fibers: Somatic sensory receptor; dorsal root ganglion neuron.

primary somatic sensory cortex: Participates in somatic sensations, principally mechanical sensations and limb position sense; corresponds to cytoarchitectonic areas 1, 2, and 3; located in the postcentral gyrus.

primary vestibular afferents: Innervate vestibular hair cells; terminate primarily in the vestibular nuclei and cerebellum.

primary visual cortex: Participates in visual perceptions; located in the occipital lobe.

projection neurons: Cortical pyramidal neurons that project their axons to subcortical sites.

proopiomelanocortin: A large peptide from which β-endorphin is cleaved.

proprioception: Sense of the position of the body; usually that of a limb or one limb segment relative to another.

propriospinal neurons: Spinal interneurons that interconnect neurons in different segments; also termed intersegmental neurons.

prosencephalon: Most rostral brain vesicle; gives rise to the telencephalon and diencephalon, which are the forebrain structures.

prosopagnosia: Inability to recognize faces.

proximal limb muscles: Muscles that innervate the shoulder or hip.

pruritic: Related to itch.

pruritic receptor: Sensory receptors responsible for the sensation of itch; activated by histamine.

pseudoptosis: Partial dropping of the eyelid.

pseudounipolar neurons: Neuron type that has a single axon and few or no dendrites in maturity (e.g., the dorsal root ganglion neuron).

pterygopalatine ganglion: Peripheral ganglion containing the cell bodies of parasympathetic postganglionic neurons that innervate nasal and oropharyngeal mucosal glands and lacrimal glands.

ptosis: Abnormal lowering or drooping of an organ or a part, especially a drooping of the upper eyelid caused by muscle weakness or paralysis.

pulmonary aspiration: The presence of food or consumed fluids in the lungs.

pulvinar nucleus: Major thalamic nucleus that has diverse projections to the parietal, temporal, and occipital lobes; involved in perception and linguistic functions.

pupillary constriction: Reduction in pupil diameter.

pupillary dilation: Increase in pupil diameter.

pupillary light reflex: Closure of the pupil with visual stimulation of the retina; used to test midbrain function in comatose patients.

pupillary reflexes: Changes in pupil diameter that occur without voluntary control; usually occur together with other ocular reflexes.

Purkinje layer: Location of Purkinje cell bodies.

Purkinje neuron (or cell): Output neuron of the cerebellar cortex; makes GABAergic inhibitory synapses on neurons of deep cerebellar nuclei and vestibular nuclei.

putamen: Component of the striatum; important in limb and trunk control.

pyramid: Tract on ventral surface of medial medulla; contains descending cortical axons, including the corticobulbar and corticospinal tracts.

pyramidal neuron (or cell): Cortical projection neuron class with characteristic pyramidal-shaped cell body.

pyramidal decussation: Where pyramidal cell axons from the motor and premotor areas cross the midline; located in the medulla.

pyramidal signs: Motor impairments that follow lesion of the corticospinal system.

pyramidal tract: Location of descending motor control pathway that originates in the motor and somatic sensory areas.

quadrigeminal bodies: Another name for the superior and inferior colliculi.

quadrigeminal cistern: Portion of the subarachnoid space that overlies the superior and inferior colliculi.

radial glia: Type of astrocyte that plays a role in organizing neural development; form scaffold for neuron growth and migration.

radicular arteries: Segmental arteries that supply the spinal cord, together with anterior and posterior spinal arteries.

radicular pain: Pain localized to the distribution of a single dermatome or several adjoining dermatomes.

raphe nuclei: Contain serotonin; located along the midline throughout most of the brain stem.

rapidly adapting: Response characteristic of neurons to a sudden stimulus in which a brief series of action potentials decrement rapidly to few or no action potentials.

Rathke's pouch: An ectodermal diverticulum in the roof of the developing oral cavity from which the anterior and intermediate lobes of the pituitary develop.

receptive membrane: Portion of a neuron's membrane that contains receptors sensitive to neuroactive compounds or a particular stimulus.

red nucleus: Plays a role in limb movement control; gives rise to the rubrospinal and rubroolivary tracts.

reduced myotatic reflexes: A condition in which the strength of muscle stretch or tendon reflexes are diminished.

regional neuroanatomy: Examines the spatial relations between brain structures within a portion of the nervous system.

relaxation times: In magnetic resonance imaging, the times it takes protons to return to the energy state they were in before excitation by electromagnetic waves.

relay nuclei: Contain neurons that transmit (or relay) incoming information to other sites in the central nervous system.

release-inhibiting hormones: Chemicals that inhibit the release of a hormone from the anterior pituitary gland; usually neuroactive compounds secreted into the portal circulation at the median eminence.

releasing hormones: Chemicals that promote the release of a hormone from the anterior pituitary gland; usually neuroactive compounds secreted into the portal circulation at the median eminence.

REM sleep: Abbreviation for rapid eye movement characterized by dreaming, low limb and trunk muscle tone, and low-amplitude high-frequency electroencephalographic activity.

reproductive behaviors: Relatively stereotypic behaviors between members of the same species that lead to a reproductive act; in animals, the hypothalamus plays an important role in promoting reproductive behaviors, often in response to pheromones.

restless legs syndrome: A disorder in which patients experience abnormal sensations in their legs that prompt the urge to move their legs to quell the sensation; abnormal sensations and movements are more common during rest and sleep than during activity.

reticular formation: A diffuse collection of nuclei in the central (medial) portion of the brain stem that play a role in a variety of functions, including regulation of arousal, motor control and vegetative functions.

reticular nucleus: A thalamic nucleus that projects to other thalamic nuclei; plays a role in regulating thalamic neuronal activity.

reticulospinal tract: Descending motor pathway that originates from the reticular formation, primarily in the pons and medulla, and synapses in the spinal cord.

retina: Peripheral portion of the visual system that contains photoreceptors as well as interneurons and projection neurons for the initial processing of visual information and transmission to several brain structures; develops from the diencephalon.

retinitis pigmentosa: Disease in which breakdown products accumulate at the pigment epithelium of the retina.

retinohypothalamic tract: Axons of retinal ganglion cells that project to the suprachiasmatic nucleus; information in this tract is used to synchronize circadian rhythms to the day-night cycle.

retroinsular cortex: Location of a vestibular cortical area; junction of the posterior insular cortex with the cortex on the lateral brain surface.

retronasal olfaction: When molecules travel from the oropharynx to activate olfactory neurons in the olfactory epithelium.

Rexed's laminae: Thin sheets of neurons in the spinal cord, which are clearest in the dorsal horn; they are significant because neurons in different layers receive input from different afferent and brain sources and, in turn, project to different targets.

rhinal sulcus: Rostral extension of the collateral sulcus, which separates the parahippocampal gyrus from more lateral temporal lobe regions.

rhodopsin: Photopigment in rod cells.

rhombencephalon: Most caudal primary brain vesicle; gives rise to the pons and medulla.

rhombic lip: Portion of the developing pons that gives rise to most of the cerebellum.

rhombomeres: Segments in the developing pons and medulla; eight in total.

rigidity: Condition in patients with Parkinson disease in which there is resistance to passive movement about a joint; sometimes there are phasic decreases in this resistance, termed cogwheel rigidity.

rod bipolar cells: Retinal interneurons that transmit signals from rod cells to ganglion cells.

rods: Photoreceptors for vision under low light conditions (scotopic vision); located away from the macula portion of the retina.

rostral: Toward the nose.

rostral interstitial nucleus of the medial longitudinal fasciculus: Plays a role in control of vertical saccades.

rostral spinocerebellar tract: Transmits information about the level of activation in cervical spinal interneuronal systems to the cerebellum; thought to relay internal signals from motor pathways, via spinal interneurons, to the cerebellum.

rostrocaudal axis: From the nose to the coccyx; the long axis of the central nervous system.

rostrum: Any beak-shaped process; also used to describe the oral and nasal region.

rubrospinal tract: Projection from the magnocellular portion of the red nucleus to the spinal cord.

Ruffini's corpuscle: Type of mechanoreceptor; distal process of large-diameter myelinated afferent fibers (A-β).

saccades: Rapid, darting movements of the eye from one site of gaze to another.

saccadic eye movements: *See* saccades.

saccule: Vestibular sensory organ (or otolith organ) sensitive to linear acceleration.

sacral: Spinal cord segment; there are five in total.

sagittal: Anatomical or imaging plane that is parallel both to the longitudinal axis of the central nervous system and to the midline, between the dorsal and ventral surfaces.

scala media: Inner ear fluid compartment.

scala tympani: Inner ear fluid compartment.

scala vestibuli: Inner ear fluid compartment; conducts pressure waves from the tympanic membrane to the other fluid compartments.

Schaefer collaterals: Collateral axon branch of neurons in the CA3 region of the hippocampus that synapse on neurons in the CA1 region.

schizophrenia: Psychiatric disease characterized by disordered thoughts, often associated with hallucinations.

Schwann cells: Glial cells that form the myelin sheath around peripheral axons.

sclera: Nonneural cover over the eye.

scotoma: Blind spot.

seasonal affective disorder (SAD): Form of depression during periods when days are short and nights are long.

secondary auditory areas: Cortical areas that process auditory information from the primary area.

secondary somatic sensory cortex: Cortical areas that process somatic sensory information from the primary area.

segmental interneurons: Neurons whose axons remain within a single spinal cord segment.

segmental: Pertaining to the segmental organization of the spinal cord.

semantic memory: Memory and knowledge of facts, people, and objects, including new word meaning.

semicircular canals: Vestibular organs sensitive to angular acceleration; there are three semicircular canals, each sensitive to acceleration in a different plane.

semilunar ganglion: Contains cell bodies of primary trigeminal sensory neurons.

sensory: Related to any of a wide range of stimuli from the environment or from within the body.

sensory cranial nerve nuclei: Process sensory information from the cranial nerves.

sensory homunculus: Form of somatic sensory representation in the postcentral gyrus (primary somatic sensory cortex).

septal nuclei: May participate in assessing the reward potential of events; receives input from the hippocampus and projects to the hypothalamus and other areas; located in rostral portion of the cerebral hemispheres.

septum pellucidum: Forms the medial walls of the anterior horn and part of the body of the lateral ventricle.

serotonergic: Neurons that use serotonin as a neurotransmitter.

serotonin: Neuroactive compound; also termed 5-HT (5-hydroxytryptamine).

short circumferential branches: Supply ventral portions of the brain stem away from the midline; primarily from the basilar artery.

sigmoid: S-shaped.

sigmoid sinus: Dural blood sinus that drains the transverse sinus and flows into the inferior petrosal sinus; located bilaterally.

six layers: Describes laminar pattern of neocortex.

skeletal somatic motor: Neuron class in which axons synapse on skeletal muscle that derives from the somites.

skeletomotor loop: Basal ganglia circuit that engages the motor and premotor areas.

slowly adapting: Response characteristic of neurons to an enduring stimulus in which a prolonged series of action potentials decrement slowly or not at all.

small-diameter axons: Afferent fibers that are sensitive to pain, temperature, and itch (i.e., histamine).

smell: One of the five major senses.

smooth pursuit eye movements: Slow eye movements that follow visual stimuli.

soft palate: Caudal, arch-shaped, portion of superior oral cavity formed by muscle.

solitary nucleus: Contains neurons that receive and process gustatory and viscerosensory information and project to other brain stem and diencephalic nuclei, including the parabrachial nucleus and the thalamus.

solitary tract: Where the central branches of gustatory and viscerosensory axons collect before synapsing in the solitary nucleus.

somatic: Related to the body.

somatic motor systems: Pathways and neurons that participate in limb and trunk muscle control.

somatic sensory: Body sense; includes pain, temperature sense, itch, touch, and limb position sense.

somatic skeletal motor column: Motor nuclei in the spinal cord that contain motor neurons that innervate somatic skeletal muscle.

somatotopy: Organization of central sensory and motor representations based on the shape and spatial characteristics of the body.

somites: Para-axial mesoderm that organizes development of muscles, bones, and other structures of the neck, limbs, and trunk.

spastic paralysis: Condition in which the presence of spasticity produces an inability to voluntarily control striated muscle.

spasticity: Velocity-dependent increase in muscle tone; occurs after damage to the corticospinal system during development or in maturity.

spina bifida: Neural tube defect; failure of the caudal neural tube to close, producing impairments in lumbosacral spinal cord functions.

spinal accessory (XI) nerve: Cranial motor nerve that innervates the sternocleidomastoid muscle and parts of the trapezius muscle.

spinal accessory nucleus: Contains motor neurons whose axons course in the spinal accessory (XI) nerve to innervate the sternocleidomastoid muscle and parts of the trapezius muscle.

spinal border cells: Neurons that contribute axons to the ventral spinocerebellar tract.

spinal cord: Major division of the central nervous system.

spinal nerves: Mixed nerves present at each spinal segment.

spinal tap: Colloquial term for lumber puncture in which a needle is inserted into the lumbar cistern to collect a sample of cerebral spinal fluid; most commonly used for diagnostic testing.

spinal trigeminal nucleus: Portion of the trigeminal sensory nuclear complex within the medulla and caudal pons; contains the caudal, interposed, and oral subnuclei; involved in diverse trigeminal functions, the most important of which are pain, temperature, and itch.

spinal trigeminal tract: Pathway in which trigeminal afferent fibers course before synapsing in the spinal trigeminal nucleus.

spinocerebellar tracts: Paths transmitting somatic sensory information from the limbs and trunk to the cerebellum for movement control.

spinocerebellum: Portion of the cerebellum that plays a key role in limb and trunk control; includes the vermis and intermediate hemisphere of the cortex and the fastigial and interposed nuclei.

spinomesencephalic tract: Transmits somatic sensory information from the limbs and trunk to the midbrain.

spinoreticular tract: Transmits somatic sensory information from the limbs and trunk to the reticular formation.

spinotectal tract: Transmits somatic sensory information from the limbs and trunk to the dorsal midbrain; term often used interchangeably with spinomesencephalic tract.

spinothalamic tract: Transmits somatic sensory information from the limbs and trunk to the thalamus.

spiral ganglion: Where the cell bodies of auditory primary sensory neurons are located.

splenium: A bandlike structure.

stapes: One of the middle ear ossicles (bones); essential for conducting changes in air pressure from the tympanic membrane to the oval window; attaches to the oval window.

stellate cells: In the cerebellum, inhibitory interneurons located in the molecular layer; more generally, a class of small multipolar neuron in the central nervous system.

stem cells: Multipotential cell that can develop into nerve, glial, or other cell types.

stenosis: An abnormal narrowing or contraction of a body passage or opening.

sternocleidomastoid muscle: Flexes the head and rotates head to opposite side.

straight sinus: Drains the inferior sagittal sinus and certain veins; empties into the confluence of sinuses; located where the falx cerebri and tentorium cerebelli meet; located on midline.

stria (or stripe) of Gennari: Band of myelinated axons in layer 4B of the primary visual cortex; axons interconnect local areas of cortex for visual stimulus processing.

stria medullaris: Pathway that courses along the lateral walls of the third ventricle; contains axons from the septal nuclei to the habenula.

stria terminalis: C-shaped pathway from the amygdala to portions of the diencephalon and cerebral hemispheres; also contains neurons.

striasome: An anatomical compartment of the striatum that contains patch-like distributions of particular neurochemicals (e.g., acetylcholinesterase; encephalin).

striatal cell bridges: Places of continuity of the caudate nucleus and putamen that span the internal capsule.

striate cortex: Another term for the primary visual cortex based on the location of the stria of Gennari.

striatum: Component of the basal ganglia; comprises the caudate nucleus, putamen, and nucleus accumbens.

subarachnoid space: Between the outer portion of the arachnoid and the pia; where cerebrospinal fluid accumulates over the surface of the brain and spinal cord.

subcommissural organ: A circumventricular organ; located near the posterior commissure.

subdural hematoma: Hemorrhage of blood into the potential space between the dura and the arachnoid.

subdural space: Potential space between the dura and the arachnoid.

subfornical organ: One of the circumventricular organs; region in which the blood–brain barrier is absent; axons project to magnocellular neurons of the paraventricular nucleus.

subgenual cortex: Located ventral to the genu of the corpus callosum; associated with clinical depression and is a target of brain stimulation for intractable depression.

subiculum: Component of the hippocampal formation.

submandibular ganglion: Contain postganglionic neurons that innervate the oral mucosa and the submandibular and sublingual glands.

submodality: Category of a sensory modality, such as color vision, bitter, or pain.

substance P: Neuroactive compound; present in neurons that process painful stimuli.

substantia gelatinosa: Laminae II and III of the dorsal horn; process pain, temperature, and itch.

substantia nigra pars compacta: Portion of the substantia nigra where neurons contain dopamine and project widely to the striatum.

substantia nigra pars reticulata: Portion of the substantia nigra where neurons contain GABA and project to the thalamus primarily.

substantia nigra: Component of the basal ganglia; comprises the pars reticulata and the pars compacta.

subthalamic nucleus: Basal ganglia nucleus involved in limb control; when damaged, can produce hemiballism; part of the indirect basal ganglia circuit.

sulci: Grooves.

sulcus limitans: Groove that separates developing sensory and motor structures in the spinal cord and brain stem.

sulcus: Groove.

superior cerebellar artery: Supplies rostral pons and cerebellum; long circumferential branch of the basilar artery.

superior cerebellar peduncle: Tract that primarily carries axons from the deep cerebellar nuclei to the brain stem and thalamus.

superior colliculus: Plays a key role in controlling saccades; located in the rostral midbrain.

superior ganglion: Of the vagus and glossopharyngeal nerves, contains cell bodies of somatic sensory afferent fibers.

superior oblique muscle: Depresses the eye when the eye is adducted and intorts the eye when it is abducted.

superior olivary nuclear complex: Involved in processing incoming auditory signals; especially important for horizontal localization of sounds.

superior olivary nuclei: Auditory relay nuclei predominantly important in the horizontal localization of sounds.

superior parietal lobule: Important for spatial localization.

superior petrosal sinus: Dural sinus; drains into the sigmoid sinus.

superior rectus muscle: Elevates the eye.

superior sagittal sinus: Dural sinus; drains into the straight sinus.

superior salivatory nucleus: Contains parasympathetic preganglionic neurons whose axons course in the intermediate (VII) nerve.

superior temporal gyrus: Involved in hearing and speech.

superior vestibular nucleus: One of four vestibular nuclei; located in the pons.

supplementary eye field: Cortical eye movement control center located primarily on the medial wall of the frontal lobe; involved in more cognitive aspects of saccadic eye movement control.

supplementary motor area: Portion of the medial frontal lobe important in the control of eye movements.

supporting cells: Provide structural and possibly trophic support for taste buds.

suprachiasmatic nucleus: Hypothalamic nucleus important for circadian rhythms; center of the biological clock.

supraoptic nucleus: Contains magnocellular neurosecretory neurons; secretes oxytocin and vasopressin into the systemic circulation in the posterior pituitary gland.

supratentorial: Referring to the brain above the tentorium cerebelli.

Sylvian fissure: Separates the temporal lobe from the parietal and frontal lobes; also termed the lateral sulcus.

sympathetic nervous system: Component of the autonomic nervous system.

sympathetic preganglionic neurons: Sympathetic nervous system neurons that are located in the central nervous system and synapse on sympathetic postganglionic neurons and cells in the adrenal medulla.

synapses: Specialized sites of contact where neurons communicate and where neurotransmitters are released; comprise three components—presynaptic axon terminal, synaptic cleft, and postsynaptic membrane.

synaptic cleft: Narrow intercellular space between the neurons at synapses.

syringomyelia: Cavity.

T1 relaxation time: Proton relaxation time related to the overall tissue environment; also termed spin-lattice relaxation time.

T2 relaxation time: Proton relaxation time related to interactions between protons; also termed spin-spin relaxation time.

tabes dorsalis: Degenerative loss of large-diameter mechanoreceptive fibers; associated with end-stage neurosyphilis.

tarsal muscle: A smooth muscle that assists the actions of the levator palpebrae muscle; under control of the sympathetic nervous system.

tastants: Chemicals that produce tastes.

taste: One of the five major senses.

taste buds: Gustatory organ, which consists of taste receptor cells, support cells, and basal cells, which may be stem cells for replenishing taste receptor cells.

taste receptor cells: Component of taste buds; transduce oral chemicals into gustatory signals.

tectorial membrane: Component of the organ of Corti; stereocilia of hair cells embed within the tectorial membrane.

tectospinal tract: Projection from the deep layers of the superior colliculus to the spinal cord.

tectum: Most dorsal portion of the brain stem; present only in midbrain in maturity.

tegmentum: Portion of the brain stem between the tectum and the base; present throughout the brain stem; Latin for cover.

telencephalon: Secondary brain vesicle that gives rise to structures of the cerebral hemisphere; derives from the prosencephalon.

temporal hemiretina: Temporal hall of the retina.

temporal lobe: One of the lobes of the cerebral hemisphere.

temporal pole: Most rostral portion of the temporal lobe.

tentorium cerebelli: Dural flap between the occipital lobes and the cerebellum.

terminal ganglia: Parasympathetic ganglia that contain postganglionic neurons; receive input from the vagus nerve; located on the structure their axons innervate.

thalamic adhesion: Site of adhesion of the two halves of the thalamus; said to be present in approximately 80% of individuals; in humans, no axons decussate in the thalamic adhesion.

thalamic fasciculus: Tract in which axons from the deep cerebellar nuclei and part of the internal segment of the globus pallidus course to the thalamus.

thalamic radiations: Axons of thalamic nuclei that project to the cerebral cortex.

thalamostriate vein: Follows C-shaped course of caudate nucleus and stria terminalis.

thalamus: Major site of relay nuclei that transmit information to the cerebral cortex; component of the diencephalon.

thermoreceptors: Primary sensory neurons sensitive to thermal changes.

third ventricle: Component of the ventricular system; located between the two halves of the diencephalon.

thoracic: Spinal cord segment; there are 12 in humans.

tonotopic organization: Or tonotopy; where sounds of different frequencies are processed by different brain regions; sounds of similar frequencies are processed by neighboring brain regions, while sounds of very different frequencies are processed by brain regions that are farther apart.

tonsillar: Relating to a tonsil, especially the palatine tonsil.

touch: One of the five major senses.

tractography: An MRI approach (diffusion MRI) to identify the locations of tracts based on information about the local directions of brain water diffusion; a commonly used tractography method is diffusion tensor imaging (DTI).

transcranial magnetic stimulation (TMS): Noninvasive brain stimulation technique in which a pulse of magnetic energy is use to activate neurons; repetitive TMS (rTMS) uses a series of pulses.

transient ischemic attack (TIA): Brief cessation of cerebral blood flow to a local brain region that produces transient dysfunction of the area; dysfunction lasts for a period of minutes to hours.

tract: Collection of axons within the central nervous system.

transverse plane: Perpendicular to the longitudinal axis of the central nervous system, between the dorsal and ventral surfaces.

transverse sinus: Dural sinus that carries blood into the systemic circulation.

trapezius muscle: Contains several functional regions that support the weight of the arm and act on the scapula.

trapezoid body: Site of decussation of auditory fibers; the ventral acoustic stria.

tremor: Trembling or shaking movement.

trigeminal ganglion: Location of cell bodies of all trigeminal afferent fibers except those afferents innervating muscle spindle receptors; also termed semilunar ganglion.

trigeminal lemniscus: Tract in which axons from the main trigeminal sensory nucleus ascend to the thalamus.

trigeminal mesencephalic nucleus: Contains cell bodies of primary sensory neurons innervating stretch receptors in jaw muscles.

trigeminal motor nucleus: Contains motor neurons that innervate jaw muscles.

trigeminal (V) nerve: Mixed cranial nerve containing sensory axons that innervate much of the head and oral cavity and motor axons that innervate jaw muscles.

trigeminocerebellar pathways: Projection from spinal trigeminal nuclei to the cerebellum.

trigeminothalamic tract: Projection from spinal trigeminal nuclei to the thalamus.

trochlear (IV) nerve: Cranial nerve that contains the axons of trochlear motor neurons, which innervate the superior oblique muscle.

trochlear nucleus: Contains motor neurons that innervate the superior oblique muscle.

tubercles: A round nodule or eminence that marks the location of an underlying nucleus or cortical region; cuneate and gracile tubercles are located on the dorsal medulla and the olfactory tubercle is located on the ventral surface of the basal forebrain.

tuberomammillary nucleus: Hypothalamic nucleus; contains neurons that use histamine as a neurotransmitter; diverse projections to activate forebrain neurons.

tufted cells: Olfactory bulb projection neurons.

tympanic membrane: Ear drum; oscillates in response to environmental pressure changes associated with sounds; coupled to middle ear ossicles.

uncal herniation: Displacement of the uncus medially due to an expanding space-occupying lesion above the cerebellar tentorium.

uncinate fasciculus: Association pathway interconnecting frontal and anterior temporal cortical areas.

uncus: Bulge on the medial temporal lobe; overlies the anterior hippocampal formation and amygdala.

unipolar neuron: Neuron with a cell body and axon but few dendrites.

urination: Release of urine from the bladder.

utricle: Vestibular sensory organ (or otolith organ) sensitive to linear acceleration.

vagus (X) nerve: Mixed cranial nerve; contains axons of branchiomeric motor neurons that innervate laryngeal and pharyngeal muscles, parasympathetic preganglionic fibers, gustatory and visceral afferent fibers, and somatic sensory afferents; located in the medulla.

vascular organ of the lamina terminalis: Circumventricular organ; located in the rostral wall of the third ventricle.

vasopressin: Neuroactive peptide that also acts on peripheral structures, including promoting fluid reabsorption in the kidney; also termed antidiuretic hormone (ADH).

venogram: Radiological image of veins.

ventral: Toward the abdomen; synonymous with anterior.

ventral acoustic stria: Decussating auditory fibers; the trapezoid body.

ventral (anterior) commissure: *See* ventral spinal commissure.

ventral (or anterior) corticospinal tract: Pathway for control of axial and proximal limb muscles of the neck and upper body.

ventral amygdalofugal pathway: Output pathway from the basolateral and central nuclei of the amygdala.

ventral anterior thalamic nucleus: Part of the motor thalamus; receiving primarily information from the internal segment of the globus pallidus of the basal ganglia; projects to cortical motor and premotor areas.

ventral cochlear nucleus: Concerned with processing the horizontal sound localization; division of cochlear nucleus.

ventral column: Portion of spinal cord white matter medial to the ventral horn; contains primarily descending fibers for controlling axial and proximal limb musculature.

ventral horn: Laminae VIII and IX of the spinal gray matter; location of neurons for somatic motor control.

ventral lateral thalamic nucleus: Part of the motor thalamus; receiving primarily information from the deep cerebellar nuclei; projects to cortical motor and premotor areas.

ventral medial nucleus (of the hypothalamus): Participates in appetitive behaviors, such as feeding.

ventral pallidum: Output nucleus of the limbic circuit of the basal ganglia; located ventral to the anterior commissure.

ventral posterior lateral nucleus: Division of the ventral posterior nucleus where information from the dorsal column nuclei is processed.

ventral posterior medial nucleus: Division of the ventral posterior nucleus where trigeminal information is processed.

ventral posterior nucleus: Thalamic nucleus for processing somatic sensory information; projects to the primary somatic sensory cortex.

ventral root: Where motor axons leave the spinal cord.

ventral spinal commissure: Where axons of the anterolateral system decussate; located ventral to lamina X and the central canal.

ventral spinocerebellar tract: Transmits information about the level of activation in thoracic, lumbar, and sacral spinal interneuronal systems to the cerebellum; thought to relay internal signals from motor pathways, via spinal interneurons, to the cerebellum.

ventral striatum: Consists of the ventromedial portions of the caudate nucleus and putamen and the nucleus accumbens.

ventral tegmental area: Contains dopaminergic neurons that project to the ventromedial portion of the striatum and the prefrontal cortex; located in the rostral midbrain.

ventricles: Dilated channels within the ventricular system; contain choroid plexus.

ventricular system: Cavities within the central nervous system that contain cerebrospinal fluid.

ventricular zone: Innermost layer of the developing central nervous system; layer from which nerve cells are generated.

ventrolateral medulla: Contains neurons that participate in blood pressure regulation through projections to the intermediolateral cell column.

ventrolateral nucleus: Principal motor control nucleus of the thalamus; receives cerebellar input and projects to primary and premotor cortical areas.

ventrolateral preoptic area: Important in promoting REM and non-REM sleep, through inhibitory connections with other hypothalamic nuclei and brain stem nuclei that promote wakefulness.

ventromedial hypothalamic nucleus: Important in regulating appetite and other consummatory behaviors; receives input from limbic system structures.

ventromedial posterior nucleus: Thalamic nucleus important for processing noxious stimuli; projects to the posterior insular cortex; caudal to the thalamic region that processes viscerosensory information.

vergence movements: Convergent or divergent eye movements; ensure that the image of an object of interest falls on the same place on the retina of each eye.

vermis: Midline portion of the cerebellar cortex; plays a role in axial and proximal limb control.

vertebral arteries: Branch from the subclavian artery; two vertebral arteries converge to form the basilar artery.

vertebral canal: Cavity within the vertebral column within which the spinal cord is located.

vertebral-basilar circulation: Arterial supply to the brain stem and parts of the temporal and occipital lobes.

vertigo: The sense of the world spinning around or that of an individual whirling around.

vestibular ganglion: Location of cell bodies of primary vestibular neurons; also termed Scarpa's ganglion.

vestibular labyrinth: Fluid-filled cavities within the temporal bone within which the vestibular organs are located.

vestibular division of CN VIII: Component of CN VIII that supplies the semicircular canals, utricle, and saccule.

vestibular nuclei: Major termination site of vestibular sensory fibers.

vestibulocerebellum: Portion of the cerebellum that receives a monosynaptic projection from primary vestibular axons; processes this information for eye movement control and balance; includes primarily the flocculonodular lobe.

vestibulocochlear (VIII) nerve: Contains afferent fibers that innervate the auditory and vestibular structures of the inner ear.

vestibuloocular reflex: Automatic control of eye position by vestibular sensory information.

vestibulospinal tract: Axons that originate from the vestibular nuclei and project to the brain stem.

vibration sense: The capacity to detect and distinguish mechanical vibration of the body.

visceral: Related to the internal organs of the body.

visceral (autonomic) motor fibers: Axons of autonomic preganglionic or postganglionic neurons as they course in the periphery.

visceral motor nuclei: Contain autonomic preganglionic neurons.

viscerosensory: Related to the sensory innervation of the internal organs of the body.

vision: One of the five major senses.

visual field: The total area that is seen.

visual field defect: Loss of vision within a portion of the visual field.

visual motion pathway: Originates primarily from the magnocellular ganglion cells of the retina and projects to V5 and ultimately to regions of the posterior parietal cortex.

vomeronasal organ: Peripheral olfactory organ important for detecting pheromones; well-documented as a functional structure in animals, but its function in humans is controversial.

Wallenberg syndrome: *See* lateral medullary syndrome.

Wallerian degeneration: Deterioration of the structure and function of the distal portion of an axon, when cut; also termed anterograde generation.

Wernicke's area: Important for understanding speech; located in the posterior superior temporal gyrus (area 22).

what pathway: Corticocortical circuits important for identifying an object using vision, touch, or sound.

where-how pathway: Corticocortical circuits important for identifying the location of an object using vision, touch, or sound and use of that information to help direct limb or eye movements.

white matter: Location of predominantly myelinated axons.

working memory: The temporary storing of information used to plan and shape upcoming behaviors.

zona incerta: Contains GABA-ergic neurons that project widely to the cerebral cortex; nuclear region of the diencephalon.

Answer Key

■ CHAPTER 6 REVIEW QUESTION ANSWER KEY

1. C	3. D	5. C	7. D	9. C
2. C	4. B	6. A	8. D	10. A

■ CHAPTER 7 REVIEW QUESTIONS ANSWER KEY

1. A	3. D	5. C	7. A	9. C
2. A	4. D	6. B	8. B	10. D

■ CHAPTER 1 REVIEW QUESTIONS ANSWER KEY

1. B	3. C	5. C	7. C	9. C
2. B	4. A	6. A	8. A	10. C

■ CHAPTER 8 REVIEW QUESTIONS ANSWER KEY

1. A	3. C	5. C	7. A	9. D
2. B	4. D	6. B	8. B	10. C

■ CHAPTER 2 REVIEW QUESTIONS ANSWER KEY

1. C	3. C	5. D	7. C	9. B
2. D	4. B	6. A	8. C	10. C

■ CHAPTER 9 REVIEW QUESTION ANSWER KEY

1. D	3. C	5. A	7. C	9. A
2. A	4. B	6. B	8. B	10. D

■ CHAPTER 3 REVIEW QUESTIONS ANSWER KEY

1. C	3. E	5. D	7. B	9. D
2. E	4. B	6. A	8. C	10. D

■ CHAPTER 10 REVIEW QUESTIONS ANSWER KEY

1. A	3. C	5. D	7. A	9. A
2. B	4. C	6. B	8. C	10. D

■ CHAPTER 4 REVIEW QUESTIONS ANSWER KEY

1. B	3. D	5. B	7. B	9. C
2. D	4. C	6. B	8. B	10. A

■ CHAPTER 5 REVIEW QUESTIONS ANSWER KEY

1. B	3. B	5. C	7. A	9. C
2. D	4. B	6. D	8. D	10. A

Index

Figures are denoted with an *f* following the page number.

Printed in the USA
CPSIA information can be obtained
at www.ICGtesting.com
CBHW080014010724
10847CB00015B/181